Healthcare Informatics *and* Information Synthesis

To Marlene

and our incredible daughters
Lori Lynn and Julie Wynne

Healthcare Informatics *and* Information Synthesis

Developing and Applying Clinical Knowledge to Improve Outcomes

JOHN W. WILLIAMSON • CHARLENE R. WEIR
CHARLES W. TURNER • MICHAEL J. LINCOLN
KEELY M.W. COFRIN

Sage Publications
International Educational and Professional Publisher
Thousand Oaks • London • New Delhi

For information:

Sage Publications, Inc.
2455 Teller Road
Thousand Oaks, California 91320
E-mail: order@sagepub.com

Sage Publications Ltd.
6 Bonhill Street
London EC2A 4PU
United Kingdom

Sage Publications India Pvt. Ltd.
M-32 Market
Greater Kailash I
New Delhi 110 048 India

Printed in the United States of America

Library of Congress Cataloging-in-Publication Data

Williamson, John W., 1931–
    Healthcare informatics and information synthesis : Developing and
applying clinical knowledge to improving outcomes / by John W. Williamson,
Charlene R. Weir, and Charles W. Turner.
        p. cm.
    Includes bibliographical references and index.
    ISBN 0-7619-0824-2 (c)
    1. Medical informatics. 2. Outcome assessment (Medical care) I.
Weir, Charlene R. II. Turner, Charles W. III. Title.
R858 .W585 2001
362.1'0285—dc21   2001006680

This book is printed on acid-free paper.

02   03   04   05   06   7   6   5   4   3   2   1

Acquisition Editor:	Heidi Van Middlesworth
Production Editor:	Sanford Robinson
Copy Editor:	Gillian Dickens
Proofreader:	Jamie Robinson
Editorial Assistant:	Ester Marcelino
Typesetter:	Tina Hill
Cover Designer:	Sandra Ng

Contents

STAGE III: DATABASE VALIDATION

STAGE IV: INFORMATION ANALYSIS AND SYNTHESIS

List of Tables

List of Figures

List of Forms

NOTE: You may reproduce these forms without requesting permission.

List of Chapter Appendixes

List of Abbreviations

AAHP	American Association of Health Plans
AAP	American Academy of Pediatrics
ABC	ABC relevance-coding convention
ACP	American College of Physicians
AHCPR	Agency for Health Care Policy and Research, now AHRQ (U.S.)
AHEC	Area Health Education Center (U.S.)
AHRQ	Agency for Healthcare Research and Quality, formerly AHCPR (U.S.)
AMIA	American Medical Informatics Association
AMA	American Medical Association
APA	American Psychological Association
AR	Absolute risk
ARR	Absolute risk reduction
BES	Best evidence synthesis
BMI	Body mass index
BMJ	*British Medical Journal*
BUN	Blood urinary nitrogen
CABG	Coronary artery bypass graft
CAHPS	Consumer Assessment of Health Plans® (U.S.)
CBA	Cost-benefit analysis
CDC	Centers for Disease Control and Prevention (U.S.)
CD-ROM	Compact disk read-only memory
CE	Continuing education
CEA	Cost-effectiveness analysis
CEBM	Centre for Evidence-Based Medicine (U.K.)
CER	Control event rate
CI	Confidence interval
CLAS	Computerized laboratory alerting system
CME	Continuing medical education
CPG	Clinical practice guidelines

CODS	Center for Organization and Delivery Studies (U.S.)
CONQUEST	Computerized needs-oriented quality measurement evaluation system
CONSORT	Consolidated standard of reporting trials
CPG	Clinical practice guideline
CPM	Confidence profile method
CPM	Critical path management
CPS	Clinical pharmacokinetic system
CRD	Centre for Reviews and Dissemination (U.K.)
CRG	Collaborative review groups
CRR	Control relative risk
CUA	Cost-utility analysis
DRG	Diagnosis-related group
DSS	Decision support systems
DST	Decision support technology
DVA	Department of Veterans Affairs
E. Coli	*Escherichia coli* [bacteria]
EBOC	Evidence-based on call (U.K.)
EBR	Evidence-based recommendation (U.K.)
EER	Experimental event rate
EP	Extramural programs (U.S. NIH)
EPC	Evidence-based practice center (U.S.)
ERR	Experimental relative risk
ES	Effect size
FDA	Food and Drug Administration (U.S.)
FERRET	Federal electronic research and review extraction tool (U.S.)
FN	False negative
FNR	False-negative rate
FP	False positive
FPR	False-positive rate
FTP	File transfer protocol
GI	Gastrointestinal
GUI	Graphical user interface
HCFA	Health Care Financing Administration (U.S.)
HCT	Historically controlled trial/health care technology
HCUP	Healthcare cost and utilization project (U.S.)
HELP	Health Evaluation through Logical Processing
HHS	Department of Health and Human Services (U.S.)
HII	Health Improvement Institute (U.S.)
HITI	Health Information Technology Institute, Mitretek, Inc. (U.S.)
HLM	Hierarchical linear model
HMO	Health maintenance organization
HRQLY	Health-related quality-of-life year
HSR	Health services research
HSR&D	Health Services Research and Development Service (U.K.)
HSRPROJ	Health services research projects in progress, AHRQ (U.S.)

HTA	Health Technology Assessment
ICD-9	*International Classification of Diseases—9th Revision*
ICD-9 CM	*ICD-9, Clinical Modification*
ICMJE	International Committee of Medical Journal Editors
INAHTA	International Network of Agencies for Health Technology Assessment (Sweden)
IOM	Institute of Medicine (U.S.)
ISI	Institute for Scientific Information (U.S.)
ISO	International Standards Organization
ISP	Internet service provider
JAMA	*Journal of the American Medical Association*
JAMIA	*Journal of the American Medical Informatics Association*
JCAHO	Joint Commission on Accreditation of Healthcare Organizations
LAN	Local area network
LC	National Library of Congress (U.S.)
LDS	Latter Day Saints, i.e., Mormons (U.S.)
LHNCBC	Lister Hill National Center for Biomedical Communications (U.S.)
-LR	Negative likelihood ratio
+LR	Positive likelihood ratio
MCO	Managed care organizations
MEDTEP	Medical Treatment Effectiveness Program (U.S.)
MEPS	Medical Expenditure Panel Survey (U.S.)
MeSH	Medical subject headings, NLM (U.S.)
MI	Myocardial infarction
NAMCS	National Ambulatory Medical Care Survey (U.S.)
NAP	National Academy Press (U.S.)
NCBI	National Center for Biotechnology Information (U.S.)
NCHS	National Center for Health Statistics (U.S.)
NCI	National Cancer Institute (U.S.)
NCID	National Center for Infectious Diseases (U.S.)
NCQA	National Committee on Quality Assurance (U.S.)
NEJM	*New England Journal of Medicine*
NGC	National Guideline Clearinghouse (U.S.)
NGT	Nominal group technique
NHANES	National Health and Nutrition Examination Survey (U.S.)
NHIC	National Health Information Center (U.S.)
NHS	National Health Service (U.K.)
NHS R&D	National Health Service Research & Development Programme (U.K.)
NICE	National Institute for Clinical Excellence (U.K.)
NICHSR	National Information Center on HSR and HCT (U.S.)
NIH	National Institutes of Health (U.S.)
NIOSH	National Institute for Occupational Safety and Health (U.S.)
NIS	Nationwide Inpatient Sample (U.S.)
NISO	National Information Standards Organization (U.S.)
NLM	National Library of Medicine (U.S.)
NNH	Number needed to harm

NNT	Number needed to treat
NPV	Negative predictive value
OCR	Optical character recognition
OIR	Office of Intramural Research, NIH (U.S.)
OMB	Office of Management and Budget (U.S.)
PERT	Program evaluation and review technique
PORT	Patient Outcomes Research Team, AHRQ (U.S.)
PPV	Positive predictive value
PR	Proportional reduction
PRO	Professional Review Organization, HCFA (U.S.)
QALY	Quality-adjusted life year
QI	Quality improvement
QM	Quality management
QUICK	Quality information checklist
R&D	Research and development
RAM	Random access memory
RCCT	Randomized controlled clinical trial
RCT	Randomized clinical (controlled assumed) trial
ROC	Receiver operating characteristic
RR	Relative risk/relative risk ratio
RRR	Relative risk reduction (not relative risk ratio)
SD	Standard deviation
SES	Social economic status
SF-36	Short Form 36-item health survey
SGHT	NHS Standing Group on Health Technology (U.K.)
SGJ	Structured group judgment
SID	State Inpatient Database (U.S.)
SK	Streptokinase (thrombolytic drug)
SP	Simulated patients
SPSS	Statistical Package for the Social Sciences
STD	Sexually transmitted disease
TIMI	Thrombolysis in myocardial infarction, NIH (U.S.)
TN	True negative
TNR	True-negative rate
TP	True positive
t-PA	Tissue-type plasminogen activator (thrombolytic drug)
TPR	True-positive rate
U.K.	United Kingdom
UMLS	Unified Medical Language System®
URL	Universal resource locator
VISTA	Veterans Integrated System Architecture (U.S.)
WAN	Wide-area network
WHO	World Health Organization
WORD	Welsh Office of Research & Development (U.K.)
WWW	World Wide Web

Foreword:
How to Read This Book

In deciding who should read this book, we have stated that our primary audience is healthcare professionals interested in synthesizing information for clinicians and for those involved in quality improvement. The intended purpose of such a synthesis is for developing resources to facilitate immediate application to improve healthcare outcomes. However, because basic principles for producing a synthesis are presented, they can be applied to any medical or healthcare subject matter, from basic research to the applied health sciences. The specific procedures and tasks may vary slightly depending on subject matter and the limitations of resources. However, this book is sufficiently flexible that it can meet the needs of a wide variety of different healthcare disciplines with varying levels of resource constraints.

In deciding how to read this book, we have provided several guides to help you learn the fundamentals of producing a relevant, sound, cost-effective, and understandable synthesis. First, we define *information synthesis* as a concept; second, we explain how this volume is two books in one; third, we explain our reading aids and style conventions, including our denotation of jargon; and fourth, we describe our synthesis data collection forms. Finally, you will see that this foreword models the basic formatting style and layout of our book as a whole.

What Is an Information Synthesis?

To get started, it is first necessary that you review exactly what we mean by the term *information synthesis*.

INFORMATION SYNTHESIS

In our terms, an *information synthesis* is a systematic review of research, adhering to a formal scientifically based protocol, which in this book will apply to a health-related topic. This protocol facilitates defining the topic within a theoretical framework (model), developing a relevant document database, selecting and validating a research data set, aggregating and synthesizing the results, and disseminating the synthesis in a form that facilitates ready application, in this context, to improve healthcare outcomes in the community.

Currently, there are many synonyms that approximate this concept, including *systematic reviews, validated reviews, critical reviews, expert reviews, evidence-based reviews, quantitative reviews* (e.g., meta-analyses), and *qualitative reviews* (e.g., ethnographic synthesis). Note that some authors use the term *overview* as a synonym for *review*.

Our basic assumption is that information syntheses are as important as original research and must be conducted with similar, if not more, rigor. This book will help you learn about recently developed scientific review methods to ensure a product of relevant, valid, mature, and understandable information that can be applied immediately for healthcare outcome improvement.

Two Books in One

This book integrates two separate dimensions of information synthesis: One is conceptual and the other is procedural. We decided against having a separate volume on each, as we judged it best for each of the five stages to have concepts presented immediately before procedures, so that our conceptual framework will be fresh in the readers' minds when they implement our or any variation of our task-by-task suggestions.

Concepts

The chapters indicated in Figure F.1 cover the following concepts: principles, issues, state of the science, and other considerations related to systematic reviews in the health sciences.

These chapters, or sections of chapters, provide the conceptual framework necessary to understand the what, why, and so-what for developing systematic literature reviews. These considerations are scattered throughout the book for an important

Review of Concepts of Information Synthesis

(Chapters, Sections, and Appendixes by Stage)

Introduction p.___

Chapter 1. Introduction: Healthcare Information Synthesis ___

Stage I: Planning and Preparation ___

Chapter 2. Synthesis Planning Prerequisites and Conceptual Issues ___

Appendix 2.1 Scientific Group Consensus Processes ___

Stage II: Database Development p.___

Chapter 5. Conceptual Issues in Database Development ___

Stage III: Database Validation p.___

Chapter 8. Data Extraction and Coding ___

Section B. Procedures for Extracting and Coding Data ___

Chapter 9. Principles of Information Validation ___

Appendix 9.1. Criteria Sets for Validating Individual Research Studies (1977-2000) ___

Stage IV: Information Analysis and Synthesis p.___

Chapter 12. Basic Statistics for Quantitative Synthesis ___

Appendix 12.1 Contingency Table Statistics ___

Chapter 13. Conceptual Aspects of Meta-analysis ___

Stage V: Complete and Evaluate Synthesis Report p.___

Chapter 17. Applying Synthesis Results for Healthcare Outcomes Improvement ___

Chapter 18. Evaluation and Refinement of Synthesis Report ___

Appendix 18.3 Criteria Sets for Validating Systematic Reviews (1977-2000) ___

Figure F.1. Presentation of Conceptual Aspects of Book

reason. Prior to each procedural section or chapter, we introduce the concepts, which you can skim to become familiar with the content and its importance, and then you can move on to the step-by-step procedures that should be studied in detail. If you have trouble with a procedure, you can go back to the concept section or chapter to better understand the framework of that particular procedure.

Procedures

The chapters or sections of chapters in Figure F.2 usually indicate step-by-step procedures for beginners in the world of information synthesis.

These procedures are often accompanied by a brief explanation of the tasks we suggest you might apply. Many of these tasks relate to forms that can be used as a checklist or used to record important information and data. Often a figure in the text will illustrate and explain a completed form; the actual blank form, which you may copy and apply, is usually at the end of the chapter. These forms are recommended templates for electronic versions that you might digitize and revise to meet your needs.

Text Orientation Guides

Definitions, Cautions, and Explanatory Notes

Throughout the text, you will find notes that provide important information. There are three major types of information presented. The first provides warnings or cautions about a point that might easily be misunderstood or a procedure that, if done incorrectly, could cause considerable extra work; the second describes important concept definitions for terms in this book; and the third provides notes regarding information such as how we calculate a false-positive rate, together with a rationale for a specific convention.

Jargon and the Use of Quotes

With the advance of scientific technology, there is always a need for jargon terms that professionals in the field readily understand; however, those outside the field may find these confusing. The same is true in the advancing field of information synthesis where there are many concepts that, as yet, have no simple common terms to use. To help you cope with such jargon, we use double quotation marks for commonly understood terms in a specialized field and single quotation marks for our

Step-by-Step Procedures

(Chapters, Procedures, and Appendixes by Stage)

Figure F.2. Presentation of Procedures in Book

own jargon or special use of terms. After using these notations several times, we assume you have the idea, and from then on we use the terms without quotes.

The remainder of the reading aids are standard to every scientific text. They include the table of contents, glossary, list of abbreviations, list of tables, list of figures, list of forms, list of appendixes, list of references, , and the standard alphabetical subject index. However, in this book, we do add a compendium of Internet sources and universal resource locator (URL) addresses. We also include several appendixes that provide greater detail on topics in the text. For example, the text lists the major training goals for a synthesis project team. The appendix provides suggested training exercises that might help the team more rapidly achieve those training goals.

Synthesis Data Collection Forms

This set of forms to facilitate your synthesis project is designed for many of the procedures suggested in this book. Some of these forms are fill-in-the-blank types, and some are checklists to remind you of important functions or products you should have compiled at a particular point. As we will continually remind you, these are starter forms for you to digitize and revise to meet your special needs. They are not stone tablets from on high. If they seem useful, feel free to replicate them.

Acknowledgments

Dr. George Miller, Dr. Paul Sanazaro, and Dr. Kerr White inspired and facilitated the conceptual formulation of much of this work, which became subject matter for two courses the senior author taught at the Johns Hopkins School of Hygiene and Public Health. Subsequently, Dr. Homer Warner and Dr. Reed Gardner both helped inspire revision of the book within a framework of medical informatics, a field of science that provides the theory and the tools that make information syntheses possible.

The senior author joined the Department of Veterans Affairs and owes a debt of gratitude to Dr. Peter Goldschmidt (former head of the Veterans Affairs Office of Health Services Research and Development) for providing ideas and partial funding for this project at that time. The authors are also indebted to the former Under-Secretary for Health, Dr. Kenneth Garthwaite, for helping secure additional funding to continue this work. More recently, the senior author owes much gratitude to his supervisors, Dr. Robert Cullen and Dr. Robert Means, for their support and patience for the time spent on this book while in the Veterans Affairs (VA) Employee Education Service.

We are also, again, grateful to Dr. Peter Goldschmidt, an early pioneer on the subject of information synthesis, for his cogent review of our 1988 manuscript that literally sent us back to the drawing boards to rework the entire book and to add a major section explaining how this work could help those who need to develop a quality synthesis but have little time or funding. We thank Dr. Michael O'Conner, who is also in the VA's Employee Education Service, for his thorough review of the 1988 manuscript in which he provided many helpful suggestions.

In addition, the authors wish to express appreciation to the following individuals for their contributions: Marlene Williamson for her substantive and editorial contributions between 1998 and 2001 and Susan Tripp, while in the VA's Salt Lake Regional Medical Education Center, who dedicated many hours of her time in copyediting the revised version of this book in 1998-1999, with input and dedicated support from our administrative associate, Evelyn Cope.

Finally, we owe much gratitude and appreciation to our spouses and children for their patience and understanding while we put in so many hours during nights and weekends at their expense. Their generous emotional support during this time truly made the book possible.

CHAPTER 1

Introduction

Healthcare Information Synthesis and Informatics

Our purpose in writing this book is to help both nonexpert and experienced health literature reviewers to produce more relevant, valid, and immediately applicable 'information syntheses' for improving healthcare outcomes. To achieve this purpose, we set forth the premise that 'healthcare informatics' is the essential foundation for both the development and application of these information syntheses. Indeed, without the science and tools of informatics, you will find it all but impossible to accomplish the ultimate goal of more immediate improvement of community healthcare outcomes in all of their many dimensions.

We will focus on fundamental procedures for compiling, validating, and synthesizing a database of research information for healthcare decision support. Throughout this book, informatics principles and tools will be described and used to help achieve our purpose.

When clinicians make medical decisions, they often rely on an implicit mental "synthesis," or integration, of knowledge from their formal education and practice experience. Unfortunately, most practitioners lack the time and skills necessary to adequately keep up with current or past literature in their own field, let alone that of healthcare informatics, quantitative sciences, and systematic review methods

(Mulrow & Cook, 1998; Williamson, German, Weiss, Skinner, & Bowes, 1989). The current emphasis on "evidence-based" medicine requires that objective, scientifically valid knowledge is easily available and applicable by the practicing clinician (Bero et al., 1998; Davidoff, Haynes, Sackett, & Smith, 1995; Guyatt, Drummand, & Hayward, 2001a, 2001b; Guyatt, Meade, Jaeschke, Cook, & Haynes, 2000; Mulrow & Cook, 1998; Sackett & Haynes, 1997; Sackett, Rosenberg, Gray, Haynes, & Richardson, 1996; Sarasin, 1999). We provide step-by-step, "how-to" instructions for producing sound, clinically applicable research syntheses. Our intended audience is a broad range of health professionals, from house staff and other graduate students to medical specialists and researchers, as well as to those who write health science articles for the lay public. However, in terms of quantitative synthesis processes, our major emphasis is for healthcare professionals who have some basic research or statistical training and who are personally interested in learning how to conduct and apply clinically relevant and valid meta-analyses. We also wrote this book for professionals who may not intend to develop systematic reviews themselves but would like to understand the basic principles for evaluating such syntheses for application in practice, whether clinical or administrative.

We anticipate that this book will provide ideas, understanding, and resources to accomplish much of the difficult task of compiling, validating, and synthesizing sound information for immediate healthcare improvement applications. This first chapter is an introduction to the book and is divided into the following sections:

INTRODUCTION: HEALTHCARE INFORMATION SYNTHESIS AND INFORMATICS

- A. Fundamental goals of this book
- B. Basic concepts: 'information synthesis' and 'healthcare informatics'
- C. Organization of this book
- D. Information synthesis methods literature
- E. Synthesis evaluation criteria
- F. Potential contributions of this book

Section A. Fundamental Goals of This Book

Three fundamental goals are woven throughout this book. No one chapter focuses specifically on these goals; rather, they are integrated into the content of all chapters at many levels of abstraction.

Help Beginners Value the Use of Synthesis and Informatics Concepts and Tools

Our first fundamental goal is to help beginners value the use of information synthesis and healthcare informatics concepts and tools. We emphasize the concept that any single research study, however sound it may be, is but one step toward eventually achieving solid knowledge on which clinical decisions can be based. We also propose that an understanding of the modern field of healthcare informatics, both conceptually and procedurally, is the foundation on which systematic reviews must be developed and applied in the community. For a historical background of the field of medical informatics, see Collen (1995).

Our book will facilitate an understanding and step-by-step approach for coping with the issues and controversies characteristic of the current state of health science information synthesis technology. In recent years, due to application of the theory and tools of informatics, the size of the field of systematic reviews has mushroomed. Most public and private organizations related to science information are finally establishing **Internet** sites; furthermore, even the traditional sources of information are making their material available online.

Requests for systematic reviews of the medical literature are coming from organizations, practitioners, and consumers throughout the world. In the United Kingdom, over the past 25 years, both government (National Health Service) and private groups (e.g., the Cochrane Collaboration) have recognized this fact and have expended substantial funds to meet this growing need. In the past decade, U.S. groups as diverse as physician professional organizations (e.g., American College of Physicians), drug manufacturers (e.g., Abbott Pharmaceuticals), and government agencies (e.g., the U.S. Agency for Healthcare Research and Quality [AHRQ]) are developing resources to meet this same challenge. More important, over the past 25 years, the U.S. government (e.g., the National Library of Medicine) and multiple private organizations have recognized that healthcare informatics will be the key for developing future knowledge, facilitating its coding, compilation, dissemination, and application to improve care outcomes throughout the world. MEDLINE is but one example, among many, of this pioneering work.

A major purpose of this book is to facilitate understanding and application of the fact that the integration of these two rapidly developing scientific fields (i.e., information synthesis and healthcare informatics) will be the foundation on which the improvement of the outcomes of future clinical practice will depend.

Although there is increasing agreement among authors in the field as to the fundamental principles and resources for performing a systematic review, several important issues remain controversial. A major issue is related to improving methods for reducing **bias** in both research and syntheses. For example, we propose that the single most serious source of bias in current reviews relates more to the literature search process than to review planning, validation, synthesis, write-up, or dissemination. We will illustrate how the theories and tools of informatics are fundamental for coping with these issues.

We will both document and discuss these conceptual issues and suggest task-by-task guidelines to illustrate how you might better manage these complex problems. In addition, throughout this work, we will refer you to other experienced review experts who go into greater depth on various subjects discussed. We will suggest other resources to help beginners become interested and active in this field. We will challenge the more experienced systematic reviewers to consider new and unique ideas for systematic reviews and informatics applications. We will suggest that future development of sound healthcare knowledge will depend on synthesizing not only empirical data but also qualitative information and intuitive experience of both providers and consumers.

Provide a Primer to Help Develop Informatics-Based Syntheses

The second fundamental goal is to provide step-by-step procedures to assist authors in producing a valid and replicable 'information synthesis.' For each stage of this book, we include chapters to explain conceptual factors, describe procedural tasks, and evaluate essential processes and products of this endeavor. Equally important, we will refer you to other resources, manuals, and collaborative teams who are at the forefront of methods development in this exciting and rapidly developing technology.

The primary audience for this book consists of such groups as students of the healthcare professions, health services researchers, providers of clinical services, quality management professionals, clinical administrators, and science writers for lay publications on health subjects. Such individuals are often charged with the task of compiling relevant and valid information for what might range from a postgraduate dissertation to guidelines for immediate healthcare use to developing medical care policies based on the best available knowledge. Because our book presents both the conceptual principles and the necessary step-by-step instructions for implementation, it should help authors and their staffs more easily identify, retrieve, and synthesize sound data and related information.

A fundamental lesson that you will learn from this book is that it is all but impossible to develop, let alone disseminate and apply, systematic reviews if you are not familiar with healthcare informatics, especially the resources available on the Internet. For example, informatics will teach us to understand basic knowledge structures essential for classifying, storing, retrieving, and applying digital data and information required in clinical practice at the time and place it is immediately needed. Procedurally, being able to use appropriate informatics equipment, such as a modern scanner, can save countless hours inputting information from paper copy. For at least the next decade, much, if not most, of needed full-text information will be found on paper, usually on the shelves of a library. Nevertheless, during this next decade, the number of online full-text documents, including both articles and books, will grow exponentially. In February 2000, there were more than 500 electronic medical journals on the Internet that linked to PubMed, one of the major search engines of the National Library of Medicine. In the 4 months after that time, the number increased to more than 900, and as of September 2001, there are more than 2,146 such journals. For documentation, see (last updated September 2001) www.ncbi.nlm.nih.gov/entrez/journals/loftext_noprov.html.

One of the contributions of this book is to provide such synthesis prerequisites such as direct Universal Resource Locator (URL) addresses of the more relevant and productive Web or other Internet sites. This resource can save you many hours of browsing to obtain the information you need. We will not only provide these healthcare information addresses as we go but also, in the back of this book, provide a compendium of these valuable resources. This compendium provides a master file of important sites within the framework of the organizations that sponsor and finance them. Within this context, you should be able to improve on your efforts to keep up with the constantly changing URL addresses and Web sites.

Again, although the intended audience is beginners or inexperienced authors, much of our content focuses in greater depth on quantitative syntheses and may be of interest to researchers and authors who are more experienced. To understand the quantitative synthesis material, readers should have some knowledge and experience with simple statistics, research principles, and research design. Chapters 12 and 13 provide a brief review of some of the statistical concepts necessary to understand and use the quantitative techniques of meta-analysis (Chapter 12 is meant as a review only). Before statistically analyzing data from the literature, those readers with little or no research background should consult with a statistician or research methodologist experienced in developing meta-analyses.

Facilitate Use of Synthesis
Results by Clinicians and Consumers

A third fundamental goal is to identify practical means for integrating the results of information syntheses into healthcare applications. Again, the field of informatics will be essential in facilitating this goal. Use of "evidence-based" knowledge in electronic practice guidelines, computerized expert systems, and rapid interchange of clinical knowledge and data such as imaging results are all common clinical needs requiring informatics tools.

Traditional reviews are not adequate to support "evidence-based" electronic clinical decision-making resources at the bedside. The question answered in the traditional reviews may not be the same as the one facing the clinician, or the population on which the research study was done may not be the same as the patient population of the clinician. A major focus of this book is to provide some necessary concepts, methods, and tools to make important links between evidence from sound scientific research and its use to improve clinical practice and healthcare outcomes.

A closely related challenge is to help authors of lay publications, particularly on the Internet, write health science information syntheses that will discriminate sound facts and ideas from those that are unsound or actually self-serving propaganda. (This topic will be discussed in Section B, Chapter 17.) Effective distribution to the lay public of valid healthcare information is critical. It was a shock to the senior author of this book when participating in a conference for science writers, lawyers, and health personnel at Harvard's Kennedy School of Government to note that lawyers and health science journalists seemed far more interested in learning how to identify sound healthcare information in medicine than were the physicians. You may be surprised at the different professional and lay groups, other than clinicians, that may need and will use your syntheses.

Section B. Basic Concepts: 'Healthcare Information Synthesis' and 'Healthcare Informatics'

Before proceeding further, it is important to understand how we use the terms *health science information synthesis* (hereafter abbreviated to *information synthesis*) and *healthcare informatics.* In the boxes below are descriptions of these concepts, both of which must be integrated if the purpose of this book is to be realized.

Understanding Our Concept of Information Synthesis

HEALTHCARE INFORMATION SYNTHESIS

In our terms, a *healthcare information synthesis* is a systematic review of scientific research on a health-related topic, adhering to a formal protocol. This protocol facilitates defining the topic within a conceptual framework (model), developing a relevant document database, selecting and validating a research data set, aggregating and synthesizing the results, and finally disseminating the synthesis in a form that facilitates ready application to improve community healthcare outcomes.

Currently, there are many synonyms that approximate this concept: *systematic reviews, validated reviews, critical reviews, expert reviews, evidence-based reviews, quantitative reviews* (e.g., meta-analyses), and *qualitative reviews* (e.g., ethnographic synthesis). Note that some authors use the term *overview* as a synonym for *review.*

We conceptualize two major categories of reviews: *traditional* and *systematic.* What distinguishes them is the rigor with which they are conducted, the detail by which their review methods are described, and whether their documentation is sufficiently thorough to facilitate editorial evaluation, updating, and replication. There can be exceptionally well-done traditional reviews and very poor systematic reviews. If done well, both of these categories have value, although they serve different purposes.

A traditional review usually focuses on questions that are more global and descriptive; it does not attempt to select all primary studies that represent an entire international field of inquiry, however narrowly defined. Sometimes, whole topics are covered, as in a textbook. Other times, the review is a summary of the author's knowledge in an area. The emphasis may often be on "background knowledge" and consists more of an overview of what is generally known on a topic or rather a formal summary of data and findings. In healthcare, textbook chapters that present known causes of a disorder and its epidemiology, clinical manifestations, diagnosis, treatment, and prognosis are in this category.

A systematic review, in contrast, usually has a more focused topic. The focus is on *foreground knowledge* or new information synthesized as a result of the review process. Rigorous, scientifically based rules are followed using a protocol to select, appraise, and integrate studies. Formal statistical pooling of results may be done. The goal is to minimize bias and help improve reliability and accuracy of conclusions. Within the general category of systematic reviews, two subtypes can be conceptualized. The first is called a *qualitative* and the second a *quantitative* review.

In a **qualitative review**, the methods used are expected to be systematic, but the primary studies under investigation are qualitative, ethnographic, or observational. This area of research has its own rigorous system of analysis, but the focus is interpretative rather than explanatory. Authors attempting to synthesize qualitative literature must be systematic and rigorous in their approach, but the protocols and rules are different than for a quantitative synthesis. We do not provide more than a brief introduction to qualitative methods in this book, but in Chapter 2 we do discuss one of the largest subcategories, a meta-ethnographic approach. In this field, questions usually addressed by qualitative researchers might include the following: "How do patients experience adjustment to liver transplants?" "What are the perceptions of couples who are infertile?" and "How do family caregivers adjust to the declining health of a loved one?"

The second type of systematic review is the quantitative review, which involves some form of statistical analysis. In this book, we emphasize meta-analysis and refer to it as any attempt to pool quantitative data from several primary studies. As with all systematic reviews, quantitative reviews are quite explicit regarding project planning, searching the literature, assessing the quality of the database compiled, and synthesizing and writing the results. Questions that can be answered by a quantitative review include the following: "Which is the better treatment?" "Which diagnostic test is more accurate?" and "What is the evidence that lack of exercise is a risk factor for heart disease?" They are questions that have as their goal improving the "power" of an inquiry by combining data from several empirical primary studies. They may provide either an estimate of a population parameter (e.g., the average survival time after the first acute myocardial infarction [MI]) or a conclusion regarding the best treatment and its use (e.g., how soon, after an acute MI is diagnosed, must thrombolytics be given) for achieving the best outcome.

Understanding Our Concept of Healthcare Informatics

Today, conducting an information synthesis without use of informatics theory and tools (computer hardware and software) is laborious, if not impossible. It is a function of synthesis preparation to consult an informatics specialist and to use up-to-date, user-friendly computer tools and software. Such help will prove essential for planning, implementing, evaluating, and applying your project in the community. One example of the contribution of informatics theory and methods is the development of online bibliographic databases such as MEDLINE (in 1964). Likewise, there is substantial value in the new field of knowledge engineering in informatics. Also of value are clinical applications (e.g., a computerized expert system to manage use of presurgical prophylactic antibiotics that has proven to save lives and monetary cost).

But what is healthcare informatics? A simplistic and narrow definition would have you believe that informatics involves only the use of computers in healthcare. We favor a broader conceptualization, built on the one reported by Stead (1998):

HEALTHCARE INFORMATICS

Healthcare informatics is a computer-related science that deals with the multiple dimensions of health information, such as its structure, semantics, relationships, acquisition, validity, storage, acquisition, and use to improve healthcare outcomes.[a] This concept is much more complex than the mere use of computers in medicine. It involves information models, Unified Medical Language System (UMLS), compilation, and use of relevant and valid data, and it encompasses both theoretical and applied sciences.

Medical informatics has been the traditional term used to describe this field. We prefer the term *healthcare informatics,* which is more generic because there are many new subdivisions of informatics in the health field. For example, nursing informatics is growing and flourishing, social work informatics has been developed, and administrative informatics has probably been around longer than any. Most of these areas have established formal academic programs where education, training, and advanced degrees can be obtained. However, we do recognize and respect the fact that *medical informatics* was the initial field that led the way and, with its many new branches, is revolutionizing healthcare as we know it.

a. This concept builds on that of Stead (1998).

By this definition, healthcare informatics is central to information synthesis, particularly focusing on information structure, validity, acquisition, and use. In the past three decades, there has been unbelievable progress in this field, which has provided a foundation for the modern technology of health science "information synthesis."

Section C. Organization of This Book

This book identifies five stages, each representing a conceptually separate phase for producing an information synthesis or a systematic review. (These stages usually overlap chronologically.)

INFORMATION SYNTHESIS DEVELOPMENT STAGES

Stage I.   Planning and preparation

Stage II.   Database development

Stage III.   Database validation

Stage IV.   Information analysis and synthesis

Stage V.   Synthesis report completion and evaluation

The five basic stages of this book reflect the fundamental steps of any basic research process, starting from problem formulation, collection of data, data analysis, write-up, and application (Cooper, 1998). For each stage, we provide a discussion of the associated terms, principles, and considerations. We follow these theoretical sections with a more detailed step-by-step description of how to accomplish the procedures and tasks appropriate to each stage. In addition, we provide relevant forms and tools for conducting, reporting, and applying an information synthesis.

In healthcare, there are a wide variety of research designs for the varied functions of medical practice. Epidemiological studies are critical for establishing local population á priori probabilities (prevalence rates of population characteristics). These data are essential for accurate diagnoses. To what extent can a physician trust local city or county health statistics? To what extent can epidemiologists trust death certificate information? Research designs to answer such questions will be somewhat different from a controlled trial testing the efficacy of a specific treatment. Experimental studies (e.g., double-blind, randomized, controlled clinical trials) are necessary to establish evidence of causal relations. However, such designs do not readily apply to the validity of descriptive health statistics, prognostics, or technology assessments. Therefore, you, as a potential author of a systematic review, will require familiarity with a broad range of information and research tools. There will be certain review functions that are common to all information syntheses, however different in content. The following stages describe those functions.

Stage I: Planning and Preparation

In this first stage, we describe concepts and procedures for developing your synthesis topic and plan and preparing for its implementation. These include defining your synthesis goals, organizing resources and staff, planning a budget, and developing an initial search strategy. Emphasis is placed on developing a conceptual model. We emphasize three prerequisites to planning that involve understanding: (a) the synthesis constraints of your resource availability in terms of informatics tools, funding, and time; (b) the variety of synthesis designs you may choose from; and (c) the "state of the science" information essential for developing a topic and theoretical model for your synthesis project.

Stage II: Database Development

In the second stage, we introduce the theoretical principles associated with identifying and compiling a relevant database of articles that represent different schools (i.e., invisible colleges) of research thought on your topic. In our judgment, the usual procedures for compiling a representative database for either a traditional or a systematic review are most likely the weakest link in the review process. This problem has been almost impossible to manage until this new era of computerized bibliographic databanks, focused research topic registers, and, by means of the Internet, international access to a growing body of important materials. We will emphasize strategies for coping with this problem.

We discuss the importance of developing a systematic coding scheme for maintaining content relevance and avoiding "topic drift." Identifying reliable criteria for relevance is particularly important because these procedures allow you to manage the **information overload** problems that often impair synthesis of medical literature. We emphasize procedures for deciding when you can terminate your information search (e.g., understanding and applying "file drawer" analysis statistics). Finally, we present illustrative tables, tools, and forms to assist you in being more efficient and thorough in implementing the above-mentioned search procedures.

Stage III: Database Validation

In the third stage, we review the current perspectives on judging the scientific validity of relevant articles in your database and indicate the fundamental principles involved in that process. We present a brief overview of the recent development of more detailed and sophisticated criteria for evaluating research methods in the materials you retrieve. We illustrate the procedures of data extraction and coding in preparation for validation. We introduce the concepts of quantitative, qualitative, and heuristic validity, discussing the relative importance of each. We present an illustrative validation instrument of our own, to be considered by readers as an initial template to facilitate validation of the individual studies in your database. We emphasize validation of quantitative research in preparation for meta-analysis. (In Appendix 9.1, we provide examples of validation criteria sets for evaluating individual research studies—criteria that have evolved between 1977 and 2000.) Finally, we will stress the estimation of the heterogeneity of your database as a whole. Ignoring this step can pose one of the more common threats to the validity of your results and conclusions.

Stage IV: Information Analysis and Synthesis

In the fourth stage, we suggest important factors in selecting the type of synthesis most suitable to your needs. Different synthesis models are required for qualitative, as opposed to quantitative, systematic reviews. Also included are a brief overview of basic statistical concepts (Chapter 12), a presentation of the issues involved in performing a meta-analysis (Chapter 13), and step-by-step examples illustrating the seven different methods by which effect sizes are computed and synthesized (Chapter 14).

Overall, one of the major goals of any synthesis process is to identify the consistencies and inconsistencies in similar research literature on a particular topic

(Cooper & Hedges, 1994, chap. 1). From the consistencies in the research findings, you might establish generalizations that can be applied to all of the studies. In such a quantitative analysis, however, you might discover many inconsistencies in the research results, which is one of the major challenges in trying to explain the variability of results from seemingly similar investigations (Cooper & Hedges, 1994). The procedures described in Stage IV are designed to help you identify, understand, and, it is hoped, manage the consistencies and inconsistencies in research on a particular topic.

Stage V: Synthesis Report Completion and Evaluation

In the fifth and final stage, we review the principles and procedures for producing, evaluating, and applying your final product. We provide guidelines and detailed forms for writing and using your synthesis. Chapter 17 focuses on applying your synthesis results in clinical practice. The complexities of statistical results of research are addressed, and a lexicon of basic terms is provided to make results more understandable and useful. Finally, we review fundamental issues in effecting behavioral change and diffusion of innovation. We discuss five modalities for effecting behavioral change in the community, emphasizing the advantages and disadvantages of each.

In each stage, we use clinical examples whenever possible and focus on issues unique to clinical and healthcare research and literature. By presenting a meta-analysis in a step-by-step format in this book, we hope it will become a useful and practical tool for interested and qualified clinicians, health administrators, or beginning researchers. Also, this book should be helpful to these groups to identify a well-documented health science information synthesis, as opposed to a poorly documented one.

Section D. Information Synthesis Methods Literature

The history of information synthesis methodology is quite long and parallels the development of research methods and instrumentation. You will learn that the Cochrane Library (United Kingdom) provides access to one of the most complete and growing methodological databases on this subject. In this section, we review a few pertinent highlights of the history of information synthesis methods and present the major issues facing authors of information synthesis today.

Evolution of Information Synthesis Methods

Early Review Problems. Although information synthesis activities occurred in the first half of the 20th century (e.g., Yates & Cochran, 1938), the methods of review remain problematic. Published guides for combining study results were written by Yates and Cochran (1938) and Mosteller and Bush (1954). The latter article, which focused on combining effect sizes, stimulated the push toward quantitative reviews in the social sciences. Feldman (1971) reported his work confirming the wide variation in results of primary data studies. Taveggia (1974) described six common problems in literature reviews ranging from inadequate searches to invalid reporting of results.

In the healthcare field, the senior author of this book performed several traditional literature reviews to identify expected posttreatment functional patient outcomes to provide quality improvement standards for 10 disease entities (Williamson, Alexander, & Miller, 1968). The literature proved sadly lacking in relevant studies that produced usable data. Because most clinicians are forced to make decisions under conditions of uncertainty, Williamson proposed building on sound research data that did exist and filling in the gaps by harvesting the implicit knowledge and experience of groups of experts to facilitate consensus development on 'best practice.' His group developed and applied structured group judgment methods (e.g., modified nominal group and Delphi techniques). Manuals (Emlet, Davis, & Casey, 1971; Emlet, Williamson, et al., 1971) on the topic of *Alternate Methods for Estimating Health-Care Benefits and Required Resources* presented 42 alternative methods to achieve team consensus for synthesizing information. The major difference between these methods was (a) whether these judgments were made in total uncertainty (21 variations) or (b) whether they used the best available research findings and whatever other hard facts that might exist (21 methods). These approaches involved structured group judgment of experts, often with participation of consumer representatives.

Williamson's (1977) book, *Improving Medical Practice and Health Care: A Bibliographic Guide to Information Management in Quality Assurance and Continuing Education,* outlined basic steps in developing an information synthesis that dealt more directly with the problems of relevance, availability, and validity of literature and use of data for healthcare quality improvement. Goldschmidt (1986) developed these ideas even further when he published his paper, titled "Information Synthesis: A Practical Guide." Brook was directly influenced by these ideas in his work with the RAND Corporation. His studies of healthcare appropriateness were early examples of what we now call information syntheses. For example, see his analysis of the literature related to acute medical care of the elderly (Brook et al., 1989).

Jackson (1980) studied 36 reviews from prestigious journals and found that only one adequately reported search procedures. Basic problems with reviews and information syntheses have continued to be noted into the present time. From the 1970s to the early 1990s, the number of methodologically valid review articles in the medical literature was small (Fleiss & Gross, 1991; Halvorsen, 1986; Mulrow, 1987; Williamson, Goldschmidt, & Colton, 1986). For example, in a 1987 review of meta-analyses of randomized controlled trials, only 25% addressed all six of the predetermined quality criteria (Chalmerset al., 1987). Mulrow (1987) found that of 50 reviews, only 17 satisfied three of eight criteria, and only one satisfied six of the eight.

Subsequent Methodological Developments. Researchers responding to these critiques have developed formal methodological solutions. Glass (1976) has been credited with naming the new field of "meta-analysis" after he used this term in his guidelines for doing a quantitative synthesis in the behavioral sciences. Light and Pillemer (1984) have also proposed formal techniques for evaluating the variation of results of primary studies (original data research) that would contribute to the evolution of information syntheses. Following Glass's lead, Cooper (1989, 1998) and Rosenthal (1984) have written comprehensive guidebooks on the processes of performing an information synthesis. Subsequently, the term *meta-analysis* has been widely accepted. Hedges and Olkin (1985) and Hunter and Schmidt (1990) greatly expanded this body of literature with their comprehensive books on the subject of meta-analysis.

Cynthia Mulrow (1987) wrote a journal article, titled "The Medical Review Article: The State of the Science," that described methodological progress up through the 1980s. The recent *Handbook of Research Synthesis* (Cooper & Hedges, 1994) is a comprehensive compendium on research synthesis methods written by leading authors in the field, coming from both the behavioral and psychosocial fields.

In the late 1980s and early 1990s, information synthesis methods were published that relate to health technology assessment and guideline development (Goodman & Baratz, 1990; Marcus, Grover, & Revicki, 1987; Wortman & Yeaton, 1987).

Thomas C. Chalmers (who passed away in 1995) had a distinguished research career and was one of the more avid investigators who focused on the methodological issues of randomized controlled trials. During the last two decades of his life, he dedicated his work to the improvement of quantitative review methods, being associated with more than 200 articles published on this subject during that period. We will heavily emphasize his contributions that led to the recent (1998) organization of the Thomas C. Chalmers Centre for Systematic Reviews that is located in Canada. (See their Web site at the following address [this home page was last updated December 1999]: www.cheori.org/tcc.)

The Cochrane Collaboration. In our judgment, the single most significant development in the chronology of the healthcare information synthesis evolution occurred in February 1992, with National Health Service (NHS) funding of the first formal "Cochrane Centre" in the United Kingdom. The purpose of this organization was "to facilitate the preparation of systematic reviews of randomized controlled trials of healthcare." The reference for the above quote and an interesting chronology of the Cochrane Collaboration are available at the following URL address (last updated November 2000): www.cochrane.org/cochrane/cchronol.htm.

This organization was inspired by the writings of A. L. (Archie) Cochrane (1972), particularly his monograph on *Effectiveness and Efficiency,* which stressed the importance of randomized clinical trials as the foundation on which the improvement of healthcare should be based. The senior author of this book was asked to write a review of this treatise (Williamson, 1973). The work of this Collaboration has grown, flourished, and influenced so many others throughout the world who contribute to this field of systematic reviews and review technology that we consider them the preeminent world leaders of this field today. A few major contributions include the following:

1. registers of controlled clinical trials;

2. development of Cochrane Centres throughout the world;

3. library index to complete systematic reviews or abstracts of reviews from their own "Centres" and possible others, which they have evaluated and continue to provide access to updates and references, particularly to the growing methods technology of this field;

4. development of a sophisticated educational program and multiple valuable training aids, such as their handbook;

5. an international conference series;

6. evolving their entire enterprise on an informatics base, with Internet links worldwide.

The education and training materials this group provides without cost on the Internet include *The Cochrane Reviewers' Handbook, The Cochrane Reviewers' Handbook Glossary,* and *The Cochrane Manual,* among many others. These may be among of the most thorough and meaningful methods materials of which we are aware.

As of January 2001, the Cochrane Collaboration listed 15 Centres throughout the world, encompassing 50 health-problem collaborative review groups (CRG) and 10 subgroups. One would hardly go astray starting any systematic review literature search by contacting and collaborating with this group. See the Cochrane

Collaboration's home page at the following Internet address (last updated December 2000): hiru.mcmaster.ca/cochrane/default.html.

However, the Cochrane group is making another contribution that, as yet, seems to remain implicit. That contribution is integrating this field with the tools of healthcare informatics. You can sit in your office and, by means of the Internet and licensed access to the Cochrane Library, benefit from their growing data and information banks. Thus, this collaboration of international centers has digitized their remarkable compilation of systematic reviews, together with their reviews of these reviews, and made them available electronically to professionals throughout the world.

Recent Technological Methods Development. In 1997, two journal articles provided a brief outline of the basic steps of a systematic review or meta-analysis. For beginners, these are cogent materials to help them understand an overview of synthesis methods as of the mid-1990s. The first is an article by Lau, Ioannidis, and Schmid (1997), titled "Quantitative Synthesis in Systematic Reviews." The second is an article by Egger, Smith, and Phillips (1997), titled "Meta-Analysis: Principles and Procedures."

Mulrow and Cook (1998) have contributed to recent clinical healthcare synthesis methods by their anthology, available in softcover, titled *Systematic Reviews: Synthesis of Best Evidence for Health Care Decisions.* This is a collection of separately authored chapters on healthcare information synthesis procedures. They have assembled a noteworthy group of contributors to provide many helpful "how-to" methods and suggestions. It is a well-integrated work that provides more methods detail of the state of the science of systematic review technology in the mid-1990s.

H. Cooper (1998) published an updated softcover edition of his *Integrating Research: A Guide for Literature Reviews* (2nd ed.) and renamed it *Synthesizing Research: A Guide for Literature Reviews* (3rd ed.). This updated volume introduces the use of electronic technology and emphasizes how important the Internet is for developing systematic reviews. He also notes the difference this informatics technology makes in identifying "invisible colleges" of colleagues. He contrasts the traditional approach with the new electronic approach by use of "computerized list management programs . . . called listservs, listprocs, or Majordomos . . . or through newsgroups" (Cooper, 1998, pp. 46-49). He covers each of our five stages in a succinct manner, providing a brief overview of this new synthesis technology.

In 1998, Arlene Fink published her book *Conducting Research Literature Reviews: From Paper to the Internet.* This is the first work we have seen that gives emphasis to the integration of synthesis and informatics technology. However, her content focus seems rather broad. She makes a particularly salient point in stating that "the scholarship and research on which you base the review come from individuals' diverse professions including health, education, psychology, business, finance, law, and social services" (Fink, 1998, p. 3). In five chapters, she covers the basic five stages of a synthesis, with three of those chapters being devoted to database development. Each chapter has subchapters devoted to validation of methodological quality, especially reliability and validity. We agree with her implication that database development is likely the weak link in the field of systematic reviews and thus deserves the most attention. In her final chapter, she delves into methods for descriptive and meta-analytic reviews with brief but cogent coverage.

The above three books illustrate important contributions to the rapidly maturing field of information synthesis technology. Together with Cooper and Hedges's (1994) classic *The Handbook of Research Synthesis,* you would have four recent references of highly relevant material to supplement our book.

Metaxis. Metaxis is a product of Update Software, Inc. that provides a CD-ROM step-by-step guide to facilitate planning and development of systematic reviews. From this site, you can also link to such ancillary software as ACLUSTER for coping with the complex statistical issues of design and analysis of cluster randomization in clinical trials. Cluster analysis is a more advanced method that may not be very relevant for beginners. Such resources represent but a few examples of a growing body of advanced methodological developments for conducting systematic reviews. The Web site for Metaxis (last updated ??, copyright 2001) is www.update-software.com/ metaxis/.

See Everitt, Landau, and Leese (2000) for the reference to their book *Cluster Analysis* (4th ed.) and the following Web site for access to their software ACLUSTER (last updated ??, copyright 2001): www.update-software.com/acluster.

Clinical Problems in Coping With Scientific Literature

Regardless of the kind of synthesis chosen or the type of product produced, a systematic review allows clinicians to cope with three major problems associated with improving healthcare by using the scientific literature.

Information Overload. The past decade has seen a veritable explosion in the number of medical information sources. Although online bibliographic databases make the task of accessing these sources easier, many clinicians do not have easy access to, or are not familiar with, the workings of such electronic resources. For example, many healthcare professionals assume that a MEDLINE search alone will provide adequate coverage of most relevant topics, but this assumption has been shown to be mistaken (Dickersin, Hewitt, Mutch, Chalmers, & Chalmers, 1985; Haynes et al., 1985; Marson & Chadwick, 1996; McDonald, Taylor, & Adams, 1999; Poynard & Conn, 1985; Woods & Trewheellar, 1998). Great care must be taken to ensure that a literature search is both comprehensive and cost-effective. In Stage II (Chapters 5 and 6), we present techniques and strategies for conducting a more adequate information search.

Another important step in the synthesis process is to determine which of the many hundreds of articles located are relevant to the topic being synthesized and will provide a homogeneous population of studies. Authors of syntheses may mistakenly assume that readers can easily discern their implicit relevance criteria. However, some studies have shown that judgments of relevance for any specific set of articles may differ in terms of how documents are to be used (Cuadra & Katter, 1967) and in the order of presentation of documents (Eisenberg & Barry, 1988). Even experts within a field do not necessarily agree on which articles are relevant for a specific synthesis (Cooper & Ribble, 1989).

Once the relevant articles have been identified, integrating them into a valid synthesis is also difficult. One aspect of the information overload problem is simply the difficulty inherent in synthesizing the results of a diverse group of publications. In his seminal article on meta-analysis, Glass (1976) commented on the importance of a formal synthesis procedure by saying, "Before what has been found can be used, before it can persuade skeptics, influence policy, affect practice, it must be known. Someone must organize it, integrate it, and extract the message" (p. 4). Cooper and Rosenthal (1980) demonstrated the effects of a nonsystematic approach to information synthesis by comparing the conclusions of researchers who performed the traditional narrative synthesis to a similar number who performed formal meta-analyses on the same topic. The two groups of researchers made directly opposing conclusions about the scientific findings. Without a formal, systematic method to integrate findings, the knowledge inherent in a field of study can easily be lost.

As the above discussion implies, effective handling of information overload requires detailed attention to the cognitive tasks of searching for relevant publications, deciding on relevance, and organizing and integrating the resultant information—an effort that is often difficult (Orwin, 1994). Effective performance of these tasks requires use of a systematic process based on sound scientific principles. Unfortunately, some clinicians may simply give up the attempt at doing a synthesis and settle for reading a single article from a well-respected journal, then immediately and prematurely apply it to practice. Williamson et al. (1989) reported a survey of a random, stratified sample of U.S. primary practitioners and their opinion leaders. More than two thirds of practitioners claimed the volume of literature was unmanageable and thus, personally, did not even try to use it.

We believe this book presents the entire synthesis process in a way that helps the clinician and novice researcher deal effectively with the information overload problem. Specific procedures are presented to help organize the steps of planning and conducting a more comprehensive search.

Information Validity. Once relevant publications have been located, discerning which of their findings are valid and usable becomes the next most important issue.

Numerous problems arise in evaluating the validity of information from primary sources. Many research articles published in peer-reviewed journals contain serious scientific flaws or biases that limit the applicability of their findings (Oxman & Guyatt, 1988; Williamson et al., 1986; Wortman, 1994). For example, Devine (1984) examined the effects of psychoeducational interventions on outcomes in surgical patients; he found that only 4 of 105 studies were sufficiently free from methodological flaws to be used. Most studies in the health field have designs that limit their scientific credibility (e.g., pretest/posttest studies that fail to indicate causal relationships because they have no control groups). Because theoretical foundations are not attended to, studies on similar questions may have vastly different research methods, sampling characteristics, and even operationalized variables. For example, the blood level of carbon monoxide or the number of cigarettes per day may measure smoking. If primary studies using different measures for the same variable are mixed, synthesis is impossible. Even randomized controlled trials can suffer from serious threats to validity; these studies often have significant attrition or crossover rates (i.e., patients in the control group end up in the experimental group, and vice versa), sometimes as high as 30% (e.g., Wortman & Yeaton, 1987). They may also suffer from improper or inadequate operationalization of the independent variable (Orwin, 1994; Sechrest, West, Phillips, Redner, & Yeaton, 1979). The inferences from such studies are unusable in clinical practice because they fail to demonstrate causality.

These validity issues create interpretative problems that are relatively invisible to clinicians. Most researchers and clinicians have little formal training in the quantitative sciences and thus lack the skills to adequately evaluate scientific validity. However, with training, considerable practice, and expert feedback, they can improve their skills in this area. In a recent study examining agreement among reviewers of review articles, the authors found good agreement between statistically trained clinicians and research methodologists (Oxman et al., 1991), indicating that to apply the results of research effectively to practice, systematic procedures must be used to assess the validity of primary research studies. In this book, we present these procedures in sufficient detail to allow the beginner to make appropriate estimates regarding the soundness of research information.

Integration Into Practice. Formal information syntheses, as generally performed, often contain significant restrictions in application of their findings to clinical practice. Recently, this deficiency was made even more apparent when the Agency for Healthcare Research and Quality (AHRQ) attempted to implement its charge from the U.S. Congress to develop and disseminate clinical practice guidelines. An essential step in implementing this charge was to determine the availability of empirical evidence for all steps in a guideline. Across almost all guideline development efforts, the AHRQ found the available scientific evidence too incomplete and too general to be applied to the necessary specific questions in a clinical practice guideline (Shekelle & Schriger, 1996). In all cases, expert panel opinion was required to bridge the gap.

There are several major limitations for applying the results of formal information syntheses in practice. The first limitation is that the results may not be meaningful for clinical decisions. A significant statistical test showing a large average effect size may not provide clear guidance about what to do. In other words, a statistically significant effect is not necessarily clinically significant. Second, the questions addressed in most meta-analyses are too broad, and the answers might not apply to the specific patient class that is under the care of a specific clinician. For example, a meta-analysis may be conducted on the efficacy of aspirin in reducing the risk of an acute myocardial infarction, but the population involved in the study may be so diverse that the results are not interpretable in terms of the 48-year-old female patient with diabetes who is actually in front of the provider. Third, the information, even if it were interpretable, is often not available at the time needed, and the questions asked are often the "easy" ones (e.g., the efficacy of a single drug or the average age of onset of certain diseases). However, more complicated questions, such as the role of patient preference in successful outcomes or the impact of drug dosage levels on patient compliance, inform practice at a deeper level. All of these issues are addressed throughout this book, ranging from how relevance criteria are selected to how results are reported to how the hazards of scientific propaganda can be avoided. A final chapter of this book outlines some specific recommendations for applying synthesis results to improve practice outcomes.

An effective synthesis, to be used in clinical practice, needs to address the above limitations. In other words, authors of research synthesis should report their results in a manner meaningful to the practicing clinician. They need to address questions that are comprehensive, as well as specific enough, to be useful to a clinician making decisions about an individual patient in a particular setting. They need to embed their findings in the larger framework of complicated, multidimensional patient care. They need to include, as part of their findings, specific methodologies for dissemination. Finally, authors of syntheses need to address questions beyond those that are available simply because they can be measured easily. Expanding the usual emphasis of a research synthesis in this way may involve developing new methodologies and applications. In any event, making this link to the practicing clinician is essential.

In general, however, there are many related publications where authors have developed systematic procedures for conducting formal information syntheses. The state of the science in this field has greatly expanded, including the development and popularity of meta-analysis. All of these methods are useful to the extent that they assist the reader and the author to cope with the basic information management problems of information overload, information validity, and integration into practice.

Section E. Synthesis Evaluation Criteria

Before beginning any project, it is important to have in mind how the project is to be evaluated. We emphasize four general criteria by which an information synthesis can be judged. How each of these criteria is applied will depend on the type of synthesis conducted. Although they seem general, together they provide a comprehensive overview of the quality of the synthesis itself. We propose, for purposes of healthcare outcome improvement, that every information synthesis should be adequately documented, clinically significant and applicable, scientifically sound, and cost-effective.

This section defines the major terms that will be applied to an overall evaluation of each stage, as well as in the book as a whole. Some of these terms are the author's jargon (e.g., 'meta-validation'); however, many are standard terms from the research literature.

Criterion 1: Adequately Documented

Adequate documentation is essential for applying the remaining three criteria for evaluating each stage of your synthesis, as well as for your report as a whole. Lack of adequate documentation can make the difference between a high-quality review and a product that is completely unusable. The adequacy of documentation is likely one of the best means of distinguishing a traditional review from an information synthesis (or a systematic review). In evaluating each stage, different criteria will be emphasized depending on the subject matter. If you intend to publish your synthesis, the amount of methods detail you can include may vary in terms of the publisher's editorial policy and the size of the article or monograph. However, at a minimum, enough methods information should be provided to allow (a) a reviewer to make an editorial decision to accept or reject your manuscript, (b) an author to update your review, and, ideally, (c) a colleague to replicate your work, as with any scientific research study. At the end of every stage, in our evaluation chapters we review what should be documented. In addition, Appendix 18.3 provides criteria for evaluating systematic reviews—criteria that have evolved between 1977 and 2000.

Criterion 2: Clinically Significant and Applicable

CLINICAL SIGNIFICANCE

We define *clinical significance* to be the extent to which scientifically valid healthcare information can be applied to a defined population, to help improve their health status and quality of life within a relatively short timeframe. This concept has two dimensions: (a) clinical importance and (b) clinical information maturity, as elucidated below.

Clinical Importance. This concept relates to the amount of benefit a given intervention (e.g., prevention, diagnosis, or therapy) might have in a population. We define **healthcare benefit** (assuming benefit outweighs cost plus harm) as the extent of outcome improvement accomplished per person, multiplied by the number of people in the population who might be helped. For instance, a life-saving intervention (e.g., removal of an early malignant melanoma) for a few people might yield the equivalent benefit of symptom relief (e.g., reduction of severe arthritis pain) for a much larger proportion of the population. In the long run, clinical importance is a value judgment that can be made by any healthcare provider or consumer. In the context of developing an information synthesis, the project team and the likely readers must determine for themselves the clinical importance of information content in an article or synthesis.

Clinical Information Maturity. Clinical information maturity is a concept that indicates the extent to which research content is sufficiently developed for immediate application to healthcare outcomes improvement in clinical day-to-day practice. This concept encompasses adequate evidence of efficacy, safety, cost-effectiveness, and acceptability of the information or intervention to both providers and consumers.

Often this determination is made informally by general acceptance and use but should be made more formally, such as by an independent panel of clinical experts. Such a group would identify meta-validated evidence to confirm efficacy, safety, and cost-effectiveness (compared to older interventions for the same purpose) and acceptability to both providers and consumers of healthcare. "Acceptability" encompasses such factors as ethical, religious, affordability, and potential pain or harm that might be involved. Review groups making these "information maturity" judgments are often sponsored by institutions developing practice guidelines, consensus statements, and now, more frequently, systematic reviews.

Information maturity can be thought of as a dimension ranging from idea construction, to single empirical studies with high-quality designs (as in randomized controlled trials), to knowledge synthesis, to assessment of impact (e.g., outcome improvement) in real-life settings. Healthcare journals often report immature clinical knowledge (i.e., information not ready for application by community practitioners). Only after many studies evaluate and confirm the impact of selected interventions in real-life settings will sound evidence be available regarding efficacy, safety, cost-effectiveness, and acceptability of healthcare interventions.

Criterion 3: Scientifically Sound

In this book, we will restrict our definition of *scientific soundness* to four variables: internal, external, construct, and statistical validity.

Internal Validity. Internal validity refers to the probability that the independent variable could, believably and logically, have caused the dependent variable. The logic of the conclusion is based on the extent to which competing explanations can be ruled out. As a meta-analysis is basically descriptive research, many possible factors can threaten its conclusions. Often, studies are not randomized, nor populations selected systematically, nor included studies proven homogeneous. Also, there are often large variations in the way treatments are implemented. Determination of internal validity is based on evaluation of (a) the processes for selection of studies, (b) the quality of studies, and (c) the use of systematic synthesis methods for such purposes as estimating heterogeneity of studies included and conducting sensitivity analysis.

External Validity. External validity refers to the extent to which you can generalize your findings from a sample of literature to the universe from which that sample was drawn. In other words, external validity is how "representative" your sample of research studies is of the spectrum of evidence from the different schools of thought on your topic. Theoretically, you can conceptualize a worldwide universe of research on any subject. A reviewer could compile a citation pool of all studies ever done on that topic and then draw a random sample of studies from that pool. A synthesis of data from those studies could then be generalized to that universe. Unfortunately, this is not ideal, cost-effective, or even possible. As shown in Chapters 5 and 6, a number of methods attempt to crudely approximate an adequately representative and balanced sample of articles from which to synthesize. Every effort must be made to avoid the potential biases in study selection.

Construct Validity. Construct validity is the extent to which the synthesis content reflects your research question(s), your scientific model, or the theoretical framework of your study. Population definitions need to be accurate and precisely defined, specific treatment procedures and care processes identified, and measurement methods valid. If care is not taken to correctly attend to definitions of variables (both the independent and the dependent variables), then the population of studies sampled and synthesized may be so heterogeneous that subsequent conclusions could be meaningless. Most important, the independent variable (treatment variable) should be precisely defined in the relevance criteria to ensure that a synthesis across studies is interpretable.

Statistical Validity. Statistical validity is essential if a quantitative synthesis is going to be done. This area of validity includes having enough power (sufficient sample size) to address biases and unreliability of measurement methods, as well as retrieval and synthesis processes. Systematic tests for heterogeneity between studies should always be done, as well as sensitivity analyses to demonstrate the degree to which the findings are robust and resistant to small threats to statistical assumptions.

At the end of each stage, we include a chapter to facilitate your validation of the procedures and results from the chapters included in that stage. Only those aspects of these four overall criteria that pertain to a particular stage are applied.

Criterion 4: Cost-Effective

The purpose of this criterion is to compare the healthcare outcome improvement value achieved for the cost expended. Outcome enhancement can be accomplished by either reducing the cost or increasing the value gained. For example, in evaluating the cost of your completed synthesis, can you estimate how many unnecessary costly purchases or wasted personnel time might, in the future, be avoided? Or on the other hand, what topic might be selected for a subsequent synthesis that would yield greater value for the cost? Every information synthesis should be budgeted realistically in terms of affordable time and dollars. If money and time are scarce, then a "review of reviews" can be conducted quickly with little financial cost. Conversely, if resources are abundant, a more complete search can be conducted along with a more elaborate data extraction, validation, and synthesis process. Though often neglected, meeting this criterion should demonstrate the important advantage of keeping fiscal and time records for better management in future synthesis projects. For example, if such management is not done during Stage II (data gathering), there is a serious risk that you might run out of funds before completing your analysis and synthesis, let alone your manuscript preparation.

Section F. Potential Contributions of This Book

This book builds on and extends previous information synthesis technology publications by reviewing and updating both conceptual and procedural developments in the fields of systematic reviews and healthcare informatics. We propose that these two fields must be understood and integrated for building new knowledge structures, synthesizing data from sound scientific studies, and facilitating its application for improving the outcomes of healthcare in the community. Although we emphasize use by beginners, there is much valuable material for use by the more experienced authors of validated reviews as well. To illustrate, for those interested in writing a quantitative synthesis, we discuss several important conceptual issues and provide a step-by-step approach in terms of seven variations of a meta-analysis. Overall, we suggest and discuss three basic contributions of this book for enhancing future systematic reviews.

The term *net benefit* seems to have been popularized by the Cochrane group but was well defined by Eddy (1990) in his article "Comparing Benefits and Harms: The Balance Sheet." Most medical interventions have some risk of harm that must be estimated and compared to the likely good they will do. Though the term is related to the jargon of fiscal accounting, it is important to recognize that "harm" may include but is not equivalent to financial "cost." For example, Barratt et al. (1999) include "cost and inconvenience" in their list of potential harms to people having a positive screening test result. The terms *benefit* and *harm* are both outcomes involving *values* as perceived by the patient and/or the care provider. Thus, you must conceptualize for both the healthcare consumer and the provider a crude quantitative difference in perceived benefit, minus harm, with the result divided by cost. Hence the concept "net benefit" (Barratt et al., 1999; Guyatt, Sackett, & Cook, 1994). This is somewhat analogous to formal cost-benefit analysis, if all factors are quantified in dollars (in the United States, for example). If benefit and harm remain in conceptual terms as opposed to fiscal terms, it is analogous to the more formal cost-effectiveness analysis.

Enhanced Net Benefits for Healthcare Providers, Researchers, and Educators

We are specifically orienting this work to those who are new to the modern technology of information synthesis and healthcare outcomes improvement. These people are often involved in developing brief papers or other scholarly writings in healthcare and will find many suggestions for identifying and building on sound, "evidence-based" information. Quality management professionals will find this book useful for establishing a knowledge synthesis foundation for producing guidelines and protocols for practice and appropriately applying new research findings in practice settings. Practicing clinicians, residents, interns, and other health professionals not interested in developing a synthesis themselves will find this book useful for helping them become better consumers of scientific information, keeping up with sound medical literature, and avoiding scientific propaganda. For those of you not interested in developing an original synthesis, there are simple indicators that you can learn from this work to help you discriminate sound scientific reviews from those that are questionable and potentially misleading.

On the negative side, healthcare practitioners can be confused with the jargon of the quantitative sciences. For example, the term *operationalize* is exceedingly important for delineating synthesis variables but may not be understood by the caregiver. Likewise, researchers may be annoyed by such concepts as "invisible colleges" for any topic. Identifying such "colleges" can be expensive and time consuming. On the other hand, not including them may result in a biased report of only one point of view. This book can also help you better communicate quantitative results of research by introducing you to more precise terminology and referring you to authoritative sources for developing a conceptual understanding of these concepts.

Enhanced Net Benefits for Authors of Healthcare Consumer Information

Equally important, this book can be of value to science writers who produce information for consumers of healthcare. Such authors frequently need to identify and interpret articles from many scientific sources. Corporate, mercantile, and political personnel flood healthcare consumers with information (too often misinformation) to influence their opinions, decisions, and expenditures. Authors of lay publications can use this book to develop an understanding of the principles for recognizing, as well as producing, sound information to help consumers. These writers can contribute much to help the public improve their lifestyle, become more discriminating in their purchases, and particularly be more effective in selecting and working with healthcare providers.

On the negative side, unless you, as a writer, are familiar with much of the jargon of healthcare and research, these chapters could prove somewhat inexplicable. For example, understanding the critical concept of a homogeneous database for ensuring a sound synthesis could be puzzling. Your writing could prove misleading if such concepts are not fully understood and communicated. Even more complex is the concept of "effect size" and its computation and pooling. This is the heart of meta-analysis and, if not done validly, may easily render the results misleading, if not worthless (Bailar, 1998).

Enhanced Net Benefit for the Population as a Whole

In the not too distant future, as the fields of information synthesis and healthcare informatics become integrated, we predict numerous net benefits for improving the health of populations wherever they may be located. This accomplishment will require information syntheses to support the development of computerized clinical guidelines and the implementation of computerized decision support systems. All individuals responsible for developing and applying public policy to improve healthcare will require immediate online "evidence-based" information to facilitate critical policy decisions. The development of relevant, scientifically trustworthy information syntheses, available by teleinformatics technology, will likely become the major factor in facilitating the nation's improvement of health status and quality of life. To contribute, in some small way, to this future is the ultimate reason we have written this book.

On the negative side, the national development of the required teleinformatics infrastructure will be slow and expensive.

TELEINFORMATICS INFRASTRUCTURE

We use the term *teleinformatics* to indicate an overall integrated network of informatics hardware, software, and interconnecting links, eventually by fiber-optic cable and satellite. With this infrastructure in place, it can be used to transmit digital data (clinical, economic, and research), text, images, and audio and tactile messages, locally or internationally. By applying "evidence-based" information (e.g., in valid guidelines), we judge this infrastructure essential for effecting substantial future population outcomes improvement.

Teleinformatics technology is maturing, but issues of leadership, collaboration, and politics will have to be resolved before this dream becomes a reality (Lundsgaarde & Williamson, 1987). In addition, until there is a more universal set of standards and an "open architecture" for hardware and software design, we will continue to experience substantial investment in noncompatible, overlapping systems that may result in great waste and block more rapid enhancement of the net benefit of the healthcare informatics system as a whole.

Summary

This first chapter introduces the science of healthcare information synthesis and healthcare informatics for facilitating population outcomes improvement. Our fundamental goals are to help authors who are inexperienced at reviewing, validating, and synthesizing literature, as well as experienced authors who want to review principles and new developments in this growing technology. Busy clinicians will not likely want or be prepared to develop needed skills required to produce sound systematic reviews. Consequently, they must depend on professionals who can develop these resources and facilitate their dissemination and use in the community.

We review the basic conceptual meaning of the terms *information syntheses* and *healthcare informatics*. It is essential that you, as well as other scientists and reviewers, recognize their critical value for developing and applying sound new healthcare knowledge in the future. There is a major difference between a traditional and a systematic review—a difference that must be understood and applied. Informatics tools will be the foundation for both developing and applying future systematic reviews to improve healthcare outcomes in the community. It is hoped that this book will both augment and help you identify the growing body of requisite informatics and information synthesis, knowledge, and resources that is and will be available in the future.

Next, this chapter provides an overview and introduction to the step-by-step procedures for implementing the five stages of an information synthesis. You will see that these stages are similar to those for conducting primary research and include defining the question; conceptualizing a model; collecting, validating, and combining the data; writing up the results; and evaluating the final product.

Then we describe a brief evolution of information syntheses methodology and the issues that are always present in this growing field of technology. These issues center on the ever-present problems of information overload, information validity, and information applicability to healthcare. We mention two appendixes that provide a brief listing of criteria that have evolved between 1977 and 2000, one set for validating individual research studies for synthesis and the other for validating systematic reviews themselves.

Next, we identify the basic criteria for evaluating each synthesis development stage, as well as assessing your synthesis as a whole. These criteria include (a) adequacy of documentation to allow evaluation and replication, (b) clinical importance to ensure value, (c) scientific soundness to ensure validity, and (d) cost-effectiveness to ensure practicality.

Finally, we discuss the potential contributions of this book for improving healthcare outcomes in the population. These will require the integration of new knowledge of systematic reviews and informatics and its application in the community to ensure the continuing improvement of population health.

PLANNING AND PREPARATION

CHAPTER 2

Synthesis Planning Prerequisites and Conceptual Issues

T he work and effort put into the planning stage of a systematic synthesis will be the most important determinant of the quality of the final product. This chapter will be presented in seven sections. The first three will discuss three prerequisites that should be met to ensure successful planning; the final four will present theory and considerations for developing the synthesis model and plan itself.

SYNTHESIS PLANNING PREREQUISITES AND CONCEPTUAL ISSUES

Prerequisites
  A. Information synthesis and resource constraints
  B. Informatics and Internet background
  C. Alternative synthesis designs to consider

Conceptual issues
  D. Formulation of synthesis topic and model
  E. Synthesis audience and their needs
  F. Linking synthesis to healthcare outcomes improvement
  G. Final project planning issues
  Appendix 2.1. Scientific group consensus process

Introduction

Before you start planning, three prerequisites must be considered: (a) your available resources, especially in terms of informatics tools, as well as finances and available time; (b) knowledge structures, concepts, terminology, and values (e.g., priorities) that can provide clues to the 'state of the science' in your field of interest, as well as availability of potential funding resources; and (c) the type of synthesis design that can be accomplished within your resource constraints and within the context of the current state of the science of your subject area. Each of these prerequisites will be discussed below.

CAUTION

All three prerequisites in Sections A, B, and C need to be reviewed before you start your formal planning process. You will find that these requirements are so integrated that what you might decide after covering one may be altered or reversed after reviewing the other two.

In terms of systematic synthesis designs, there are a number of possibilities that range between qualitative and quantitative. On one extreme (qualitative research), descriptive rather than empirical data are required. These include study designs for investigations that focus on interpretation and observation—namely, hermeneutic, phenomenological, and ethnographic types of inquiry. "Data" from qualitative studies are rarely available in the form of numbers, and the questions are not causal in nature. Systematic hypothesis testing is rarely done for research in this discipline. Although it is not the purpose of this book to present formal procedures for doing qualitative syntheses, we will briefly describe this type of synthesis design.

On the other extreme (quantitative syntheses), empirical data are essential, and the questions asked frequently involve ruling out evidence of causality by accepting the null hypothesis. We judge that the most rigorous research design for this purpose is the randomized controlled clinical trial or, more briefly, **randomized controlled trial** (RCT). We further judge that the **meta-analysis**, if done well, is likely the best quantitative synthesis design. However, numerous other research questions cannot be answered by a meta-analysis of RCTs. For example, "How accurate are psychological tests for identifying clinical depression in pregnant women?" Also, for many multivariate questions, synthesis of quasi-experimental studies might be more appropriate. Finally, if RCTs are not suitable to your topic, you may have to fall back on less rigorous research designs or even scientific consensus methods, building on whatever hard data might be available. These alternative quantitative syntheses can still provide useful information for immediate decision making.

Section A. Information Synthesis and Resource Constraints

One of the more important challenges in conducting an **information synthesis** is to balance your need for informatics resources, funds, and time with the reality of what is feasible within your budget constraints. It is often advisable to consider what resources might be available before you select a synthesis design or a topic for your project. Our discussion will focus on two premises regarding time, fiscal, and informatics resources that seem feasible to obtain. The first premise concerns developing a synthesis for immediate (within months) decision purposes and/or under circumstances of scarce fiscal and informatics resources and tight time deadlines; the second premise concerns developing a major systematic review under circumstances of abundant informatics, fiscal, and time resources.

Overview of Potential Expenditures Required

The first prerequisite can be explored by asking, "What are your current resource constraints for developing a systematic synthesis?" To answer this question, your inquiry might focus immediately on informatics constraints. Do you have access to an adequate computer with substantial random access memory (RAM) of at least 64 megabytes, hard drive capacity (at least 5 gigabytes), and a fast microprocessor or chip (over 300 megahertz)? Do you have an adequate scanner for digitizing small-font reference lists in books and articles? Do you have Internet connections, preferably with a cable modem and a good browser? Do you have software for word processing, technical research data processing, and perhaps meta-analysis effect size processing? Most of these functions can be managed with a word processor and a spreadsheet, although the programming may be somewhat tedious. Finally, is there an available university medical center department of healthcare informatics and a good medical library for consultation?

Next, what available funding do you have to hire research assistants and staff to find the hardcopy information for your synthesis? (Relatively few complete documents are online at present.) Administration of a synthesis rapidly becomes a complex operation, so a project manager is essential, even if the author(s) must fill this need. There will be Internet charges, the usual printer ink and paper (by the reams), and occasional, potentially expensive technical service charges for maintenance and troubleshooting.

CAUTION

We advise that you be careful about the use of "900" area code numbers when seeking technical help. The reason is that many firms may charge you by the minute at full technician rates while you wait on the phone for their service personnel to become available. On the other hand, many will not charge you at all if their technicians cannot help you.

With software technicians, there are several levels of expertise. The first person who screens your call will likely be at Level 1. If this person cannot help you, ask for a Level 2 or higher professional with whom to consult, especially if you may have a "deep usage problem." This is a jargon phrase for an extremely complex issue that may not be manageable without reprogramming the software.

There are many Internet addresses where you can get the same help from an online technical service. If you, or your local medical library, do not have the above informatics tools, your budget will possibly be $5,000 or more (April 2001) merely for basic hardware and software of adequate capacity and quality to manage your synthesis needs.

Finally, in this resource category, your most precious commodity will be time. Synthesis projects take a substantial effort if you expect to have a high-quality product. As authors, you will spend countless hours on the phone or Internet trying to network with colleagues worldwide who might have an interest in your topic and at least be willing to give referrals to others, if not agreeing to participate themselves in completing an occasional Delphi questionnaire or other online structured group judgment process. All such arrangements require time. If you have had any experience writing scientific articles or books, you will understand that producing a final manuscript is a major process and could take longer than your database development, depending on the quality of your documentation and the complexity of your subject matter.

Premise 1: Managing With Sparse Resources

Unfortunately, most healthcare decisions today are made under work conditions requiring personnel to do more and more with fewer and fewer resources. Obtaining sound, up-to-date, scientific information for facilitating critical decision making is an increasingly serious problem made worse by resource constraints. Illustrative questions that may require up-to-date, valid information to answer are the following: (a) For a patient with acute myocardial infarction, what are the consequences of a time delay between onset of pain and receiving anticoagulant therapy? (b) How cost-effective is the installation of a complete digital imaging system (X-rays, CAT scans, MRIs, pathology slides, still photographs, and real-time video) in a 400-bed hospital? (c) What serum serotonin reuptake inhibitors (SSRIs) have the fewest side effects, based on at least 5 years' follow-up data from postmarketing studies? (d) What is the most effective way to reduce nausea and vomiting among patients undergoing chemotherapy (Devine & Westlake, 1995)? (e) What is the comparative accuracy of endoscopy, versus an upper gastrointestinal barium X-ray series, for detecting the source of bleeding when a patient has black tarry stools? (f) Is aerobic exercise an effective way to reduce resting blood pressure in women? Often such questions need to be answered, and various primary data studies reveal conflicting results. With little time, and less quantitative expertise for interpreting raw clinical data, however well peer reviewed, what is the overworked practitioner to do?

Moreover, professionals other than healthcare practitioners also need sound information. A common example where such information is required under severe fiscal constraints is a graduate student conducting a dissertation project. Also, clinical and administrative decisions often require sound information that must be obtained under conditions of tight time deadlines. Developing a sound scientific background for a large grant proposal often must also be accomplished under both fiscal and time constraints.

Although the purpose of this book is to provide both synthesis and informatics theory and procedures to facilitate a review closer to a gold-standard review, we also recognize the many information needs where a major systematic review is not feasible. The remainder of this subsection will focus on theoretical strategies for compiling relevant and scientifically sound information under conditions of limited time, money, and informatics resources. What we recommend is development of some form of mini-synthesis to meet such needs.

What Is a Mini-Synthesis? We conceptualize this term as follows.

MINI-SYNTHESIS

A 'mini-synthesis' is a brief information synthesis of information syntheses that can be developed with minimal resource expenditure. To produce a mini-synthesis, the same principles may be followed as for a major "systematic review," but instead of developing and validating your own database, you systematically evaluate and synthesize information from available reviews that have implemented these steps for you. The final product is usually a narrative, analytic 'review of reviews.' If possible, structured group judgment consensus methods, using volunteer regional or national experts, will lend greater credibility to your final result.

It is always possible that one or more individuals could develop a synthesis without outside fiscal support, trained staff, or much time. Under these circumstances, you require (a) basic informatics hardware, software, and skills; (b) a focused topic and conceptual model; (c) a literature search limited to only other "systematic reviews" or traditional reviews, if necessary; (d) explicit criteria for assessing the methodological rigor of retrieved reviews; (e) a consensus synthesis by e-mail or telephone of two or more volunteer topic experts; and (f) a narrative write-up and concurrence with your conclusions by your consultants. Henceforth, we will term these brief "systematic reviews" as *mini-syntheses*.

Mini-Synthesis Advantages. The main advantages of a mini-synthesis are savings in time and expense and the potential to meet urgent decision needs with information of far greater acceptability than might otherwise be possible. Your first and best strategy will be retrieving existing systematic reviews, recognizing current content limitations, and recognizing a likely exponential increase in their production as time passes. In this case, requisite synthesis tasks (e.g., relevance coding, validation coding, analysis/synthesis, and documentation) are already completed. Again, this assumes there are systematic reviews available on your topic.

If such reviews are not available, your second strategy might be to extrapolate from nonsystematic but meta-validated reviews (i.e., those that have been assessed by two independent groups of qualified reviewers) or traditional reviews such as the Lange series, the Yearbook series, or reliable primary articles or abstracts from sources such as the American College of Physicians (ACP) Journal Club. These materials have the advantage of being readily available and cover a wide clinical content, especially in the subspecialties.

Mini-Synthesis Disadvantages. The main disadvantage of producing a review under the premise of resource scarcity is that with little or no funds and a tight timetable, you may be minimally successful in achieving a representative and valid database. The reason for this problem is that there are not many systematic reviews on most topics; as yet—the content coverage is growing rapidly. Another disadvantage is that you must assess the scientific rigor of each synthesis included. If methods documentation is incomplete, you will have to trust the synthesis skills of the author(s). A worse problem will be the temptation to obtain a haphazard sample of peer-reviewed but non-meta-validated primary articles reporting studies that have not been replicated or analyzed for information maturity in practice. Such a sampling procedure may yield information that most likely will be seriously biased.

Informatics Resources for Mini-Syntheses. The best sources of **meta-validated information** are peer-reviewed journal articles that are reevaluated by a specialty panel to determine whether they at least meet minimum criteria of scientific soundness, if not cost-effectiveness, safety, and net benefit. As with any systematic review, it is

---

TABLE 2.1 Illustrative Online Sources (May 2001) of Systematic Reviews
             for Mini-Syntheses

---

1. Cochrane Collaboration Library—United Kingdom: www.update-software.com/cochrane.htm

2. Agency for Healthcare Research and Quality Evidence-Based Practice Centers (EPCs)—United States: www.ahcpr.gov/clinic/epc/

3. Centre for Evidence-Based Medicine—United Kingdom: cebm.jr2.ox.ac.uk

4. Thomas C. Chalmers Centre for Systematic Reviews—Canada: www.cheori.org/tcc/index.htm

5. National Guideline Clearinghouse—United States: www.guideline.gov/body_home_nf.asp?view=home

6. Centre for Reviews and Dissemination—United Kingdom: www.york.ac.uk/inst/crd/welcome.htm

7. National Health Services HSR&D Centre for Health Technology Assessment—United Kingdom: www.soton.ac.uk/~hta

---

NOTE: See Compendium for more complete list of Web sites.

---

essential that you have available informatics resources, such as the Internet. Most medical libraries will let you use their hardware, software, and expertise to meet this basic requirement. Furthermore, you may obtain consultation from a growing number of academic centers that focus on healthcare informatics. These centers are listed at the following Web site (last updated April 2001): www.nlm.nih.gov/ep/curr_inst_grantees.html.

By means of the Internet, you can directly contact relevant information banks that will get you started with your mini-synthesis or major systematic review. Table 2.1 illustrates a few of these sources most relevant to systematic reviews and provides Internet addresses by which you can contact them. Our compendium at the back of this book provides a much more comprehensive annotated listing of such sites and suggests ideas to help you keep up with this rapidly growing and changing technology.

1. The Cochrane Collaboration Library (now available online from Update Software, Inc.), with headquarters located in the United Kingdom, is probably the single best source of both content and methods information related to systematic reviews. It has a growing worldwide network of 15 centers contributing to its program. In terms of its materials, for example, as of May 2001, this library lists 1,081 complete systematic reviews, 1,993 abstracts of quality-assessed systematic reviews, 2,187 abstracts in its health technology assessment database, 3,407 references to information syntheses methods literature, and more than 307,870 studies in its controlled trials register. It has even developed a new database of methodology reviews

that will be another important contribution to the development of this exploding technology. The United Kingdom is rapidly developing new centers for development and dissemination of these information syntheses, most of which have collaborated in some way with the Cochrane group. In the United States, groups such as the ACP and its *Annals of Internal Medicine* are developing collaborative relationships with these same information synthesis pioneers.

2. The U.S. Agency for Healthcare Research and Quality (AHRQ) has launched an initiative to promote evidence-based reviews immediately applicable to daily practice in everyday care. At present, more than 12 evidence-based practice centers (EPCs) have been funded and are producing clinically relevant and rigorous information syntheses. As of March 2000, they list the titles of 56 systematic reviews being developed, of which 40 have been completed and with summaries, and many have full reports available by linkage from their Web site.

3. The Centre for Evidence-Based Medicine (United Kingdom), sponsored by the National Health Service (NHS) research and development group, can be readily identified. It has been heavily influenced by the Cochrane group and is related to the publication of five different evidence-based journals. It emphasizes information regarding efficacy and cost-effectiveness of healthcare.

4. The Thomas C. Chalmers Centre for Systematic Reviews (Canada) is one of the more recent review centers (founded in 1998) that has become available. Tom Chalmers is one of the world's leading figures in randomized control trial methodology. During the last decade of his life, he dedicated his career to meta-analysis, being associated with the publication of more than 200 papers on this subject during this time. As of December 2000, its Web site listed about 20 titles, but it would seem that this group will now be far more productive. Being based on Tom Chalmers's values and philosophy, the quality of its systematic reviews will likely be superb.

5. The National Guideline Clearinghouse (NCG) is sponsored by the AHRQ, together with the American Medical Association and the American Association of Health Plans. To qualify for inclusion in its collection, a guideline must be based on approved systematic reviews (i.e., information syntheses). These guidelines provide a rich collection of validated information and methods for immediate application to health outcomes improvement.

6. In the United Kingdom, the Centre for Reviews and Dissemination (CRD), again sponsored by the NHS, is another valuable source of information for systematic reviews. It focuses on content directly related to improving healthcare in the NHS. For example, it also emphasizes information regarding efficacy and cost-effectiveness of healthcare. The CRD both produces and evaluates systematic reviews in-house and commissions selected academic and qualified healthcare professionals to do likewise. It is based at the University of York in England and collaborates with the Cochrane group.

7. In the United Kingdom, the Health Technology Assessment (HTA) program, initiated by the NHS Department of Research and Development, is another good source of synthesis-related information. Its database is available through the NHS Centre for Reviews and Dissemination described above. Its purpose is "to ensure that high-quality research information on the costs, effectiveness and broader impact of health technologies is produced in the most efficient way for those who use, manage and work in the NHS." Many, if not most, of their publications are systematic reviews (or information syntheses, in our terminology).

Other Information Resources for Mini-Syntheses. If you still cannot find reviews that qualify for inclusion, you may have to rely on nonsynthesis meta-validated reviews (e.g., peer-reviewed primary research reports that have received a second review by a specialty panel). One of the better examples of such a publication is the American College of Physicians' *ACP Journal Club.* It systematically screens articles that have already been peer reviewed, performs a second validation analysis in terms of research design, checks on information maturity for immediate community application, and reports the results in an easy-to-read one-page abstract. This is one of the few instances where the reader can likely trust an abstract as reporting sound information, due to the rigorous process by which the complete articles are selected for abstraction.

Many other meta-validated sources, although not as well analyzed and documented, provide information substantially more trustworthy than raw, isolated journal articles, even though peer reviewed. Sources include the Lange series of reviews (e.g., *Current Medical Diagnosis and Treatment*), the Yearbook series (e.g., *Yearbook of Medicine*), and the *Scientific American Review of Medicine.*

The Lange series was formerly published by Appleton & Lange, but in June 1999 they were acquired by McGraw-Hill and distributed through "Prentice Hall Health"™, Blacklick, Ohio. They have teams of nationally recognized experts in the different primary and specialty fields who update these books annually. To learn more about these publications, use the following Web address: www.books.mcgraw-hill.com/medical/appleton/.

However, with recognized sources such as those above, it is still important to check the publisher's editorial policy and its information review process. It is especially critical to determine whether it uses explicit relevance and validation criteria to assess the research studies it considers for inclusion. Our book, as well as other sources we will describe, may help you know what to look for to ensure the quality of such publications (see Chapter 3, Appendix 3.2).

Premise 2: Managing With Abundant Resources

If you have abundant resources, you have a much greater range of possibilities in terms of topics, questions, and depth of coverage. If you contemplate a major synthesis, we assume that you plan to obtain a grant or contract support for a team effort to complete your project. We suggest that reading Stage I of this book can be helpful in conceptualizing and developing a grant application in any area of the healthcare field, especially health services research and quality improvement. If your grant is for developing a systematic review and is awarded, then the material in Stages II through V of this book can help you produce a sound and publishable information synthesis.

In the preplanning phase of your synthesis project, we assume that you, as senior author, are a professional in the healthcare area and/or have a vital interest in this subject. For example, if you are not a healthcare provider, you might be a journalist having a fundamental interest in obtaining relevant and valid scientific information for communicating to the public, or a lawyer preparing for a major medicolegal case. We further assume that your purpose, as author, for developing this review is to assist your target readers to apply your results to improve healthcare outcomes either directly or indirectly. We also assume that you have identified one or two interested and qualified colleagues who are willing and able to make the time commitment necessary to ensure the success of your project.

The major advantage of this second premise, which assumes adequate resources, is that you will be able to obtain a representative and validated database from primary data articles as well as available systematic reviews on your topic. Also, if a meta-analysis is planned, you should be able to manage the many flaws and threats to validity that you might face in the current literature (e.g., missing data, or a heterogeneous database of research studies).

The main disadvantage of such a well-funded project is, like all enterprises, that you may spend more time and money than you budgeted. Careful planning and built-in monitoring of systems can help hedge against this ongoing hazard. One of the more common reasons for overspending is inadvertent "topic drift," occurring in the early stages of a synthesis. If the topic changes substantially, much previous work may have to be repeated, resulting in unnecessary costs and lost time.

In reality, it is rare that either situation (very few or unlimited resources) is the case. By careful planning and applying systematic methods, budgets can usually be met with minimal loss of validity or integrity. Establishing a representative database, on the other hand, may be more of a problem.

NOTE

In much of this book, we will assume that your synthesis will be a team effort and that you will have adequate funds, informatics resources, and time available, closer to what is described in Premise 2. Thus, many of our suggestions will refer to a more ideal level of synthesis development. However, we usually make clear at all stages how the procedures could be modified to meet resource limitations.

Section B. Informatics and Internet Background

Introduction

In Stage I, reviewing background information related to your general area of interest can prove helpful to a variety of tasks, from your topic formulation through to final synthesis project planning and planning evaluation. Not only will this information facilitate more creative thinking about your topic, but it will also prove invaluable later when you map your database search strategy and scope.

Healthcare informatics will clearly provide you the most meaningful tools for rapidly accomplishing this purpose of compiling background information. The U.S. National Library of Medicine's Unified Medical Language System® (UMLS) project, for example, is continually building better knowledge structures to facilitate digitization, translation, and worldwide Internet communication of healthcare information. Using these knowledge structures, new and more effective search engines and browsers are being built. Net sites (including the Web) are being developed by most major organizations, from the World Health Organization down to local community-integrated health systems. Next, the Internet will facilitate your rapidly becoming familiar with the values and priorities in various areas of potential synthesis development. By seeing research projects and other systematic reviews that have been funded, are ongoing, or are completed, you can discover what various groups have been judged to be important in the recent past. By reviewing new information from health services research investigations and by noting current funding priorities, you can discover where resources might be available to facilitate your planning. Without funding, your review project will be of limited contribution and perhaps of lesser quality in terms of representing work in your area, let alone ensuring a high level of scientific quality and adequate documentation of your efforts.

Knowledge Structures, Concepts, and Nomenclature

A valuable prerequisite to planning your synthesis is to review important knowledge structures, concepts, and nomenclature. For purposes of information storage and retrieval, the capability to recognize synonyms and jargon in one vocabulary and translate them into that of another is a major problem, especially when foreign languages are involved. One of the most important research and development programs dedicated to managing this problem is the National Library of Medicine's (NLM's) Unified Medical Language System (UMLS). See its home page at www.nlm.nih. gov/research/umls/.

UMLS provided the groundwork and tools for developing NLM's two major search engines—Internet Grateful Med® and PubMed, among many other applications. Access to UMLS is free to all qualified registered licensees. For those who may be interested in understanding this seminal development, contact this resource at the "2000 UMLS Documentation" page; the Web site (updated February 2000) is www.nlm.nih.gov/research/umls/UMLSDOC.HTML.

At a much higher lever of application, the NLM's Medical Subject Heading's (**MeSH**) "tree structures" provide a useful classification of healthcare knowledge structures. Each search engine, browser, or database may have its own tree structure, knowledge relationships, and terminology.

Thus, it is important to understand the informatics tools and search nomenclature for your area of interest. This can be found under "Search Terms," "Indexes," "Directories," or "Glossaries" at these Internet sites. One of the most relevant glossaries for information synthesis terminology is that produced by the Cochrane Collaboration. It lists most of the major terms and concepts related to a systematic review technology, particularly quantitative. This source can be linked from its Reviewers' Handbook 4.0 "Contents" page (updated March 2001) by clicking on "Glossary" at the following Web site: www.cochrane.dk/cochrane/handbook/handbook.htm.

A similar reference of terms for the field of informatics is the U.S. National Library of Congress series titled "Library of Congress Brief Guides to the Internet." This series includes an authoritative glossary to be found at the following address: lcweb.loc.gov/loc/guides/glossary.html.

For the novice, the Consumers Union (1999) publishes an annual *Home Computer Buying Guide* that provides an authoritative introduction to informatics tools and vocabulary.

As a final example, the AHRQ provides a helpful glossary for the field of quality improvement, titled "Health Care Quality Glossary," at www.ahcpr.gov/qual/hcqgloss.htm.

Values or Priorities in Areas for Potential Synthesis

Another type of background information that can be accessed on the Internet is material having listings from which values (e.g., priorities) can be inferred. This is roughly analogous to identifying the editorial policy of a publisher. Again, the Cochrane Collaboration Reviewers' Handbook provides what is perhaps the most relevant set of criteria (of its values) for identifying topics for systematic review. This source can be found by linking from the above-mentioned handbook "Contents" page to Section 3.0 ("Developing a Protocol") and then to Section 3.2 ("The Background for a Review").

Another example of a listing indicating values is the United Kingdom's NHS Research and Development (R&D) Health Technology Assessment (HTA) program, which has an annual listing of research priorities for health services research and development (HSR&D) studies. In this case, the values represent a consensus of its "Standing Group on Health Technologies" or (for 1999) the HTA program director.

Likewise, the U.S. AHRQ has a listing of its priority topics, listed under the heading of "Topic Nomination and Selection," initiated by agency leaders who select broad areas for synthesis research and within which they seek nominations from relevant professional associations, health plans, providers, and others who might see their solicitation notice in the U.S. Federal Register. It lists its priority criteria as well as previous systematic reviews it has completed or on which it is working.

Perhaps the listings of most immediate interest are the research funding priorities in your field of interest. This type of information is easily accessible on the Net. You can find what current priorities are for soliciting grants and contracts applications, as well as lists of grants and contracts funded in the past 5 years or so. For example, the following Web site provides direct research priority information related to grants and contract funding: www.nlm.nih.gov/ep/extramural.html.

Another illustrative source of priorities information is the AHRQ extramural funding program, labeled "Funding Opportunities," index page; it also includes sections on "Contract Solicitations," "Grant Announcements," and "Policy Notices" about which programs have been deactivated and which areas are receiving greater emphasis, as well as "Future Year Commitments on AHRQ Grant Awards." This Web site is (last updated ??) www.ahcpr.gov/fund/.

This same agency disseminates a "fact sheet" titled "Health Services Research Projects in Progress" (HSRPROJ). "[HSRPROJ] contains descriptions of research in progress funded by federal and private grants and contracts for use by policy makers, managers, clinicians and other decision makers. It provides access to information about health services research in progress before results are available in a published form." The Web site for this quote (last updated December 1998) is www.nlm.nih.gov/pubs/factsheets/hsrproj.html.

Sources of Salient Health Services Research Information

Numerous areas of health services research have produced much valuable background information for information syntheses. Although this material may be somewhat premature for use in practice, it can be invaluable heuristically to generate topics for syntheses, criteria, and measurement instruments and leads to mature information for improving healthcare outcomes. We encourage you to make use of such investigative material as background information to conceptualize meaningful topics for systematic reviews. The following research areas might serve this purpose.

TABLE 2.2 Information Synthesis Topic Ideas From Patients'
Diagnostic Questions

1. What has happened to me? (health problem/preliminary diagnosis)
2. Why has it happened? (etiology)
3. What is going to happen to me in the short term? The long term? (prognosis)
4. What are you going to do to me? (examinations, tests)
5. Why are you doing this rather than something else? (diagnostic options)
6. Will it hurt or harm me? (invasive procedures needed)
7. How and when will you know what the tests mean? (diagnostic process)
8. When and how will I know what the tests mean? (feedback of diagnostic results)
9. How much will this cost? Will my insurance cover it? (economic outcomes)
10. How certain will you be about what my problem is? (diagnostic probability)

Research on consumers' perceptions of healthcare is a valuable source of ideas for systematic reviews. One of the better examples is the Consumer Assessment of Health Plans® (CAHPS), sponsored by the AHRQ together with Harvard University, RAND, and the Research Triangle Institute. Their questionnaire alone took several years to develop and validate. The results of this 5-year project should be a rich source of ideas for systematic reviews. Overview information about the project can be found at the following Web site: www.ahcpr.gov/qual/cahps/dept1.htm.

Examining issues from the patient's frame of reference is reinforced by Counsell (1998), who, in relation to formulating topics for systematic reviews, stated, "The most relevant questions are often asked directly or indirectly by patients" (p. 67). The Bayer Institute for Health Care Communication (1995b, p. 43) has specified a standard set of questions that most patients want to know from their physicians, whether the patients ask them or not. See Tables 2.2 and 2.3 for a list of these questions in relation to patient diagnosis and patient treatment, respectively.

Clinicians view these same questions in a somewhat different light because they are more invested in making an accurate diagnosis as a basis for establishing an effective therapeutic plan, an accurate prognosis, and an economic projection of costs and potential revenues. Either patients' or clinicians' point of view could make an appropriate topic for a synthesis.

Research on information that clinicians use is another relevant source of synthesis ideas. Many of these studies are direct observation or ethnographic studies of clinical practice to identify information needs of various healthcare professionals. To our knowledge, the classic work in this field related to physicians is that of Peterson, Andrews, Spain, and Greenberg (1956), titled *An Analytical Study of North Carolina*

TABLE 2.3 Information Synthesis Topic Ideas From Patients'
                  Therapy Questions

---

1. What are the treatment or prevention options available? (available interventions)
2. What are the relative benefits or risks of harm from each? (net benefits)
3. How certain are you regarding these benefits and risks? (therapeutic efficacy)
4. How many patients have you treated with my problem? (personal competence)
5. What type and for how long will I experience disability? (treated prognosis)
6. How much and how long will I experience pain or discomfort? (treated prognosis)
7. When will I be able to get back to my major life activities? (treated prognosis)
8. Where, by whom, and for how long will I be treated? (care resource availability)
9. What will the treatment cost me, and will my insurance cover it? (economic risks)
10. What will be my final outcome, and how certain are you? (treated prognosis)

General Practice—1953-1954. A Science Citation Search (Sci-Search) of this work could bring you up to date on the major clinical observational studies of this type. Williamson et al. (1989) completed a national survey of U.S. primary practitioners as to their information needs. Other examples include Smith (1996), who wrote a review that cited two direct observation (ethnographic) studies of clinical practice— namely, Osheroff et al. (1991) and Forsythe, Buchanan, Osheroff, and Miller (1992). Smith's review elucidates important points about doctors' questions and information needs. Gorman, Ash, and Wykoff (1994) asked whether the medical literature can answer the questions physicians ask. Ely, Osheroff, Ebell, et al. (1999) reported their survey and their new taxonomy (Ely, Osheroff, Gorman, et al. 2000). The AHRQ has developed an index of relatively mature information that physicians might require; the data are available from various U.S. government sources. The Web site (last updated ??) is www.ahcpr.gov/clinic/.

Research on medical errors provides current and highly relevant information for identifying subject matter for systematic reviews for the health professions. A recent study by the Institute of Medicine (IOM) of the National Academy of Science on the subject of medical errors provides vital information for immediate use to identify topics for information syntheses. Based on this study, IOM estimates that up to 96,000 preventable deaths may occur in hospitals alone each year. Further information regarding research on medical errors, as of February 2000, can be accessed through the following Web site (last updated February 2000): www.ahcpr.gov/errors.htm.

We also recommend reading the report on the IOM study given by John Eisenberg (director of the AHRQ) to the subcommittee of the Senate Appropriations Committee on December 13, 1999. The Web site is www.ahcpr.gov/news/stat1213.htm.

An older Web site summarizes information on medical errors and includes strategies for coping with these serious problems. At that time, AHCPR (now AHRQ) estimated that "about 180,000 preventable deaths occur each year across all healthcare sites" (AHCPR Pub. No. 98-P018). Any one of the topics mentioned in this document could be the focus for a synthesis. This reference can be found on the following Web site (last updated April 2000): www.ahcpr.gov/research/errors.htm.

Research on quality improvement provides another relatively mature source of healthcare information that can be rich, heuristically, for generating ideas for systematic reviews. Numerous online databases can be most useful in this area. The AHRQ recommends the following projects and databanks as exemplary:

CAHPS—Consumer Assessment of Health Plans®

Foundation for Accountability—discussion paper and abstracts on measuring "quality" in several health conditions; also see Wilson and Goldschmidt (1995) for an especially thorough quality management glossary developed in collaboration with Australian and U.S. quality improvement leaders.

HCUP QI—Healthcare Cost and Utilization Project Quality Indicators. The following Web address will provide a summary of this resource, HCUP quality indicators, a fact sheet, and many other such topics (last updated ??): www.ahcpr.gov/qual/.

CONQUEST—The Computerized Needs-Oriented Quality Measurement Evaluation System is an especially valuable resource for identifying ideas for information syntheses. "CONQUEST is a software tool that uses a common structure and language to help users identify, understand, compare, evaluate, and select measures to assess and improve clinical performance. CONQUEST is comprised of two data bases—one for clinical performance measures and one for conditions." The CONQUEST database (as of March 1999) contains 1,197 clinical performance measures and includes information on 57 common or costly clinical conditions affecting the general population, such as arthritis, asthma, cancer, cataracts, depression, diabetes, gallbladder disease, heart attack, hypertension, and pregnancy. The Web site for the fact sheet describing this resource (last updated March 1999) is www.ahcpr. gov/qual/conquest/conqfact.htm.

Finally, *research on health economics* is an HSR subject worth mentioning in terms of identifying salient topics for information syntheses. The following two sites are pertinent: MEPS and HCUP.

MEPS (Medical Expenditure Panel Survey) "is a United States nationally representative survey of healthcare use, expenditures, sources of payment, and insurance coverage for the United States civilian non-institutionalized population, as well as a national survey of nursing homes and their residents. MEPS is cosponsored by the Agency for Health Care Policy and Research (AHCPR) and the National Center for Health Statistics (NCHS). This survey is designed to yield comprehensive data that estimate the level and distribution of health care use and expenditures, monitor the dynamics of the health care delivery and insurance systems, and assess health care policy implications." The Web site for this reference and access to MEPS (last updated February 2000) is www.meps.ahrq.gov/.

HCUP is another source of synthesis topic ideas in the area of healthcare economics. Its database is managed in the Center for Organization and Delivery Studies (CODS). It has two databases that contain inpatient information for hospitals: (a) the Nationwide Inpatient Sample (NIS), which includes inpatient data from a national sample of about 900 hospitals, and (b) the State Inpatient Database (SID), covering inpatient care in community hospitals in 22 states (this represents more than half of all U.S. hospital discharges). HCUP's objectives are to (a) obtain data from statewide information sources, (b) design and develop a multistate healthcare database for health services research and health policy analysis, and (c) make these data available to a broad set of public and private users. Further information on HCUP can be accessed at the following Web site address (last updated April 2001): www.ahrq.gov/data/hcup/hcupnet.htm.

Section C. Alternative Synthesis Designs to Consider

At this point, we will assume you have made two major decisions: (a) to develop a systematic synthesis as opposed to a traditional review and (b) to develop a complete information synthesis as opposed to a mini-synthesis of reviews. Now you have to decide what type of synthesis would be most appropriate, ranging from a formal qualitative synthesis through several quasi-quantitative methods to a meta-analysis or, at the other extreme, a formal quantitative synthesis.

In preparation for making your own selection of a design for a systematic review, we discuss several options.

Introduction

The method for synthesizing primary research is determined by the availability of resources, the overall purpose of the synthesis itself, the type of question being asked, and the kind of data available. Readers may automatically assume that a formal quantitative synthesis, or meta-analysis, is the best (and perhaps only) method for synthesizing primary research articles. Many times, such a conclusion is not warranted. Even for empirical research reporting experimental data from randomized controlled trials (RCTs), there are several design variations from which you might choose. In other cases, primary studies do test formal hypotheses, and the data are reported in numerous investigations. However, the study designs may be of poor quality, or the actual number of studies may be few. Or, the purpose of the synthesis may not be to simply test a hypothesis across studies but rather to review theoretical, policy, or methodological issues. In either of these cases, a modified meta-analysis, called "best evidence synthesis" (BST), may be the best approach.

Occasionally, the primary studies are empirical and the quality acceptable, but the quantity of data reported is very low. Sometimes, only significance values are reported. In these cases, quantitative techniques such as "vote counting" and combining of significance levels may be used. Although these procedures are less desirable, they are sometimes necessary.

We will describe several systematic synthesis methods that range from formal qualitative to formal quantitative approaches. The emphasis here is to introduce the reader to issues involved in choosing a synthesis method, not to provide step-by-step instruction. (Specific procedures are described for the meta-analysis only, and these are in Chapters 13 and 14.) However, because all of these methods are systematic, regardless of the type of synthesis to be applied, Stages I (developing a plan), II (establishing a database), III (validating individual studies), and V (preparing and evaluating synthesis manuscript) will be quite similar, if not identical.

Formal Qualitative Syntheses

There is very little work on the topic of synthesizing qualitative literature. Noblit and Hare (1988) have written a book called *Meta-Ethnography,* and much of what is presented below is derived from that publication.

Logistical Premise. According to Noblit and Hare (1988), synthesis of qualitative studies should be interpretative rather than aggregative. In other words, studies examining the same topic of interest should be gathered together for the purpose of creating a deeper interpretation, not to "sum up" the results. A deeper understanding can be described as the "interpretive explanation," a type of explanation that is holistic, historical, contextual, and personal (related to the people involved).

As a goal of a qualitative synthesis, the interpretive explanation might often mean giving up the notion of comparability between studies. Studies may be selected because they appear to use a common metaphor or occur at the same time, or for any number of other reasons. It is not necessary in this type of synthesis to choose studies that all examine the same population or attempt to answer the same question. In fact, establishing relevance criteria for selection is done not up front but rather after selection.

Process of Meta-Ethnographic (Qualitative) Synthesis. The actual process of a meta-ethnographic synthesis is to effectively translate qualitative studies into each other. The translation process is the heart of the meta-ethnographic synthesis. It consists of comparing the metaphors and concepts and their interactions with the metaphors and comparisons of other studies. This activity is much like treating the studies as analogous to each other. The themes, organizers, and concepts of each study are attended to carefully, and then the study is examined in terms of the themes, organizers, and concepts from another study. The result is a clearer understanding not only of each study but also of which metaphors "work" across many studies, which concepts and metaphors appear to be contradictory, or which set of metaphors relates to each other in a linear direction.

Relationships Between Metaphors. Each type of relationship between metaphors constitutes a method of synthesis in meta-ethnography. The first type of relationship is called "reciprocal translations" and involves discussing how each study can be explained by the other's metaphors and concepts. The second type of relationship is a "refutational synthesis" and is characterized by differences between interpretations. These differences can either be explicit, where the authors point out how they are interpreting the situation differently than others, or implicit, where they are identified only through the process of translation. The third type of relationship is called a "lines of argument" synthesis. As studies are translated into each other, the relationship between their respective metaphors and basic concepts appears to suggest a whole, larger than the sum of the parts. This kind of activity can be described as theorizing, in that identifying a latent structure is a basic aspect of the activity. This integrating and abstracting activity is accomplished through constant comparisons between studies, comparisons that eventually reveal the larger structure.

The above description of qualitative synthesis is by no means complete. However, it should provide the reader with a feel for the kind of activity involved in doing a synthesis of qualitative work. The guiding rule here is to honor the basic principles underlying qualitative research in the process of conducting a synthesis. If this approach is of interest, see the book by Noblit and Hare (1988), *Meta-Ethnography.*

Vote Counting

There are three types of empirical evidence usually available from original articles. Bushman (1994) refers to them as *Type 1* data (data that can be used to calculate effect sizes), *Type 2* data (data providing information concerning the statistical significance of the hypotheses being tested), and *Type 3* data (data that only report the direction of statistical significance). When available, the first type of data provides a more compelling basis for synthesizing the results across studies. However, you may have access only to data of the second or third type and, as a result, will not be able to compute effect sizes.

Vote Counting as a Concept. **Vote counting** is a procedure for determining whether the majority of studies in a domain provide evidence to support, contradict, or provide no evidence concerning a research hypothesis (Glass, McGraw, & Smith, 1981; Light & Smith, 1971). In the synthesis process, you count how many articles report data that are consistent with each of these three outcomes. That is, each study would be treated as if it provided a vote in favor or against the hypothesis. The final decision would depend on the number of articles that fall into each of the three categories (i.e., support, contradict, or are neutral). Often you can see this approach used informally in many narrative syntheses when the authors conclude that "most" of the evidence is consistent with (or contradicts) the hypothesis. Explicit procedures for conducting a vote-counting synthesis using the sign test and other methods are described in detail by Bushman (1994, p. 193).

Advantages of Vote Counting. The quantity, quality, and type of data reported by empiric research vary considerably. Ideally, you would want experimental data, such as that reporting effect size of the magnitude of the relationship between one variable (independent; e.g., penicillin) and another (dependent; e.g., meningiococcus). The advantage of the vote-counting approach is that it provides useful information in situations where you discover that some or most of the research articles in your database do not report the type of data needed to calculate effect sizes. In this circumstance, there may be value in making preliminary inferences from a procedure such as a "sign test." Bushman (1994) describes a useful approach for performing a vote-counting method, and we recommend that you read his chapter if you confront this problem.

Disadvantages of Vote Counting. Three major problems occur in vote counting (Bushman, 1994). First, the procedure ignores sample size, and the likelihood of a statistically significant effect is greater with larger sample sizes. The reason for concern is that small sample size studies alone might have too little power to reject the null hypothesis, but the vote-counting procedure gives too much weight to small sample size studies compared to large sample size studies (Light & Smith, 1971). A second problem is that vote counting ignores the differences in the effect size obtained in each study. Hence, a very small negative effect is given the same weight as a very large positive effect (Glass et al., 1981). Third, the vote-counting procedure has relatively low statistical power for detecting any effects whatsoever (Bushman, 1994; Hedges & Olkin, 1985).

Combining Significance Levels

The Concept of Combining Significance Levels. You may be able to combine significance levels when there is not sufficient data to calculate effect sizes for some of the studies in your database. For example, suppose some of the original authors did not report enough within-condition information such as standard deviations, sample sizes, or statistical test values for significance. However, the authors of the studies in your database might have reported the significance levels (probabilities or *p* values) associated with tests of significance. These *p* values represent the probability of observing a given test statistic given that the null hypothesis is true; that is, these values are the probability of a Type I error (of incorrectly rejecting the null hypothesis). These *p* values can be directly combined. If you decide to pursue this approach, we recommend that you examine a chapter by Becker (1994), in which she presents several useful techniques in combining significance levels.

The Initial Procedural Step. The first step in this approach is to decide which type of sampling distribution is appropriate for the data; typically, this is the standard normal distribution. Next, the exact *Z* score value on a standard normal distribution that would be associated with a given *p* value is determined. Suppose that a two-tailed test of significance for a study in your data set has a *p* value of .05. The standard normal *Z* value for this *p* value is 1.96. You can use tables of the standard normal distribution to estimate a *Z* score for most *p* values. You would obtain the *Z* score for every study and then combine the results using Formula 2.1. The value of *k* in the formula is the number of studies to be combined, and *i* refers to the specific study.

$$\bar{Z} = \sum_{i=1}^{k} z_i / \sqrt{k} \qquad (2.1)$$

Determining Statistical Significance. We can determine whether this value is statistically significant by comparing the obtained value to the value required to reject the null hypothesis at a particular significance level, typically $\alpha = .05$. If you found that the absolute value of the observed mean Z is greater than the threshold value of $\bar{Z}_{1-\alpha/2}$, then you would reject the null hypothesis.

Becker Method for Combining Studies. Becker (1994) also presents a method for combining studies using the logs of the significance levels. Computing the natural log of the probability values associated with each study performs this procedure. If you sum these values and multiply by (–2), you obtain a χ^2 value with $2k$ degrees of freedom, where k is the number of studies being combined. You multiply by the minus sign because the log of a decimal is a negative number, and the multiplication converts the result to a positive number (Formula 2.2).

$$\chi^2 = -2 \sum_{i=1}^{k} \ln(p_i) \qquad (2.2)$$

Advantages and Limitations of Combining Significance Levels. These procedures are relatively easy to follow. Because combined procedures represent nonparametric analysis, they can be more appropriate than effect size approaches when your database studies do not satisfy the stricter assumptions of parametric analysis (Becker, 1994). However, whenever the studies satisfy the assumptions of parametric analysis, these procedures are relatively unsatisfactory. That is, effect size methods provide all the information that can be obtained from the significance level approach. In addition, the effect size approach also provides information about the size and the strength of effects.

Best Evidence Synthesis

The first stages of "best evidence syntheses" (BES) are identical to that of a meta-analysis. (Do not confuse this synthesis design concept of "best evidence" with the concepts of evidence-based technology, which is applied in a very different context.) Developing the model for the question, creating the synthesis plan, and conducting the search strategy to establish a synthesis database are conducted identically regardless of the validation and synthesis procedures to be applied to the information compiled. To understand a BES, you need to recognize how it differs from the usual meta-analysis. Overall, BES is an attempt to make up for some of the limitations of a meta-analysis, especially the tendency to be "typically mechanistic, driven more by concerns about reliability and replicability than about adding to understanding of the phenomena of interest" (Slavin, 1995, p. 11; see also Slavin, 1986). This reminds us of the similar tension (if not an inverse relationship) between internal and external validity, or between diagnostic false-negative and false-positive rates. The following five factors explain the main difference between a BES and a traditional meta-analysis.

Question Specificity. BES does not aim to include all relevant studies but only those few that are the clearest examples of the question to be tested. The method requires strict adherence to specific questions. As a result, both independent and dependent variables can be narrowly defined, with a resultant increase in clinical and theoretical relevance. For example, if the topic is the relationship between patient-doctor communication and outcomes, both of these variables could be defined more explicitly and perhaps even more narrowly than a regular review or meta-analysis would require. The review could be narrowed to address only time spent with the patient and compliance as outcomes. A narrow focus can increase the clinical applicability and reduce study bias.

Study Selection. Conceptually, BES uses rules of evidence in a manner similar to that of the legal field, wherein a piece of evidence is applicable as long as there is nothing better. However, when a piece of evidence appears that is more valid than the previous one, then the previous one is no longer admissible. R. E. Slavin at Johns Hopkins (1995) uses the example of determining legal authorship. A typed copy can be evidence, but if there is a handwritten copy, the typed copy no longer functions as "evidence" and so is discarded. Similarly, three or four very well-done studies may provide "better" evidence than six or eight poorly done studies. By focusing on the methods and results of those four very well-done studies, even in a narrative form, the overall field of investigation is more enriched.

Validity Assessment. Defining the synthesis as "best evidence" requires closer attention to measuring the scientific quality of single studies than is usually suggested for meta-analyses. Slavin (1995) recommends that quality criteria not be based on standards developed independently of the chosen topic (see also Chalmers et al., 1981) but rather be uniquely customized by experts for the specific topic at hand. Quality criteria should focus on designs that minimize bias (for the specific question) and not necessarily include all aspects of reliability and validity. In the topic under investigation, areas of the most potentially troubling bias should be identified and applied to the selection process. For example, most researchers view correlational studies as containing significant bias because groups are not randomly assigned. However, not all correlational studies have a large bias if the independent variable is not correlated with confounding factors that are themselves correlated with the outcome to be measured. Understanding these relationships requires an in-depth understanding of the field of inquiry.

Slavin (1995) also suggests that external validity should weigh as much as internal validity when evaluating studies. Many studies create an artificial context by randomizing individuals in such a way that the results are not applicable in any real-world setting. For example, in a study examining the acceptance of an information system, physicians were randomized on whether to use the system or not to use it (Rotman et al., 1996). However, the new system did not perform all of the functions required, making it necessary for the physicians to use the old system concurrently. Not surprisingly, the usage of the new system declined remarkably (and early) over the course of the study. Thus, this study could not evaluate the stated hypothesis regarding real-world acceptance of the new system. In fact, the study had very little real-world value as it failed to test the question asked, even though it started with a randomized controlled trial design.

Effect Size Synthesis. For the synthesis itself, pooling of effect sizes may or may not occur. If there are enough relevant studies to make an aggregation of effect sizes statistically reasonable, they may be pooled. However, small sample sizes or too many studies in which the data are incomplete should not be grounds to abandon the synthesis. As Slavin (1995) notes, "Pooled effect sizes should be reported as adjuncts to the literature review, not as the primary outcome." Both pooling of effect sizes and subsequent analyses should be based on theoretical grounds, not solely on statistical exigencies.

Presentation Depth. The body of the BES paper is a systematic discussion of the relationship between variables in a causal model rather than a summary of statistics. The discussion uses effect sizes to describe and illustrate the theoretical analyses. In some cases, the only difference from a traditional narrative review may be the inclusion of effect sizes in the discussion of each individual paper. In other cases, there will be a systematic pooling of effect sizes across studies as in any meta-analysis, but the studies themselves will also be explored conceptually in much more detail.

Formal Quantitative Synthesis (Meta-Analysis)

Earlier in Section C, we presented examples of less rigorous quantitative analyses, each of which can be useful in certain circumstances. We judge that meta-analysis may be one of the most sound methods of increasing research power and reducing bias in experimental research. Consequently, the following discussion focuses on meta-analysis (conceptualized in the box below).

META-ANALYSIS

We conceptualize meta-analysis as the statistical study of pooled research results from many individual studies, following the prototype of Glass (1976). This type of systematic review is a subset of the general category of quantitative syntheses.

Jeng, Scott, and Burmeister (1995) provide a more detailed definition: "Meta-analysis is a methodological tool that applies statistical methods and scientific strategies to limit bias and to allow appraisal and synthesis of results from relevant studies on a specific topic."

The goal of a meta-analysis is to provide a more effective integration of multistudy results to answer a research question better than can be accomplished in a traditional nonsystematic review (Glass, 1976). To conduct such a synthesis, a formal, quantitative representation of the meta-analytic model is needed. Constructing this model requires an understanding of the basic principles of statistical analysis and hypothesis testing, which we review in Chapter 12. However, there have been "step-by-step" guides for developing a quantitative synthesis such as the materials available from the Cochrane collaboration (see the compendium at the end of this book) and other publications such as Egger et al. (1997) and Lau et al. (1997).

In Chapter 14, we present computational procedures for implementing a meta-analysis. We demonstrate seven variations of these methods using different types of statistics, such as correlation coefficients, differences in means, proportions, and odds ratios. As an extension of the differences in proportions, we demonstrate the use of quality-weighted procedures that give higher quality studies greater weight in the analysis. We also demonstrate the use of fixed and random effects models. Our approach is based on the work of Shadish and Haddock (1994).

If you elect to do a meta-analysis, you need to choose a design from the seven variations of a meta-analysis listed below.

SEVEN VARIATIONS FOR IMPLEMENTING A META-ANALYSIS

1. Combining study effect size differences in correlation coefficients
2. Combining study effect size differences in means
3. Combining study effect size differences in proportions
4. Combining study effect sizes using a quality-weighted approach
5. Performing random rather than fixed effects meta-analyses
6. Combining study effect size differences in odds ratios
7. Combining study effect size differences in odds ratios with small sample sizes (Mantel-Haenszel)

In Chapter 14, for each of the variations, we describe nine basic implementation tasks as applied to each particular design.

At this point, you should be familiar with a variety of systematic synthesis methods, ranging from qualitative to quantitative, that might be used when you start your formal synthesis planning in the next section of this chapter. The design most appropriate for your project will depend on your resource availability and the topic you finally choose.

Section D. Formulation of Synthesis Topic and Model

Conceptualization of Synthesis Question or Topic

Implicit Questions in Your "Problem Space." In our judgment, the formulation of questions for a research synthesis, just as for a research study, is an intuitive inductive process that takes place in a "problem space."

PROBLEM SPACE

Problem space is the implicit mental construct of your synthesis or research questions or problems at hand. It includes associated concepts and variables, your ideas about how these elements relate, and the overall context in which they become defined in your own mind before they are recorded in explicit form.

This function of formulating explicit concepts from implicit ideas in our minds is at the heart of most creativity. There is no formula you can follow to make this happen. However, we theorize that this process can be facilitated.

Explicit Question Formulation. To facilitate original question formulation, the effort expended in meeting the three prerequisites (Sections A, B, and C above) will prove valuable. It is important to have requisite "apperceptive knowledge" or background information and nomenclature, as suggested in Section B. At least a brief familiarity with the research and developments, as well as terms and jargon in your field of interest, will prove of great help in the more formal conceptualization process of planning. You will have to use inductive skills to recognize or formulate explicit assumptions, theories, concepts, ideas, and improvement hypotheses in the domain of your question. You will have to decide which theories, concepts, and ideas are most relevant for a given patient population. In formulating these ideas, working with a group of colleagues may be much more successful than doing this alone. It is helpful to understand and be able to apply structured group judgment methods such as brain-storming, nominal group technique (NGT), or Delphi. Such methods can provide a rich source of original creative ideas and prove far more cost-effective for topic formulation than traditional committee processes. In our experience, experts often find these structured consensus methods intriguing, as well as a valuable personal learning experience. All of this should facilitate the creative process of formulating explicit questions. (Further detail on conducting a modified nominal group technique is in Appendix 2.1.) A helpful reference on formulating topics for systematic reviews is Counsell (1987, 1998); see also Lundberg, Paul, and Fritz (1998).

Establishing Priorities of Potential Synthesis Questions. The next important consideration for your synthesis question is establishing priorities among several possible alternative topics. It is generally agreed that the final application of your review, if successful, should achieve the most net benefit for the time and effort you invest. What will be the population net benefit (e.g., in quality-adjusted life years [QALYs]) or health status for these alternative synthesis topics? (In terms of health status, Ware [1998] uses a more accurate phrase: "health-related quality of life years" [HRQLYs].) What resources, especially in time, dollars, and expertise, would be required for each? Establishing priorities is an excellent focus for using structured group judgment (i.e., systematic consensus development methods). Murphy et al. (1998) have written an exceptional review of such methods as applied to clinical guidelines.

Wording Your Synthesis Questions. Finally, clinically relevant questions should be worded concretely and explicitly to imply how they might be answered (Oxman, Sackett, & Guyatt, 1993). The more precise your terminology, the easier it will be for your reader to infer your criteria of inclusion and exclusion. Later, when you develop your synthesis model, you will be able to provide the specific details necessary to more thoroughly define your criteria of relevance. In our judgment, the most functional format for stating a synthesis question is in the form of testable improvement hypotheses. This type of wording makes the purpose of your review that of finding sound evidence for or against your hypothesis, rather than merely exploring available information on your topic (Light & Pillemer, 1984, p. 26). Exploratory synthesis question wording makes it difficult to set bounds of inclusion and exclusion and far more difficult to come to closure.

Understand "Problem Space" and "Working Theories"

Once you have a topic, it is essential that you place it in context. *Context* refers to the implicit aggregate of concepts known as the "problem space" and "theoretical framework." Without such a framework and clarification, the meaning of your findings will be difficult and subject to misinterpretation. You can establish the context by specifying (a) why the question is important, (b) to whom the findings will be relevant, and (c) what the relevant theories are on the topic. For example, the real meaning and importance of the finding that dogs salivate when a bell rings indicating food could only be appreciated when it was realized that these results supported theories of associative learning. Similarly, studies that examine the role of communication between the patient and the provider can best be interpreted if one is focusing on patient outcomes, patient consumer advocacy, legal ethical issues, or testing theories of psychology. Sometimes, the theoretical framework is formal and explicit; however, more often it is implicit and assumed. Bringing implicit assumptions forward for inspection will do a great deal to improve your methodology.

Aspects of Model Development

Your "project model" will outline the question, identify the conceptual variables involved in the question, and specify possible cause-and-effect relationships. Development of a model makes clear any assumed or implicit theory behind your question. Definition of action goals and strategies at each stage will be much easier to accomplish with an explicit working model. For these reasons, we emphasize model development as one of the most important initial steps in planning your synthesis project. Many synthesis experts assert that this step is one of the more critical elements of synthesis activity (Cooper, 1998; Goldschmidt, 1986; Hall, Tickle-Degnen, Rosenthal, & Mosteller, 1994).

SYNTHESIS "PROJECT MODEL"

A "project model" is an explicit description of a small aspect of your detailed, implicit "problem space" that is associated with your original synthesis question or topic. A project model, as defined here, is a verbal, written, or graphical representation of a theoretical relationship between variables. Your model outlines the question, identifies conceptual variables involved in the question, and specifies possible cause-and-effect relationships.

Regardless of the origin of the question, a model should be developed. Adequate scientific explanation requires that the "contingencies or circumstances that lead to an event or relationship be identified" (Becker & Schram, 1994, p. 359). In many ways, a model has the goal of all theory, and that is to provide an adequate "explanation" of a phenomenon.

Formal models provide important benefits for all types of syntheses. In a traditional narrative synthesis, a formal model helps authors to address the relevance of methodological and theoretical issues. In a quantitative synthesis, developing a formal causal model helps you avoid limiting findings to simple questions only (main effects) and allows the inclusion of a variety of variables important to practice. Developing a conceptual model initially greatly enhances the usefulness and quality of a meta-analysis.

In the early planning stages of your project, you should make a formal model to ensure that the following information is quite clear: (a) the variables directly and indirectly involved in the question, (b) the direction of relationship between variables, and (c) the causal character of those relationships (see Cook, Guyatt, Laupacis, & Sackett, 1992; Eagly & Wood, 1994; Miller & Pollock, 1994; Shadish & Sweeney, 1991).

Definition of Model Variables. Definition of variables is the heart of model building, as this activity "fleshes out" the full meaning of the topic or question. Asking, in general, how patient-provider communication affects patient outcomes appears on the surface to be a clear question. However, once you formalize the definition of each of those variables, you begin to see how a variety of interpretations of the same variable could easily occur. You could be asking how the length of time spent with a patient (one measure of communication) affects hospitalization rates and lengths of stay (two measures of patient outcomes). Or, you could be asking how provider warmth (another measure of communication) affects functional status (another measure of patient outcomes). As you can see, variable definition and clarification is very important.

The two most important classes of variables are *dependent variables,* the variables that are the outcomes or events of interest, and *independent variables,* which affect the dependent variables. For example, an independent variable named "psycho-educational care" might determine the values of the dependent variables called "depression" and "anxiety" (Devine & Westlake, 1995). Each of these variables must be defined in a precise, measurable way. The process of defining variables in a precise, measurable way is called *operationalization.*

OPERATIONALIZATION

This term refers to the process where the conceptual variable is structured into specific behavioral and measurable events. Variables must be defined at a level of precision that is both usable and yet conceptually congruent with the underlying construct. (Precision of estimates indicates a narrow confidence interval, i.e., being sharply or narrowly defined.)

This task is as difficult for the author of the synthesis as it is for the researcher of a primary clinical study. In our previous example, psychoeducational care is the independent variable. It can be defined as "provision of some type of behavioral or cognitive counseling focused on developing skills or changing thoughts and behaviors" (Devine & Westlake, 1995, p. 1373). Other definitions include supportive listening, or information about living with cancer. Even within each of these definitions, there may be differences in how measurement (or manipulation) is done.

Similarly, the dependent variables of "anxiety" and "depression" must be measured rigorously. Anxiety could be measured through the use of a standardized test such as the Profile of Mood States (POMS) or the Multiple Affect Adjective Checklist (MAACL) (Devine & Westlake, 1995). Depression can also be measured through the use of standardized tests such as the Beck Depression Inventory (BDI). As an author of an information synthesis, you must decide on the level at which the definitions are sufficiently broad to capture the full meaning of the variables and yet not risk the problem of comparing "apples and oranges." Only a thorough and comprehensive process of model building will provide a clinically useful and meaningful information synthesis.

Finally, as part of the process of variable definition, you must specify the underlying assumptions you hold regarding the distribution of the variables of interest. By *distribution,* we are referring to beliefs about how these variables may vary. Do values on this variable make up a continuous normal distribution? Or do values on this variable only occur at certain points, discreetly defined, such as threshold levels for anemia or other physiological measures? In other words, you must construct a random or a fixed effects model.

RANDOM OR FIXED EFFECTS MODEL

A *fixed effects model* assumes that the levels of the independent variable (e.g., dosages of drugs, types of treatments, or time spent with patient) exactly reflect the universe of possibilities.

A *random effects model* assumes that the levels of the independent variable are randomly sampled from a universe of levels. The result is an ability to generalize to all levels of an independent variable (and to all studies in a domain).

An example of a fixed effects model would be a study in which the levels of the independent variable being assessed are assumed to exhaust all of the possible levels. For example, the types of psychoeducational care (active listening, information, counseling) are all the interventions of interest. This specification eliminates a source of variance or uncertainty in the data analysis that does not need to be statistically controlled. Strictly speaking, however, it would not be possible to liberally generalize to other types of studies or studies with different "operationalizations" (forms or

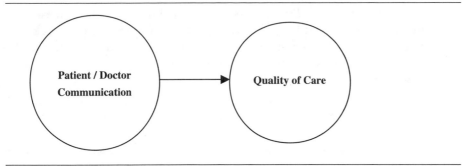

Figure 2.1. Model: Relationship of Patient-Doctor Communication and Quality of Care

manipulations) of the independent variable. In other words, it would not be possible to generalize to other types of psychoeducational care. Fixed effects analyses have been the basis of most meta-analyses in the past and are easier to perform.

In a random effects model, you can generalize to all levels of an independent variable (and to all studies in a domain); however, you also have to estimate variance or uncertainty from an additional source, namely, the universe from which the levels of the independent variable were sampled. In the case of an information synthesis, this approach assumes that studies differ randomly in terms of study characteristics and in terms of effect sizes.

The practical implication of using random versus fixed effects models for the information synthesis process depends on the stage. At Stage I, the impact is greatest when developing criteria for study relevance. If you assume a fixed effects model, then only those studies that are very similar in how the independent variable is operationalized would be considered relevant. If you assume a random effects model, you may be more liberal in defining what studies are relevant. At Stage IV, the synthesis stage, this decision makes a very large impact on the formulas used to combine effect sizes.

Delineation of Model Structure. There are many types of models, so you may want to limit yourself to the traditional models found in theory development. In clinical practice, the use of quality management (QM) models is common, such as the Pareto charts or the "fishbone" diagrams (see Wilson & Goldschmidt, 1995). Other common models familiar to clinicians include clinical pathways and decision analysis. The choice of a model will depend on your experience with the different types, your audience, and whether your goal is to test a hypothesis or to do an overall description of an area of concern. Often a simple model structure will be sufficient. In Figure 2.1, we have presented the simplest of model structures identifying two variables, patient-provider relationship and healthcare improvement, linked by an arrow indicating that the direction of effect is from the former to the latter.

Specification of Relationships Between Variables. Model development delineates the relationship between variables, ideally including both the direction of the relationship and its character. Research methods experts break down independent variables into two classes, called mediators and moderators, based on a specific type of relationship with the dependent variables.

MODERATOR AND MEDIATOR VARIABLES

Mediator variables are those factors that likely cause the relationship between the independent and dependent variable (e.g., increased knowledge about possible side effects of chemotherapy leads to lower levels of anxiety).

Moderator variables are those factors that change the relationship between the independent and dependent variable (e.g., the above relationship between knowledge and outcomes is only true for less severely ill patients). In other words, severity of illness moderates the relationship between patient-doctor communication and healthcare outcomes.

Mediator variables are those factors that are believed to cause the treatment to be effective; in other words, they specify the mechanism by which the independent variable affects the dependent variable (Baron & Kenny, 1986).

As an example of a moderator variable, a researcher may believe that decision support computer software will improve the quality of care. The researcher may further propose that the mechanism by which the decision support software has that effect is both by increasing the knowledge of providers and by helping them to value themselves as being more responsible for the patient's care. In this example, knowledge and responsibility are the mediator variables; the decision support computer software increases knowledge and responsibility, which in turn leads to improved quality of care. Furthermore, the researcher may believe that the impact of decision support on the quality of care occurs only for relative novices in an area, and there is little or no impact on experts. In this case, clinician's skill level is a moderating variable; the positive impact of the decision support computer software is restricted to novice practitioners.

Using our ongoing example, improved information about chemotherapy side effects may positively affect anxiety when the patient is not severely ill, but when the patient is very ill, then differences in information may have little relationship with the quality of care. In this example, severity of illness moderates the relationship between provision of information and anxiety. However, severity of illness does not cause or mediate the relationship. Moderators are important if you are to understand the conditions under which the treatment may be differentially effective (Baron & Kenny, 1986). Moderator variables may include setting, patient acuity, practitioner

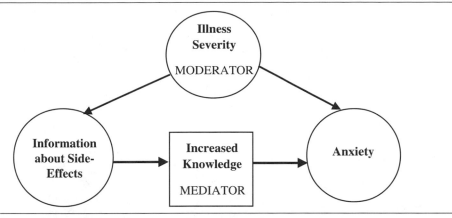

Figure 2.2. Model: Effect of Moderators and Mediators of Information and Patient Anxiety

training, or gender. Figure 2.2 shows the expanded model with the addition of mediators and moderators.

Another important aspect of the relationship between variables is defining the problem in terms of whether you are interested in a univariate or multivariate question.

UNIVARIATE AND MULTIVARIATE QUESTIONS

Univariate questions focus only on one independent variable and one dependent variable.

Multivariate questions consider how a group of independent variables, when considered together, affects one or more dependent variables.

A univariate question focuses only on one independent variable and one dependent variable (e.g., the relationship between information and anxiety). In other words, there is only one relationship that is of concern.

A multivariate question considers how a group of independent variables, when considered together, affects one or more dependent variables (e.g., provision of information combined with relaxation techniques interact to reduce anxiety). Commonly, both mediators and moderators are considered in a multivariate question. A multivariate approach, in general, provides a richer and more complete explanation because most phenomena are determined by multiple factors. However, multivariate quantitative syntheses can sometimes be more difficult to conduct because you may not be able to find a sufficient number of primary studies that include all the variables you want to examine.

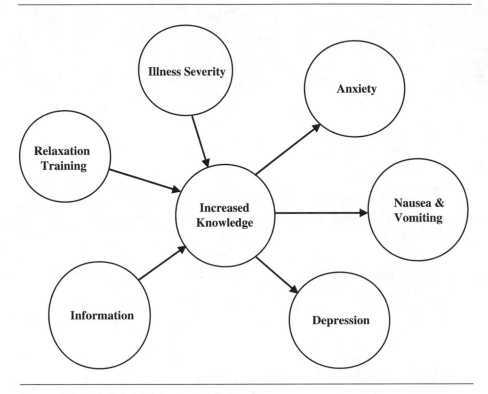

Figure 2.3. Model: Multivariate Relationships

In other cases, however, a multivariate approach is necessitated by the nature of the question. For example, when considering the impact of two different clinical protocols (A and/or B) on the quality of care, it is essential to control for severity of illness in some fashion. Controlling for a moderating factor (severity of illness) while looking at the relationship between the two protocols of interest is a multivariate approach. These types of models are abundant in the literature. As you can see, by including mediators and moderators and using a multivariate approach, model building in information synthesis allows you to see patterns across studies and to conceptualize the question of interest in a larger context, thus improving both understanding and prediction. Figure 2.3 demonstrates a multivariate model that may be used to model the question regarding the relationship between psychoeducational care and patient outcomes.

In Figure 2.3, the construct "psychoeducational care" is operationalized two ways. The first is "information," meaning that the patient receives information about living with cancer. The second is "relaxation training," which involves training the patient in relaxation techniques so he or she can better maintain a calm state.

Knowledge about the cancer and how to cope with it (the mediator) is then hypothesized to increase. As a result of increased knowledge, we see improvements in the healthcare outcome measures of anxiety, depression, and physical symptoms.

A final aspect of specifying the relationship between variables is to state, á priori, if the question is to be descriptive or inferential.

DESCRIPTIVE OR INFERENTIAL QUESTIONS

A descriptive synthesis question simply asks about the aggregated findings regarding the relationship between two or more variables. In this case, the goal is to count how many Y (e.g., HIV) patients are in Z (e.g., California) population in a specified period of time. This is a classic epidemiological descriptive measure of prevalence.

An inferential synthesis question tests a hypothesis and asks whether a given finding is significantly different from what would be expected by chance. In this latter case, the goal is to generalize the findings to the larger population and come to a conclusion that the difference is statistically significant (i.e., not due to chance alone).

Examples of descriptive syntheses include prevalence estimates or the kinds of coping strategies used by infertile couples. Studies that look at the natural history of disease or describe the kinds of symptoms associated with a disease are all descriptive in nature. Syntheses for these kinds of questions may not necessarily need to use quantitative techniques.

In contrast, inferential questions ask about what is the cause of disease (by testing two or more possible explanations) or what are the best treatments. Controlled clinical trials are usually used for these kinds of questions to ensure adequate scientific control. The purpose is to be able to generalize the results, with some certainty, to a larger population. Quantitative synthesis techniques are almost always used in these areas.

In summary, this section (topic/question formulation) proposes that a critical step in an information synthesis is a systematic method to formulate and prioritize potential synthesis topics and then develop the conceptual framework within which your synthesis question will be answered. We propose that the best way to specify a clear question is to conceptualize a topic abstracted from your implicit "problem space" and then develop a model to make explicit and define the variables involved with that topic, as well as to establish the relationships between those variables. The end results of this approach are clear and precise question(s) as well as a sound working model for developing your synthesis plan. Although the topic definition or problem formulation will change throughout the synthesis development, the change will

TABLE 2.4 Sources and Illustrative Questions for a Clinical Information Synthesis

Source of Questions	Examples
Quality improvement team	Reducing operating room delays
	Developing the best admission procedures
	Assessing appropriate antibiotic usage
Clinicians	How is insulin production affected in this patient who takes a large variety of medications?
	Would this epileptic patient on Dilantin have a toxic reaction to antidepressant medications?
	What is the most effective management of a 50-year-old patient with early Alzheimer's disease?
Guideline development	What is the best way to select an antibiotic(s) to treat a *Pseudomonas aeruginosa* infection?
	What is the best way to manage an endogenous cholesterolemia?
Editorial peer review	How do we judge methods adequacy of a meta-analysis?
	How do we judge adequacy of an article's bibliographic methods documentation?
Clinical research	What are the long-term side effects of Viagra?
	How can we diagnose pancreatic carcinoma earlier?

produce greater yield and clarity if the process begins with a clear understanding of the "problem space" and conceptual framework.

Section E. Synthesis Audience and Their Needs

To adequately focus a synthesis, you must specify the readership you will be addressing. By understanding the audience, you will be able to direct the review to their needs, language level, and conceptual understanding. Table 2.4 describes several potential end users of your synthesis, followed by questions they may want answered.

Below we offer a more detailed description of specific classes of end users, each with unique information requirements that must be kept in mind when planning an information synthesis project.

Healthcare Providers

This group includes all the various health professions such as nurses, doctors, clinical psychologists, social workers, and occupational and physical therapists. Because they are individuals who directly care for patients, they need information to be available at the time of decision making in a form that is easy to understand and immediately applicable. Special attention should be given to make the synthesis question clinically relevant and the results applicable in practice. For example, statistical significance is often irrelevant to decision making at the bedside. Rather, differences that are clinically significant should be emphasized. Evidence tables, short summaries, and specific recommendations may be the best forms in which to put information synthesis results.

Healthcare Improvement Professionals

This group of individuals has the responsibility for looking at care across time, patient populations, and service areas. They may have responsibilities for implementing systems for assessment and monitoring patient outcomes. Often, members of a quality improvement staff are the individuals in an institution responsible for answering to outside accreditation agencies (e.g., the Joint Commission on Accreditation of Healthcare Organizations [JCAHO]). The most urgent need of these professionals is access to assessment and improvement interventions that have been tested for both reliability and validity. These interventions are ready for immediate implementation. For these individuals, information synthesis results may be most useful in terms of evidence tables or graphs, with a special emphasis on the degree to which the intervention has been tested across populations and settings. In addition, of particular concern would be the details of an implementation with a preference for the independent variable (the treatment) being implemented in the same way across studies.

Researchers (Clinical and Health Services)

Researchers require detailed levels of documentation and rigorous compliance with the rules of research design and practice. They are less concerned with the practical implications and issues of implementation than they are with the theoretical ramifications. Often, questions are conceptually based, meaning that there is less need for a concretely defined independent variable (the treatment) or clinically relevant dependent variables. Multivariate and theory-testing questions are more desirable. Usually the output is a traditional publication. If your synthesis is geared to a research audience, be sure that you thoroughly document the methods and carefully articulate how this research activity adds to the body of knowledge in the particular field of study.

Policy Analysts and Administrators

Policy analysts usually require syntheses with a much broader scope. The questions they ask are often broader (e.g., What is the impact of a community physician shortage on the quality of care?) than questions asked by providers or researchers. The context of the questions also tends to be oriented more to a general population (e.g., all age groups and all disease groups). Questions can be formed at a general level but must still remain relevant to the practical world. In addition, there is greater emphasis on economic factors. Citing literature that stresses cost-effectiveness requires review and editing by experts in this domain. Writing for administrators may require a different frame of reference, with careful consideration of issues relating to generalizability and applicability.

Professional Educators

Professional educators are concerned with capturing the essential principles in a synthesis and determining the applicability to practice. Implications for the educational process should always be addressed. Often, the focus of questions in this arena covers both the "why" and the "how." Frequently, information from a synthesis is not sufficiently detailed to infer specific practices. Expert group judgment may be needed to bridge the gap between results from a review and what is needed for instructional purposes. In addition, the review must very carefully identify both what is known and what is still left to be determined. Issues of dissemination (methods by which information is presented) are of high importance to educators. Some information is best delivered to adult audiences in the form of role-playing and videos rather than as written or lecture material.

Science Writers for Lay Audiences

Writing state-of-the-science reviews for lay audiences requires that syntheses meet strict communication effectiveness standards. For example, lay readers need a well-written glossary of frequently used basic terms and a clear definition of any acronyms appearing in the text. We suggest that the most essential materials to be communicated to lay audiences are how results will directly affect their lives. In addition, writing should be at a much simpler level than is usually necessary when communicating to fellow scientists. Detailed methods sections are not required. Pretesting material on lay readers familiar with the topic may help ensure that the writing is at a proper level. Graphical illustrations are also useful and should be made easy to interpret.

Section F. Linking Syntheses to Healthcare Outcomes Improvement

The ultimate purpose of healthcare, let alone a synthesis, is to improve outcomes, defined in the broadest sense, for both consumers and providers. The degree of improvement is not compared to "no treatment" but rather compared to "usual care" (acknowledging that, in certain instances, outcomes might be better if care were withheld). If authors of information syntheses in the health field do not understand that their efforts must ultimately result in healthcare outcome improvement, their syntheses are unlikely to have the positive impact they might have wished. **Healthcare improvement professionals**, especially, must understand outcomes and their relationship to care processes and structures. Other target readers must at least be aware of the concept of healthcare outcomes, even if their needs are somewhat remote to the ultimate purpose of all mature (immediately applicable) healthcare information. To understand this concept, we need to recognize what an outcome is and how information syntheses might use this concept to improve the final results of healthcare.

Introduction to Healthcare Outcomes

We introduce this concept by asking three deceptively simple questions:

What Are Healthcare Outcomes? In any context, the term *outcomes* is abstract and refers to the results of any process and structure measured at one point in time. We use the plural of the term *outcome* to remind you that there are multiple outcomes of any care episode—health status, economic status, and satisfaction of either the patient or the provider, to name but a few. In healthcare, *outcomes* is a multidimensional concept that is especially complex and does not relate well to mechanical or industrial outcomes. Thus, it is important to recognize the multiple interacting and often intangible factors that are encompassed by the concept of outcomes in a healthcare context.

Healthcare outcomes can be measured at different levels of specificity, ranging from a molecular level to an individual level to the total world population. In this book, we apply this term at many levels but place our emphasis at the local-to-national population level, measured in terms of health status and quality of life.

Why Are Outcomes Important? The goal to which all providers are oriented is optimal health. Healthcare improvement professionals analyze outcomes in a specific setting to deduce process or structure changes that might result in outcomes improvement. Health services researchers develop and verify new methods and technologies (e.g., computer expert systems and guidelines) to be used by clinicians and quality improvement personnel. Educators and trainers help healthcare staff apply these new technologies by a variety of learning modalities to improve self-learning and care results. Outcome-centered thinking is a paradigm, or worldview, that links together the worlds of research, education, and clinical practice to improve the results of healthcare.

What Is Healthcare Outcomes Improvement? Healthcare outcomes improvement is both a model of healthcare and a paradigm of thought. We introduce the basics for understanding this idea and define the dimensions of outcomes as well as our concept of the relationship between Donabedian's (1966) "structure, process and outcome." Outcomes improvement necessarily integrates measures of all three assessment foci.

In this same regard, we describe the healthcare quality improvement cycle. Many have described different forms of this basic cyclic quality improvement model; however, they all have three elements in common, as shown below.

Dimensions of Healthcare Outcomes

Outcomes Content. In terms of content, we conceptualize eight generic families, or clusters, of healthcare outcomes, as shown in Figure 2.4. Each of these eight clusters has a different denominator population for sampling, different types of instruments required for data gathering, and different barriers and biases threatening valid assumptions and inferences.

The column heading "Consumers" encompasses anyone who may, either now or in the future, require care or who is currently receiving care (i.e., patients). The column heading "Providers" encompasses the entire range of personnel required to operate a healthcare system, such as clinicians, administrators, manufacturers, suppliers, third-party payers, purchasers, and regulators. The row heading "Health"

	Consumers	Providers
Health		
Economic		
Satisfaction		
Other		

Figure 2.4. Healthcare Outcome Clusters

includes the physical, mental, emotional, vocational, recreational, and social well-being of either the consumer or provider. The row "Economic" refers to fiscal effects both for the consumer and the provider. For the consumer, this includes the overall out-of-pocket costs and earnings loss. For the provider, it is the balance of revenues and expenditures. The row labeled "Satisfaction" involves the consumers' or patients' positive or negative perceptions regarding the care received; with providers, it involves working conditions, job satisfaction, and burnout. Finally, the row "Other" includes such factors as the ethical, medicolegal, educational, or even religious outcomes of care for either the consumer or the provider.

Levels of Social Aggregation. Within each generic outcome family, a synthesis can focus on any level of **social aggregation**, ranging from the individual level to the institutional, community, regional, national, and international levels. Each of these levels requires different measurement instruments and sampling techniques. For example, the sampling base at the individual level might be a patient log by a certain physician; at the institutional level, the aggregate of all patients admitted to a hospital; and at the international level, you would theoretically require a listing of populations in all nations.

Structure-Process-Outcome Relationships. Each outcome is a cumulative result of a series of preceding actions (processes) by healthcare providers using certain material resources (structure). This quality assurance focus on structure, process, and outcomes was conceptualized by one of the leading pioneers in the field, Avedis

Donabedian (1966). This triad of assessment and improvement factors, by the way, has caused debate and controversy for several decades as to which is more important to assess. We take the stance that they are all important and must all be assessed at one time or another. However, what makes the most sense to us is to start with an unacceptable outcome and work back to deduce process and/or structures that must be changed to result in improvement of the original outcome(s) targeted. Some of these actions greatly affect the outcome(s), and others have only a minor impact. One method for establishing cause(s) of a targeted outcome is looking at the relationship between structures, processes, and outcomes. If each cell of the eight-cell 2 × 4 matrix (Figure 2.4) is considered the final or ultimate result of care, then it is possible to conceptualize lower levels of processes and/or structures that are causally linked to those final outcomes. If it is difficult or impossible to measure the final outcomes, then you must fall back and use surrogate outcomes if this is feasible. These are lower-level care results that have intermediate to high predictive validity for estimating the final outcomes. "Drilling down" the causal chain of the hierarchy, starting with any of the eight final generic outcome clusters, can identify lower-level outcomes.

Healthcare Outcomes Improvement Cycle

All healthcare improvement activities go through essentially the same basic problem-solving processes.

Establish Priorities of Improvement Hypothesis. A judgment is made regarding which problem or question has the highest priority or potential for healthcare improvement. In healthcare, we conceptualize two major domains of improvement hypotheses, determined by the direction of clinical logic. The first consists of improvement in diagnostic outcomes; the second consists of improvement in therapeutic outcomes. This framework provides a practical focus for establishing a comprehensive spectrum of quality improvement (QI) topics to consider.

*Test the Top-Priority Hypothesis (Initial **Outcome Assessment**).* To test the top-priority hypothesis, measurements are taken to determine if the problem really exists and to assess its severity and extent. At this point, an achievable improvement threshold is estimated, below which additional effort will be required to meet or exceed that threshold. This threshold level serves as a goal to determine the rest of the outcome improvement process and a standard by which success is measured.

Deduce Cause of Problem and Develop Improvement Plan. Causes of the problem are deduced and improvement hypotheses generated through a number of methods. These methods include group processes, screening the literature, or consulting experts. In this step, you will cycle back to identify other causes if early ones do not seem correctable or if improvement interventions are not affordable. When it seems clear that practical changes of care processes and/or structures will affect outcome improvement, a systematic plan of solving the problem is developed. When the plan is complete, the cycle ends and you go on to implement the plan.

Implement Plan to Improve Outcomes. The above improvement plan is implemented over the period of time judged necessary to have a measurable effect. Preliminary or partial data collection may be necessary to determine this point in time and move on to the next step.

Reassess Outcomes and Recycle If Needed. The impact of the intervention is now formally assessed, comparing the results to the baseline. This process is repeated until the desired goal is reached (Williamson 1978a, 1991). Once you are sure the initial improvement is achieved, a monitoring schedule is put into place to ensure that the improvement is maintained. It is important to realize that if the improvement threshold is not met (i.e., the improvement hypothesis cannot be proved), it may be because either the related care needs enhancing or the threshold is unrealistic (unattainable). In the latter case, the target threshold is lowered to a more achievable level.

Understanding this cycle assists the clinician and reviewer to identify areas where more information is needed and where **application to practice** has the highest priority. Questions for an information synthesis can arise out of any one of these steps. For example, synthesizing information that will help determine priorities for healthcare quality improvement activities is possibly just as valuable a contribution to healthcare as is a synthesis on the most efficacious treatment. This model can also result in education of care providers, especially if their improvement goal is unrealistic, and can stimulate study of other systematic reviews for more convincing evidence, if necessary and practical. Also, this model can help educate health science writers to the importance of including information synthesis evidence in their reports.

Section G. Final Project Planning Issues

For final project planning, there are five important considerations to understand.

Authorship Issues

Synthesis Authorship Qualifications. With a topic in mind, you can start to formulate the responsibilities of a team that will work with you to produce this systematic review. When recruiting coauthors, there are at least four qualifications required of individuals accepting coauthorship. The requirements should be stated in any job descriptions or recruiting materials you generate.

First and foremost, each potential author should have a major interest in the subject matter, so the project will be self-motivating and provide a sense of discovery. Second, each author should have the background knowledge and skills to make a contribution to the success of your project. Third, each potential author should have the opportunity to devote the time and energy to get the job done and gain a sense of pride as the tedious multiple drafts evolve into a quality product. Fourth, authors should be willing to comply with an explicit set of rules regarding order and level of contribution. In general, they should be willing to meet the requirements for authorship of the International Committee of Medical Journal Editors (ICMJE, 1997; 2000).

Avoiding Potential Authorship Problems. When qualifications are not explicit, understood, and agreed on, authorship squabbles can easily arise in the preparation of the final manuscript. Research findings indicate that authorship disputes are rapidly increasing for lack of such agreements and commitments (Wilcox, 1998). This is sad because there are international consensus standards for authorship, agreed on by most medical journals and publishers (see Hoen, Walvoort, & Overkebe, 1998; ICMJE, 1985, 1997; see also www.icmje.org [updated May 2000]).

For example, one of the more serious problems is the failure of authors to meet the commonly accepted criteria of authorship. One study found that about 1 in 4 of 200 American medical journal publications had authors not meeting these criteria (Shapiro, Wenger, & Shapiro, 1994). A subsequently published British study sent questionnaires to first authors of all papers published in five consecutive issues of a peer-reviewed general medical journal. Results indicated that of 84 authors, 53 (almost two thirds) did not fulfill the criteria of authorship (Goodman, 1994). These findings were confirmed by a survey of 1,179 articles from the *Annals of Internal Medicine,* the *Journal of the American Medical Association* (*JAMA*), and the *New England Journal of Medicine,* reported in Flanagin et al. (1998). The results found a substantial proportion of articles in which authors made little or no contribution to the studies. Equally interesting, even when authors know and agree with international criteria for authorship, there is often a gap between what they state and what they actually do (Bhopal et al., 1977). These are serious breeches of ethical and professional conduct about which journals, such as *JAMA,* are trying to increase awareness. As mentioned by Shapiro et al. (1994), some journals are now requiring detailed statements from each author detailing his or her individual contributions to the paper.

Often professionals glibly agree to participate and then lose interest or find the time requirement far greater than anticipated or affordable. The major task of producing a quality manuscript is writing, rewriting, and rewriting draft after draft. A quality book can require well over 12 to 15 redrafts (a redraft being a substantial change in outline, or addition or deletion of whole paragraphs or sections) per chapter, and often far more than 5 copyedit drafts. Furthermore, even when a book manuscript is accepted and submitted for publication, there is still a considerable amount of additional work to be done that the whole team must share. After many redrafts, outside reviewers or your own team will still find major errors that have to be corrected, and many additional redrafts must be done to produce a quality product. Surprisingly, the more unsophisticated your reader, the more redrafts have to be done to ensure communication effectiveness. This experience in producing a manuscript for publication is a real test of commitment for the author and coauthors, and the amount of work required is often a major surprise.

The following suggestions for authorship might prove of value in your own work (Morton, 1999).

INTERNATIONAL COMMITTEE OF MEDICAL JOURNAL EDITORS

Guidelines on Authorship

1. Each author should have participated sufficiently in the work to take public responsibility for the content. Participation must include: (a) conception or design, or analysis and interpretation of data, or both; (b) drafting the article or revising it for critically important intellectual content; (c) final approval of the version to be published. Participation solely in the collection of data does not justify authorship.
2. All elements of an article (a, b, and c above) critical to its main conclusions must be attributable to at least one author.
3. A paper with corporate (collective) authorship must specify the key persons responsible for the article; others contributing to the work should be recognized separately (see Acknowledgments and other information).
4. Editors may require authors to justify the assignment of authorship.

Acknowledgments of Contributions that Fall Short of Authorship

1. At an appropriate place in the article (title page, footnote, or appendix to the text; see journal's requirements) one or more statements should specify: (a) contributions that need acknowledging but do not justify authorship; (b) acknowledgments of technical help, (c) acknowledgments of financial and material support, and (d) financial relationships that may constitute a conflict of interest.

2. Persons who have contributed intellectually to the paper but whose contribution does not justify authorship may be named and their contribution described—for example, "advice," "critical review of study proposal," "data collection," "participation in a clinical trial." Such persons must have given their permission to be named.

3. Technical help should be acknowledged in a separate paragraph from the contributions above.

4. Financial or material support from any source must be specified. If a paper is accepted it may also be appropriate to include mention of other financial relationships that raise a conflict of interest, but initially these should be outlined in the cover letter.

SOURCE: Numeration is ours; otherwise quoted verbatim from International Committee of Medical Journal Editors (1985, 1997, 2000).

Staff Management and Training. An essential part of planning is to incorporate the practical issues of managing staff. This includes training, tracking, and communication. At every step, the appropriate staff must be trained. Training may range from a short meeting explaining procedures to special required training seminars. Tracking staff requires that attendance, time on the job, and workload be recorded and monitored. It is one thing to plan for staff to perform a certain function; it is another to ensure that they actually do. Finally, means of communication have to be agreed on. These could be as simple as exchanging phone numbers or e-mail addresses or as elaborate as having formal face-to-face or teleconference meetings. Ensuring that all of these functions are at least brought to awareness in the planning process will prevent many errors, missed opportunities, and redundant effort.

Documentation Needs

For every section, there will be essential requirements for documentation. Some items need to be documented only during the process, such as which articles were retrieved, ordered, or ignored out of every search. Other items must be kept as part of the synthesis report, such as the number of citations found for each source screened. An essential part of planning each stage is to identify what has to be documented and what are the most efficient mechanisms for accomplishing this documentation. Understanding documentation needs can best be understood by reading the evaluation chapters for each section in this book. These chapters have, as their content, a complete documentation checklist appropriate for each stage. Together, these checklists provide a good overview of the information you will need to record for the complete information synthesis process.

Maintenance of Scientific Rigor

As stated above, an information synthesis is a form of research. As a result, every effort should be made to conduct the process with as much validity and reliability as possible. Attending to this issue in the planning stage will prevent backtracking and redundant work. Rules for reliability and validity have been described in the introduction as well as outlined in the evaluation chapter at the end of each stage. In general, it is important to pay the closest attention to sampling issues, data accuracy and consistency, and scientific procedures. In situations where there is limited time and money, preserving validity will maintain synthesis quality.

Project Management Integration

This dimension of planning focuses on the big picture. It is important to ensure that some tasks be completed before beginning others, that resource use is integrated with personnel availability, and that critical timelines and dependent paths are identified. There is an abundant number of available software for project management such as MacProject, Program Evaluation and Review Technique (PERT) software, or Critical Path Management (CPM) software. If you plan a large, complex synthesis, using such tools will be invaluable. If you decide not to do a complete project management plan, it is still essential that you identify the tasks critical to the timeline and list the resources associated with each task.

Summary

This chapter on synthesis planning is divided into two parts. The first part discusses three prerequisites to be met before formal planning begins. These are (A) information synthesis and budget constraints, (B) background information on the Internet, and (C) information synthesis design options to consider. The second part discusses theoretical considerations for the synthesis planning itself. These are (D) formulation of synthesis topic and model, (E) synthesis audience and their needs, (F) linking synthesis to healthcare outcomes improvement, and (G) final project planning issues.

In Section A, we explain the importance of understanding your resource constraints prior to getting into the processes of synthesis planning and preparation. If you have limited time and fiscal resources but require a brief systematic review for immediate clinical decisions, you might consider a mini-synthesis of completed reviews, hopefully those that are systematic. On the other hand, with abundant time and resources, you can consider a more definitive synthesis and plan a more comprehensive approach. Your own situation will usually be somewhere in between those extremes.

In Section B, we consider the different types of background information that might be helpful in formulating potential synthesis topics. This includes established principles, recognized theories, concepts, and nomenclature used in your general field of interest. We emphasize how some studies in health services research provide rich ideas to help you in developing explicit synthesis topics.

In Section C, we discuss the various types of systematic synthesis designs that might be appropriate, considering your resources and subject interest. These types range from a formal qualitative synthesis, at one extreme, through to a vote-counting approach, on to a formal quantitative synthesis (such as a meta-analysis), at the other extreme.

Understand that you may go through several cycles of rethinking any of the three prerequisites for planning your synthesis project. The topic you finally establish may require rethinking of your needed resources or the type of synthesis that seems appropriate. Or the type of synthesis of most interest might require rethinking your resources and your topic.

In Section D, we explain the importance of formulating a priority problem/question that has potential for achieving healthcare outcomes improvement. Based on this subject, you must then specify a theoretical model and improvement hypothesis within which you will compile evidence that might subsequently be applied to assessment and improvement activities. This model should include explicit variable definitions, both for the independent and dependent variables. It should specify the structure of the model in terms of moderators and mediators and their overall relationship. Finally, the model should specify the overall nature of the question, that is, either descriptive or inferential (hypothesis testing). Models assist in problem specification and help guide continuing synthesis work.

In Section E, we emphasize the importance of specifying your audience and identifying their unique needs. A range of six categories of potential readers is listed and described, and a few of their potential improvement needs are illustrated. When planning your project, you must keep in mind the clinical context of how your evidence will ultimately be used to test your healthcare improvement hypothesis.

In Section F, we discuss your basic premise: the improvement of healthcare outcomes. Keeping this orientation in mind may facilitate appropriate evolution of your topic and project framework. We briefly define outcomes and discuss their importance in conceptualizing and applying an information synthesis. Next, we explain several important dimensions of this outcome concept, including generic functions for assessing and improving the final results of healthcare.

In Section G, we present several theoretical considerations for finalizing your project implementation preparation. We present background material for authorship qualifications and potential problems in this area. Finally, we list and discuss several final aspects of planning and preparation for project implementation in Stage II.

APPENDIX 2.1
Scientific Group Consensus Process

Sackett (1997), in his commentary "A Science for the Art of Consensus," points out how many biases can threaten the consensus processes. Murphy et al. (1998) have written a monograph on this topic and summarize the evidence, as of 1987, of the strengths and weaknesses of structured group processes. We suggest that such formal processes, incorporating the best available expertise and scientific data, can facilitate a systematic review in nearly all of its stages. The following example highlights a few of its applications.

Developing science information synthesis by consensus methods assumes that a priority topic has been determined by another group, based on criteria of healthcare need, incorporating patient preferences, funding, and political considerations as well. This topic selection team also establishes the key issues for resolution by a panel of experts on the topic subject matter. This second panel (used in this example) is appointed to establish the best evidence on the key issues and make recommendations for their management in community practice.

In our judgment, the most rigorous validation process is conducted by a consensus panel consisting of quantitative (those, in the aggregate, having expertise in research methodology, statistics, and epidemiology) and qualitative professionals (those having expertise in clinical research, community practice, including a consumer advocate). For additional discussion on the value, or lack thereof, of consensus methods, see Sackett (1997), Murphy et al. (1998), and Wortman, Smyth, Langenbrunner, and Yeaton (1998). This consensus team systematically establishes the best evidence (published or nonpublished) related to the topic and then determines what level of consensus (range 51% to 100%) they agree to achieve on the key issues that constitute their charge. Before the process starts, the panel may establish a higher minimum level of consensus on information to be reported to the scientific community or to the public.

We judge the most rigorous and cost-effective process to be a modified nominal group technique (NGT) using a panel of only 9 to 13 individuals. Given a specific topic and vital issues related to this topic, the panel might follow the following validation process. First, with consultation from outside, panel members would (a) identify a representative database of articles (published and nonpublished) on the assigned topic that, it is hoped, has a first level of validation, such as editorial peer review; (b) conduct an independent methods validation of each article using explicit criteria related to the research design of that study (only the most methodologically sound investigations would be used to provide evidence for discussion); (c) read those scientific reports and complete a brief worksheet, weighting their judgment as to the aggregate evidence for each critical issue (e.g., the efficacy and/or health risk of a new intervention); (d) engage in an "open-interaction" discussion of those issues when the group seems most disparate and possibly when someone challenges a high agreement; and (e) prior to adjournment, submit their independent worksheets showing their revote on weights for each issue. An additional round may be required, if feasible, to improve the consensus reached on any item. Whatever statistical consensus the group reaches by the time of adjournment stands. If the consensus is low, additional research might be indicated because the current material would be considered premature for distribution to the public, let alone the scientific community.

CHAPTER 3

Procedures for Synthesis Planning and Preparation

In Chapter 2, you became familiar with several conceptual ideas and terms related to synthesis planning. The importance of recognizing your time and fiscal restraints was emphasized and illustrated at two extremes—few or abundant resources. For most of this book, we will assume you have abundant fiscal resources and sufficient time to complete a synthesis closer to an ideal. Understanding the limits of what is achievable, you must develop your own project plan in terms of what is realistic.

PROCEDURES FOR SYNTHESIS PLANNING AND PREPARATION

A. Formulate topic by group consensus
B. Establish a project plan
C. Obtain informatics resources
D. Recruit and train project staff
E. Organize project files
F. Finalize preparations
Appendix 3.1   Suggested search team training exercises
Appendix 3.2   Rationale for ABC relevance-coding convention

Procedure A: Formulate Topic by Group Consensus

Conceptualizing your synthesis topic (or question) is of fundamental importance and often neglected in many "how-to" manuals on information synthesis. For this reason, we provide in-depth suggestions on how this process might be accomplished. Any approach to topic/question formulation depends on such factors as the type of healthcare provider targeted, the setting where he or she works, and a judgment as to subject matter where there is potential for substantial healthcare net benefit not currently being realized.

How meaningful your topic/question ultimately proves to be, in terms of improved outcomes, depends on the method you use for its formulation. We suggest that this task is sufficiently important to your entire project that it is worth the effort to organize a priority panel, which uses a structured group judgment approach, to establish your project focus. This focus will determine qualifications of the synthesis project team you will later recruit.

Remember, the following procedures represent more of an ideal approach than many can afford or for which they have enough time. If you have severe time constraints, you might just complete the first procedure and skip the priority panel. Even better, you could have a single priority panel meeting to obtain a crude consensus on a promising topic. Best of all would be to follow all of the procedures outlined below.

Task 1: Establish Area of Synthesis Topics From Personal Interests

Because you are the senior author of this project, you are responsible for establishing the general topic/question area that is of major interest to you personally and your coauthors as a whole. Consequently, the subtasks of Task 1, Procedure A are your responsibility. The priority panel you select and the project staff you recruit will all contribute to formalizing a specific topic within the area of your interest and, it is hoped, theirs.

Conceptually, as described in Chapter 2, your initial thought processes are implicit and take place in what cognitive psychologists term ***problem space***. By the end of Task 1, your implicit ideas will become an explicit, recorded topic/question area.

Think of a General Topic Area of Personal Interest, to Get Started. It will be an advantage if the topic/question concept is in your own area of expertise. Develop some crude boundaries of inclusion and exclusion for this area of interest. For example, suppose you have an interest in presurgical educational interventions. You might list contrasting criteria of inclusion and exclusion such as surgery, not medicine;

educational versus pharmaceutical; outpatient, not inpatient; and elective versus emergency.

Quickly Generate Key Words That Frame This Topic Area. Off the top of your head, record several words or concepts that might express your topic idea in more detail. To illustrate, in the above example regarding educational interventions for surgery, you might include elective surgery, education, anxiety reduction, recovery (not hypnosis), diagnosis, trauma, or attitudes.

Use Above Key Words to "Flesh Out" Characteristics of Your Area of Interest. For example, browse Tables 2.2 to 2.4 in Chapter 2 of this book for important dimensions of your topic that have not yet come to mind. For additional ideas, check health condition codebooks such as the *International Classification of Disease,* the U.S. National Library of Medicine's MeSH headings, directories, and tree structures. As a starter, Table 2.1 lists several exceptional Internet sites encompassing systematic reviews that you might screen (see the Internet compendium at the back of this book for a much more complete listing of relevant URL addresses listed by their sponsoring organization).

Write a Concise Description of Your Topic Area. Because your next task is to recruit a priority-setting panel to select a topic, you will need a brief description of your topic area and its boundaries to explain to potential recruits. Again, describe both inclusions and exclusions of your question or topic. It is helpful if, at this point, you conceptualize several illustrative improvement hypotheses that might be tested by your synthesis.

IMPROVEMENT HYPOTHESIS

An *improvement hypothesis* is a convention for wording a synthesis topic or question in a way that implies how it might be tested empirically. The wording frames the result of the test in terms of healthcare outcomes improvement.

For example, if acute myocardial infarction (MI) suspects are screened in an emergency room and, if positive, receive thrombolytic medication within 1 hour of entry, the death rate, extent of myocardial necrosis, and functional disability can be substantially reduced from what might otherwise be expected. Consequently, the improvement hypothesis concept might be as follows: "Changing the process and structure of emergency room management of acute MI suspects will result in reduced mortality, disability, dissatisfaction, and fiscal losses." As in all research, if this topic is selected for study, each of the terms will have to be specifically defined and operationalized (e.g., variables measured and change factors implemented). Note that, at this point, variable quantification and projected extent of improvement will be rather crude. Usually much more information will be needed before more precise estimates can be made.

Task 2: Recruit a Sponsor, Recruit a Priority Panel, and Schedule an Initial Workshop

Theoretically, you are going to establish a group "problem space" where ideas will be generated and tested implicitly within the minds of the group members, explicitly in the open group discussion step, and then implicitly in the item weighting steps. The result becomes a group synthesis of ideas expressed as a list of topics/ questions that will have potential for being structured as improvement hypotheses.

Recruit a Healthcare Organization Project Sponsor. Working with leaders of a sponsoring organization can provide both credibility and access to needed resources. Perhaps a sponsor's most important function is to facilitate recruitment of required priority panel experts. In our presurgical education example, your nearest academic medical center Department of Patient Education, a local nursing association, and even a county or state medical association might be candidates for being sponsors of your synthesis project.

Develop a Balanced List of Expertise Required for Your Panel. These experts will be key for helping you further develop your topic. You may require panel members such as clinicians, administrators (especially fiscal officers), a professional organization leader, and one or two patient advocates. Using the above presurgical education example, your panel might consist of a surgeon, two nurses (one being a leader of the local nursing society), a general internist, a doctor of patient education, your administrator and comptroller, and lay members of two different families who have cared for surgical patients. We consider these lay members "experts" in understanding the family point of view.

Recruit a Panel of 7 to 11 Qualified Experts. Ideally, there are many advantages for recruiting your team by a two-step process (Emlet et al. 1971). First, recruit a group of qualified professionals to nominate colleagues they know, from experience, to have exceptional judgment. This group can be as small or as large as you choose; however, the more the better. Second, recruit a team of 7 to 11 experts, from those nominated, who agree to participate. This two-step process is especially important for involving practitioners whose behavior may have to change to effect **outcomes** improvement. We have had considerable success with this approach in national studies of Veterans Affairs (VA) physicians (Goldman, Weir, Turner, & Smith, 1997; Smith et al., 1996).

On the other hand, you can do a traditional phone or personal contact recruitment of experts, with input from your sponsoring organization. The risk is that you will achieve much less "buy-in" for the project, possibly have a less qualified panel, and perhaps experience less panel participation.

Schedule a 2-Hour Priority Panel Workshop. This subtask might require more time and effort than you expect, given everyone's heavy schedules. This meeting will be conducted using structured group judgment (SGJ) methods to ensure both effectiveness and efficiency in the use of the group's time. The product of this meeting will be the three topic/questions that receive the highest priority weights as potential improvement hypotheses to be tested by application of your synthesis. The panel will not meet again for the final decision until a month later, after a **mini-synthesis** has been completed for each topic. If resources do not allow this luxury, the final meeting can be scheduled within a few days or even hours, giving the group time to rethink its original judgments.

Schedule a 1-Hour Final Decision Meeting. This session will be relatively brief because the panel will have previously read the executive summaries of the mini-syntheses for each of the three leading topics. A quick revoting and possible discussion by the panel should result in selection of the final topic.

Task 3: Familiarize Panel With Structured Group Judgment Consensus Methods

Review Several Articles on Structured Consensus Methods. As a project leader, you should be aware of the rationale and methods of structured group judgment consensus methods (e.g., Aldag & Fuller, 1993; Delbecq, Van de Ven, & Gustafson, 1975). Browsing any of the references listed after the note box might help you accomplish this task.

NOTE

In the first meeting, you should demonstrate only one type of structured group judgment consensus method, namely, modified nominal group technique (NGT). This approach is the one we have found most effective to use for topic selection. NGT requires that your team meet face-to-face, and it will take about 1 to 2 hours, at most. You will discover that you can accomplish more in that time than an "open-interactive" committee might do in 2 days.

Murphy et al. (1998): "Consensus Development Methods and Their Use in Clinical Guideline Development" (book)

Counsell (1998): "Formulating Questions and Locating Primary Studies for Inclusion in Systematic Reviews" (book chapter)

Lundberg, Paul, and Fritz (1998): "A Comparison of the Opinions of Experts and Readers as to What Topics a General Medical Journal (*JAMA*) Should Address" (*JAMA* article)

Smith (1996): Information in Practice (editorial)

Smith (1996): "What Clinical Information Do Doctors Need?" (*BMJ* article)

Williamson (1978b): "Formulating Priorities for Quality Assurance Activity: Description of a Method and Its Applications" (*JAMA* article)

Delbecq et al. (1975): "Group Techniques for Program Planning: A Guide to Nominal Group and Delphi Processes" (monograph)

Delbecq and Van de Ven (1971): "A Group Process Model for Problem Identification and Program Planning" (*JABS* article)

Pertinent information can be abstracted from any of the above sources. See the reference section in this book for complete citations.

Send Panel Members a Printed Introduction to Your Project and SGJ. You should write a one- or two-page document briefly explaining your synthesis project. Mention the unique methods you will use to elicit needed consensus on synthesis topics that will most likely result in outcomes improvement if applied in practice. In particular, you might stress that (a) extensive research over the past 50 years has been done to develop and evaluate structured group consensus methods such as nominal group technique and Delphi, (b) these methods take far less time than the traditional "open-interaction" committee meetings, (c) the consensus topics developed by these means will more likely be accepted by others, (d) these topics will more likely motivate participation to implement an information synthesis project, and (e) this project is important to the sponsoring organization. This introduction should be sent to the panel members several days before the first consensus meeting.

Conduct a Demonstration of a Modified NGT at the First Meeting. You should demonstrate the modified NGT at the beginning of the first meeting. You will require three panel members for this exercise, and you can use any topic relevant to your setting.

1. *Establish a field of study.* For example, in a primary care facility, your question for this demonstration panel might be the following: What primary care problem do you consider having the most potential for outcomes improvement by developing an information synthesis? You might mention that this synthesis would be the basis for developing a computerized guideline for the facility. Let the group know that the consensus process steps will be self-evident as the demonstration goes on, so you need not explain them before the exercise.

2. *Generate initial topic ideas.* Next, the mini-panel should be given 2 minutes to silently record on paper several topic ideas that come to mind. Then you would have a 3-minute round-robin listing of up to two best items from each of the three panel members. The topics would be printed on a flip chart or on a blank transparency, enumerated by alphabetic letters, items a, b, c, and so on. Allow up to 2 minutes for the panel members to ask each other for clarification of unclear items. Judgmental statements arc not allowed at this point.

3. *Weight each nominated topic for improvement potential.* After clarification, each participant silently records the sequential letters of the items as seen on the flip chart and weights (not ranks) each one on a scale of 1 to 5, or 1 to 10, whichever you choose. Five (or 10) is high, indicating those items as having the most potential for achieving outcomes improvement at an affordable cost. A team member could weight all of his or her items as 5 (or 10) by this method. The weights for each item, together with a median weight, are then recorded on the chart for all to see.

4. *Evaluate the two leading topics.* During the next 3 minutes, the "mini-panel" openly discusses only the two top weighted items, articulating either or both the strengths and weakness of each. Any major barriers to implementing the implied project or applying the resulting systematic review should be made explicit at this time. This would also be the opportunity to mention any important resource availability or any project facilitators as well.

5. *Select final topic.* The demonstration session ends after each of the three panel members silently reweights the two top items on his or her paper, which is then handed to you, the leader. You then determine the median weights and identify the leading topic.

This is the quickest means for your priority panel to learn what they will be expected to do in the remaining time of this initial consensus workshop. Overall, this demonstration can be done in about 15 minutes if you, as leader, understand or have had experience with the NGT process.

Task 4: Conduct Initial Priority Consensus Workshop

Use Modified Version of NGT. As mentioned in the article by Williamson (1978b), we judge that weighting nominated topics is more meaningful than merely ranking them.

Establish the Lowest Acceptable Threshold of Topic "Weight." First, the panel must agree on the lowest acceptable threshold of weights to be considered, using a scale of 0 to 10. For example, if a threshold is set at 7.5, and the highest topic weight is 4.8, all items would be unacceptable. If the highest topic weight is 7.9, and the remaining topics are all below 6.0, only one topic would be considered. If all topic weights are above the threshold of 7.5, all might be considered, although most likely the top three would be selected.

Establish the Lowest Acceptable Level of Consensus. This level could be as low as 51% or as high as 100%. A reasonable level might be 67%, but that depends on the consequences for whatever topic is involved. In our example, if five topics are weighted above 7.5, and this was accomplished with a 70% consensus, the top three of that five likely would be used in Task 5.

Select Up to Three Leading Topics. The main problem that might occur in making this selection is when more than three topics have weights that seem "statistically" identical. This finding is roughly analogous to empirical data having overlapping 95% confidence intervals. Again, panel judgment should prevail as to which three are selected (see Ashton, 1986).

Task 5: Complete a Mini-Synthesis on Up to Three Leading Topics

The purpose of this task is to establish sound evidence for or against the leading topics. This information will facilitate selecting the most promising topic for your synthesis project.

Assign Panel Members to Do a Mini-Synthesis on Two to Three Leading Topics. Often, the member who nominated the topic that was noted among the top three might be sufficiently involved to accept this assignment. As senior author, you need to be sufficiently familiar with the tasks involved to provide assistance in selecting members for an assignment.

Search Only for Systematic Reviews and/or Meta-Validated Information. A mini-synthesis can be done from one's home using the Internet and possibly the telephone. Each assigned panel member should spend approximately 8 hours only, over the span of 1 month, to complete this assignment. With new electronic bibliographic technology, the risk is that the assigned panel members will find this job so exciting that they will spend even more time for their own interest. See Chapter 2, Table 2.1 for the initial Net addresses where you might start such a search.

Use the Short "AC" Form of Relevance Coding. Because a mini-search is often an expedient way to "pick only the low-hanging fruit," so to speak, it is appropriate to make a rapid dichotomous judgment of whether or not to retrieve a complete document. Relevance judgment will be based on placing either an "A" (retrieve) or a "C" (do not retrieve) on citations and abstracts.

Complete "Final" Product: A Brief Documented Narrative Synthesis. Each of the assigned panel members should produce a one-page report on his or her assigned topic and attach the single best review found. Perhaps only three questions should be answered by each mini-synthesis: (a) How mature is the research field for this topic (e.g., availability of systematic reviews)? (b) What is the probability that a formal synthesis would produce sufficient net benefit to make this project worth the effort? (c) Does the sponsoring organization have adequate interest and resources to support one formal systematic review on this topic if it has the highest priority?

Task 6: In a Second Meeting, Select One Topic for the Synthesis Project

Each panel member should prepare for this second meeting by reading the one- to two-page narrative mini-syntheses. At this point, there should be sufficient evidence, combined with the priority panel's experience and best judgment, to select a single "best" topic.

In the Second Meeting, Vote Again on the Three Best Topics. When the priority panel convenes, take an immediate vote on the three topics to see if there is a clear consensus that a project on that topic should be implemented. If there is no consensus, or a poor one, discuss whether any of the topics might be salvageable for a formal project. Finally, have the panel revote, weighting each topic.

If a Topic Is Selected, Dismiss the Panel and Prepare for Project Implementation. If the above task is successful, then you must prepare to implement a formal synthesis following the next stages described in this book. Part of this preparation will be to seek funds for this purpose. Perhaps the sponsoring organizations would be sufficiently interested to fund the project themselves. Other sources could include government or private funding groups that might be interested in your project (e.g., the U.S.

Agency for Healthcare Research and Quality or the Robert Wood Johnson Foundation). The National Library of Medicine also provides grants for developing such syntheses.

If No Topic Is Acceptable, Further Team Discussion Is Required. If the priority team cannot agree on an acceptable topic/question for project implementation, the panel must discuss what steps to take next. One possibility might be to select another topic from the top three for additional exploration. A second possibility might be to select a new topic altogether for you, as senior author, to explore yourself. Another possibility might be to disband the priority panel altogether and start over.

Formulate One or More Improvement Hypotheses From the Selected Topic. These hypotheses should be subjects for testing by means of a formal information synthesis and its subsequent application in the community. Such hypotheses should facilitate stating your questions in terms that are answerable (Straus & Sackett, 1998, p. 340) and lead to more specific descriptions, denoting inclusions and exclusions. This information should also be included in your "final" report to your sponsor. You are now ready to go on to Procedure B.

Procedure B: Establish a Project Plan

Initial planning and preparation for the overall project is a difficult but crucial function. It will require abstract conceptualizations as well as detailed work scheduling and budgeting. It requires that you be familiar with your topic, its inclusions and exclusions, before moving on to other tasks of preparation, such as recruiting your coauthors and staff. With an adequate understanding of your subject, you can initiate your project by applying the following six tasks to complete project planning and preparation.

Task 1: Establish Synthesis Purpose and Goals

Completing Form 3.1 will provide an initial concept of your overall synthesis project, including purpose and significance. Figure 3.1 illustrates a completed example.

FORM 3.1: EARLY SYNTHESIS PLANNING FORM (Illustrative Copy)

Date: 2 Apr 01

Initials:　sc

Identification:

Synthesis title: Anticoagulant Guidelines for Acute MI Patients

Authors and staff:

PI:	Susan Cornwal	Assistant:	Lois Fenway	Secretary:	Gilbert Ames
Co-PI:	Albert Johns	Assistant:	Cory Anderson	Clerk:	Lou Sims
Co-PI:	Heinrich Berns	Other		Other	

Synthesis Focus:

Topic: Effectiveness of guidelines for administering anticoagulants to acute MI patients in terms of mortality and cardial damage.

Purpose and Goals: To develop an information synthesis of studies measuring the average time from admission to a community hospital emergency room to administration of anticoagulants for acute myocardial infarction patients. To calculate the net benefit of guideline implementation for patients.

Target Audience: Physicians in general medicine, ER staff, administrators, and relevant consumers

Significance: Potential saving of lives and reduction of cardiac damage in survivors

Product: A published paper for dissemination to target audience

Figure 3.1. Completed Form 3.1: Early Synthesis Planning Form

IMPORTANT NOTE

The forms we offer in this book are only suggested ideas to help you get started. You should adapt these to your own needs as they prove helpful. You may find it necessary to develop an entirely different format for your planning forms. Subsequent synthesis stages will accommodate whatever planning documents you choose. We assume that you will make an electronic copy of these tools to provide formatting flexibility and reproducibility.

In Form 3.1, under the first major heading ("Identification"), the title should be brief and descriptive. Remember that in electronic bibliographic printouts, this title will be the reader's only clue (unless an abstract is also included) to the content of your synthesis. As we will explain in Stage V, it is important to mention in the title or subtitle that your work is an information synthesis or a meta-analysis, if this is the case. Some authors are using terms such as *validated review, systematic review,* or *evidence-based review* to describe what we call an "information synthesis."

Under the heading "Authors and Staff," record the names of the individuals who are finally on your team. Be sure you understand the format that the potential publisher requires.

The second major heading of Form 3.1, "Synthesis Focus," consists of three items.

In the first item, "Topic," describe in greater detail what your title covers. The second item, "Purpose and Goals," should be a single sentence describing your overall intended contribution to be achieved by this project. Then list several specific goals that must be met to achieve your purpose. The goals can vary substantially, depending on your purpose and the audience targeted by your synthesis. For example, the goals of a literature synthesis developed as part of a grant proposal will be different from the goals of a more complex synthesis on the same topic intended for publication to help quality improvement professionals. Later, objectives and methods will be recorded in more detail. The third item describes your "Target Audience," or readers. For purposes of this book, readers are usually health services researchers, quality management (QM) professionals, graduate students, or possibly lay science writers who communicate with the public. For example, QM professionals might apply your synthesis to develop a computerized guideline. Recall that the purpose of our book is to help clinicians effect direct healthcare outcomes improvement in community practice. Thus, you record a brief statement of your target audience and how they will likely use your final synthesis. It is conceivable that this audience may change as your synthesis project develops; however, it is necessary to have a specific readership in mind at the outset to guide early decisions regarding synthesis goals, outcomes to be assessed, and the scope of the search.

The third major heading, "Significance," concerns the likely healthcare net benefits that should be achieved, directly or indirectly, by your synthesis if it is successful. *Net benefit* requires weighting the likely accomplishments against the likely losses. These benefits could range from improved healthcare structures, or care processes remotely related to final patient health outcomes, to interventions having an immediate impact on the patient's or consumer's health status and quality of life. The adverse effects might be such factors as increased health risk, financial expenditures, and complications.

Finally, in the fourth major heading, "Product," state the form of your final synthesis, whether it is a formal paper for a conference presentation, part of a grant proposal, a peer-reviewed journal article, a book, an Internet site, or a software program. The type of product selected must match the needs of, and be accessible to, the proposed audience. For example, the consensus syntheses produced by the National Institutes of Health (NIH) are reported in small booklets that can be quickly read by busy physicians who would rarely read a complete report. These provide a synthesis of major research literature systematically integrated with the knowledge and experience of practitioners. NIH panels usually consist of nationally or internationally recognized experts on the specified topic. Thus, the clinician does not have to be concerned about detailed methods and discussions from all of the papers encompassed but can rely on the selection and validation rigor of the panel. The final product is a small booklet presenting a distillation of the consensus conclusions. The assumption is that it will be the responsibility of other scientists, not the practitioner, to critique the research reports encompassed and the NIH consensus methods applied.

Form 3.2 helps you develop your plan in greater detail by specifying limits of search scope (e.g., language, bibliographic dates, extent of retrieval effort, recommended search sources). Figure 3.2 illustrates a completed example.

Search resources include such items as computer hardware, software, electronic bibliographic databanks, Internet addresses, people sources, and acceptable information types (e.g., articles, books, and letters to the editor).

As your project progresses, planning forms will be essential documentation to remind you of such details as your initial topic, concepts, search scope, and **relevance criteria**, among other factors. This information will also be essential for your evaluation of the quality and cost-effectiveness of the products of each stage.

Task 2: Develop an Explicit Synthesis Model

This task will help you delineate the topic of your synthesis as well as the causal model you are proposing. We suggest four specific subtasks to assist in model building and to help ensure clarity of the question or topic you have selected.

FORM 3.2 SEARCH PLANNING AND UPDATE (Illustrative)

Iteration #: ___5___

Date: __19 Nov 98__

Initials: ___TS___

Topic: Treatment of mastitis during lactation

Scope of the Search:

Languages

__X__   English only   _____ All languages

__X__   English translations of non-English documents

_____ Foreign language papers (specify): _____

_____

Time frame

_____ Screen bibliographic indexes from: __1995__ to __1998__

_____ Obtain documents produced from: __1990__ to __1998__

Extent of Retrieval Effort

_____ Only local community colleagues, schools, libraries

__X__   Retrieve nearby national literature (e.g., United States and Canada)

_____ Retrieve international literature, (e.g., European libraries)

__X__   Contact nearby experts (e.g., United States, Canada)

_____ Contact distant experts (e.g., Western Europe, Japan)

Recommended Search Sources

__X__   Computerized bibliographic indexes (e.g., MEDLINE)

__X__   Internet (World Wide Web)

__X__   People sources (colleagues, authors)

__X__   References listed in relevant documents

_____ Organizations (e.g., academic or professional)

_____ Funding sources (e.g., National Institute of Health)

_____ Paper indexes (e.g., Index Medicus)

Checklist of Information Types

__X__	Published primary data articles	_____	Draft manuscripts
__X__	Books, book chapters, syllabi	_____	Educational manuals
_____	Conference proceedings	_____	Audiovisuals
__X__	Editorials, letters to the editor	_____	Newsletters
_____	Dissertations, printed reports	__X__	Internet material
_____	Abstracts	_____	Studies in progress
_____	Policy papers, editorials, essays	_____	News media
_____	Other (specify):		

Contact several community OB-GYN specialists

Cancel previous request for dissertations and abstracts

Figure 3.2. Completed Form 3.2: Search Planning and Update Guide

Define Both Dependent and Independent Variables. The first activity, specifying the conceptual definition of the independent and dependent variables, is essential to ensure both validity and replicability of the synthesis. This level of definition needs to be precise, behavioral, and measurable. Another way of expressing the concept of defining variables precisely is to say that they are "operationalized," indicating that they are measurable. For example, you may believe that introducing a computerized patient record will improve patients' satisfaction with their care because response time for providing care would be faster and continuity of care substantially improved. Before you begin an "information synthesis" to summarize the findings in the literature, you would need to define what you mean by "patient satisfaction." You might believe that it is the quality of the patient-doctor relationship that is important, or you might be more interested in the quality of communication or the amount of information exchanged. Whichever you choose, you must decide what you will accept as reasonable representations of the concepts you are assessing. You might include studies that survey and interview patients regarding their satisfaction with their care and exclude studies that ask patients how much they learned or those that videotape the patient encounter to assess the quality of information exchange. The synthesis research question then needs to be defined using these specific conceptual and operational variables.

In other cases, rather than decide to focus on one specific "operationalization," you may want to examine a more robust definition of the constructs of interest. Therefore, it may be appropriate to rename the variables at a broader level of analysis that is a more sensible conceptual integration. For example, you are interested in examining the impact of computerized medical records, but you want to include both those used with provider order entry and those used with clerk entry from paper. If you later discover many related studies that examined electronic medical records with imaging and special communication devices, you may then want to change focus. All of these variables may come under a broad conceptual definition of electronic medical records and could be included in your information synthesis.

Specify Form of Overall Causal Model. A second synthesis modeling activity is revising the causal model that links variables together in a cohesive, meaningful structure. The causal model you develop may be simple or complex, depending on the type of question you are asking and the goal of your information synthesis. A simple model may specify a single one-directional effect, such as the effect of a regular exercise program on glucose control among diabetic patients. Other information synthesis models may be more complex. You may propose variables that interact in a bidirectional fashion or that do not have a simple linear relationship but instead have a curvilinear relationship (such as that between anxiety and performance).

Specify Moderators That Affect the Scope of Relationship Between Dependent and Independent Variables. Another essential part of model development and topic/question specification is to stipulate the scope of the relationship between the independent and dependent variables. *Scope* refers to the degree to which the relationship between the independent (treatment) variables and the dependent (outcome) variable differs across settings, populations, situations, and time. These latter factors are moderators because the relationship between the independent and dependent variables is modified by the presence of these factors. They help specify the time, place, and context where the independent variables may have the most influence. Examples of moderators include the type of hospital or clinic, the age group of the patients, and the time of year when studies are done. The refined questions for your synthesis should include questions regarding prospective moderators (Hall et al., 1994; Shadish & Sweeney, 1991). Moderators are likely to come to light once you assemble your data set and begin coding the data. At this point in your synthesis, you may find it necessary to augment your moderators, depending on what you find in the literature. In this planning stage, however, it is vital to specify the initial set of moderators you will include in your synthesis model.

Delineate Mediator Variables, Known or Suspected, That Affect the Causal Relationship Between Dependent and Independent Variables. Finally, an effort should be made to make explicit any questions regarding the underlying causal structure. Understanding causality means specifying potential mediating variables. Again, mediating variables are those believed to cause the relationship between the independent variable (the treatment variable) and the outcome. For example, it may be that you know of many articles examining the relationship between patient-provider communication and patient compliance (and perhaps patient anxiety), and there are already several meta-analyses on these issues. However, there are no systematic syntheses on the underlying causes of this effect, so you decide to focus on the role of anxiety. You hypothesize that the major result of a good patient-provider relationship is to diminish the patient's anxiety, which then leads to improved compliance, which in turn leads to better outcomes. The question for your synthesis will then focus on the potential mediating properties of anxiety on patient compliance and less on the outcomes themselves.

Task 3: Outline Synthesis Methods and Work Schedule

The synthesis methods will be specified in some detail in the "procedures" part of each stage. These methods will be very different, depending on which stage you are implementing. If you have outlined your plan using project management software (likely some variation of the program evaluation and review technique [PERT]), the program will require that each person be given a specific work assignment to accomplish the goals and objectives for each stage.

Task 4: Formulate Criteria for a Successful Product

There are numerous criteria in the literature for evaluating a successful information synthesis. Whether or not you meet these standards depends heavily on how well you conceptualize your model, or project theoretical framework, and the detail in your final plan. In this book, we suggest that you maintain a basic framework of four criteria that we described in Chapter 2—namely, the following:

SYNTHESIS EVALUATION CRITERIA

a. Adequate documentation
b. Clinical significance
c. Scientific soundness
d. Cost-effectiveness

Task 5: Establish Project Budget and Timetable

Now that you have a model and a work plan, you have much of the needed information to develop a reasonable budget and timetable, which you can fill in on Form 3.3. See Figure 3.3 for an illustration of this same form with the timetable filled in as a Gantt chart.

This task involves allocating required personnel time and dollars. These costs will typically include salaries for research assistants (including additional staff who may have to be hired to evaluate article validity), search costs for online references and/or interlibrary loans, book purchases, software and hardware expenses, clerical costs, and photocopying expenses. A synthesis can be performed at many different levels of detail and involves interesting, though potentially distracting, tangential subject matter. A clear guide to resource allocation helps to ensure that you accomplish your goals while you stay within the constraints of available resources. The budget and timeline also ensure that each important task receives adequate attention as deadlines approach.

Task 6: Outline Responsibilities of Authors and Staff

Senior Author. The most important person in an information synthesis is the senior author—you. As the person responsible for the project, you will oversee management of the synthesis team, set priorities, and delegate to a team participant the responsibility (under your supervision) for the day-to-day project management. You will be responsible for obtaining necessary financing, writing much of the manu-

FISCAL BUDGET

Indicate total hours and dollars of staff effort projected for entire synthesis project.

Position	Initials (Name)	Hours	Salary Code	Project Total $	Position	Initials (Name)	Hours	Salary Code	Project Total $
Principal Investigator					Asst.				
Co-PI					Asst.				
Co-PI					Sec.				
Other					Other				

	Personnel $	Consults $	Computer $	Books $	Supplies $	Telephone $	Graphics $	Copying $	Other $	GRAND TOTAL $
Project Costs										

TIMETABLE

Indicate span of time for completing each of the five stages.   (NOTE: Schedule illustrates a completed Gantt Chart)

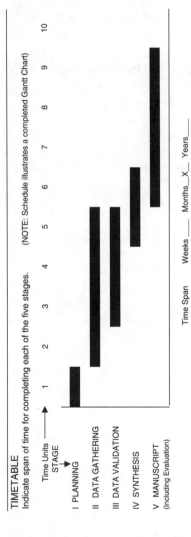

Time Units → STAGE

1   2   3   4   5   6   7   8   9   10

I   PLANNING

II   DATA GATHERING

III   DATA VALIDATION

IV   SYNTHESIS

V   MANUSCRIPT
(Including Evaluation)

Time Span   Weeks ____   Months _X_   Years ____

Figure 3.3. Illustrative Budget and Timetable Planning Form

script, approving contributions from coauthors, and making arrangements for its publication. As the first author, it is up to you to oversee the writing of the synthesis itself and to ensure that the coauthors stay on track, keep on schedule, and maintain adequate standards of quality. You also need to arrange for independent reviewers to critique your manuscript as you go. With their feedback, you must then ensure that coauthors participate in the multiple manuscript revisions (usually more than 12). If for any reason coauthors cannot, or will not, assume ancillary responsibilities, you, as senior author, will have to assume their responsibilities as well as your own. You need to do the final review and approval of the manuscript before submission for publication.

Coauthors. The coauthors share much of the senior author's responsibility for planning, implementing, and evaluating the overall project. Subspecialty areas of the manuscript may be delegated to certain qualified coauthors. If for any reason ancillary staff cannot fulfill their responsibilities, coauthors have responsibility for seeing that the work gets done.

Staff. The staff you hire accomplish most of the routine work. (Remember that we are assuming you have ample funds for hiring staff. If you do not, it is the responsibility of the authors and coauthors and whoever they might find to donate time.) In general, staff tasks include the following:

1. inputting data, maintaining documentation files, and retrieving needed information (this requires advanced secretarial help);

2. setting up computer equipment and providing maintenance and troubleshooting when necessary (part-time experienced hardware/software expert);

3. retrieving and relevance-coding citation-abstracts and complete documents (a database development team [Stage II]);

4. making preparations for Stage III database validation (research methodologists and statisticians familiar with your healthcare topic).

Later in this chapter, we explain procedures for hiring, training, and using staff talent for cost-effective project activity in producing a health science "systematic review." At that point, more detailed responsibilities will be discussed.

Procedure C: Obtain Informatics Resources

Development of an information synthesis is a labor-intensive activity. Prior to the advent of medical informatics, this function was rapidly becoming impossible for busy clinicians (Williamson et al., 1989). Imagine going to a medical library and having to pull out multiple drawers of reference cards and then searching the library for the documents that seemed relevant, having no idea whether or not they were scientifically sound. The information explosion (or for clinical use, often the misinformation explosion) of the medical literature discourages busy clinicians from even attempting to search the literature. What is worse, determining the soundness of the scientific information they do find is often a more technical task than they can manage.

Today, conceptualizing and planning a synthesis project topic, let alone conducting a systematic review itself, without the use of computer hardware and software is laborious, if not impossible, for producing a sound product. It is a vital function of preparation to obtain the most up-to-date, user-friendly software packages that are essential to planning, implementing, and evaluating your project. Medical informatics has been coming to the rescue, especially with the onset of MEDLINE in 1964. (Recall Chapter 1, Section A for an introduction to the field of medical informatics and its crucial role for information synthesis development.)

Here in Procedure C, we do not include basic word-processing, spreadsheet, and audiovisual slide-making packages. The need for this software goes without saying. Everything, from early planning notations through to the final manuscript, will depend on this technology. We assume that most readers are aware of standard word-processing packages, as well as those clustered with spreadsheet technology (e.g., Microsoft Excel) and audiovisual software such as Microsoft PowerPoint. (These three are usually packaged together in software such as Microsoft Office.) We mention Microsoft only because it has been the basis for most of our experience. Many other competitors are as good or better for many of these purposes. Building on your present computer platform, you have undoubtedly already purchased your own equivalent of Microsoft Office. Thus, we will not get into any technical detail on this subject.

We emphasize six basic tasks of synthesis development in which informatics theory and resources are essential and available. We briefly introduce specific software and hardware (the latter restricted to scanners) needed.

Although it is not our intent to discuss each of the above factors in depth, these topics do provide a starter list for you to consider in planning and purchasing informatics bibliographic software and/or hardware.

Resource 1: Project Planning Software

There are many software packages for flowcharting your project (e.g., MICRO-GRAFX's FlowCharter, among others). We suggest use of a PERT-type software package as the most efficient way to make an overall layout of your total project. For more details, see the following Web site: www.robertluttman.com/Week4/page5.htm.

Critical path method (CPM) is another variation of PERT that, though originally slightly different, is now almost identical to PERT. There are many variations on this classic technique. Such software permits planning all tasks and provides a means of tracking your project, identifying trends, and letting you know if you are off schedule or over budget. It includes means for fiscal and time accounting, possibly saving the expenditure for specialized financial accounting software. These PERT-analogous programs will also calculate a "critical path" for functions that, if not done on time, will hold up other functions down the line. This program provides an excellent means for planning and implementing a major project.

Resource 2: Digital Scanning Hardware and Software

In bibliographic management, one of the more difficult functions is that of inputting reference data. We have noted that direct electronic input of data is more accurate than manual typing, especially of long bibliographies or reference lists. However, scanners and voice recognition hardware and software are rapidly developing and will likely provide a more accurate and rapid means of inputting nondigital data and text, such as book reference lists.

One immediate solution might be use of a high-quality scanner, one that has at least 98% accuracy. A flatbed scanner with optical character recognition (OCR) software that can read 8-point print with a maximum optical density of 3.4D (your best measure of resolution with scanners) and claims $1,200 \times 2,400$ dots per inch (dpi) can be purchased for around $500 or less (December 2000). By this means, photocopied articles, documents, and reference lists can be accurately entered electronically. However, as with manual typing, scanning does produce errors, depending on the font size, print style, and type of paper, not to mention the quality of the scanner and OCR software. Consequently, careful copyediting will always be essential, even if scanning accuracy is claimed to be better than 99%.

Another possibility that is currently available is the use of bibliographic software that searches and imports directly from Internet sites. For example, END-NOTE allows the user to initiate a simple search directly from the desktop that searches and downloads directly into the bibliographic database the citations from PubMed.

Resource 3: Electronic Bibliographic Data Management Software

Because bibliographic data management is at the heart of your project, it is essential that you select appropriate computer hardware and software (including an adequate scanner) to complete these tasks accurately and efficiently.

The most important resource will be Internet hardware and software and electronic bibliographic data management software. For this purpose, you require a basic computer package, a modem, and an Internet service provider (ISP). For a major information synthesis, direct fiber-optic cable connection is essential to provide the bandwidth necessary for rapidly downloading software upgrades, bibliographic data, and complete documents. Using a telephone modem Internet connection is helpful but will quickly prove frustrating as you wait and wait to download the information you need. For managing electronic bibliographic information, once it is acquired, we have had the most experience using ProCite®, with its accompanying software package ProCite Bibliolinks®. However, many others can be considered and should be researched.

Unfortunately, for many years to come, it will be necessary to manage paper documents, especially books, complete journal articles, and printed reference lists. Because it is too costly to use hand-typed information input into the computer, especially long reference lists in very fine print, scanning technology becomes another necessity. Fortunately, this field has progressed far enough that, with prices dropping rapidly, scanning now seems practical.

Overall, bibliographic information management is quite complex and requires a number of specialized functions. The following box provides a brief listing of a few more essential tasks that you must be able to manage. We will provide much more detail later in Stage II to both explain principles and outline procedures and tasks for your guidance.

BIBLIOGRAPHIC MANAGEMENT FUNCTIONS

Task 1:   Finding Internet bibliographic data resources
Task 2:   Inputting hardcopy citation-abstracts and whole text
Task 3:   Creating bibliographic files in multiple styles
Task 4:   Creating file space for adding multiple codes and notes
Task 5:   Profiling "references in references"
Task 6:   Analyzing whole-text documents
Task 7:   Sorting on multiple parameters (e.g., authors, dates)
Task 8:   Feedback on missing data (e.g., relevance codes)
Task 9:   Retrieving bibliographic information
Task 10:   Downloading references to other programs

Although it is not our intent to discuss each of the above tasks in this chapter, the above list might give you a start for planning and purchasing informatics resources for bibliographic data management. Throughout this book, we also provide direct Uniform Resource Locator (URL) Internet addresses to guide you directly to the sources we judge to be relevant for information synthesis development and application.

Resource 4: Research Data Management Software

Most of the statistical computations you need for a synthesis can be programmed into a standard spreadsheet. There, you can type in data for automatic computation and analysis. More complicated data management software may be needed for large and/or complex quantitative synthesis projects. In managing empirical data from primary research studies that are compiled for quantitative syntheses, the numerical data will require different types of computations and statistical processing. Numerical data require different types of factors for consideration in an information synthesis. The following is a brief list of five major prerequisites of software required to manage empirical research data.

RESEARCH DATA SOFTWARE PREREQUISITES

1. Inputting digital and nondigital data
2. Data manager to store, clean, organize, sort, count, and provide easy input to statistical software
3. Statistical software to accomplish the analyses you require
4. Specialized meta-analysis hardware for synthesis purposes (e.g., adjusting for obvious biases)
5. Easy outputting to word processing and other software to produce research reports electronically on computer disks, Internet files, and traditional hardcopy

---

Depending on your subject area of interest, it is likely you will need to augment this list to meet your own particular needs. We have had the most success with Microsoft's ACCESS (www.microsoft.com/office/access/default.htm).

This program allows links across various data tables and construction of new data tables, if needed, on an ad hoc basis. Fields can be redefined at any time in the data entry process and new fields created. The order of fields can be easily modified either in the database itself or on entry forms. This flexibility allows for new changes in coding procedures if, for example, an additional category of patients has to be added because they were discovered in a few of the articles. In addition, ACCESS allows data of any format to be easily transferred into either text or spreadsheet files for further analyses in a statistical program, such as Statistical Package for the Social Sciences (SPSS), or meta-analysis programs, such as FAST*PRO. ACCESS also includes commands that compute simple scores such as means and standard deviations of the data, performs "if-then" statements to select data, and creates plots of selected variables.

On the negative side, ACCESS is a very complex program with a rather long learning curve to be able to use its advantages. If you do not have the inclination to acquire and invest the time in learning a new program, any spreadsheet will do the job, without all of the bells and whistles of a more powerful program.

Also important are the functional attributes of software you should keep in mind when purchasing packages for use with research data that involve **effect size**. Although there are many brands available, there are four requirements for information synthesis work:

Manual and Digital Input of Data. The database management system should allow for easy manual and/or electronic data entry. Spreadsheets, such as Excel, can be set up in matrices corresponding to distinct items and categories within items. Data can be typed in readily to these software programs. Database management software, such as ACCESS or Paradox, allows manual and digital input to multiple files that are linked formally and allow for embedded and hierarchical data.

Data Verification and "Cleaning." Database management systems also allow for the creation of on-screen forms composed of a group of separate "fields," with each field corresponding to a variable. The organization and placement of these fields on the screen can be created in such a way that makes data entry easier by allowing for default entries, incorporating short descriptions of items, and highlighting important items. Desirable but not necessary is the ability of the database management system to do internal quality checks, including checking data for expected number of digits, type of variable (alphanumeric or numeric), and expected quantitative value.

Data Analysis and Cross-Linkages. The system needs to provide an easy method for analyzing data from multiple points of view. That means that the software should allow for multiple linkages between data. For example, we may want to sort by year of publication and look at correlations within two groups of articles.

Electronic Input and Export of Data. The database management software should allow for easy electronic input and export of data to and from other applications. Information stored in a word-processing document or a spreadsheet should be easily transferred to this software. To facilitate meta-analytic work, the database management software should be able to import information from the bibliographic software. Important information that will be transferred includes date of publication, name and location of author(s), and the complete citation. Electronic transfer methods reduce errors. Similarly, article status information will need to be moved from the database management software to the bibliographic software containing the master file. This information includes items such as retrieval status, code names, and coding status.

Resource 5: Meta-Analysis Computational Software

Meta-analysis, as it has been implemented in the past, is not the answer to a scientist's prayer. Like many other tools, it has serious flaws. According to Bailar (1998), "Meta-analysis simply does *not* work very well in practice," (emphasis added). (John C. Bailar III, M.D., Ph.D., is a former statistical editor of the *New England Journal of Medicine* and currently is a professor at the University of Chicago.) Furthermore, Feinstein (1995), in an article titled "Meta-Analysis: Statistical Alchemy for the 21st Century," emphasized the negative aspects of meta-analysis. In developing information reviews of any type, especially quantitative syntheses, we cannot afford to dismiss the criticisms, however caustic, of these highly respected experts. Advanced computer software is one of the resources that will help us address such issues more efficiently and validly. The following are some of the better meta-analytic computational software programs.

ES®. Source: Assessment Systems Corporation, 2233 University Avenue, Suite 200, St. Paul, MN 55114. Web site address for product description (as of April 2000): www.assess.com/ES.html.

In our experience, ES is one of the most useful tools for conducting a meta-analysis. It calculates effect size estimates for more than 50 different kinds of circumstances. As the authors of this software note, researchers frequently make errors in estimating effect sizes when they extract data from complex research designs (e.g., multifactorial and multivariate designs or repeated-measures designs). William Shadish, the primary author of the software system, is one of the leading scholars in meta-analysis. This software system, with its alternative calculation possibilities, reflects its perceptive and robust design. We have found this system easy to use. You will find the user manual especially useful.

ES provides effect size estimates for a variety of "change scores" problems and for various 2×2 tables with dichotomous outcomes, including odds ratios. The program also provides estimates for analysis of covariance designs and for multivariate analysis of variance designs. The program can accommodate designs with unequal sample sizes as well as differences in within-cell variances for the treatment and control conditions. Furthermore, ES permits the user to convert effect size estimates between d (mean difference) and r (correlation) estimates. Because this program is not intended to provide a full meta-analysis (i.e., it does not include methods for combining effect sizes), you may want to obtain another program that actually combines the data. The program should be able to import data from other software sources and produce files of effect size estimates that can be exported to other statistics programs.

StatXact®. Source: Cytel Software Corporation, 675 Massachusetts Avenue, Cambridge, MA 02135. The Web address for product description (as of April 2000) is www.cytel.com/products/statxact/statxact1.html.

The Web address for product review is www.cytel.com/reviews/reviews.html.

The StatXact software system provides a test of the several types of odds ratio problems. The system performs both an exact (Zelen, 1971) and an asymptotic test (Breslow & Day, 1980) of homogeneity of odds ratios across K studies. It also performs both exact tests and an exact confidence interval (Mehta, Patel, & Gray, 1985), or an asymptotic test, and computes an asymptotic confidence interval for the common odds ratio across the K studies. The program can combine data for categorical, rather than dichotomous, outcomes. This system is closely related to the SPSS system, and transfer of data between SPSS and StatXact is rather easy.

Egret®. Source: Cytel Software Corporation, 675 Massachusetts Ave., Cambridge, MA 02135. The Web address for product description (as of April 2000) is www.cytel.com/products/egret/egret1.html.

This software package performs analyses on a binary outcome variable for multiple studies using either fixed or random effects models. In the fixed effects case, Egret treats the data in various strata, and the results are examined as stratified $2 \times k$ tables. The tests of homogeneity are licensed from the Cytel Software, so these results are the same as for StatXact. In the random effects logistic regression, an assumption is made that the effect of exposure variables is constant across studies, but each of the individual studies contains an unmeasureable random component that adds variability to estimates. Egret® estimates four different regression equations to model these various effects. Three of the models are appropriate for examining a single feature of a study. The fourth model is useful when the investigation provides a comparison between two conditions (as in comparing treatment and control conditions). The software system provides conditional and unconditional logistics, Cox proportional hazards, and Poisson, exponential, and Weibull regression models. The system also provides an analysis of 2 x k tables and Kaplan-Meier estimates. According to Hasselblad et al. (1995), this package is well known for its level of user-friendliness and for its excellent graphics (www.apcatalog.com/cgi-bin/AP?ISBN= 012230621X&LOCATION=US&FORM=FORM2).

This package provides software to perform a meta-analysis using the confidence profile method (CPM). The software provides a wide variety of modeling possibilities, including random and fixed effects analyses using many different effect size measures and assuming different types of underlying population distributions (Weibull, log normal, Poisson).

HLM 4. Source: Developed by Anthony Bryk, Stephen Raudenbush, and Richard Congdon; distributed by Scientific Software Inc., 7383 N. Lincoln Ave., Suite 100, Lincolnwood, IL 60712-1704. The Web address for product description (as of April 2000) is www.ssicentral.com/product.htm#la2.

This software package performs a hierarchical meta-analysis. The package is designed to perform **hierarchical linear models** and can be used to perform calculations in a wide variety of meta-analysis problems.

A recent release has an excellent graphics user interface (GUI) and "help" screens for developing meta-analytic models. The hierarchical linear model (HLM) program provides parameter estimates for Level 4. In this HLM approach, an analysis is performed at each level and is represented by its own submodel. Parameter estimation can be performed using empirical Bayes, generalized least squares, and maximum likelihood estimates. HLM also provides reliability estimates of parameter values, as well as enabling the simultaneous testing of multiple parameters. The software can model the effects of biases through the use of regression procedures. The system provides least squares and empirical Bayes' residuals for use in further analyses.

The program is also well suited for some types of nonnormally distributed data (Poisson or Bernoulli distributions). It accepts input data from various statistical packages, such as SAS, SPSS, BMDP, and SYSTAT.

Consider Traditional Software Programs. If you do not have access to any of the above software programs, you can achieve most of the analyses using relatively traditional software with spreadsheet and database programs such as Excel and ACCESS. You can also use any of a variety of statistical software programs such as SPSS, SAS, BMDP, or S-PLUS. Although these programs enable you to perform most meta-analyses, they are not specifically designed for a meta-analysis, so you have to create many of your own specific command files and diagnostic procedures. You will need to create effect sizes for each of the studies in your data set. If the research designs are at all complicated, then you may need to use special software to assist you in these calculations.

Resource 6: Fiscal and Time Management Resources

It is essential to document accounts of monetary expenditures, as well as each team member's weekly estimate of work time on your synthesis project. These accounts will be referred to frequently, especially during the Stage II information search. Immediate corrective action must be taken if these data indicate that you are consuming your fiscal or time budget too rapidly in this or any other stage of your project.

We have found PERT-analogous software programs to be the most efficient method for keeping fiscal and time data. For a description of PERT, see the Net site in Resource 1.

If you cannot obtain such planning software, there are many financial management programs on the market (e.g., Intuit's Quicken, which can provide ledgers for fiscal and time accounting). These programs facilitate complex budgeting formats that can warn you about potential cost overruns during any of your project stages. By recording your fiscal and time data into such software, it can automatically calculate personnel costs in both hours and dollars and can be readily transferred to other software for more complex analyses. However, if all else fails, there is always the quill pen and green eyeshade.

Procedure D. Recruit and Train Project Staff

The major tasks that are completed in Procedure D require astute decisions and considerable effort on the author's part. These tasks are specifying qualifications for recruits, recruiting the project team, and training the project team.

Task 1: Specify Qualifications for Recruits

Before your project is completed in Stage V, you will need two work groups for three overlapping procedures—namely, (a) Stage II database development, (b) Stage III validation of relevant database articles, and (c) Stage IV implementation and validation of the synthesis and its conclusions. At this point, we only discuss your search team because they should be recruited immediately and trained prior to Stage II, when you implement your project plan.

With the basic five-step search-iteration procedure in mind (in Task 1, Procedure F of this chapter), you should recruit a search team, which, in the aggregate, has at least the following qualifications. (Note that we stress noncognitive characteristics and skills as being of the highest importance. Responsibility and persistence, in a team member, for example, can make the difference between success and failure.)

Specify Noncognitive Skills. The most important traits that you will require in candidates (in the aggregate) for synthesis staff positions are noncognitive. For example, because a major task in screening most information sources involves contacting people, having good interpersonal relationships and communication skills is essential. Your team members will be talking to librarians, contacting experts on your topic, requesting technical help on informatics matters, and getting along with other colleagues who may be willing to participate. When the senior author was at the Johns

Hopkins School of Hygiene and Public Health, he learned that a surveyor with a good "telephone personality" had substantially higher response and completion rates on telephone surveys than those who did not have these skills.

This subtask also includes many other noncognitive skills that are essential. For example, a good sense of humor and enthusiasm can help the whole team deal with the inevitable frustrations and stress that will be involved. Being willing to admit mistakes that always happen is another valuable trait. Honesty, integrity, responsibility, and persistence go without saying. The most practical measure of these traits must be obtained from forthright colleagues who have known these individuals over a span of time.

Specify Health Science Information Search Skills. Experience in screening or searching health science information sources is an essential skill for your team members. Also required is skill in identifying and compiling lists of possibly relevant 'citation-abstracts' from various information sources, whether they be electronic, people, or paper. The team must have skill in analyzing and relevance-coding citation-abstracts and complete articles; this skill may determine both the quality and cost-effectiveness of your synthesis database. Remember that most of the information you will obtain will likely be from paper sources, so your team should have experience hand-searching journals, books, and reports. Recall that the qualifications you judge essential must apply to the team as a whole and not necessarily to each recruit.

These team recruits may be graduate students, trained research assistants, experienced medical librarians, or other trained information specialists. If budgetary restrictions prevent you from hiring certified health science information specialists, you might recruit trained research assistants or qualified local undergraduate or graduate students. Obviously, these individuals will require additional training and more supervision than professional "searchers." However, they might work for course credit or use your material for their own papers or dissertations in lieu of a salary.

Specify Computer Hardware and Software Skills. This is another important skill that the candidate must have and for which you may not be able to afford the time to train him or her if these skills are inadequate. Internet skills are particularly essential. To do reviews of modern science literature requires judgment proficiency in accessing computerized bibliographic databanks, databases, and individual citations obtained from sources such as PubMed. Team members must also be able to use bibliographic management software (e.g., ProCite for downloading "A" or "B" relevance-rated citation-abstracts and for maintaining your **master list** of project references). Furthermore, the team should be able to use research data management software for storing and retrieving needed data for analysis and for statistical computation programs. If a meta-analysis is to be your final product, you will require other sophisticated software (e.g., FAST*PRO). Team members with previous experience in large electronic information-retrieval projects probably will be familiar with these, as well as with less mainstream methods for information retrieval.

Specify Relevance-Coding Capability. Assessing the relevance of citations based on systematic coding criteria is a responsibility that requires a moderate level of topic familiarity (such as direct clinical experience and an understanding of the jargon in that topic area). Listed citations must be rated (relevance-coded) to establish priorities for retrieval of complete articles. Thus, establishing whether the candidate has these skills or is able to quickly catch on to the idea is important to determine to avoid considerable future rework.

Specify Document Retrieval Experience. Candidates need experience in using bibliographic management software when later downloading "A+" through "B" relevance citations into your electronic master list. Retrieval personnel will generally photocopy articles or book chapters, check out needed books from the library, perhaps make book purchases, and submit interlibrary loan requests. Because documents and books accumulate rapidly, these personnel must have appropriate organization skills for retrieving and filing these materials. However, these people do not require the discriminating coding skills that are so critical for members of the team who do **relevance coding**.

Overall, Task 1 is primarily aimed at determining the qualifications of the candidates. They will have formal training and tutoring as the project progresses. However, if their judgment skills prove lacking, after several training attempts, they should be considered for clerical or other routine tasks if you recruit them at all.

Task 2: Recruit Project Team

Although Stage II is likely to be the most labor-intensive part of your project, the number of staff required depends on the complexity of your topic and the richness of the literature to be screened. With many simple projects, the authors can do the library work and information processing themselves. However, we recommend one or two research assistants to help make more efficient use of the author's time and to participate with the author in interactive processing of concepts to help produce a higher quality product. With larger, more complex validated reviews that have adequate grant support, clerical staff should also be hired to manage word processing of the multiple copyedited drafts, to organize and manage electronic and paper bibliographic files, and to keep the fiscal and time ledgers up to date.

Develop Candidate Pool. To develop your pool of candidates, local university graduate schools are a good place to start. Be sure to develop a list that includes both students now in training and those who have recently graduated. The latter group will likely still be struggling to find jobs and might have both the time and the interest to work with your team. Because such individuals vary widely in terms of temperament, personality, and professional judgment, it goes without saying that talking to people who have had longitudinal experience with the candidate is likely one of the best ways to develop your short list. Requisite skills (such as with computers) can always be checked in person before or after your interview with the candidates.

Screen Candidate Pool. You probably have had experience screening candidates for a job. The subtle cues of their interpersonal communication skills under stress must be noted and correctly interpreted. As you well know, your gut feeling is likely your best indicator as to whether or not this person will fit in with your other staff members. However, there are several judgment skills that you may want to check during the screening process.

For example, to make a quick check of a candidate's relevance-coding ability, a series of citations or complete articles can be given him or her to code. Naturally, a brief orientation to the task is required. If individuals are not familiar with your topic field, perhaps two or three rounds of having them code the materials in private, then obtaining feedback from you (or other staff), and then trying again will provide some evidence as to their judgment and learning ability.

As another example, you might test candidates for skills in using the library. They could be assigned to retrieve citations you already know are at an A+, A, A–, B, or C relevance level. Again, it might require two or three rounds of this task before you feel comfortable as to whether or not they qualify.

Make Your Final Selection. With the above information acquired from each candidate, the final decision will be a judgment call by the senior author. It may help to have a brief nominal group consensus meeting with staff and any available consults to identify and weight the strengths and weaknesses of each candidate. For a small project, such formality is likely "gilding the lily."

Task 3: Train Project Team

Training may be constrained by a small budget and a short time frame. However, all teams must have topic familiarity because each subject is usually associated with a unique context, jargon, and relevance cues. Even professional information scientists must train briefly for each new search to become familiar with its language, design, and specific conventions to be applied. Finally, it is important that the team fully understand the author's synthesis purpose, goals, audience, and ultimate product use.

If funds are difficult to obtain, the author(s) is often forced to recruit a team with rudimentary search skills. These teams may require substantial training, practice skills exercises, and frequent feedback from the author(s) and other team members. Training exercises should be tailored to the group so they are able to accomplish the following training goals:

SEARCH TEAM TRAINING GOALS

Goal 1:   Become familiar with synthesis topic, model, and plan
Goal 2:   Learn search procedures, especially search iterations
Goal 3:   Understand the ABC convention for relevance coding
Goal 4:   Develop skills to identify, retrieve, and relevance-code literature
Goal 5:   Develop skills in leading team coding calibration sessions
Goal 6:   Develop skills in search documentation and filing
Goal 7:   Develop skills for managing electronic and paper files
Goal 8:   As a team, understand and be able to use informatics tools, especially
          the Internet, as required for your synthesis

See Appendix 3.1 at the end of this chapter for suggested learning experiences you might use to help your team achieve these eight training goals.

Procedure E.   Organize Project Files

Task 1: Prepare Search Documentation Tools

Electronic and paper search documentation tools used to plan, prepare, and conduct a systematic literature review (i.e., synthesis) are listed below. Computer software for such purposes will be discussed later. We suggest that all paper forms in this book can be readily converted to electronic form, given the appropriate hardware and software. Although these tools may seem rather compulsive in nature, they will provide your map and compass to avoid being drowned in a sea of paper and bytes.

Forms for Evolving Project Plan.   Blank forms (Forms 3.1, 3.2, and 3.3) at the end of this chapter are for developing the initial and all subsequent revisions of the search plan. Form 3.1 (synthesis planning framework) will likely remain stable unless your topic substantially changes. It outlines your synthesis focus in terms of purpose, goals, and target audience.

Form 3.2 (search planning and update guide) outlines your search scope and strategy, including language, time frame, extent of your retrieval effort, revised priorities for screening selected search sources, new information modalities, and subsequent search facilitation information. The information on this form will likely change with each iteration of the search as new leads are found. Figure 3.2 illustrates Form 3.2 completed for the fifth iteration of a search.

Form 3.4 outlines specific new bibliographic databanks to screen, experts to contact, bibliographies and key articles to screen, and new descriptors or relevance criteria to apply (new relevance criteria would be listed only in the first three to five iterations at most). Figure 3.4 shows this same form as it would be when completed.

The content of these three forms is reviewed and changed, if warranted, in Step 5 of every iteration, which provides the leads for Step 1 of the subsequent search iteration.

These plans (completed forms) accumulate from each search iteration and are stored chronologically in a special electronic or paper plan file.

Electronic Citation Printouts and Photocopied Reference Lists. These lists of citations are from sources such as the library, where scanning technology is not available. These hardcopy documents provide another valuable tool to guide your literature review in each search iteration. They are, in a sense, forms to be completed by recording handwritten relevance codes on all listed citations compiled by your search team.

Relevance Cue Logs. These electronic logs are used to list all cues (e.g., investigators, key words, journals, or other bibliographic sources) you identify during your search activity. For an overall framework, we will use ABC relevance-coding convention, as listed in Table 3.1.

See Appendix 3.2 for a discussion of our rationale for the ABC convention. We suggest that you use electronic word-processing software for recording cues, having a separate field for each of the five relevance levels: A+, A, A–, B, and C. Each field then has space denoted for inclusions and for exclusions. Form 3.5 shows the format for developing blank cue sheets for each relevance level. Figure 3.5 illustrates the same form when filled in—in this case, only for the A+ level.

Form 3.5, at the end of this chapter, can be used as a model for your electronic relevance cue logs for the remaining levels A, A–, B, and C. These logs are for recording **key words**, descriptors, subject jargon, phrases related to your topic, key authors, publishers, journals or books, and especially "fugitive literature" sources. You can use the information on the relevance cue logs to derive your formal relevance criteria list, as well as to guide you in screening various sources of information that have been

SEARCH LEADS FOR NEXT ITERATION (Illustration)

Iteration #: _____

Date: _____

Initials: _____

Topic: _____

Electronic bibliographic database(s) to screen: _____

_____

_____

Key expert(s) to contact: _____

_____

Best available bibliography: _____

_____

_____

_____

Best "A+" review or "A" article: _____

_____

_____

_____

_____

Descriptors/key words: _____

_____

_____

_____

Notes:

_____

Figure 3.4. Illustrative Form 3.4: Leads for the Next Search Iteration

TABLE 3.1 ABC Convention for Relevance Coding

A+   **Criterion:** Review article is on your exact or similar topic.

   Action implications for: *Citation*—include in master list and retrieve document; *Document*—Relevance-code article (including references), retrieving those of A+, A, and A–, and, if data prove valid, include in your synthesis.

A   **Criterion:** Reference is to a single research study on your topic.

   Action implications for: *Citation*—include in master list; *Document*—retrieve complete document and relevance-code (including references) and, if data prove valid, include in your synthesis.

A–   **Criterion:** Reference is to content not likely appropriate but may provide leads to other important citations or information sources.

   Action implications for: *Citation*—include in master list; *Document*—retrieve complete document, relevance-code, and screen for leads to other important information. Document validation is not warranted because the data are likely peripheral to your topic.

B   **Criterion:** Reference is to questionable content not likely needed.

   Action implications for: *Citation*—include in master list; *Document*—do not retrieve unless time and money allow or if more relevant sources are not found.

C   **Criterion:** Reference is to content clearly not appropriate.

   Action implications for: *Citation*—do not include in master list; *Document*—do not retrieve.

identified. These logs will grow and evolve as the search continues, accumulating important new cues and deleting nonproductive ones. As each list is completed during an iteration, these logs, or forms, will be stored in a special computer file developed for this purpose.

   These relevance criteria logs are usually not included in your final synthesis product; however, they should be available for colleagues on request.

Relevance Criteria List. This electronic criteria list distills the most productive terms (e.g., formal index descriptors, authors' key words, and other valuable cues) culled from your relevance cue logs. For example, the first MeSH descriptors can be filled

RELEVANCE CUE LOG—A+ CUES

Date: ___20 Aug 99___

Initials: ___BR___

Page ___1___ of _3_

Topic: Validated quality-of-life measurement instruments

Instructions: Specify any cues to be included or excluded in terms of descriptors, key words, topics, jargon, phrases, sources, investigators, journals, organizations, or other leads to an A+ review on above topic.

Inclusions:

1. Ware, J. E.; Bjorner, J. B.; or La Puma, J.

2. Berzon, R. A., et al. (1993). Quality of Life Bibliography and Indexes: 1993 Update. *Quality of Life Research* 4:53-74

3. Serials: "Medical Outcomes Trust," "Report on Medical Guidelines and Outcomes Research," "Medical Care" 4. MeSH Descriptors: "Review," "Quality of Life," or "Health Status"; Key words: "Quality-of-Life Years"; SF.36 Health Status Measurement Instrument

etc.

Exclusions (other than A, A–, B, and C log category inclusions ratings):

1. Future directions for measuring quality of life

2. Statistical models for validating quality-of-life instruments

etc.

Figure 3.5. Illustrative Completed Form 3.5: A+ Relevance Cue Log

in on Form 3.4 (iteration search leads) and again on all subsequent updates of synthesis plans in Step 5 of each iteration. New descriptors are accumulated on this form until they prove productive or nonproductive of needed studies. The same is true with other key words and specific inclusion and exclusion terms that are recorded on Form 3.5 (relevance cue logs) until their value is determined. (Note that references shown on this form are in the reference list of this book, namely, Berzon, Simeon, Simpson, Donnelly, & Tilson, 1993; Berzon, Simeon, Simpson, & Tilson, 1992; Bjorner & Ware, 1998; La Puma & Lawlor, 1990; Ware, 1998; also see Racezk et al., 1998; Ware, Keller, Hatoum, & Kong, 1999.) Those cues that prove productive will be formalized into relevance criteria. These relevance criteria lists (electronic or paper) are important documentation forms to be given to each member of the search team when he or she carries out individual search assignments. Such criteria must be stabilized in the early iterations and remain fixed for the rest of the database development.

Software for Calibration and Data Storage. These documentation tools are important for recording all calibration data, including that from individual raters and the consensus ratings for the team as a whole. Much, if not most, of these data will be Kappas, together with the original individual worksheets and team collation forms. Individual data will usually be in paper form and later recorded into an electronic spreadsheet (e.g., Excel or ACCESS) that performs the required computations (see Table 10.1 for these calculations). This software also facilitates development of data files to be fed into the validation and synthesis operations.

Formatted Electronic Master List of Citation-Abstracts With Codes. A complete electronic list of all A and B relevance citation-abstracts will be your most valuable tool for managing your database. We suggest use of electronic bibliographic management software (e.g., ProCite® and Bibliolink®, mentioned in Task 3, Procedure C of this chapter). Such software will improve the cost-effectiveness of both your search filing and retrieval effort for citation-abstracts, as well as the collateral coding required. These databases allow for electronic downloading of entire citation lists, with or without abstracts, or for manual input of individual citation-abstracts from nonelectronic sources. In addition, many bibliographic software packages allow for custom fields where you can record special documentation codes. For example, these codes can indicate progress in the retrieval status of complete documents for each A+, A, or A– citation, specifying whether the document was obtained, is still in process, or is unavailable. You can also record a citation count for any complete document reference list, together with a profile of its relevance codes (i.e., the number of A+, A, A–, B, and C references), as shown in Table 3.2.

TABLE 3.2 An Illustration of a Relevance Profile (Skewed to the Left)

A+	A	A–	B	C
14%	40%	27%	10%	9%

NOTE: n = 100 citations. Shows the proportion of citations at each relevance level in the total citation count.

This profile can be valuable in confirming or casting doubt on the relevance of the articles whose references were thus coded.

Later, validity codes will be added to each reference file in the 'master list' to indicate the scientific soundness of complete documents. During this preparation, your main task is to obtain the bibliographic software, become adept at using it, and prepare your citation file formats for all material you wish to include.

Electronic Fiscal and Time-Accounting Records. Form 3.3 provides a low-cost example of a do-it-yourself fiscal and time-accounting form you can develop on a spreadsheet. However, there are many financial management software packages you can purchase (e.g., Intuit's Quicken or Microsoft Money) that can provide automated ledgers for fiscal and time accounting. We suggest any of the many variations on the classic PERT model. These programs make it simple to record fiscal and time data for each of the many layers of your project's operation and provide powerful tools for managing your synthesis.

Search Statistics Compilation Forms. The specific counts compiled from your search documentation forms will be important for the final Stage II evaluation—that is, the number of citations screened, the profile of how many were relevance rated (A+ to C), and how many of the high-relevance citations were followed to retrieve their complete documents. Other statistical counts include trend analyses of **interrater reliability** and precision rates, along with citation-abstract false-negative and false-positive rates, as calculated in calibration sessions for each search iteration (see Petersen & White, 1989, for examples of these search statistics).

You may choose to record other statistics in each citation file of the master list. For example, you can keep a profile of the type of documents found (books, monographs, journal articles, technical reports, unpublished studies, electronic data, and other information modalities).

Task 2: Organize Database Storage Files

IMPORTANT NOTE

In nearly every information search, despite modern informatics tools and resources, you will find yourself drowning in paper. This material will consist of documents such as computer citation-abstract printouts and retrieved and photo-copied documents (original hardcopy books, photocopied journal articles, book chapters and technical reports, and reference lists photocopied prior to scanning).

Consequently, you must be prepared for the fact that for the next decade, most of the information you seek will be in hardcopy, on the shelves of libraries, and in the file drawers of numerous colleagues. One of the better resources to help you cope with this reality is the *Cochrane Hand Search Manual,* which outlines strategies, procedures, and quality control methods. Although they focus on RCTs the principles described have much wider application. Part I of this resource is available at the following Web address (last updated April 1999): hiru.mcmaster.ca/cochrane/cochrane/hsmpt1.htm.

Consequently, before starting your initial search, you must develop an organized set of storage files for these different types of electronic and paper products accumulated during this database development procedure.

The first and most important group of documents to store are the complete journal articles or technical reports (usually photocopied at the library) you retrieve because their citation-abstract was given an A+, A, or A– relevance rating. Many journals are now available in digital form, so their reference lists can be downloaded into special files for this purpose. However, unless obtained through a medical library, these online journals can be very expensive and, as yet, will provide rather limited coverage of the material you require. For many years to come, a trip to the library will be essential. Many modern medical libraries even have scanning capability. You insert a 3.5-inch floppy disk into the copier and then copy an original paper document as usual, which will result in a hardcopy and also a digitized copy downloaded to your disk. If you do not have your own scanner, this new capability may be a lifesaver.

A second set of documents to store are citation-abstract digital files or printouts, from electronic bibliographic databases, or digital listings downloaded from the

Internet or other such sources. This information, with your recorded relevance codes, will be needed for your search documentation and evaluation analyses.

The third group of paper documents to file could include your coded hardcopy citation printouts, any photocopied bibliographic reference lists, paper relevance cue logs (see Form 3.5 to illustrate an A+ cue log), completed hardcopy spreadsheets, and possibly fiscal and time-accounting ledgers if scanners and electronic software are not used. However, the more of these materials you can obtain in digital form, the more accurate your counts will be.

As you can see, there are many clerical tasks required for any information synthesis. These tasks include location of the primary studies at the library, writing up requests for interlibrary loans, photocopying articles, scanning reference lists or photocopied documents, entering citations into bibliographic management software, filing, data entry, and other such tasks. Because most of these tasks require minimal training, though moderate intelligence, these staff can be undergraduate students who have an interest in working on a research project. The advantage of using undergraduates is that they can often work for course credit instead of wages, thus freeing up money in the budget for other costs. At the same time, the learning rewards for them will likely be useful throughout their careers. Once you have identified the staff you need to complete your synthesis project, they, like the authors, can be listed on the Synthesis Planning Form 3.3 together with their salary codes for automatic budget calculations.

Procedure F: Finalize Preparations

Task 1: Operationalize Search-Iteration Procedure

The basic search strategy we suggest throughout Stage II (the next stage) is multiple applications of a five-step search iteration. There will be multiple iterations required to build your database of relevant studies. Initially, you will complete three to four iterations to begin Stage II. These initial rounds end when your relevance criteria have stabilized. The second group of iterations will consist of 10 to 12 or more iterations, ending when the synthesis database is complete, which marks the termination of Stage II. The final iterations will conclude your compilation of studies when you decide it is reasonable to terminate your search.

The fundamental concept of an iteration is important for you to understand. Below we list the five basic steps that make up a single iteration. Following these steps will help maintain the consistency of your search. It will help you recognize exactly where you are in the search, including which references have been processed and which have not. If you must discontinue your synthesis for a time, completing an iteration before you stop will facilitate your becoming quickly oriented to where you previously stopped. Finally, completion of each iteration provides a resting point while you analyze the following: the results of the previous five steps in terms of number of citation-abstracts screened and complete articles retrieved, interrater reliability and precision rates and trends, and the decision of whether to continue the same search scope and direction or make alterations before starting the next iteration. Note that "A" indicates A+, A, or A–, individually or in combination.

Step 1: Compile and Relevance-Code New Citation-Abstracts; If Rated "A," Retrieve and Code Complete Documents. In Stage II, your initial iteration uses the search plan from Stage I to search, retrieve, and relevance-code citation-abstracts that were obtained.

Note that in Step 1 of subsequent iterations, you will implement the revised plan from Step 5 of the preceding iteration. When implementing your initial one or two iterations, we suggest you restrict your search to readily available local sources. Furthermore, we suggest that you restrict the yield of these early rounds to no more than 25 citations to simplify your learning task. You will, rather quickly, compile a small, manageable bibliographic database for screening.

Step 2: Relevance-Code References in Complete Documents Obtained; If Rated "A," Retrieve and Code Documents Cited. You can establish priorities for retrieving other complete documents cited in these "references in references." These relevance ratings of references will be more accurate and have greater precision than those from electronic database printouts (or downloads) because in document references, you can check the context of the citation (similar to but much better than "key word in context" indexes). Next, relevance-code each new document you retrieve. In relevance-coding new reference lists during these early iterations of your search, it is again helpful to augment your team with one or two consultants who are expert in the content of your topic. Their ratings will be aggregated with those of the team later in the calibration session. Discussion of the resulting coding differences may be an enlightening experience for all.

Step 3: Conduct Team Calibration Session, Calculate Interrater Reliability and Precision Rates, Analyze and Improve Poor Results. In the initial iterations, it is especially important to calculate interrater reliability and citation-abstract precision rates. For calculating interrater reliability, we usually use a **Cohen's Kappa statistic**, which is a measure of team coder agreement that controls for chance (Table 10.1 in Chapter 10). At this point, we also suggest you calculate your citation-abstract precision rates, as explained in Appendix 3.1, Goal 5. For a more detailed discussion of relevance-coding precision and recall rates, see Chapter 5.

Also, in these initial iterations, your team must establish a lowest acceptable threshold for analyzing the results of these calculations. In our judgment, a Kappa lower than 0.70, or a precision rate below 60%, is usually not acceptable. However, your team must establish these threshold values to use for the remainder of your synthesis. In other syntheses on new topics, these threshold values may vary according to the circumstances.

During the coding process, the raters should discuss the source of all disagreements. For example, one or two team members may have seriously misunderstood the wording of one or more relevance criteria. Fortunately, such problems are often easily corrected unless there is a fundamental conceptual issue that needs to be resolved for everyone. In the early iterations of your search, this step will greatly improve the clarity of your relevance codes and the cost-effectiveness of your search as a whole. Such discussions might also result in adding new cues to the relevance cue logs and possibly new relevance criteria, which you can add to your formal list if your criteria list has not stabilized.

Once your list of relevance criteria has stabilized, all subsequent iterations will apply these same criteria. It is always possible that you may later identify new, highly significant relevance criteria. In such cases, you must decide whether adding these criteria, which will require recoding all previous citation-abstracts and complete documents, is worth the high expense required for such rework. The closer you are to finalizing your search database, the less likely such a task will be worth the dollar and time expenditures required.

Step 4: Update Search Documentation Forms, Calculate Search Statistics for This Iteration, and File All Materials. This step is important in all iterations because subsequent assessments, including that by the publisher, will depend on having detailed documentation of your search procedures. To complete this task, you must first update all of your search documentation forms. These include electronic bibliographic printouts (or downloads), photocopied reference lists from complete documents retrieved, relevance cue logs, the formal 'relevance criteria list,' completed calibration forms, your electronic master list, and the fiscal and time ledgers.

Calculate your search statistics in each iteration and include items shown as follows:

CALCULATE SEARCH STATISTICS FOR EACH ITERATION

(a) Citation-abstracts coded divided by total to be screened
(b) Documents retrieved divided by the total (A+, A, A–) citation-abstracts coded
(c) "References in references" coded divided by the total to be coded
(d) Relevance profiles of citation-abstracts and documents
(e) Team calibration results (interrater reliability and precision rates)

Note that these individual iteration statistics will be compared across several iterations for purposes of trend analysis. At the end of Stage II, they will be aggregated for a final overall evaluation. If you are doing a rapid synthesis with a tight deadline and a limited budget, these statistics could be optional if you understand the risk this may mean for the soundness of your final conclusions. However, if the results of your work might influence life-or-death decisions, being obsessive is essential and will improve the validity and likely cost-effectiveness of your product.

In another example, "profiling" bibliographic reference lists has many benefits that would be lost if search statistics were not compiled and analyzed (see Table 3.2). If a profiling analysis reveals an increasing proportion of B or C citations, the direction of your search may be drifting and might require considerable reworking to get back on track. On the other hand, if the profile indicates a high proportion of relevant citation-abstracts or documents, you are on track and should continue as you are doing. Finally, you should file these documentation forms and search statistics in their appropriate electronic or paper storage areas.

With this updated documentation at hand, you can move on to the final task of the iteration.

Step 5: Revise the Search Plan and Prepare for the Next Iteration.   The last task of each iteration is to revise your search plan based on the results of the previous iterations. This revised plan will be implemented as Step 1 of your next iteration. By far, your most important task in the initial rounds is to revise your formal search criteria. Remember that these criteria must remain stable throughout the remainder of your database development. For all subsequent iterations, you will, however, continually revise your search strategy and scope as needed.

At this point, you should prepare your new list of citation-abstracts that were given an A+, A, or A– code, in preparation for your next search iteration. If your interrater reliability statistics, or precision rates, are trending down or are close to your threshold, it might be necessary to have a relevance criteria review session in preparation for the next iteration.

If your initial screening of an electronic database produces a paucity of studies with no reviews on your topic, it might be necessary to seek help from a medical librarian to analyze your search descriptors and search logic. This same person can provide help in revising your search plan. If, with this help, you still find very little research on your topic in subsequent iterations, you will need to broaden the scope of your information sources to be screened or, worst-case scenario, select a different topic and start again.

If your initial electronic search yields a rich harvest (i.e., several hundred citations, including many reviews and bibliographies), you might consider narrowing the scope of your synthesis. This is especially important if you are working under tight budget and time constraints. Having mastered an understanding of the search-iteration strategy, together with your practice skills training, you should be ready to finalize preparation for implementing your actual project.

Task 2: Revise Project Plan and the Work Assignments as Needed

In completing the tasks of planning and preparation for implementing the synthesis project, you will have a project plan based on the author's best judgment. Recall that this information was recorded on Form 3.1 with the title, purpose, targeted readers, benefits, and product. On Form 3.2, you fill in greater detail regarding starting your search in Stage II and for changes in each iteration thereafter as needed. On Form 3.3, the budget and timetable Gantt chart are recorded. On Form 3.4, for each iteration, authors record their judgment of the project search leads in terms of electronic bibliographic databanks, experts to contact, best bibliographies and articles, and descriptors or key words. Finally, on Form 3.5, you record relevance cues for each of the five levels of relevance. Figure 3.5 illustrates such a form for only A+ cues. Of importance is your revised synthesis research model (the original one was developed in Chapter 2) illustrating your updated variables, including mediators and moderators, and a diagram indicating anticipated causal relations between the dependent and independent variables.

These elements require a brief review by the project manager in preparation for assigning Stage II work tasks, products, and due dates.

Task 3: Provide Leads to the Search Team for Initiating Search

The authors should have a fair idea of where the search team might get started as they begin to build the database and develop their search skills. The material from the synthesis topic formulation process should provide a rich source for this purpose. If a mini-synthesis was compiled, as suggested for the final topic, you will have a list of colleagues to contact, electronic and paper reviews to screen, and possibly relevant bibliographies or reference lists to provide needed leads. Form 3.4 provides a worksheet to facilitate listing these and other helpful ideas for your search.

For example, the author might suggest searching an electronic bibliographic database. Because PubMed on the Internet provides free access to MEDLINE, and Internet Grateful Med provides free access to 14 other National Library of Medicine (NLM) bibliographic databases, including MEDLINE, this is a logical place to start. More detailed suggestions on how to use these databases are explained in Chapter 5, Section D.

The author should be able to suggest one or two key experts in the field of the synthesis project. The members of the search team need to develop experience in contacting these individuals and eliciting needed leads (e.g., bibliographies, key articles, or other experts to contact). Search staff might also ask the expert if he or she would consider being a reviewer of your work later when an early draft of the synthesis is completed.

If the author knows a good bibliography on the chosen topic, the team can get off to a quicker start. Better yet, a systematic review on your topic is the most helpful because it not only provides bibliographic material but serves as a model for learning about the organizational structure of an information synthesis. If these are not available, a single article on your subject is important to show your team exactly what it should be looking for. Finally, provide several relevant MeSH descriptors or other key words for starting a MEDLINE search.

Products of the Procedures in Chapter 3

Personnel. You need a qualified, trained, and initially calibrated project team; the names, telephone numbers, and e-mail addresses of quantitative and qualitative research experts for future consultation; and access to medical informatics specialists, medical librarians, and other health science information professionals.

Medical Informatics Resources. You will have purchased the needed hardware and software to conduct a synthesis. Assuming you have requisite computers with sufficient RAM and hard-drive memory, the only hardware left to be purchased will be a quality digital scanner. The scanner will save literally weeks of typing and ensure comparable accuracy when inputting such information as references from books, articles, and bibliographies. You will have investigated the computer software you need for each of the six basic functions in which informatics resources are most required.

Search Resources. The search resources you will have developed will include (a) a Stage I search plan, specifying a strategy and scope to initiate your search; (b) forms for developing your relevance cue logs; (c) a form for recording your relevance criteria list; (d) calibration data forms and spreadsheet statistical programs for calculating interrater reliability and search precision rates, together with the threshold values for analyzing results; and (e) an electronic master list for downloading, storing, and retrieving relevance-coded citation-abstracts. We also suggest that profiles of relevance-coded "references in references" found in each retrieved document be recorded in the corresponding citation-abstract file of the master list.

Storage Files. You will need (a) an organized set of computer disks or external hard drives for master list and other electronic data storage; (b) files for storing hardcopy database materials, such as coded citation printouts and coded photocopied reference lists; (c) shelves for storing books, monographs, and technical reports; (d) files to store search statistics and any preliminary analyses completed using such data (e.g., trend graphs for team search precision ratings); and (e) files for storing the successively revised search plans completed in Step 5 of each search iteration.

Summary

In Procedure A, we provide rather detailed structured group judgment methods to formulate a topic/question to be the focus of your synthesis. The basic question is written as an "improvement hypothesis" to be tested by the synthesis project and its subsequent application in the community. To hedge against getting off on the wrong track, we suggest that a mini-synthesis be accomplished for each of the top two to three selections for your final topic. Only by focusing on meta-validated information (e.g., completed systematic reviews) can you finish such a project in less than a week. Based on all information, the priority team selects a final topic to be the subject matter or question for your overall information synthesis project.

In Procedure B, we provide ideas and suggestions for developing your synthesis plan, which, it is hoped, will be the focus for the next four stages of your synthesis project. Starting with Form 3.1, you provide an explicit statement of such factors as your synthesis purpose and goals. Then you complete Form 3.2 to "flesh out" other important details of your plan. On Form 3.3, you indicate your budget and timetable. Next, on Form 3.4, you record relevant search descriptors, key words, and other terms to facilitate implementation of your Stage II search. On Form 3.5, you list cues that might provide leads to A+ information, for example, a systematic review on, or close to, your topic. You also prepare similar cue sheets for each of the remaining A, A–, B, and C levels of information. Next, develop a causal model depicting your dependent and independent variables, together with highly relevant mediators and moderators that might affect your final synthesis conclusion. Finally, we discuss four overall assessment criteria to be used to evaluate the progress of your synthesis project at the end of each stage.

In Procedure C, we suggest that certain informatics resources are essential for conducting a cost-effective synthesis that will meet suggested quality criteria. There are six major functions of a systematic review for which informatics tools (computer hardware and software) are required. These include project planning software, Internet capability, bibliographic management software, and scanning hardware and software. If your goal is a meta-analysis, you will require computational software to manage effect sizes from the individual studies in your database.

In Procedure D, we provide suggestions for recruiting and training project staff. We discuss qualifications for the staff members to facilitate building your project team. The specific functions this team must accomplish are outlined. An eight-goal training plan is suggested, with details shown in Appendix 3.1.

In Procedure E, we provide suggestions for developing some simple tools to facilitate your search documentation. We also describe database storage files you should prepare before starting your search. We emphasize that, currently, most of the substantive information you require will be in paper form such as bound journals and books. To better cope with this reality, we recommend that you become familiar with the *Cochrane Hand Search Manual,* especially if you are seeking randomized controlled trials.

In Procedure F, we discuss three important tasks required to help finalize your project preparations. The first task is to operationalize the five-step iteration process applicable to any literature search. The second task is to manage the evolution of your topic and plan as your search progresses. The third task is to acquire leads from the information you compiled in generating and evaluating your final topic, which will be the subject focus of your information synthesis.

At first you might feel overwhelmed by the work that needs to be done in planning an information synthesis. Actually, most of these tasks are relatively simple and will provide an efficient, systematic process that soon becomes routine. Whether it be a mini-synthesis requiring only a week or two of work or a full synthesis requiring many months of effort, we urge you to use a systematic approach based on an explicit protocol.

At this point, you should be ready to do a brief evaluation (Chapter 4) of the quality and cost-effectiveness of your Stage I planning and preparation effort. If this assessment shows acceptable results, you are ready to implement your project plan.

APPENDIX 3.1
Suggested Search Team Training Exercises

Before initiating your data-retrieval effort, an essential goal is to train the search team you have recruited. The training goals listed below are followed by suggestions you might consider for customizing these learning exercises to meet the needs of your team.

TRAINING GOALS FOR PROJECT SEARCH TEAM

Goal 1:   Become familiar with synthesis topic, model, and plan
Goal 2:   Learn search procedures, especially search iterations
Goal 3:   Understand the ABC convention for relevance coding
Goal 4:   Develop skills to identify, retrieve, and relevance-code literature
Goal 5:   Develop skills in leading team coding calibration and consensus sessions
Goal 6:   Develop skills in search documentation and filing
Goal 7:   Develop skills for managing electronic and paper files
Goal 8:   As a team, understand and be able to use informatics tools, especially the Internet, as required for your synthesis

Goal 1: Become Familiar With Synthesis Topic, Model, and Plan

Training begins with search preparation. To achieve this goal, you must help your team to understand the basic elements of a search plan (see Forms 3.1, 3.2, 3.3, and 3.4). Team members should study a copy of your initial plan before participating in their first training workshop. Senior staff should explain the rationale and assumptions for selecting this search topic, the synthesis goals and methods, and especially initial relevance criteria and search parameters. They should identify the intended readers and their likely need for this review, describe the intended final product (e.g., a journal article or technical report), and describe the likely impact this work will have on improving healthcare outcomes. Each team member, in turn, attempts to explain to another member his or her own concept and interpretation of these items. During this exercise, agreements and misunderstandings among team members can be identified and corrected before implementing the initial search in Stage II.

Goal 2: Learn Search Procedures, Especially Search Iterations

Five Stages of an Information Synthesis. The team must develop an understanding of the procedural framework for an information synthesis. Members should learn that each synthesis plan, overall, involves five independent but overlapping stages.

FIVE STAGES OF AN INFORMATION SYNTHESIS

Stage I: Planning and preparation
Stage II: Database development
Stage III: Database validation
Stage IV: Data analysis and synthesis
Stage V: Complete and evaluate synthesis report

A training exercise to help your team understand this might consist of a meeting where each member writes down his or her understanding of each of these stages. After they complete this task, each reads the explanation of the procedures to the instructor and other team members. The instructor might then ask the group to critique that explanation and fill in anything that was left out or correct any concept that seems to be incorrect.

Learning the Five Steps of a Search Iteration. Next, the team should understand our model for literature searches, which encompass multiple iterations of a standard five-step process. These iterations start and end in Stage II, when your database is all but completed. After that time, only a few serendipitous references might be added if they are sufficiently important. Later we explain ideas for streamlining these steps, as the team becomes more skilled and able to maintain consensus from iteration to iteration.

FIVE STEPS OF A SEARCH ITERATION
(Core Functions of Every Search Cycle)

1. Compile and relevance-code new citation-abstracts; if rated A+, A, or A–, retrieve and code complete documents.
2. Relevance-code references in complete documents obtained; if rated A+, A, or A–, retrieve and code documents cited.
3. Conduct a team calibration session, calculate interrater reliability and precision rates, and analyze and improve poor results.
4. Update search documentation forms, calculate search statistics for this iteration, and file all materials.
5. Revise search plan and prepare for the next iteration.

A training exercise similar to the previous one in Goal 2 might be conducted to achieve an understanding of the **five steps of a search iteration**.

Goal 3: Understand the ABC Convention for Relevance Coding

This goal can be met using practice skills exercises as in Goals 1 and 2 and using a copy of Table 3.1. The instructor could introduce the workshop by explaining the rationale of the **ABC convention for relevance coding** (see Appendix 3.2).

The training exercise requires duplication of a number of sets of complete articles, one being given to each member to independently relevance-code each citation, citation-abstract, and complete document. Next, in a calibration session, the individual ratings are displayed for the team to analyze. When team members seriously disagree as to a relevance rating for any citation, discussion of the differences may help clarify their understanding. Repeated calibration sessions should help the team learn to apply the ABC convention.

We also suggest that the team have some experience with the short form of the ABC relevance-coding approach. This form is indicated for relevance coding when there are time deadlines or under conditions of sparse resources. We will later discuss the mini-synthesis where such rapid coding is essential. We term this short form as an *AC* convention that can accommodate rapid dichotomous decisions.

A = (A+, A, A–) of the long form = (retrieve complete document)

C = (B, C) of the long form = (do not retrieve complete document)

Goal 4: Develop Skills to Identify, Retrieve, and Relevance-Code Literature

Ideally, these training sessions should include a tour of an academic medical library and instruction from a medical librarian on how to find and copy articles efficiently. Then each trainee should independently identify, retrieve, and relevance-code a sample of five documents from a new citation list that the instructor provides. Each trainee should have a different list of five.

Next, the team should meet with the author(s) to review and compare their search strategies and their retrieval and coding results. In this way, the team can learn from one another, as well as from more experienced searchers, such as the author(s), who can provide both substantive and methods feedback to each trainee.

Finally, your coding team should apply the skills learned in Goal 3 to relevance-code all citations listed in each A+, A, or A– rated complete document. The profile of consensus ratings for each document should then be entered into the master list. If a document has few A+, A, or A– relevance-coded citations and many that are C level, you might question the relevance of that document as a whole. On the other hand, if many A and few C references are found, you might have greater assurance that you are on the right track in your database development.

Relevance profiling consists of counting and recording the number of A+, A, A–, B, or C citations in a given data resource file, as shown above in Table 3.2. In this example, the profile (or distribution) indicates 81 As, compared to 19 Bs and Cs. This distribution indicates that this search seems to be going well.

Search precision rates will be indicated by the relevance profile of the complete articles or documents. If this profile is skewed to the right, it indicates low precision because all of these articles were retrieved because their citation-abstracts were A+, A, or A–. If a substantial proportion of final articles prove irrelevant, additional training of the search team would be indicated. Low precision yields many false-positive documents and wastes time and resources. One other interesting point is that the proportion of A+ documents is a crude measure of the research maturity of this field. If there are no reviews at all, you may wonder if any had been written; if they were written, they might have been missed by your search team.

Profiles are needed for the citation-abstracts on such materials as electronic citation-abstract printouts, complete documents, or references in references. If these profiles reveal a skew to the right, it usually indicates the search might be off track. A skew to the left likely indicates that you are doing well. The meaning of either skew must be inferred because this is not a direct measure of where you are in your search in relation to where you want to be.

Goal 5: Develop Skills in Leading
Team Coding Calibration and Consensus Sessions

To achieve this training goal, the author should participate in a calibration session to help team members learn about measuring search precision rates and coding interrater reliability. To calibrate the trainee raters' skills, each trainee should apply the ABC relevance-coding convention to at least 25 articles. For each article, this includes a code for the citation alone, the citation-abstract, and the complete document.

First, the leader demonstrates how to calculate precision rates. To do this, count the sum of complete documents that you coded as A+, A, and A– (references verified as relevant) and divide this total by the sum of all corresponding citation-abstracts coded A+, A, and A– (references you initially judged might yield a relevant document); multiply the result by 100 to transform this figure into a percentage (the precision rate).

CALCULATING A LITERATURE SEARCH PRECISION RATE

Suppose you are searching for randomized controlled clinical trials comparing intramuscular bicillin versus oral amoxicillin for treating meningococcus pneumonia. You identify 50 citation-abstracts that you relevance-code A+, A, and A–. You retrieve the complete documents for all 50 citation-abstracts and code 40 as being of A+, A, and A– relevance for your synthesis database and 10 as Bs or Cs.

The precision rate (for searching) = 40/50 * 100 = 80%.

This rate is the same as the positive predictive value expressed in a percentage. It also equals a false-positive rate of 20% (100 – precision). (We usually define a false-positive rate of [1 – positive predictive value] as clinically more meaningful and ranging from 0 to 100 like a false-negative rate.)

Second, the leader demonstrates how to calculate a Cohen's Kappa statistic for interrater reliability in coding relevance of the citations alone, the citation-abstracts, and the complete documents. The results of the individual relevance ratings are entered into a spreadsheet that is programmed to calculate Kappa statistics, using standard formulas (Fleiss, 1981, pp. 219-232), and those shown in Table 10.1, Chapter 10 of this book. For interpreting these results, the team must agree on minimum acceptable threshold rates that indicate a successful calibration. For precision rates, this might be set at 80%; for Kappa rates, this could be set at 75%.

If the 95% (or whatever reasonable percentage) confidence intervals do not include the agreed-on team threshold of acceptability, for either the precision rates or Kappa statistics, additional training is required. The author or leader should pull 25 new articles and make a copy for each team member. Using a modified nominal group technique training session(s) (see Appendix 2.1 on details of this method), continue several rounds until the team precision rates and the Cohen's Kappas are the above agreed-upon thresholds.

Goal 6: Develop Skills in Search Documentation and Filing

This training task can be accomplished by practice skills sessions for preparing to implement iteration, Step 4. Because this procedure will be repeated for each search iteration, the major training of your team will be on-the-job. The essential skills for search documentation are also required for article validation in Stage III.

Search statistics to be calculated for results of each iteration include (a) total citation-abstracts actually coded in this iteration, divided by the total that need to be coded; (b) number of complete documents retrieved, divided by the total to be retrieved; (c) number of "references in references" coded, divided by the total to be coded; (d) a relevance profile (proportion rated at each level, A+ through C) determined and analyzed for each of the above citations, citation-abstracts, and complete documents retrieved; (e) the citation profile for total "references in references" recorded in the master list file for each citation; and (f) the results of calibration sessions in terms of interrater reliability and citation-abstract precision rates. In your master list, you have coded the type of documents retrieved, whether they are books, monographs, journal articles, technical reports, unpublished reports, or photocopied material that were compiled in that iteration. The utility of this information is that, at any time, the computer can give you a total count of technical reports retrieved, for example. If later you count the number of technical reports in your hardcopy file and find a lesser count, it is possible that a document has been misfiled, borrowed, or is missing or lost. With missing purchased books, this could be an expensive problem. Recall that most of these statistics will later be aggregated from each search iteration and the total counts used in the final documentation and evaluation of Stage II.

Goal 7: Develop Skills for Managing Electronic and Paper Files

All trainees must learn how to sort, file, and retrieve important project materials, such as handwritten relevance cue logs, hand-coded citation-abstracts on bibliographic hardcopy computer printouts (from PubMed, for example), and finance and time management ledgers. More important is managing electronic files such as the bibliographic master list, electronic lists of coded citation-abstracts and complete documents, and Internet files.

As a learning exercise, the trainees should review the subsection ("search documentation") of Section C in Chapter 5. During the initial iterations of an actual synthesis (as opposed to practice exercises), the team will soon gain experience and skills in achieving Goal 7.

Goal 8: As a Team, Understand and Be Able to Use Informatics Tools, Especially the Internet, as Required for Your Synthesis

We suggest that this goal is self-explanatory.

APPENDIX 3.2
Rationale for ABC Relevance-Coding Convention

The rationale for our ABC convention is primarily for the purpose of learning about and reducing search bias from Type I (search precision) and Type II (search recall) errors and for reducing inadequate interrater reliability rates. This information is essential to develop and maintain systematic database development. The literature search, in our judgment, introduces the most serious biases of all the procedures in a systematic review. As we understand it, Cochrane's handbook (undoubtedly one of the best of its kind) still relies heavily on implicit criterion judgments in their search procedures. The judgments are similar to our short, dichotomous A-C convention[a] (for retrieval or nonretrieval of complete documents) used in mini-syntheses when time and resources do not permit a more thorough analysis for relevance. This short coding convention loses the precision and recall of a 5-point scale, A+ through C, with its relevance cue log documentation.

Overall, we propose that the ABC convention strengthens the following procedures of a systematic review:

- Identification of invisible colleges
- Managing relevance criteria development
- Managing search logistics and prioritization
- Maintaining a search bias checklist
- Facilitating the search termination decision
- Facilitating structured group judgment consensus

The weakness of the 5-point A+ through C convention is the additional time and effort required for its implementation. Some have judged that the cost of this rigor far outweighs its benefits for information searching. Furthermore, its value is still based on intuition and anecdotal evidence. To our knowledge, replicated RCTs using the ABC convention as the independent variable and net benefit as the dependent variable have yet to be done. Admittedly, this assumption that our approach has not been validated may represent a Type II error on our part (possibly missing sound validation studies), due to our inadequate searching.

However, the advance of science is a series of proposing unique ideas, testing them empirically, and accepting, revising, or discarding them. To our knowledge, this ABC convention is still at the proposal stage. Validation studies by synthesis methods researchers will eventually determine whether the potential strengths and benefits of this ABC convention outweigh its potential cost or harm in terms of increased bias.

---

a. The short form of the ABC convention is A = (A+, A, A–) of the long form = (retrieve complete document); C = (B, C) of the long form = (do not retrieve complete document).

FORM 3.1: INITIAL SYNTHESIS PLANNING FORM

Date: _____

Initials: _____

Identification:

Synthesis title:

Authors and staff:

PI:	Assistant:	Secretary:
Co-PI:	Assistant:	Clerk:
Co-PI:	Other	Other

Synthesis Focus:

Topic:

Purpose and Goals:

Target Audience:

Significance:

Product:

FORM 3.2
SEARCH PLANNING AND UPDATE GUIDE

Iteration #: _____

Date: _____

Initials: _____

Topic:

Scope of the Search:

Languages

_____ English only   _____ All languages
_____ English translations of non-English documents
_____ Foreign language papers (specify): _____
_____

Time frame

_____ Screen bibliographic indexes from: _____ to _____
_____ Obtain documents produced from: _____ to _____

Extent of Retrieval Effort

_____ Only local community colleagues, schools, libraries
_____ Retrieve nearby national literature (e.g., United States and Canada)
_____ Retrieve international literature, (e.g., European libraries)
_____ Contact nearby experts (e.g., United States, Canada)
_____ Contact distant experts (e.g., Western Europe, Japan)

Recommended Search Sources

_____ Computerized bibliographic indexes (e.g., MEDLINE)
_____ Internet (World Wide Web)
_____ People sources (colleagues, authors)
_____ References listed in relevant documents
_____ Organizations (e.g., academic or professional)
_____ Funding sources (e.g., National Institute of Health)
_____ Paper indexes (e.g., Index Medicus)

Checklist of Information Types

_____ Published primary data articles   _____ Draft manuscripts
_____ Books, book chapters, syllabi   _____ Educational manuals
_____ Conference proceedings   _____ Audiovisuals
_____ Editorials, letters to the editor   _____ Newsletters
_____ Dissertations, printed reports   _____ Internet material
_____ Abstracts   _____ Studies in progress
_____ Policy papers, editorials, essays   _____ News media
_____ Other (Specify): _____
_____
_____

FORM 3.3: BUDGET AND TIMETABLE PLANNING

FISCAL BUDGET

Indicate total hours and dollars of staff effort projected for entire synthesis project.

Position	Initials (Name)	Hours	Salary Code	Project Total $	Position	Initials (Name)	Hours	Salary Code	Project Total $
Principal Investigator									
Co-PI					Asst.				
Co-PI					Asst.				
Other					Sec.				
					Other				

	Personnel $	Consults $	Computer $	Books $	Supplies $	Telephone $	Graphics $	Copying $	Other $	GRAND TOTAL $
Project Costs										

TIMETABLE

Indicate span of time for completing each of the five stages.   (NOTE: Schedule illustrates a completed Gantt Chart)

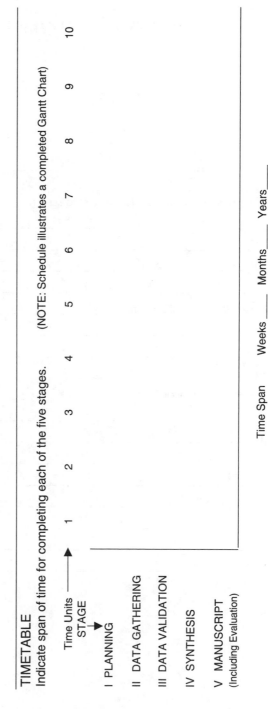

Time Units 1 2 3 4 5 6 7 8 9 10
STAGE

I PLANNING

II DATA GATHERING

III DATA VALIDATION

IV SYNTHESIS

V MANUSCRIPT
(Including Evaluation)

Time Span   Weeks_____   Months_____   Years_____

FORM 3.4: SEARCH LEADS FOR NEXT ITERATION

Iteration #: _____

Date: _____

Initials: _____

Topic: _____

Electronic bibliographic database(s) to screen: _____

_____

_____

Key expert(s) to contact: _____

_____

Best available bibliography: _____

_____

_____

_____

Best "A+" review or "A" article: _____

_____

_____

_____

_____

Descriptors/key words: _____

_____

_____

_____

Notes:

FORM 3.5: RELEVANCE CUE LOG—A+ CUES

Date: _____

Initials: _____

Page _____ of _____

Topic:

Instructions: Specify any cues to be included or excluded in terms of descriptors, key words, topics, jargon, phrases, sources, investigators, journals, organizations, or other leads to an A+ review on above topic.

Inclusions:

1. _____

   _____

2. _____

3. _____

etc.

Exclusions (other than A, A–, B, and C logs of category inclusion ratings):

1. _____

   _____

2. _____

3. _____

etc.

CHAPTER 4

Evaluation and Improvement of Stage I

In this evaluation of Stage I, your focus is on how well you have accomplished your synthesis planning and preparation. The four criteria stated in Chapter 1 are used for evaluation of each stage of this book. They are listed as follows:

EVALUATION AND IMPROVEMENT OF STAGE I

Assess and enhance:
- A. Documentation adequacy
- B. Clinical significance
- C. Scientific soundness
- D. Cost-effectiveness

Because Stage I is the planning stage of the whole synthesis project, you must keep all of the above criteria in mind when doing your final assessment. In other stages, only one or two may prove of special relevance.

Procedure A. Assess and Enhance Documentation Adequacy

Task 1: Review Adequacy of
Completed Chapter 3 Documentation Forms

Extensive documentation of both the process and the outcomes of planning is essential. The following are the names of the five forms provided at the end of Chapter 3:

LIST OF PLANNING FORMS IN CHAPTER 3

Form 3.1:   Synthesis Planning Framework
Form 3.2:   Search Planning and Update Guide
Form 3.3:   Budget and Timetable Planning
Form 3.4:   Search Leads for Next Iteration
Form 3.5:   A+ Relevance Cue Log

The completed planning forms will serve as a starting point for implementing your information search. Before moving on to the next task of this evaluation, make sure that all the items on these forms are completed, readable, and understandable. If needed, additional discussion may be necessary to clarify any items. When finished, provide a copy to all synthesis staff (authors, searchers, raters, consults) to keep them on track and focused on the same goals.

Task 2: Ask Team to Provide Suggestions for Improving Documentation Process

In Task 1, you reviewed the documentation outcome of Stage I. Task 2 is to determine what the team has learned from the documentation process so as to make it more thorough and efficient. It is important to accomplish this learning task now while the team's experience is still fresh.

Procedure B. Assess and Enhance Clinical Significance

Clinical significance in Stage I refers to the topic question and the relevance criteria. As part of the planning stage, you will have applied a group consensus method to select a high-priority topic. If this structured process worked well, you should have a topic outcome that will facilitate ultimate clinical improvement by means of your systematic review of the literature. Tasks that might be conducted in evaluating the clinical significance of your topic are as follows.

Task 1: Assess and Enhance Topic Question to Ensure an Appropriate Outcomes Framework

Synthesis questions can be phrased at many levels of abstraction and in a variety of frames of reference (i.e., models). For example, a model may be developed from the clinician's, the administrator's, or the consumer's point of view. A better way to ensure that your synthesis will be applicable in practice is to phrase the question in simple terms that a patient can understand.

QUESTIONS TO DESCRIBE INITIAL OUTCOMES

Healthcare outcome is

   (a)   a result of what process?

   (b)   experienced by what population?

   (c)   in which healthcare setting?

   (d)   under whose care?

   (e)   measured when and by what means?

At this point in your synthesis preparation, it is important to confirm that answers to these five questions make your model understandable and indicate that the links between outcomes and processes clarify what is being studied and what is not being studied. You can also consider alternative outcomes to be sure no important ones have been omitted from consideration.

Task 2: Assess and Enhance Model Outcome and Process Variables for Clinical Relevance

We suggest you assess your definitions of variables now, before you begin the synthesis. If you are an expert in the domain, this step will be readily accomplished. If not, it is important to seek expert consultation. If this preventative step is taken, much unnecessary work can be avoided. The following questions might be of help for this procedure.

SUGGESTED QUESTIONS FOR RELEVANCE ASSESSMENT

   1.   Is the dependent variable(s) a measurable healthcare outcome or process?

   2.   Can the variables be discriminated as processes and outcomes, and is the relationship between the two made explicit?

   3.   Are inclusions and exclusions in the relevance criteria defined in terms of specific outcomes of interest?

Task 3: Assess and Enhance Model Outcomes and Process Variables for Measurability

Regardless of the topic, the variables in your model need to be defined in a manner that indicates they are measurable. Many authors assume that they are describing their variables within sufficient precision, but no one would be able to replicate the measurement process. This is an appropriate time to call the author(s), who usually are glad to share them with you. Equally important is to look for evidence that these measures are sound. For example, what precision do they have? Have they been validated against an acceptable **gold standard**? Is there sufficient construct validity? If so, what was the rate of false negatives? What was the rate of false positives? If this evidence indicates the measures are acceptable, your outcome and process variables are likely measurable. If not, you may have to undertake the arduous job of developing and testing new instruments.

Task 4: Assess and Enhance the Clinical Appropriateness of the Population Defined by the Relevance Criteria

You will note that your relevance criteria define populations of interest that should be included in your synthesis. You need to expressly define these populations so they make clinical sense. For example, if it is known that the elderly respond much differently to a specific drug than younger patients, you must specify those population differences in the relevance criteria. Assess whether or not the populations encompassed by your relevance criteria may require domain expertise (i.e., a consult in that specialty). If such expertise is not available, we strongly suggest that you seek consultation from such experts at a local academic medical center.

Task 5: Assess and Enhance Literature Maturity and, If Needed, Adjust Your Synthesis Plan

Review Your Pilot Search of Internet Literature (Mini-Synthesis). You will not have a complete understanding of your field until you are much further into the search stage. At this point, you should have completed a brief Internet pilot search of the literature on your topic (see Procedure B, Chapter 3). The mini-synthesis you conducted at that time should provide sufficient information to determine how far advanced your field of inquiry may be.

Analyze the "Maturity" of Your Research Field From the Findings. You can determine the maturity of your field by noting the following indicators: (a) there will be a large number of reviews, "information syntheses," or "systematic reviews" on or close to your topic; (b) there should be many clinical trials of high quality and other studies having sophisticated and sound research designs; (c) you will find many valid and reliable measures and measurement tools; and (d) there will be a well-developed theoretical base.

If your field is less mature, you will not find the above characteristics, and you may have to reconsider your topic or prepare to do much more work gathering and validating primary data studies, as well as developing and assessing your own measurement instruments.

Understand the Categories of Research Designs. (Note: "research designs," as described here, should not be confused with "information synthesis designs," described in Section C, Chapter 2.) One relatively simple method to confirm your literature maturity is merely to count the number of studies found in your mini-synthesis that fall in the following categories:

SUGGESTED CATEGORIES OF RESEARCH DESIGNS

1. Case studies
2. Descriptive (e.g., epidemiological, prognostic)
3. Methods development (e.g., new diagnostic tools)
4. Evaluation (e.g., technology assessments, economic analyses [e.g., cost-benefit], educational programs)
5. Quasi-experimental (some randomization)
6. Experimental (randomized controlled trials)
7. Quantitative syntheses (e.g., meta-analyses of randomized clinical trials [RCTs])

Note that studies using any of the above designs may range in quality. An exceptionally well-done case study might provide more meaningful information than a faulty and misleading RCT. Furthermore, the above assessments require criteria that are usually unique to the research design. If there are inadequate data available to establish such criteria, your team may have to infer them based on their current knowledge and judgment. Expert consultation may be required for this task.

Adjust Your Plan and Relevance Criteria as Warranted. Finally, once you have determined the maturity of the field you are investigating, you may need to adjust your topic and your plan. For example, if relatively few mature articles are found, your search scope may have to be much broader. If your field is mature, then your relevance criteria can be highly specific and very focused; you will be able to define your topic in precise terms, including specific types of research designs, populations, healthcare contexts, processes, and outcomes.

Procedure C. Assess and Enhance Scientific Soundness

Scientific soundness refers to the degree to which the findings and conclusions of a synthesis are valid and reliable. Because Stage I involves little in the way of data collection or analysis, the most important scientific aspect of soundness is the logic and practicality of the model you develop.

Task 1: Assess and Enhance Causal Logic of Model

The causal model you create will serve as a guide for your information synthesis activities. The following subtasks are suggested to assess your model.

Sketch a Diagram of a Causal Model for Your Topic. To test your understanding of your topic, try to sketch a rough diagram of a causal model (e.g., see Figures 2.1, 2.2, and 2.3). In Section D, Chapter 2, we discuss the importance of model development and present a variety of model types that could be the focus of an information synthesis. In Procedure B of Chapter 3, we indicate how to develop your project model. Regardless of the type of model you choose, it should include variables that are logically related to each other. Assessment of your developed model should begin by making sure that the nature of the relationship between the variables has been made clear. In a simple model, this should include the nature of the relationship between an identified outcome variable and the variable(s) thought to create change in that outcome.

Confirm That Required Model Specifications Are Explicit. Recall that the following must be indicated:

1. Type of distribution: random or fixed effects

2. Direction of effects (one-way, two-way, etc.)

3. Type of effects (moderating, mediating, interactions)

4. Specification of multiple measurement strategies for the same conceptual variable

Record Evidence Supporting the Causal Links in Your Diagram. This subtask requires that you list whatever evidence (e.g., research citations, expert judgment) you have that supports the causal connections you have shown.

If Lacking Research Evidence, Indicate Why You Assume Causality. Your assumption could be based on experience, consultation with experts, or perhaps some vague memory of having read about meaningful evidence in the "fugitive literature."

Lacking Evidence of Causality, Delete That Link. Perhaps you could make a list of those links that do not seem to have any supporting evidence or rationale. You may later come across a sound reason why it should be in your model.

Task 2: Assess and Enhance Adequacy of Relevance Criteria

Be Sure Variables Are Defined in Concrete Terms From the Beginning. For example, patient-physician communication must be described in terms of how you expect it to be measured, such as time with the patient, subjective assessments of patient satisfaction, or amount of information conveyed.

Include Specific Definitions of Outcomes That Will Be Assessed. The most direct method to assess relevance criteria is to have a domain expert review them. If that is not possible, or if it has already been done, the synthesis team should now review them carefully and discuss any difficulties.

Ensure That Interrater Agreement Is Acceptable Before Starting Stage II. One of the best ways to uncover ambiguity is to have several people independently review a set of citations (perhaps 20) and then compare responses. Low interrater reliabilities are clues that the criteria are not written clearly. For example, the Kappa statistic should be at least 0.70.

Procedure D. Assess and Enhance Cost-Effectiveness

Cost-effectiveness assessment of Stage I will be measured by means of your fiscal and time expenditure records. These data must be assessed by comparing them with your synthesis budget. The team must decide whether the products are worth the cost. The synthesis plan should be reviewed, including items in Chapter 3, Forms 3.1 to 3.4. Every aspect of the process should be thought through ahead of time to avoid excessive expenditures, expensive last-minute adjustments, and time loss. The use of a software package using the program evaluation and review technique (PERT) will substantially facilitate this analytic task because the program reminds you to work out essential planning details. In addition, time and fiscal totals are done automatically. Regardless of the topic field or the extensiveness of the project, five areas should always be covered in your plan: calculate Stage I monetary and time expenditure totals, compare expenditures with resource budget, assess and improve adequacy of staff training, assess and improve adequacy of informatics tools and resources, and assess costs versus accomplishments ratio.

Task 1: Calculate Stage I
Monetary and Time Expenditure Totals

Budget and time frames can be created and monitored in a variety of ways. The following illustrate but two:

Program Evaluation and Review Technique (PERT)/Critical Path Method (CPM). Application of PERT software (Hofmann, 1993; Kost, 1986; Luttman & Pearson, 1995) is one of the better means of planning and evaluating the details of a project, especially fiscal and time expenditures. This approach is suited for intermediate and large synthesis projects. By this means, you establish budgets and timelines that are reasonable.

Gantt Chart Display of Time and Dollars. Figure 3.3 (Chapter 3) illustrates a Gantt chart as a far less sophisticated approach that still requires use of accounting methods and a spreadsheet. This method is suited for small, brief projects.

Task 2: Compare Expenditures With Resource Budget

PERT/CPM Totals Dollar and Hour Expenditures Compared to Your Budget. If you have not purchased needed resources by the end of Stage I, your preparation is incomplete. Budgetwise, if for some reason a purchase is not possible at the time, you need to be sure sufficient funds are set aside until the product is available. In terms of processes completed, with PERT's time-recording methods, once a product is on the "critical path," you know that your entire project may be delayed if that particular function is not completed on schedule. If your product is not on the "critical path," you may have some free time with which to improve what you have achieved to date.

Gantt Display Is Used to Analyze Your Expenditures and Budget. You will likely want to use a spreadsheet to accomplish your mathematics and graphic displays. This method is suited to small and/or brief synthesis projects. By this means, you could use the graphics that are available in spreadsheets or word-processing software. With each entry of data, you would note the change in the length of the bars displayed. Using a Gantt chart, one light bar would denote projected time or fiscal requirements for a single process, and a second darker bar would indicate the actual time or money used. Watching the relationship between the two during the process of planning and preparation gives you a rough sense of whether you are falling behind or getting ahead during that stage.

Task 3: Assess and Improve
Adequacy of Staff Credentials and Training

Review Team Credentials and Roles. We assume that by this time, you will have established a collaborative relationship with coauthors and hired staff. Make a final check to see that you have individuals to do searching, copying, filing, relevance coding, validity rating, statistical analysis, and writing. You might review your inventory of staff task assignments that need to be accomplished. (Again, PERT provides substantial help in completing this task.) The next three items might provide a framework for that review.

Reanalyze and Improve the Results of Team Training. Were members clearly superior in terms of understanding the conceptual tasks, doing relevance coding, and speaking up to be helpful to others in the training sessions? Are there tasks of greater responsibility these individuals might fulfill? Were there any who just "didn't get it" and had to be told over and over? Were there also those who were usually the outliers in calibration sessions? Were there any who could not admit making a mistake or pretended to understand critical concepts when they did not have a clue? Such individuals might be given less responsibility or let go at the end of the job probation period. To improve, you need to provide feedback and counseling.

Finally, check communication and interpersonal relationship abilities of coauthors and staff on the job. Do they get along well, or are they constantly backbiting, complaining, and disrupting the work of others on the team or, worse, insisting on having their way, even though they are clearly wrong? Do they have a pleasant telephone personality (because much work with consults and relevant authors will be done on the telephone)? Are they able to relate to consultants, librarians, and other outside individuals crucial to the project and have good writing ability for e-mail communications or correspondence? Again, to improve, you should provide feedback, counseling, role-playing exercises, and other additional training.

Prepare and Review Worksheets With Each Person. For all major work tasks, assignment sheets should have clear written statements of the job to be done, including the date due. After the staff gets started in Stage II, there will likely be discussion and negotiation required regarding the status of the literature, availability of authors to contact, and staff time constraints.

If Necessary, Establish in Writing an Expected Time Task Commitment for Certain Staff Members. Usually, most staff members will be sufficiently conscientious that this somewhat overbearing step will not be needed. However, in any project, the unexpected may happen, such as a coauthor(s) dropping out for lack of time or a staff member having to make an important unplanned trip and not arranging backup. However, if one or more staff or coauthors consistently do not keep up with their agreed-on assignments or keep claiming they had not understood the details of their commitment, and constant reminders become necessary, limits must be set. Taking the trouble to write out detailed task plans may be necessary. Then, if commitments are not kept and responsibility not taken, such individuals should be asked to withdraw from the project. If you are using a PERT planning program, remind your staff when their tasks are on the "critical path" and might delay the entire project if their assignments are not completed on time.

Task 4: Assess and Enhance Adequacy of Informatics Tools and Other Resources

One of the important tasks early in the preparation phase is to test all equipment, especially that which has been recently purchased. It might be costly to find your warranty has run out before you have used some of the equipment you purchased. For example, an expensive scanner that does not work can be a major frustration if your staff have to input "references in references" into your database by hand. When you determine that your resources and purchases are in good working order and your staff finds they can use them properly without extensive additional training, you can make an initial judgment about the value of these resources in relation to their cost.

In terms of other tangible and intangible resources, it goes without saying that it is essential that you arrange for adequate space, furniture, and equipment for each full-time staff member. Likewise, the value of having staff with good interpersonal relationship and communication skills is an important intangible value that must be factored into the accomplishments of Stage I.

Task 5: Assess Value of Costs Versus Accomplishments

When you do your final budget assessment, you and your team will have to judge the value of your staff, resources, and purchases achieved by the end of Stage I. If interpersonal relationships remain good, the next most important resource will be the time your coauthors and staff can firmly commit and, finally, the adequacy of your budgeted funds. Remember, the most time-consuming parts of the synthesis project will be data gathering (Stage II) and manuscript preparation (Stage V). We will point out later several useful controls you might apply to data gathering. However, the manuscript time requirement may come as a shock to those who have not produced a systematic review or monograph on a health science topic. Consequently, when you complete your Stage I assessment, be sure you have adequate time and dollars set aside for Stages II and IV to be completed thoroughly, so as to produce a quality product.

Finally, complete Form 4.1 (at the end of this chapter) to obtain an overview assessment of Stage I and, if possible, make improvements. If improvements are not possible, perhaps you could record these facts in a "lessons learned" diary.

Summary

This chapter provides several ideas and constructs for evaluating the development process and initial plan outcome of your synthesis. On completing these tasks, you will have a much better idea of the quality of your work in this area. As we said in the beginning of this chapter, the planning stage provides the foundation of all other work you will do on your project. Thus, it is critical that your assessment of Stage I be especially thorough. We suggest several tasks to be completed as part of this evaluation.

In Procedure A, we focus on assessing and enhancing the documentation you have compiled thus far. The products we expect for this stage include the topic statement, improvement hypothesis, the model, initial relevance criteria, your detailed plan (including related task assignments), and budget (fiscal and time) for all authors and team members. All of these products should be well documented.

In Procedure B, we evaluate the projected clinical significance of your project topic. Issues we address include ensuring clinically relevant populations, focusing on outcomes language, literature maturity, and clinically relevant and accurate measurements. We encourage using domain experts as outside evaluators at this stage to prevent problems and difficulties later. Make any improvements that seem feasible.

In Procedure C, we assess issues of the scientific or methodological soundness of your project plan. In Stage I, we expect that the logic of your model is the focus of your review criteria. In addition, the importance of clear and concrete relevance criteria is also discussed. In any event, make those enhancements required.

In Procedure D, we review methods for compiling and comparing your expenditures (fiscal and time) with your budget. We indicate that, due to lack of precision of your measurement tools, you must set acceptable limits about your budget. Finally, your team must make some crude estimate of the value of accomplishments to date. If your plan is too rough or abstract, with the tasks assigned to individuals unclear, much rework will be required, and the expenditure of time and dollars may not seem worth the cost. If this is the case, the plan must be augmented, revised, discarded, or started over with the same or a new topic.

FORM 4.1: STAGE I EVALUATION CHECKLIST

Date:

Recorder:

> **Instructions:** Complete the following checklist summarizing tasks described in Chapter 3. This form will help ensure you have thoroughly evaluated your Stage I end products.

_____ Is Form 3.1 (synthesis purpose and goals) completed?
_____ Are responsibilities of each author specified and agreed on?
_____ Is your topic question worded as an improvement hypothesis?
_____ Is the synthesis model well described? Does it include (where applicable) the following:
    ____ independent and dependent variables?
    ____ specified causal relationships between variables?
    ____ specified mediator and moderator variables?
_____ Are an adequate budget and timetable established?
_____ Is Form 3.4 (Gantt chart) completed?
_____ Are your informatics resources obtained?
    (Or has a schedule for their acquisition been established?)
    Check the following as they apply:
    ____ project planning and word processing
    ____ scanning hardware and software
    ____ bibliographic data management
    ____ research data management
    ____ meta-analysis computation
    ____ fiscal and time management

_____ Is your search team recruited and trained?

_____ Are your search documentation tools prepared?
    ____ Form 3.2 (search plan)
    ____ Form 3.3 (identified bibliographic data banks, experts)
    ____ citation printouts and copied reference lists
    ____ relevance cue logs
    ____ relevance criteria list
    ____ electronic master list
    ____ electronic fiscal and time-accounting records
    ____ search statistics compilation forms

DATABASE DEVELOPMENT

CHAPTER 5

Conceptual Issues in Database Development

At this point, you have formulated your synthesis topic; conceptualized your rationale, assumptions, model (theoretical framework), working plan, budget, and timetable; and organized a well-trained project team. Chapter 5 covers the conceptual issues to help you cope with the procedural problems of database development outlined in Chapter 6.

We divide this chapter into five sections:

THEORETICAL FACTORS IN DATABASE DEVELOPMENT

A. Bias
B. Levels of information soundness
C. Strategic search considerations
D. Generic sources of health science information
E. Fugitive literature

Section A. Bias

The most important characteristic of a **synthesis database** is that it represents a valid sample of studies conducted by researchers that balances different "schools of thought" as applied to your topic/question. Because you cannot access every research study ever conducted on your topic, we suggest you focus your effort on representativeness across schools of thought, time periods, and geographical locations. In addition, Stage II database development is mainly concerned with content relevance rather than scientific soundness (which is managed in Stage III). Bias in database development must always be considered.

Defining Databank, Database, and Data Set

SYNTHESIS DATABANK, DATABASE, AND DATA SET

Note that these terms are not to be confused with formal bibliographic data warehouses, data farms, databanks, and databases, as used by the U.S. National Library of Medicine (NLM) or the U.S. National Library of Congress (LC). We are not aware of any standardized international nomenclature for online data and information resources in healthcare.

Synthesis Databank. We use this term to signify a major bibliographic source that links to multiple databases. A databank can have its own unique **search engine** or merely link to individual database search engines, online catalogs, directories, registries, or indexes that might exist. For example, the online U.S. Department of Health and Human Services' (HHS) Directory of HHS Data Resources links to databases of all of their administrations, agencies, and centers.

Synthesis Database. We use this term to describe all information gathered, relevance-coded, and stored in your database file. Thus, all A+ and A relevance materials are included in the database that will subsequently be assessed for scientific soundness. This material can be in any form, such as articles, books, or technical reports, which may be found on paper, tape, audiovisual or electronic media, or ideas in the minds of qualified experts. Excluded are materials rated A–, B, and C. Recall that A– and B references are stored in the master file and A– citations are processed for leads to more relevant information to be added to the database.

Synthesis Data Set. We define a **synthesis data set** as the raw data culled from the relevant research studies (A+ and A citation-abstracts) in the database. This material consists of both written text and numeric data. This function is accomplished in Stage III, prior to validation of the research reports from which the data sets were abstracted.

Database Representative of What?

Theoretically, the total universe of information on your topic (both published and unpublished) is the target of your search. Initially, it would seem intuitive to have your database be that universe. However, obtaining every article or paper ever written on any subject is a costly and, for most topics, an impossible task. Even if you try to accomplish this goal, there are many difficulties that result in unacceptable biases. For most reviews, lack of resources forces a compromise that may render the data retrieved seriously flawed, if not worthless. For example, if your search is restricted to one or two electronic bibliographic databases, though convenient and affordable, this strategy will likely miss many critical articles. As a result, your data will represent a biased view of a limited number of investigators, whose articles happened to be accepted for publication in journals that happened to be indexed by those electronic sources. On the other hand, an "all-out" haphazard screening of a large number of sources may have the same result, again biased by traditional methods of searching. It is hoped that if you followed the suggestions in the Stage I planning phase of your synthesis, focusing on your theoretical framework or model, these issues of database bias may be more readily resolved.

Another bias is that of compiling a database that only represents one or two of the predominant **invisible colleges**. This issue was discussed in Stage I and may offer a means of establishing a better universe that should be represented by your search. As discussed earlier, each "silent college" has its own favorite research designs, usually coauthors who quote one another, and idiosyncratic methods and terminology. If the results are in line with the publisher's values and biases, the articles get published, indexed, and represented in reviews, systematic or not. So in answer to the question of being representative of what, we surmise that your **final data set** should represent research from a balance of invisible colleges.

Balancing Your Search Strategy

The problem of not considering a full spectrum of research information sources, particularly invisible colleges, is a serious threat to final synthesis conclusions. In our judgment, to cope with this issue, there is ample evidence that the following postulate is sound.

POSTULATE

The key to successful database development is to implement a multidimensional search strategy (e.g., checking computer, people, organizational, and paper sources of research information).

To restrict your search to only those sources that are convenient is almost certain to guarantee unacceptable bias.

Overreliance on electronic bibliographic databases can produce serious bias. Using a single large database or a single search engine will likely result in missing a substantial number of research studies you are seeking (see Adams, Power, Frederick, & Lefebvre, 1994; Bender, Halpern, Thangaroopan, Jadad, & Ohlsson, 1997; Egger & Smith, 1998; Gehanno, Paris, Thirion, & Caillard, 1998; Haynes et al., 1985; McDonald et al., 1999; Woods & Trewheellar, 1998). Restricting the scope of your search to electronic databanks, not picking up the telephone to contact people sources, or not doing a hand search of dusty library files can result in missing much important information.

Finally, be aware that electronic sources, though vital, will point you primarily to paper sources where the data are to be found (over the next decade, this will gradually change as complete books and journal articles become available in digital form). As the Cochrane Collaboration emphasizes, a successful literature search will ultimately depend on the skills you apply to "hand searches" of paper documents, such as those on medical library shelves or in author's file drawers (see the following Web address for the *Cochrane Hand Search Manual* [last updated April 1999]: hiru.mcmaster.ca/cochrane/cochrane/hsmpt1.htm).

Thus, we emphasize the importance of systematic development of a multidimensional search strategy in Stage II. Your final database will be a major determinant of the quality of your final data set and contribute much to the validity of your final synthesis conclusions. No amount of expertise in the synthesis or write-up of your project will compensate for an inadequate search that may yield a biased, nonrepresentative database of heterogeneous studies.

Publication Bias and "Funnel Plot Analysis"

PUBLICATION BIAS

Publication bias is the tendency for journals to reject studies that report null results or unique methods that reviewers may reject as being unproven. As a consequence, potentially sound and important investigations are not disseminated and remain in the realm of elusive, or fugitive, literature.

Publication bias results in a database that may be seriously skewed and may lead to questionable, if not misleading, conclusions (Begg, 1994; Dickersin, 1990; Dickersin, Chan, Chalmers, Sacks, & Smith, 1987). Easterbrook, Berlin, Gopalan, and Matthews (1991) point out that it is even less likely that small and nonrandomized studies will be published. Many scientifically sound papers, because they report negative results, might not be published and thus might not appear in your final database. Even more serious, authors may not write up their own studies that fail to reject the null hypothesis (Greenwald, 1975).

Consequently, it is especially important that you identify, analyze, quantify, and try to manage this problem (Begg, 1994; Chalmers, Frank, & Reitman, 1990; Dear & Begg, 1992). Hedges (1992) and Vevea and Hedges (1995) propose their own ideas about statistical methods for coping with publication bias. We examine the "funnel plot" and "file drawer" approach in more detail because they are often used at the present time.

Rosenthal (1979) coined the term *file drawer*, which is being recognized and applied increasingly today. A serious bias can result from the fact that a positive research result may relate to publication bias rather than the quality of the study. Articles you retrieve often tend to have a positive result and may or may not be of high methodological quality. On the other hand, negative trials may often have much higher methodological quality. A number of studies have reported this paradoxical finding (see Williamson et al., 1986, pp. 380-381).

FUNNEL PLOT ANALYSIS

A funnel display (or "plot") uses graphs to estimate the interaction of two variables (Egger, Smith, & Phillips, 1997). The x-axis represents quantitative outcomes (e.g., effect size), and the y-axis usually represents sample size. If this plot of the studies resembles a funnel, it is likely that there is no publication bias. Studies with small sample sizes will have large variability in effect sizes (the base of the funnel), and studies with large sample sizes will have much less variability in effect sizes (the top of the funnel). Failure to publish nonsignificant (negative) results would likely be a result of studies with small sample sizes and would result in a funnel missing the left side at the base (see Figures 5.1 and 5.2). Other continuous-scale moderating variables can be used instead of sample size, such as the year of publication, drug dose, or length of treatment.

Light and Pillemer (1984, pp. 63-72) were probably the first to report this concept.

Another way of identifying publication bias is by means of a **funnel plot**. Plotting effect size (x-axis) against several types of variables (e.g., sample size) is an effective method to estimate several types of bias in your database. For example, it might determine (a) whether all of your studies come from a single population; (b) publication bias; (c) temporal (historical) trends among statistical effects, such as the temporal pattern of nonsignificant findings; or (d) effects of sampling variability due

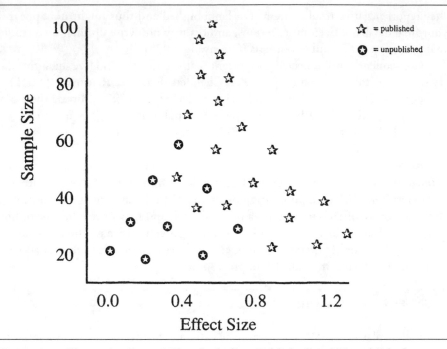

Figure 5.1. Illustrative Funnel Plot, Including Published and Unpublished Studies

to such factors as treatments, participants, or care settings. As but one illustration, Figure 5.1 provides an illustration of a funnel plot encompassing both published and nonpublished studies.

Note that the studies rejecting the null hypothesis will likely be on the right, and those not rejecting the null hypothesis will be on the left side of this plot. Also, studies with smaller sample sizes have a wide range of nonsignificant and significant effects, in contrast with those having larger samples (related to the central limit theorem). If the plot is truncated or even circular (i.e., completely random), a serious flaw such as publication bias must be considered. As an illustrative example, Figure 5.2 shows one possible configuration of the plot if all nonpublished studies are removed.

The truncated funnel plot in this figure is somewhat typical of a study having publication bias (as shown in this illustration), although this may be but one explanation; for example, methods quality may be a possible explanation. Egger, Smith, Schneider, and Minder (1997) extol the funnel plot except when the randomized clinical trial (RCT) database contains a number of small trials. Egger and Smith (1998) point out that newer statistical methods have been developed to more objectively measure funnel plot asymmetry (see also Begg & Mazumdar, 1994). Song, Eastweed, Gilbody, and Sutton (1999) recognize the value of the funnel plot but stress that the best way to minimize publication bias is to register trials when they are

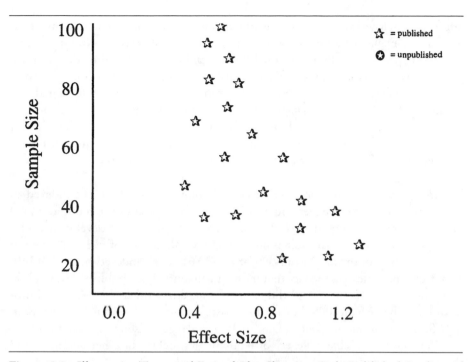

Figure 5.2. Illustrative Truncated Funnel Plot Showing Only Published Studies

being planned. Petticrew, Gilbody, and Sheldon (1999) reported on the degree to which the funnel plot is a reliable measure of publication bias in a meta-analysis. They concluded that the funnel plot may be a misleading indicator where there is significant variation in the quality of, or sample size of, research projects encompassed.

One of the more effective procedures to cope with publication bias is an intensive search of fugitive literature. By doing a file drawer analysis, you can make a crude estimate of how many negative studies will be required to overturn the conclusions from your current database. However, we do agree with Song et al. (1999) that only by registering clinical trials in the planning stage will we be able to successfully manage this serious problem.

Other Search Biases to Be Managed

In an exceptional study on bias in the location and selection of studies for meta-analysis, Egger and Smith (1998) remind us of the following issues.

Language Bias. There are three areas for which you should be aware—namely, English language bias, database bias, and citation bias. Egger (2001) and Egger and

Smith (1998) have examined these areas rather extensively and found that investigators in non-English-speaking nations usually publish positive papers in English and negative papers in their local non-English medical journals. They provide the example that over a 10-year period, 63% of trials in English were positive, compared to only 35% published in German as but one example. Moher et al. (1996) stated that inclusion of studies in all languages was essential for reducing systematic errors and increasing precision of results. However, Moher et al. (2000) studied the effect of language on results of meta-analyses and found no difference at all in terms of an estimate of benefit. We will await further study of this language bias.

Location Bias. Journals from less developed countries are often not indexed in MEDLINE or Embase. Egger and Smith (1998) found that of the 3,000 to 4,000 journals indexed by those two, only about 2% are from the less developed world. They give the example that India is one of the most productive of research papers of the developing countries, yet only 30 of the 3,861 serials indexed by MEDLINE were from India, despite the fact that most Indian journals are published in English. Nieminen and Isohanni (1999) did an interesting study titled "Bias Against European Journals in Medical Publication Databases" that is worth reading. In any event, if U.S. investigators only quote U.S. or English-language sources, they may miss existing sound "invisible colleges" of reputable researchers in other countries and thus unwittingly introduce serious bias into their own work.

Citation Bias. Studies quoted by other investigators are far more likely to be positive. In the field of cholesterol lowering, positive trials were referenced and quoted substantially more than negative trials, regardless of the size and quality of the studies involved (see Ravnskov, 1992). Hence, use of reference lists is far more likely to yield positive studies. Multiple publication bias is a result of the fact that positive studies are presented multiple times and also published and republished in many different journals under different titles. (Note: In our own experience, republications are often under different titles, as well as different journals.) Egger and Smith (1998) found multiple references reporting that the same data from different publication sources are duplicated in different meta-analyses. Furthermore, they found that many duplicate reports of multicenter trials did not have a single author in common. (Again, we reiterate the need for balanced "invisible colleges" to avoid this increasingly common problem.)

Data Availability Bias. Bias in provision of data is another unfortunate occurrence. In conducting a meta-analysis, it is frequently necessary to contact the authors to obtain critical data not included in their report. As Egger and Smith (1998) report, researchers can be very hesitant to share information such as how adequately their data were stratified.

Inclusion Criteria Bias. Again, the Egger and Smith (1998) article documents how investigators can, knowingly or unknowingly, manipulate inclusion criteria resulting in selection of positive studies and rejection of negative studies. In one instance, the authors excluded a study for having inadequate randomization yet accepted the identical study in a duplicate publication where they approved the adequacy of the randomization process.

Section B. Levels of Information Soundness

At this point, it is important to become acquainted with our concept of meta-validation, which will be referred to in the remainder of this book.

META-VALIDATED DATA OR INFORMATION

We define *meta-validated data* or *information* as that which has been assessed for relevance and scientific soundness by at least two independent panels of qualified experts, each possibly using different methods. For example, the editorial peer review process is often accepted as an initial validation review. Because the editorial peer review may be rather subjective, it is necessary to have a second, more systematic, assessment to determine if the project methods meet explicitly defined criteria customized to its research design and model.

CAUTION

Let us reiterate that the soundness of meta-validated information depends on the process used and the adequacy of documentation of that process in compiling and validating the evidence. As a consumer of scientific data, you must be sure to check for these prerequisites. (In Chapter 9, Appendix 9.1, we review evolving validation criteria developed between 1977 and 1999 for this purpose.)

Meta-Validated Systematic Reviews

This source has the highest potential for producing sound data from valid research studies. The term *systematic* refers to reviews following a rigorous protocol for planning, database development, data validation, synthesis, and write-up. However, their most distinguishing characteristic is the thoroughness of their review methods' documentation, just as with any scientific study.

Perhaps the most valuable type of information synthesis is a quantitative review. Meta-analysis is an example of this type. The main advantage of this form of review is that it has the potential to provide empirical data and information of the highest relevance and validity. Of course, this assumes that the authors are experienced and follow the principles that we and many others are trying to popularize as perhaps the most bias-free source of new knowledge. Moreover, this information, being developed in the computer age, is becoming more accessible than most traditional paper-based publications because it is often available electronically.

A serious disadvantage of online systematic reviews is that many of these syntheses are only available for a fee, for subscribing to the journal where they are published, or for being licensed as a dues-paying member of a bibliographic databank group. Consequently, reviewers may not have direct access to these most valuable electronic sources, the *British Medical Journal* being a notable exception. Another disadvantage is that, as yet, computerized content coverage is relatively small. However, the number of centers producing systematic reviews is growing rapidly, so this problem will be diminishing. This is illustrated by the worldwide network of the Cochrane Collaboration, which is not for profit and is developing information syntheses in many different nations. The new jargon they are using not only is helpful but is becoming popular internationally. For instance, such terms as *evidence based, best evidence,* or *systematic reviews* will likely become part of mainstream health services research language.

Meta-Validated Nonsystematic Reviews

Next, in order of potential value, are 'meta-validated' nonsystematic sources of clinically applicable information. Documents in these sources are usually read and interpreted by two or more individuals and reported in narrative form. Blue-ribbon panel reports, special commission reports, and consensus statements may be at this level of soundness.

Perhaps one of the better example of this type of meta-validated source is the U.S. National Institutes of Health (NIH) Consensus Development Program, whose Web address as of March 2000 is (last updated December 1999) odp.od.nih.gov/consensus/.

NOTE

NIH consensus statements, now termed "State of the Science Statements," are "systematic" in the sense that they follow a uniform protocol. Each statement usually has a brief note that states,

> Many State of the Science Conferences and Workshops adhere to the NIH Consensus Development Conference (CDC) format because the process is useful for evaluating complex issues. In the CDC format, NIH State of the Science Statements are prepared by a non advocate, non-Federal panel of experts, based on: (1) presentations by investigators working in areas relevant to the consensus questions typically during a 1-1/2-day public session; (2) questions and statements from conference attendees during open discussion periods that are part of the public session, and (3) closed deliberations by the panel during the remainder of the second day and morning of the third. Each statement is an independent report of the panel and is not a policy statement of the NIH or the Federal Government.

This quote may be found at the following Internet address (last updated ??, as checked in September 2001): odp.od.nih.gov/consensus/ta/talist.htm.

Such a statement is not the same as the detailed methods documentation of what we refer to as an information synthesis or systematic review. For example, to our knowledge, the NIH does not provide detailed documentation of the process used to select each specific panel, specify if or how explicit criteria are used, systematically validate each paper presented to the consensus panel, or document the type of synthesis process applied, especially in the closed sessions. We suspect it is likely by "open-interactive" discussion following presentations. Furthermore, the NIH does not state the level of consensus achieved other than by a "minority report" if there was serious controversy on a topic. On the other hand, with its extensive experience with consensus conferences, there may be solid reasons for its policies. Its products, nevertheless, are likely among the more authoritative available.

This is not to detract from the major value these much-needed consensus statements contribute to the scientific and clinical practice community. We rate them second highest in our hierarchy of seven value levels. We recommend that you routinely check the NIH index of such statements when you develop a mini-synthesis or are launching a major information synthesis. Its Internet address as of September 2001 (last updated ??) is odp.od.nih.gov/consensus/cons/cons.htm.

This index lists 110 consensus statements, developed since their first consensus program in 1977. The materials are indexed by subject and date. For example, clicking on the subject index listing of "Mental Health" yields 9 consensus statements. The most recent is one titled "Diagnosis and Treatment of Attention Deficit Hyperactivity Disorder, November 16-18, 1998." The documents can be downloaded to a computer file or to a printer.

Another example of nonsystematic, meta-validated reviews is the Lange Medical Series, now published by McGraw-Hill. Their expert panels update their assigned chapters once a year. This meta-validated information is published in narrative form, in categories most relevant to clinical use. For example, their *Current Medical Diagnosis and Treatment* is a classic (Tierney, McPhee, & Papadakis, 1999).

Finally, the nursing profession would value the Virginia Henderson International Library of the Nursing Honor Society of Sigma Theta Tau. This group is developing many sources of meta-validated nursing literature, called "knowledge bases." Its home page URL (last updated ??, as checked September 2001) is www. Nursingsociety.org.

There are numerous other publishers of such meta-validated material. The Yearbook series, the *Scientific American Review of Medicine,* or any of the many review journals and yearly review publications on all topics are all acceptable sources of meta-validated research articles and other information. Traditional health professional textbooks are also in this class. Although encyclopedic in coverage, their slant is usually so basic as to make them most valuable for students of the health professions and possibly for practitioners who need a basic review for Board examinations, as but one example.

Finally, the U.S. National Library of Medicine MeSH term "Review Literature" can be used to browse for reviews. Using this descriptor and the operator AND, together with the MeSH heading for your topic, should yield many reviews that might be at any level of soundness. However, this is a rather inefficient approach for identifying nonsystematic meta-validated reviews because, at present, most traditional reviews are not likely to be validated.

An advantage of meta-validated nonsystematic reviews is that their reference lists will most likely provide sound leads to valuable research reports. If you are conducting either a mini-synthesis or a thorough 'systematic synthesis,' these leads are important. Furthermore, you might check other citations by the same author of the meta-validated investigation for other studies that might be of similar quality.

Another advantage of these meta-validated nonsystematic materials over systematic reviews is the fact that they have such broad content coverage. This is due, in part, to the fact that this approach has been used for so many years in the past. Indeed, this is the modality that most clinicians and researchers in medicine know. (It is hoped that this will be changing as these professionals realize that a review must be conducted with the same rigor and documented with the same detail as any scientific study.) Also an advantage is that renowned university scientists often write them. You can at least know that their writings represent current academic thinking. These reviews are usually updated on a regular basis (e.g., the Lange series is revised every year) or augmented when new knowledge is established (e.g., NIH augments its consensus statements whenever it seems warranted).

A disadvantage of meta-validated nonsystematic reviews is that **structured group judgment techniques** may not have been used when synthesizing new research information. The synthesis process is usually "open-interactive" discussion and therefore susceptible to group bias. How often did the person with the highest reputation have his or her way based on authoritarianism rather than objective consensus of the group? Another disadvantage is that the cycle of updating (e.g., textbooks) can be as long as 5 to 10 years.

Meta-Validated Individual Research Reports

Next in potential value are individual meta-validated articles presented whole or in abstract form. These materials can be quite useful because teams of experts have already determined their relevance, validity, and often their maturity for immediate clinical practice. One of the better examples that meet most of the above criteria is the American College of Physicians' publication, *ACP Journal Club*. This review journal consists mainly of one-page abstracts of important articles that have been rigorously assessed for the methods' validity and **information maturity** (i.e., readiness for use in the community). Numerous publishers have "Advances in . . ." series of complete research reports that are considered of importance by the editors, however weak, biased, or strong their editorial selection process may be. Again, it is important to contact these publishers to learn about their editorial policy and assessment procedures regarding how they determine the relevance, validity, and maturity of the information they disseminate.

An advantage of individual meta-validated research reports is that their reference lists will most likely provide sound leads to other valuable investigations. If you are conducting a thorough systematic synthesis, these leads are important. Furthermore, you might check other citations by the same author of the meta-validated investigation for more of his or her studies that may be of similar quality.

A disadvantage of an individual meta-validated study is that, although the study itself may be sound, the cited references may or may not be valid. Only if the evaluator states that he or she formally assessed each reference for methodological soundness can you be sure. Often, you can have confidence that cited information is sound based on the reputation and judgment of the authors. However, these implicit inferences of validity may not stand up to formal scrutiny. Another disadvantage of reports at this level is the fact that you may have to screen numerous articles to find a meta-validated or quantitative report on your topic.

Direct Contact With Experts in Your Topic Field

This source of information is only as good as the knowledge and judgment of the experts you contact. However, although not meta-validated, their leads will probably be more relevant and sound than most bibliographic databanks. One of the reasons for this is the fact that they can have a brief dialogue with you to understand what you actually need before making suggestions.

The main advantage of direct contact with experts is that, based on their long experience with your topic field, they might be one of your best leads to identify Level 1 and Level 2 reviews. Furthermore, they provide two filters: one for relevance to your described needs and one for scientific soundness, based on their judgment and familiarity with individual research studies in their field. Their references to other colleagues who specialize in your topic area can be invaluable. Furthermore, they will usually tell you if they are not sure about the relevance or validity of some citations of which they are aware.

The disadvantage of individual experts is much like that described above for meta-validated single articles. In other words, experts' judgments may vary, and to some extent you must take what they say on faith. If you do not have any information about the individual's background other than that he or she wrote a relevant article on your topic, you might need to check with others before making such a contact, so you do not discover later that this person was really a "self-proclaimed" expert. You need to be cautious in accepting his or her suggestions.

Non-Meta-Validated Traditional Reviews

Most reviews you will find in the literature are the product of one or more authors who provide a descriptive analysis of relevant information they have identified and synthesized. For example, use of the MeSH heading "Review Literature" in a MEDLINE search will likely yield this type of traditional **narrative synthesis**.

The advantage of these traditional reviews is the fact that their content coverage is largely based on the many decades during which they were produced. As qualitative reviews, they might provide new and valuable insights on your subject. Equally valuable are their reference lists that might lead to new meta-validated material you have missed. Terms such as *validated review or authoritative review* or reviews by authors of other "systematic reviews" might be valuable leads from this level.

The disadvantage of these traditional reviews is their lack of methods documentation. This requires that you contact the author(s) to find out exactly how the review was compiled. This interview may prove embarrassing to both of you if the authors perceive your detailed questions to be arrogant or if the authors start to realize what an inadequate review they actually did. In such a case, the reference list of the study report may be misleading. Even worse, you may discover that the citation of an article with an exciting title turns out to be in a "science propaganda" publication. (We came across a journal of health science reviews in which every paper referred to a product the publisher was marketing.)

Non-Meta-Validated
Bibliographic Databanks or Reference Lists

Suppose your goal is not a mini-synthesis, and you have screened most information at validity Levels 1 to 5 and found very little on your topic. Your next fallback search strategy might be to browse online bibliographic databanks and retrieve printed bibliographies from research reviews and reports at any level of soundness.

One of the richest sources in this category is a "bibliography of bibliographies."

BIBLIOGRAPHY OF BIBLIOGRAPHIES

This term refers to a bibliography that only reports other bibliographies or databases on a given topic. This source can be in either electronic or paper form. These materials are often compiled and updated by medical historians in that subject area. Unfortunately, we could find no medical subject heading (MeSH) descriptor for this concept (bibliography of bibliographies) as of January 25, 2000. NLM usually uses the term *databases* or *databanks* to refer to such material. There are MeSH headings that are close: "Bibliography"; "Bibliography (PT)"; "Bibliography, Medicine"; "Bibliography, National"; "Bibliography, Statistical"; "Bibliography, Descriptive"; "Bibliometrics"; "Biobibliographies"; "Databases, Bibliographic"; and "Documentation."

An early example of a "bibliography of bibliographies" was published in the book *Improving Medical Practice and Health Care: A Bibliographic Guide to Information Management in Quality Assurance and Continuing Education* (Williamson, 1977). This "bibliography of bibliographies" lists 260 individual bibliographies from the late 1960s to the mid-1970s, including 48 annotated bibliographies (the latter encompassing nearly 1,000 articles on the subject of healthcare quality).

Current examples of some of the better electronic "bibliography of bibliographies" are the NLM, ELHILL®, and TOXNET® databanks. These cover more than 40 online databases containing about 18 million references. These could be termed "an index of databanks" or a "list of databanks." The main point, however, is that there are numerous organizations developing these lists. As of May 2001, one such NLM Web site (last updated August 17, 2001) is www.nlm.nih.gov/databases/databases.html.

In this source, "NLM provides a wide variety of resources related to the biomedical and health sciences, both past and present. The format of these resources varies: searchable databases & databanks, bibliographic citations, full text (when available), archival collections, and images."

NLM also has a "Databases & Electronic Information Sources" site that provides a list of its online databases. The contents can be found at the following Web site (last updated January 2001): www.nlm.nih.gov/databases/databases.html.

When available, these listings are among the most valuable bibliographic sources available. With the explosion of online bibliographic databases and databanks, these bibliography of bibliographies are becoming much more numerous.

Another resource of this type is the NLM Resource Lists and Bibliographies' Current Bibliographies in Medicine (last updated March 2001): www.nlm.nih.gov/pubs/resources.html.

Next in potential value are traditional bibliographies compiled by respected scientists, independent of review articles. They can be found by such means as (a) research registries, (b) pyramid telephone contacts with experts who have written or know of colleagues who have developed such materials, or (c) citations in "editorials" or "letters to the editor" in the area of information science.

Depending on the maturity of your topic's research field, you may or may not find a useful set of references to be screened. Again, the disadvantage of these bibliographies is that they are usually helpful only in terms of content relevance because most articles cited often are not validated. The responsibility will be on your shoulders to decide which references you will include and which you will reject.

While screening bibliographies, if such terms as *systematic reviews, validated reviews,* or *meta-analyses* appear in the citation, you will obviously want to obtain these documents. Usually, however, you might be screening hundreds of irrelevant citations to find those that seem worth checking further.

The advantage of these sources is that, if computerized, you can access substantial material rapidly, especially if available on the Internet. You can also identify investigators and other professionals who know people to contact. Occasionally, you might identify overlooked Level 1 or Level 2 references.

The main disadvantage of these sources is the extensive time and funds required to screen these bibliographies and reference lists. This fact alone precludes their use for mini-synthesis. For screening more thorough systematic reviews, the responsibility, again, will be on your shoulders to decide which of the studies are sufficiently sound to include and which need to be rejected. In addition, such bibliographies often do not have detailed documentation as to which descriptors were used in which databases over what period of time. Lacking such information, relevance of the citations listed may be questionable.

Obtaining such information sources electronically will be discussed in detail in Section E of this chapter, with a compendium at the end of this book.

Non-Meta-Validated Individual Research Reports

In terms of writing a mini-synthesis, this source of information is at "the bottom of the barrel" and likely should not be screened for this purpose. At this level, you will be screening "raw," probably immature, reports of single investigations, both published and unpublished.

The major advantage of this level of information is that it is readily available and useful for clinical and health services researchers and possibly for authors of systematic research reviews such as yourself. Furthermore, at this level, you can readily identify those studies that have received at least the first level of **information validation**—namely, peer review, despite the problems of this evaluation method.

The disadvantages of this level of information are the paradox: Although claiming to be the information with which practitioners should be keeping up, it is, in fact, the very information that clinicians and **quality improvement professionals** should consider avoiding (Haynes, 1990). Practitioners who do not keep up with the quantitative and epidemiological, let alone the clinical, sciences depend on experts in the field of information synthesis to evaluate relevance, validity, and maturity of research data for immediate use in community practice. This book has been written to help meet this urgent need.

Section C. Strategic Search Considerations

This section discusses the theoretical considerations for six search functions of special importance when you implement your synthesis plan: initial database compilation (the mini-synthesis), relevance-code development and evaluation, "invisible college" identification, search documentation, database management, and search termination.

Initial Database Compilation: The Mini-Synthesis

We suggest that in any literature search, your initial function should be to determine whether someone has already completed an acceptable information synthesis on, or close to, your subject. The following description explains how we use the term *mini-synthesis* and the three major reasons for producing this type of brief review.

MINI-SYNTHESIS

A *mini-synthesis* is a brief literature review based on the most readily accessible and scientifically sound information on your topic. Its purpose is threefold: (a) to confirm your team's consensus judgment regarding viability of its highest priority outcomes improvement hypotheses, (b) to provide a quick synthesis of the best evidence available to answer an important question under conditions of severely limited time and fiscal resources, and (c) to provide the initial step in building a database for a more formal systematic review under conditions of more abundant time and money.

For your initial search strategy, we suggest you successively screen the top four levels of our seven-level scale of information soundness. In screening the first and highest level, restrict your search to retrieving only meta-validated information syntheses (e.g., systematic reviews or information syntheses). The following Internet addresses are the same as those in Table 2.1 and illustrate resources where you might get started with this approach.

ILLUSTRATIVE SOURCES OF SYSTEMATIC REVIEWS
(With Internet Site Addresses)

(a) The Cochrane Collaboration Library—United Kingdom:
www.update-software.com/cochrane.htm

(b) Evidence-Based Practice Centers—United States:
www.ahcpr.gov/clinic/epc

(c) Centre for Evidence-Based Medicine—United Kingdom:
cebm.jr2.ox.ac.uk

(d) Thomas C. Chalmers Centre for Systematic Reviews—Canada:
www.cheori.org/tcc/index.htm

(e) Centre for Reviews and Dissemination—United Kingdom:
www.york.ac.uk/inst/crd/welcome.htm

(f) National Guideline Clearinghouse—United States:
www.guideline.gov/body_home_nf.asp?view=home

(g) Health Technology Assessment Programme—United Kingdom:
www.hta.nhsweb.nhs.uk/main.htm

Next, you would search for materials at Level 2, following the same principles as for "systematic reviews," but instead search for meta-validated nonsystematic reviews. A good place to start at this level would be the index for NIH consensus statements, arranged by either subject or date, at the following address (last updated ??, as checked in September 2001): odp.od.nih.gov/consensus/cons/cons.htm.

Then screen Level 3 (meta-validated individual studies). At this point, you are getting down to the "bottom of the barrel" with meta-validated information. As far as we know, the best single source of this material is the *ACP Club*. It is sponsored by the American College of Physicians and the American Society of Internal Medicine. It has explicit criteria for many different research designs that its teams use to validate information. Its results are published as abstracts you can trust. Its Web site, ACP-ASIM Online (last updated May 2001), is www.acponline.org/journals/acpjc/jcmenu.htm?idx.

Finally, search material at Level 4, contacting experts. We understand that many individuals have the expertise and experience to provide trustworthy information. However, one of the pioneers of the Delphi technique, Norman Dalkey, expresses the old adage: "n heads are better than one" (Dalkey, Rourke, Lewis, & Snyder, 1972). This bit of self-evident wisdom seems to apply in this instance. The three levels of meta-validated information mentioned above have been systematically reviewed, using explicit criteria, by two independent groups of experts to arrive at some consensus after studying many articles on their subject. A single expert, using implicit criteria applied in ways we cannot know, may be correct, but you have little confirmation other than taking his or her word on faith. In no way do we want to disparage the soundness of information at this level because it is at this level where nearly all clinical decisions are made. But, for purposes of developing a mini-synthesis or a complete systematic review, you are on safer ground if you first seek well-documented, meta-validated information at Levels 1 through 3.

Relevance-Code Development and Evaluation

Whatever the source of your information, we suggest that it is necessary to systematically code each article for relevance, based on your explicit criteria and denoted by the ABC coding convention referred to in Chapter 3, Table 3.1.

Defining Relevance Coding. This phrase indicates a judgmental process for establishing operational priorities for citations, citation-abstracts, and complete articles.

RELEVANCE CODING

Relevance coding refers to the rating of information priorities according to a standard measurement convention. In this book, we suggest the ABC convention measuring relevance in five levels: A+, A, A–, B, and C. Conceptually, these relevance ratings refer to the priority of each item (e.g., citation-abstract for further processing, such as retrieving and coding their complete documents).

The specific relevance codes for this process are explained in Chapter 3, Table 3.1.

Defining Citation-Abstract Codes. This phrase denotes our coding convention to determine which complete documents will be retrieved. This concept is explained below.

CITATION-ABSTRACT CODES

When coding the initial citation, we encourage you to rate this article title without reference to the abstract. This will permit precision, recall, and interrater **reliability** rates being computed for assessing your skill in rating titles alone. In MEDLINE, more than one in three citations you identify may not have an abstract, thus forcing you to make a relevance judgment based on the title alone. The interrater reliability, precision, and recall of such coding may prove rather poor.

However, if there is an abstract, after coding the title alone, you will next code the title and abstract as one entity. This citation-abstract combined rating of "A" (i.e., A+, A, A–) should represent your best judgment as to whether the complete article or document should be retrieved. (The term *abstract and/or citation* relevance code is a more accurate way of saying the same thing but too awkward for continual use.) However, this code will permit calculation of your team's search interrater reliability and precision but not recall, unless you also retrieve all documents that have a B or C citation-abstract rating.

Defining Formal Relevance Criteria. Developing a formal set of clear relevance criteria is a critical step in ensuring that your search will be thorough and efficient.

FORMAL RELEVANCE CRITERIA

This phrase refers to the specific kinds of information required for purposes of developing an information synthesis. Because many temporary relevance cues will be developed and tested for viability in identifying needed information, those that prove most fruitful are formalized as criteria that will likely be used throughout the rest of the database development stage. Criteria that prove misleading or nonfruitful are discarded.

Without such criteria, much time and effort will be spent weeding out the many "false-positive" citations that your search might otherwise identify. Worse, imprecise criteria can lead to your missing many essential articles required for establishing a balanced, representative database. Including your relevance criteria in the final report of your information synthesis provides an essential documentation item to which most reviewers and readers will frequently refer. This information gives other researchers a clear picture of your search scope and will help them evaluate, update, or even replicate your project.

Developing Formal Relevance Criteria. In Chapter 3, we described relevance cue logs (Form 3.5 shows only one of five levels, i.e., A+) as the mechanism we recommend to identify formal relevance criteria. During the early database development process, you will be constantly noting potential clues such as new key words, journals, authors, descriptors, or research institutions. These terms can then be used in a search to determine their yield in relevant research studies required for your synthesis. Most may prove unproductive, but many will lead to the material you need. In other words, the relevance cues are the denominator from which the numerator of formal relevance criteria is abstracted.

Evaluating Search Precision and Recall. A major advantage of the ABC relevance-coding convention is that it facilitates assessment of your **search precision** and search **recall**.

SEARCH PRECISION AND RECALL

Precision, in terms of a literature search, indicates the proportion of citations, abstracts, or complete documents that you code "A" (A+, A, or A–) that subsequently prove to be relevant at that same level. In other words, precision is the extent to which you avoid false-positive relevance ratings. This rate is equal to the positive predictive value and is important to the efficiency of your search.

Recall is the proportion of citations, abstracts, or documents in the universe of citations that your search encompassed, which are, by the gold standard, actually "A" (A+, A, or A–) and which you coded at that level of relevance. In other words, recall is the extent to which you avoid false-negative relevance ratings. This rate is equal to sensitivity and is important to the **effectiveness** of your search.

Operationally, you can crudely measure the precision and recall of your citation coding only for those references that have abstracts. (Note that citation coding is different from citation-abstract coding.) To measure precision, you use the abstract rating as a gold standard, however mediocre. Subsequently, you can estimate how many

"A" (A+, A, and A–) citations are associated with abstracts that are also rated at the "A" level of relevance. Those high-relevance rated citations (i.e., coded "A") for which, after reading the abstract, you rate the citation-abstract at a low relevance level (i.e., B or C) would be the equivalent of false positives. Likewise, to measure recall, you would determine the proportion of all those citation-abstracts you coded "A" (A+, A, or A–) that are associated with citations alone that were originally coded at that high level of relevance. Those citation-abstracts coded "A" (A+, A, and A–) that had an original citation rating of B or C would be the equivalent of false negatives.

These false-positive and false-negative citation coding rates are important because they provide a crude self-calibration of how well you relevance-code the citations alone. This will help you improve the balance of precision and recall rates that you judge optimum. Because, in the future, you will be coding so many citations having no available abstracts, this evaluation should prove valuable.

On the other hand, in evaluating for your citation-abstract relevance codes, you can calculate precision rates but not recall rates. In this case, the complete document relevance rates provide the gold standard for evaluating your citation-abstract coding precision because you can distinguish true positives from false positives. However, this only helps you save resources by reducing false-positive document retrievals. Conversely, it your precision rates are above, say, 85% to 95%, you must be concerned about missing many important documents that are false negatives. To cope with this hazard, we recommend that periodically you select a sample of citation-abstracts, then retrieve and relevance-code all complete documents in the sample. Then you can compare the proportion of "A" complete documents, with a citation-abstract previously coded as "A," to calculate recall rates to determine whether they are too low (e.g., below 65% to 75%).

"Invisible College" Identification

Russett Factor Analysis Technique. One of the earliest methods for identifying citation patterns was that of Russett (1968, pp. 7-8), as quoted by Crane (1972, p. 82). Russett's approach is a **factor analysis technique** or, in more recent jargon, a "Q-sort" method. Although his subject focus was political science, his methods are applicable to the medical or health sciences. A complex quote from his work is shown as follows:

> By factoring the matrix where citers are considered as variables and the authors cited as observations, the resulting factors identify groups of scholars who make similar choices, people who tend to read and absorb the same kind of materials.

Each citer has a loading, or correlation, with each of the major factors. The squared loading indicates the percentage of the variance (variation) in the chooser's pattern of citations that can be explained by the factor. Once we have identified the factors as groupings of choosers, it is then possible to compute factor scores to see what sources the members of a particular group commonly use. Thus each man cited has a factor score for each factor, indicating the relative contribution his materials make to the "typical" citer in the group. (Russett, 1968)

In simpler terms, Russett is indicating that clusters of investigators can be identified in any literature that seem to have a common conceptual approach or, volume-wise, make a greater or lesser contribution to the total literature. These clusters of investigators often cite the same articles for praise or for less positive comments. This latter group may represent researchers from a competing "college" that might be worth your checking.

Contingency Table Technique. The approach required to identify these "colleges" usually involves an analysis of your database of complete articles. This analysis might be a Q-sort, as used by Russett (1968), or may use a **contingency table** where the x-axis lists the same names of independent authors (in your database) as the y-axis. The intersects (cells) of this table reveal potentially common links in terms of either coauthoring or citing each other. This is another means to identify and code unique groups of researchers that might constitute different "colleges." Finally, it is helpful to contact key researchers of each "college" to identify other members of their same "college" or to obtain referrals to unrelated "colleges" of investigators interested in your topic. These professionals are also excellent sources of leads to the "fugitive literature" (i.e., published or unpublished research reports that are usually very difficult to identify and retrieve).

Pattern Analysis Technique. More crudely, invisible colleges can be discerned by briefly analyzing the references in your retrieved articles for patterns of authors. You can also identify clues to invisible colleges by referring to such sources as editorials and letters to the editor, in which researchers are quoted who disagree with the findings of specified studies. Retrieving the complete documents for such citations might help identify additional invisible colleges whose research findings might contradict those you have compiled to date.

The invisible colleges concept is useful as a framework around which you can build your information search. Identifying a representative group of unique invisible colleges of investigators is a useful means to help ensure that your "synthesis database" will be balanced and represent the differing research viewpoints on your topic.

Search Documentation

Any literature search should be sufficiently documented to (a) allow for evaluation of your manuscript, especially for publication; (b) facilitate future updating of your synthesis with a minimum of unnecessary overlap; and (c) ideally, facilitate replication of your work by independent investigators. Such documentation requires detailed records of the information sources you screened, the key words and **index terms** you included, and the search parameters applied (e.g., the time period covered and the languages included). Because of the space limitations imposed by most journals, you may not be able to include comprehensive documentation of the search methods used in the text of your manuscript. However, using appendixes or providing a footnote that such documentation is available from the author on request ensures that others can access such basic methods information. Of course, if you are publishing your synthesis as a book, or if it is designed to be an unpublished document for organizational use, all search documentation should be included in the final manuscript.

Database Management

As you locate relevant citations and references, you will need a place to record and file them. Thus, another tool to develop during your information search is a citation-abstract master list, which will provide a central place to record all relevance and validation ratings for each citation and its complete abstract if retrieved. The master list can also facilitate checking the retrieval status of each citation: (a) whether the article was located, coded, and retrieved; (b) whether the retrieval is still in process (e.g., pending interlibrary loan request); (c) whether the article was never located due to lack of search time; or (d) whether the article was not located despite a thorough retrieval effort (e.g., out of print).

Your master list may be compiled as a citation log or on traditional library index cards. In our judgment, by far the most efficient and powerful means for this purpose is through use of computerized bibliographic database management software, such as ProCite® (by Personal Bibliographic Software, Inc.), described below. This software allows direct downloading of all citation-abstracts into your file, automatic chronological enumeration of your citation entries, and automated revision of your citation style to meet different publishers' requirements.

PROCITE DESCRIPTION

ProCite is a bibliographic generator and general reference organizer to help archive Net references and other online documents. With the BiblioLink function, you can import records from hundreds of online, CD-ROM, and Internet-based services, saving time and effort while gathering information. Digital bibliographic management software has many advantages. For example, as you download each citation, these programs can automatically check for duplicate citations entered earlier. This feature ensures that each citation in your master list is unique. If desired, these software programs also allow adding codes indicating relevance of each complete document for topics not related to your current synthesis but that might be of substantial value for your other projects.

The home page for the ProCite product can be accessed through (last updated ??, copyright 2001) www.procite.com/pchome.asp.

By using related software (we use BiblioLinks®, by Personal Bibliographic Software, Inc.), the full search results can be downloaded from an electronic database to your personal file. However, additional citations (such as reference lists from retrieved articles or formal printed bibliographies) may have to be scanned in or hand-entered from a text file. In either of the latter input methods, careful checking for errors is essential.

It is possible to have ProCite automatically assign chronological numbers for each citation as it is downloaded (or entered by other means). These numbers can then be used as identifiers when searching your personal electronic information database. The listings can be formatted for instant retrieval by any of several means (i.e., by identifier number, author, title, relevance code, validity code, or free text).

Search Termination

The last task of Stage II database development is making the decision to terminate your information search. We present several theoretical issues that you might consider. Recall that the final decision to terminate your search may not be possible until later in Stage III, after effect sizes and validity ratings for each study are recorded. However, because Stages II and III usually proceed concomitantly, it may be possible during your search to make preliminary "file drawer" estimates (i.e., the number of articles with null results needed to alter your conclusions) (see Table 6.1, Procedure D, Chapter 6). Furthermore, the evaluation of your information database (see Chapter 7) may necessitate an augmented search if it reveals problems or serious omissions.

No matter when you decide to terminate your search, however, several important issues must be kept in mind. Obviously, you must balance the effects of continuing your search too long (wasting time and dollars) or stopping your search too soon (losing essential articles contradicting your conclusions that might otherwise be retrieved). In reality, however, continuing a search for too long is an error few researchers make because they seldom have the time or resources to conduct even an adequate search, let alone one that is inappropriately long. One means to determine whether your searching efforts have continued too long is by examining the number of new relevant articles that are being identified as you proceed with the search. Once your searching efforts fail to identify many new articles, or your file drawer analysis indicates it would require a large number of additional articles to overturn your tentative conclusions, you can reasonably terminate your information search.

Section D. Generic Sources of Health Science Information

In this section, we discuss the major generic information sources that you might consider when planning a database search.

Whether you choose to include all of these categories in your search effort will depend on your goals and budget. However, we urge you to include, in priority order, as many of these categories as your resources allow. Keep in mind that the more diversified the generic categories you search, the more representative and comprehensive will be your final database.

(As a memory aid, Table 5.1 provides a more detailed checklist of the above five generic reference sources that should be considered in building any database.)

Computerized Sources

From our above discussion on search strategy, it is clear that we judge computerized sources to be the best way to start your synthesis database development. The main drawback at present is that much, if not most, full-text information is still on paper, usually in medical libraries. On the other hand, PubMed of the U.S. National Library of Medicine now links to nearly 2,000 online medical journals (as of May 2001) that provide recent full-text articles electronically.

Your first effort should be to determine whether anyone has already produced a systematic review on your topic. Also, this preliminary search will provide an information background to facilitate your asking more cogent questions and talking more knowledgeably with experts when you are ready to consult 'people sources.'

The following are some fundamentals we will briefly review. Those experienced with searching the Internet should move on to the second source, people sources.

The Internet. The Internet provides a major computerized means of finding research data and information. The **World Wide Web** (WWW) is that part of the Internet that gained fame by use of a graphical user interface (GUI) with its hypertext access-

---

TABLE 5.1 Checklist of Generic Reference Sources

Computerized sources

  Electronic catalogs in libraries
  Internet
  Online search engines
  Electronic bibliographic databanks
  Online research registers
  Online journals and monographs
  CD–ROMs

People sources

  Domain specialists
  Medical librarians
  Authors of reviews (especially systematic)
  Science writers for the lay public
  Editors and publishers

Research funding sources

  Government agencies
  Private philanthropies and endowment funds
  Disease-specific fund-raising groups
  Pharmaceutical corporations

Nonfunding organization sources

  Professional societies
  Research institutes
  Private interest groups
  Corporations related to healthcare

Paper sources

  Published and printed indexes
  Published bibliographies
  Bibliography of bibliographies
  References in major references
  Printed information source catalogues
  Hard copy "fugitive literature"

---

ing format and its colorful displays on each Web site. Clearly, developing information syntheses is not a cost-effective activity if you do not have access to the Internet. Even then, many Web sites require a license for which you must pay each year. Some rather costly search engines provide access to multiple sites, each of which you would otherwise have to pay to access.

The advantage of these Web sites is that they can be accessed far more rapidly than it takes to go to the library to spend countless hours looking up a few reference leads. However, a disadvantage is that the number of such online sources for accessing complete journal articles and books is, as yet, somewhat limited, despite the fact that there are more than 500 medical serials online, with the list growing exponentially.

Online Search Engines. The first question you may ask is the following: What is a search engine? In their recent book on this subject, Glossbrenner and Glossbrenner (1999) state,

> A search engine is a tool that lets you explore databases containing the text from tens of millions of Web pages. When the search engine software finds pages that match your search request (often referred to as hits), it presents them to you with brief descriptions and clickable links to take you there.
>
> Some search engines, like AltaVista concentrate primarily on providing a powerful search capability. But the best search sites (AltaVista included) also offer a multi-level topic directory that you can browse for information on a given subject. (p. 5)

There are numerous online search engines on the Internet, particularly on the Web. A few of the more popular ones include AltaVista, Argus Clearinghouse, Deja News, Excite, HotBot, Infoseek, InfoSpace Liszt, Lycos, Yahoo, and Zip2 Yellow (see Glossbrenner & Glossbrenner, 1999, Appendix A, pp. 233-248 for details on each).

To illustrate this crucial tool for online searching, we describe two NLM search engines—namely, Gateway and PubMed.

Gateway is one of the most useful "smart" search engines for searching many of MEDLARS® multiple databanks. To quote from their Web site (updated June 2000):

> The NLM Gateway allows users to search in multiple retrieval systems at the U.S. National Library of Medicine (NLM). The current Gateway searches MEDLINE/PubMed, OLDMEDLINE, LOCATOR*plus*, MEDLINE*plus*, DIRLINE, AIDS Meetings, Health Services Research Meetings, Space Life Sciences Meetings, and HSRProj.

This quote can be found at the following Web site (last updated September 2001): http://gateway.nlm.nih.gov/gw/Cmd?GMBasicSearch.

PubMed is another search engine that allows free access to MEDLINE and other NLM databanks. To quote from the "PubMed Overview" (updated December 2, 1999),

> PubMed provides access to bibliographic information which is drawn primarily from MEDLINE, PreMEDLINE, HealthSTAR, as well as from publisher supplied citations. In addition, electronically supplied journals that are indexed selectively for MEDLINE include articles unrelated to medicine or the life sciences. Medline covers over 4000 biomedical journals published in over 70 countries. PubMed also provides access and links to the integrated molecular biology databases included in NCBI's Entrez retrieval system.

The Web site for this reference (last updated April 2001) is www.ncbi.nlm. nih.gov:80/entrez/query/static/overview.html. An advantage of PubMed is its growing linkage to nearly 400 publishers' online material (as of September 2001), including more than 2,142 electronic medical journals. The only problem is that user registration, a subscription fee, or some other type of charge may be required to access the full text of articles in some of these journals. On the other hand, at least one study indicates that (in 1994) the sensitivity (recall) and precision of the MEDLINE search engine may be questionable. Dickersin, Scherer, and Lefebvre (1994) studied the MEDLINE search engine in relation to finding known RCTs (known from other sources) in ophthalmology. They measured weighted means for precision in three studies, finding 51%, 77%, and 63%, respectively. The weighted mean for sensitivity was 8% (median 32.5%). There have since been many similar studies on many different topics, such as Adams et al. (1994). This would be an excellent topic for a systematic review of the precision and recall of similar search engines.

Electronic Bibliographic Databanks. Most libraries provide computer access to their in-house catalog of resources. However, the Internet provides international coverage. The U.S. National Library of Medicine has one of the earliest and most comprehensive bibliographic sources. Its overall system is known as MEDLARS® (Medical Literature Analysis and Retrieval System). MEDLARS comprises two major computer subsystems, ELHILL® and TOXNET®, encompassing more than 40 online databases containing about 18 million references. To access these resources without charge, link directly to the following Web address (last updated January 2001): www.nlm.nih.gov/databases/databases.html.

A major limitation of MEDLINE is that it does not include books, monographs, audiovisuals, journals, and other important reports in the NLM collection. To locate these, you must use the LOCATOR*plus* database at the following Web site (last updated ??): locatorplus.gov/.

Online Research Registers. Registers are another important and frequently updated source of research information. One of the more thorough discussions of this topic is by Dickersin (1994), who states that "all research registers of which this author [Dickersin] is aware concentrate, to a large extent, on 'prospective' registration of research at the time a project is initiated" (p. 72). We readily agree with this definition but would allow for databases of ongoing or recently completed research projects on a specific topic. As Dickersin points out, such registries are among the few resources that can help us manage publication bias. However, it is difficult to estimate what proportion of those research projects that are conducted have been actually registered. In other words, we judge that registers probably have high precision but questionable or low recall. An interesting article by Bickell and Chassin (2000) measured the sensitivity and specificity of three teaching hospital breast cancer registries. The gold standard was a quality improvement project that identified breast cancer patients in those hospitals from multiple sources. Sensitivity and specificity were in the mid-90% range. However, for follow-up of outpatients receiving radiation therapy, the gold standard identified 80% versus the 48% that the tumor registry identified. Likewise, for receipt of adjuvant systemic treatment, the rates were 78% versus 22%, respectively. Consequently, we would judge that registers are certainly necessary but far from sufficient for data collection purposes. Again, numerous studies on this topic could provide material for a systematic review of the quality of data in research registries.

The Cochrane Controlled Trials Register (1997) is among the most thorough sources for tracking RCTs. As of September 15, 2001, it listed 311,022 independent trials. This database is accessible by contacting the Cochrane Library. Its Web site (last updated ??) is hiru.mcmaster.ca/cochrane; the Library button or www.update-software.com/cochrane/.

The National Research Register (NRR) (United Kingdom) is sponsored by the National Health Service (NHS) and made accessible by Update Software, Inc. (London and San Diego). This source includes ongoing and recently completed research projects funded by, or of interest to, the United Kingdom's NHS. As of May 2001, it had more than 53,042 complete research projects in its database and 19,667 ongoing project listed. It states that its purpose is to

> identify unpublished research, particularly important to systematic reviewers of research;
>
> provide early warning on research that may lead to important research findings;
>
> improve the uptake and participation in clinical trails;
>
> identify and bring together researchers between and across related areas of research;

help avoid unnecessary duplication in research—a waste of resources as well
as potentially unethical. Records held on the NRR can include details
on the research title, research question, methodology, sample group,
outcome measures, and research project contacts.

The Web site to its home page, with Update Software linkage to product information for the above quote, as well as linkage to "Access NRR Online" to view its sub-
sidiary sites shown below (last updated 2001), is www.update-software.com/
National/nrr-frame.html.

The Register of Research Registers is a 'meta-register' sponsored by the Department of Health of the National Health Service in the United Kingdom and is
included in the NRR database. As of May 2001, it listed 69 different registries of
clinical trials worldwide. This is one of the best sites to contact regularly to keep up
with the growing number of registries in the healthcare research field.

The Register of Reviews in Progress is another registry included in the National Research Register's database. As of May 2001, it listed 318 reviews that are
ongoing.

The *meta*Register of Controlled Trials (*m*RCT) is another Web-based register of
registers, sponsored by Current Controlled Trials, Ltd., which is part of the Current
Science Group. Following a simple registration process, you can access its information free of charge. You can link to 20 healthcare-related registers encompassing
6,441 trials (as of May 2001), and the list will be growing. For example, they recently
added the U.S. Department of Veterans Affairs Cooperative Studies Program. Its
Web page can be accessed by linking through the home page of Current Controlled
Trials, Ltd. (last updated ??) at www.controlled-trials.com/home_page.cfm.

Cochrane CENTRAL Controlled Clinical Trials Register (CENTRAL/CCTR)
(United Kingdom) is one of the most complete sources of information for quantitative syntheses of which we are aware. It currently lists 307,870 references for CRTs.
If you are a subscriber to the Cochrane Collaboration, this Web site can be accessed
by clicking on its home page Cochrane Library link. After you sign in, all of its databases, including this one, are then available. The Web address of its home page (last
updated May 2001) is www.cochrane.org.

Health Services Research Projects in Progress (HSRPROJ) (United States) is one
of the more relevant registers sponsored by the U.S. Agency for Healthcare Research
and Quality. "[HSRPROJ] contains descriptions of research in progress funded by
federal and private grants and contracts for use by policy makers, managers, clinicians and other decision makers. It provides access to information about health services research in progress before results are available in a published form." The reference for this quote and access to HSRPROJ can be found (last updated December
1998) at www.nlm.nih.gov/pubs/factsheets/hsrproj.html. NLM Research Programs
is a Web site for linking to the various research centers where additional relevant

(with the possible exception of the Computational Molecular Biology databases) registries can be identified (last updated March 2000). Its Web site can be found at www.nlm.nih.gov/resprog.html.

Sigma Theta Tau Registry of Nursing Research (RNR) (United States) is a useful location for finding relevant nursing studies. It has a complete search engine and multiple links. Its headquarters is in Indianapolis, Indiana (www.stti.iupui.edu/library/).

Online Journals and Monographs. As of May 2001, the National Library of Medicine has listed more than 1,888 medical journals, which have at least one link to MEDLINE. Some (e.g., *British Medical Journal* [*BMJ*]) provide free access to all of their materials; others (e.g., *New England Journal of Medicine* [*NEJM*]) require that you subscribe to their journal to have access to their online version. Most of these have tables, color graphics, and color photographs included. When addressing their home page, many have easy-to-use indexing to all volumes back to the time they came online. (For most, this is middle to late 1990s.) The Web site (last updated May 2001) for the NLM list of online journals, which includes each year online, is www.ncbi.nlm.nih.gov/entrez/journals/loftext_prov.html.

A major advantage and a unique feature of many of these online journals are that, with the full-text article, they include references (often linked to MEDLINE or to a full online journal article), editorials, letters to the editor, authors' replies, references to other authors who have cited the paper, and augmentation (e.g., errata or updates that seem important) from MEDLINE and other journals that the publisher screened.

The main disadvantage of this technology at the present time is its limited subject coverage as of today (May 2001). However, we predict that within the next two decades, journals or even monographs published on paper will become a relic of a bygone era. Another major disadvantage is cost. Very few offer free access as the *British Medical Journal* does. To access most of these requires that you have a subscription to their paper copy or have purchased a site license, which lets you browse that journal.

CD-ROMs. CD-ROM databases can be purchased from numerous vendors and are often available at your local medical library at no cost. Once purchased, they can be used for many hundreds of searches without the fees charged by many online sources. Because the disk vendors often make this resource very expensive, individual ownership is usually not feasible. The disadvantage of CD-ROMs, other than cost, is that they are updated less frequently than online sources (sometimes only once every 6 months), so they may not include the more recent articles published during that time.

People Sources

This source of information can be thought of as databases "in people's heads." There are numerous methods for identifying individuals to contact by phone, e-mail, or in person. The following provides a few general considerations in exploring this highly valuable source of information that can be applicable to your synthesis topic.

Domain Specialists. Clinical content experts on your topic can be of substantial help in providing ideas of where to begin your search. They can give names of other experts in the field (i.e., members of their own or other "invisible colleges") and leading research programs to explore. Perhaps more important, they can point to scientifically sound information, a service that standard bibliographic indexes often cannot provide. Likewise, they can be valuable in providing leads to elusive "fugitive literature" (M. C. Rosenthal, 1994).

Medical Librarians. Your local medical librarian is another important "people source" of information. Because the available sources of information and the means to access them are constantly changing, you need a way to find the latest data. Medical librarians keep up with such changes and will be able to assist you in locating experts, searching databases, and retrieving citations. In addition, they can identify "meta-references," "lists of lists," or "bibliographies of bibliographies." These rich sources of information can save you considerable time if a large data set on a given topic has already been compiled. The following Web site can get you started by providing worldwide online linkage to medical libraries (last updated April 2000): www.lib.uiowa.edu/hardin-www/hslibs.html.

Librarians with special training and experience in health information sciences and informatics can be identified among the participants in the Area Health Education Center (AHEC) & Outreach Programs' *Health Sciences Library Directory.* The fourth edition was compiled by the Georgia Statewide AHEC Network in December 1988. You can contact your local medical librarians for more recent information about this program and those who participated in or were trained by this program.

Other Experts. You might contact authors of systematic and other types of reviews, synthesis methods specialists, science writers, editors, and publishers.

In screening "people sources," especially research professionals, it is important not to rely solely on any one group of experts. Keep in mind that members of a given invisible college will share similar perspectives and will likely refer you to their respected colleagues, usually in the same "college"; thus, you should try to locate experts from a variety of invisible colleges. One beginning approach is to ask everyone you contact if there are other researchers who disagree with their methods and/or results. Describing these differing points of view can be an important contribution to the thoroughness of your final synthesis.

Research Funding Sources

Research funding groups are good sources of information about proposed projects, as well as projects in progress and those that have been completed or published. Examples of these groups are government agencies such as the National Institutes of Health (NIH) or the Agency for Healthcare Research and Quality (AHRQ); private philanthropies such as the Robert Wood Johnson Foundation or the Henry J. Kaiser Family Foundation; corporations such as Abbott Pharmaceuticals; disease-specific groups (often of consumers) that raise research funds, such as the Muscular Dystrophy Foundation or the American Cancer Society; and others who fund formal investigations. They also maintain bibliographic databases on topics that are of high priority to them.

By personally contacting these funding groups, you can obtain valuable leads to studies and researchers or organizations that might be conducting investigations on your topic. For these reasons, this source should be a priority focus for screening in the information-gathering stage of your synthesis.

Nonfunding Organization Sources

It is helpful to brainstorm about organizations that, although not usually funding research, might have a vested interest in your topic. These include professional societies, academic departments, and consumer groups whose purpose is to provide the public with health education and information. Such organizations often have literature databases that might be of value. By contacting individual staff of these organizations, you can obtain leads to other specific literature, other experts, current investigations, or research institutions that might prove helpful. A useful way to identify and contact such organizations is by use of DIRLINE®.

DIRLINE® (Directory of Information Resources Online) is a database that focuses primarily on health and biomedical information resources, including organizations, government agencies, information centers, professional societies, voluntary associations, support groups, academic and research institutions, and research facilities and resources. Their records contain resource names, addresses, phone numbers, and descriptions of services, publications, and holdings. To learn more about this valuable database, see its fact sheet at the following Web site (last updated August 1999): www.nlm.nih.gov/pubs/factsheets/dirlinfs.html.

To access the information in DIRLINE, use the interface search engine at the following address (last updated August 1999): sis.nlm.nih.gov/dirline/.

Paper Sources

Numerous paper sources of research literature are available in most medical libraries and elsewhere. These sources have one advantage over computer sources: They are usually free of cost (if you do your own searching and copying) and relatively easy to locate. The following material will describe five paper sources of bibliographic listings and a National Library of Medicine service (Loansome Doc®) to facilitate obtaining paper copy of complete documents identified from your citation lists.

References in References. These are a unique source of bibliographic information on your topic that are usually in paper form. We explain this term as follows:

REFERENCES IN REFERENCES

We use the term *references in references* to denote those citations in the bibliography (reference list) of a complete document, such as an article or book. This type of reference is unique because relevance coding for these is usually much more accurate than that for isolated citations. With this improvement, you will likely have a much more acceptable balance between **false-negative** and **false-positive coding rates**. The reason for this is that the coder can check the context of the material where it was cited. Another reason is that this source may provide a crude validity screen as well, depending on the discriminatory skills of the author who selected these references. This approach is similar to, but more robust than, bibliographic formats called "key words in context."

Further details regarding procedures for coding "references in references" are provided in Task 2, Procedure C, Chapter 6.

Index Medicus. This is a valuable source of references, especially for older publications. It indexes medical literature from 1879 to the present and likely provides one of the most extensive paper health science bibliographies (in both length and breadth of coverage) in the English language. When the NLM started MEDLINE in 1964, it became the online version of the Index Medicus, indexing journals from 1966 to the present. (However, OLDMEDLINE now indexes articles back to the 1950s.)

Excerpta Medica. This is an old, comprehensive, paper bibliographic database covering the worldwide literature in biomedical and pharmaceutical fields; it is produced by Elsevier Science. EMBASE has been the electronic database of Excerpta Medica since 1974. This file is analogous to MEDLINE, which has been the electronic database of the Index Medicus since 1966.

Current Contents. This is another popular paper source and is a product of the U.S. Institute for Scientific Information (ISI). You can subscribe or find library copies of these serials. This source lists the weekly or monthly table of contents of leading journals. It provides one of the better means of tracking very recent literature published since your last search iteration. This should be one of the sources you check last, before your final Stage IV analysis and synthesis.

Science Citation Indexes. These are also published by the ISI. These paper reference sources can be found in most medical libraries. Although the paper sources are falling out of use due to recent computerization of bibliographic databases, they have advantages often overlooked. For example, those citations listed in the Index Medicus before MEDLINE came into existence could be the subject of a Science Citation Index search using the paper version to keep down Stage II expense.

Quality Management Periodical Lists. These are bibliographic listings of worldwide coverage for QM journals and newsletters published in the English language. One such paper information source is in the book *Quality Management in Health Care* (Wilson & Goldschmidt, 1995, pp. 695-724). The number of these QM serials has been increasing exponentially since 1970.

In addition, Goldschmidt and Liao (1998) have published *Health Care Quality Management Resources Directory—1998/99.* This is a worldwide list of English language periodicals whose primary focus is one or more aspects of healthcare quality management, including a descriptive listing of accrediting organizations throughout the world that provide standards regarding healthcare practices. This directory is published annually and covers such topics as outcomes measurement, evidence-based medicine, practice guidelines, and clinical/business reengineering. World Development Group, Inc., in Bethesda, Maryland, sponsors this directory in paper form. You can keep up with the latest developments on the following Web site: www.hii.org/.

See the compendium at the end of this book for a more detailed description of online bibliographic sources, including their URL addresses. These are organized by government agencies or private corporations that fund Web site development. In theory, these large organizations are less likely to change than the specific Web sites that they sponsor. By linking to their home pages, you can identify changes they made.

Loansome Doc®. Unfortunately, most of the original journal articles, books, and other reports you will require are available only on paper. Though online documents are becoming available at an exponential rate, for the next decade, the vast majority of literature must be copied from tomes on library shelves or other hardcopy sources. This aspect of information database development will usually require access to a good medical library and consultation with librarians or other information retrieval specialists.

Healthcare personnel can use PubMed or other electronic bibliographic databanks to list citations or other bibliographic materials to be screened. Loansome Doc was developed by the U.S. National Library of Medicine so you can obtain, without going to a library, complete paper copy of cited documents you require. The following describes this service and provides a Web site for accessing further information.

LOANSOME DOC®

Loansome Doc is a means of ordering complete medical documents over the Internet by means of a one-time registration with the National Library of Medicine (NLM) and with a local university medical library. This service is available to those using electronic databases to develop citation listings to be screened. Articles can be faxed, mailed, or picked up at a local library. There is a nominal per page fee involved.

You can learn more about Loansome Doc by e-mail (last updated May 2001): www.nlm.nih.gov/pubs/factsheets/loansome_doc.html.

Section E. Fugitive Literature

Understanding the Concept

FUGITIVE LITERATURE

Fugitive literature is that segment of the literature that is often elusive and difficult to identify or retrieve using standard search methods. Marylu C. Rosenthal recently discussed this concept in some depth (M. C. Rosenthal, 1985, 1994, pp. 85-94). She asserts that fugitive literature includes both published and unpublished reports. Published reports can be elusive because they are new studies produced after you complete your database or are in obscure journals or books that you miss. She also lists categories of nonpublished elusive information in technical reports, interim reports, unsubmitted papers or manuscripts, conference papers presented, dissertations, and rejected papers, as well as nonwritten data on computer printouts in a researcher's working notes or even in his or her head. Close synonyms of fugitive literature include **file drawer** articles, **gray literature**, or **subterranean literature**.

Importance of Fugitive Literature

Why is this concept so important to authors of systematic reviews? The major importance of fugitive literature is that, if systematically searched, it may help you cope with the frequent biases that occur in most nonsystematic reviews. For example, one source of bias is the fact that publishers often do not publish studies that accept the null hypothesis. Consequently, authors frequently do not submit these "negative" studies, having had so many rejected previously. Another major factor may be lack of adequate resources to make an intensive effort to find research that eludes conventional modes of screening. Reviewers frequently "do not know what they do not know," so if a study does not turn up after a MEDLINE search, they often assume it does not exist. This information, if found, might alter the current synthesis conclusions (Egger, 2001; McAuley, Pham, Tugwell, & Moher, 2000).

Searching the Fugitive Literature

Fugitive literature presents a challenge to both the scope and focus of your literature search. To develop a better background for coping with this difficult issue, we urge you to read M. C. Rosenthal's chapter in Cooper and Hedges's (1994) *Handbook of Research Synthesis*. In this book, she points out that it is essential to develop a specific search strategy to identify these studies.

For purposes of healthcare literature syntheses, we suggest emphasis on systematic screening of categories of "fugitive" research studies. To help you with this task, based on M. C. Rosenthal's list (1994), with a minor augmentation of our own, we have prepared Table 5.2 to indicate a variety of sources to screen for fugitive literature.

You can see that each of the above sources will require a somewhat unique procedural approach for completing your search. In Procedure D, Chapter 7, we will discuss other strategies you might consider.

Identifying Leads to Online Fugitive Literature

Several online sources can help you identify fugitive literature. Three examples are the following: Information for Researchers, SIGLE, and CPI.

TABLE 5.2 Categories of Fugitive Literature

Completed unpublished research

Technical reports (e.g., government or corporate in-house documents)
Interim reports (e.g., progress reports on research in progress)
Unsubmitted papers (e.g., reporting negative or "uninteresting" results)
Presented papers (e.g., talks at conferences or professional meetings)
Academic documents (e.g., dissertations, theses, or course papers)
Rejected papers (e.g., those not accepted for publication)

Uncompleted research

Progress reports
Requested interim reports

Elusive published research

Editorials
Letters to the editor
New publications
Obscure older publications

SOURCE: Adapted from M. C. Rosenthal (1994, p. 89).

Information for Researchers (U.S. National Library of Congress, "Frequently Requested Materials") is an important Internet site (last updated January 1999) for getting you started. Its Web site can be found at lcweb.loc.gov/rr/main/inforeas/frequent.html. It covers academic dissertations, telephone directories, U.S. congressional documents, U.S. government publications, state government publications, and United Nations documents. The main advantage of this source is the broad coverage of elusive information, improving your recall rate. The main disadvantage is the low precision of such an online search, resulting in much wasted effort retrieving complete documents that prove to be false positives.

The Library of Congress also has another index to access fugitive literature, titled "Abstracts, Indexes, and Bibliographies for Finding Citations to Periodical Articles," focusing on the general areas of the humanities and social sciences, including library science, medicine, and psychology. This Internet site (last updated September 1998) is lcweb.loc.gov/rr/main/ab_index.html.

SIGLE (System for Information on Gray Literature in Europe) is a database that covers conferences from 1981 to the present and contains more than 420,000 citations in a variety of fugitive literature. SIGLE covers all manner of scientific topics, including biology and medicine.

CPI (Conference Proceedings Index) is a good source of conference information; the British Library publishes this index. It contains 300,000 citations from 1964 to the present. Proceedings from major conferences or abstract listings often are not published as complete articles but can be clues to valuable elusive information and references.

Summary

This chapter discusses the theoretical issues related to database development. We cover five major subjects.

The first section defines a synthesis database. It suggests ways to minimize bias and optimize how representative your final information may be of the different schools of scientific thought on your subject. Finally, it postulates that the key to successful database development is to implement a multidimensional search strategy (e.g., checking computer, people, organization, and paper sources of research information).

The second section discusses levels of potential scientific soundness that might be readily identified from clues in the material itself. The implication is that information in the highest levels should be retrieved first (i.e., materials such as other systematic reviews or recent guidelines on your topic). Your relevance assumptions will be assessed here in Stage II. Your validity assumptions will be tested in Stage III.

The third section presents several logistical considerations for database development. These include (a) understanding "systematic" literature search technology by analyzing the methods and results of the mini-synthesis produced in your topic selection procedures in Stage I, (b) understanding methods of information relevance coding, (c) valuing the power of identifying invisible colleges to optimize how representative your final database may be, (d) recognizing the vital importance of the search methods' documentation, (e) exploring methods of database management, and (f) recognizing the complexity of deciding when to terminate your Stage II literature search.

The fourth section explores the range of generic sources for database development—namely, the following: (a) computer sources (e.g., Internet), (b) people sources (e.g., experts in your topic field), (c) evidence-based synthesis groups (e.g., the Cochrane Collaboration), (d) references in references (e.g., the bibliography of a systematic review), (e) research funding sources in your subject area (e.g., the Robert Wood Johnson Foundation), (f) nonfunding organizations (e.g., the National Health Information Center [NHIC in U.S. HHS]), and (g) research literature in paper sources (e.g., Index Medicus for pre-1960 literature, published by the National Library of Medicine). Note: Although most of these sources will provide citations, the substantive information and data you require will likely come from paper sources (e.g., bound journals, books, technical reports).

The fifth and final section of this chapter explores sources and strategies for searching the fugitive literature. We provide information to facilitate your understanding of this concept and emphasize the importance of identifying vital elusive information, both published and unpublished. We discuss theoretical issues regarding your search strategy and point out several illustrative online sources for you.

With the explosion of information sources in the healthcare field, it is important to be aware of a wide range of generic possibilities, yet be parsimonious about those specific ones you will spend your own scarce resources searching. In Chapter 6, we explain implementation of standard procedures for searching the literature, applying the theoretical concepts mentioned in this chapter.

CHAPTER 6

Healthcare Information Search Procedures

The key to any successful synthesis database development is careful implementation of your search plan. It is essential that you establish systematic procedures for searching, identifying, and relevance-coding citations, abstracts, and complete documents and then documenting what you actually did, including the cost. In this book, we will present detailed forms and tools to help you accomplish these tasks. Remember, as with the rest of this book, these functions, tasks, forms, and tools are merely suggested as a guide or checklist, not as rigid rules. They can be augmented or deleted, or new elements can be added to meet the needs of your own subject matter. Finally, at the end of this section, we will list the specific products that, ideally, you should have developed at the completion of your database. This chapter will consist of the following four procedures:

HEALTHCARE INFORMATION SEARCH PROCEDURES

A. Search preparation update
B. Initial search iterations
C. Subsequent iterations
D. Search termination

Procedure A. Search Preparation Update

It is possible that some time has passed since completing the procedures in Chapter 3. We suggest the authors make a final check of the staff, resources, planning, and preparation to implement this synthesis project. Procedure A consists of the following five tasks:

SEARCH PREPARATION UPDATE TASKS

1. Augment original search plan as needed
2. Determine if search team is ready to start
3. Prepare search team for "on-the-job" training
4. Review search documentation tools
5. Recheck files for search product storage

Task 1: Augment Original Search Plan as Needed

The authors should review the "big picture" and answer the following questions: Do the topic, purpose, goals, and audience and their needs require clarification? Next, review the plan for Stage II database development in greater detail. Are local materials (e.g., an illustrative A+ or A article) on hand for the search team? Are expectations for achievement in these early iterations clear and realistic? If the answers to such questions are no, make whatever last-minute plan changes seem warranted. See Figure 3.2 for an example of a completed "Search Planning and Update Guide" used at the fifth iteration of a search. (Also, recall that at the end of Chapter 3, we provide Form 3.2, which is identical to Figure 3.2, except that it is a template for your own use.)

Task 2: Determine if Search Team Is Ready to Start

The authors should ask the search team several important questions, such as, "Can you explain the ABC convention? Why is it important? What are the five steps of a search iteration? What does *citation-abstract* mean? Why is it important to our synthesis?" You may think of any number of questions based on your observations during the Stage I training experience.

Task 3: Prepare Search Team for "On-the-Job" Training

Stress that as the team progresses with synthesis development, they will learn not only about the content of the subject but also about synthesis methods—in this case, about developing and managing an adequate database. Important feedback will include such profiles as the relevance of material acquired from different generic sources of information, a bibliography downloaded from the Web, or the results of the calibration sessions when you estimate the level of group consensus regarding relevance judgments (using a Cohen's Kappa statistic). This feedback will provide a compass to help determine whether or not you are on track, so you can make corrections accordingly.

Task 4: Review Search Documentation Tools

Recall that the level of synthesis methods documentation is one of the factors that distinguish a systematic review from a traditional review. We have provided forms to facilitate this critical task of search documentation. One of the more important factors that you must continually monitor is the time and dollar expended, compared to your budget. The project manager and author(s) share this important responsibility. It would be sad to get far into Stage II database development only to discover you will not have sufficient funds for Stage III, the validation review of the data to be synthesized.

Task 5: Recheck Files for Search Product Storage

As the search commences, computer hardcopy printouts from electronic sources, complete articles, papers, books, reports, notes, and files will accumulate at a rapid rate. If the proper files for each type of document are not prepared as you proceed with your search, you may permanently lose several documents and/or spend much wasted time trying to locate a needed article or list of downloaded citations.

Procedure B. Initial Search Iterations

The main purpose of Procedure B is to initiate your formal data search, focusing on locally available sources (e.g., MEDLINE). It is prudent, especially in the beginning, to limit your harvest to about 25 citations in each iteration. These will provide substantial material to digest for relevance coding and consensus development. Next, in the final set of early iterations, the team broadens its scope and search strategy, continuing until the formal relevance criteria become stable. In contrast, after the initial iterations are completed, the remaining ones will require a major portion of your resources for the total project. Although your relevance criteria will stabilize, your search plan (both strategy and scope) will continue to evolve in each iteration as you learn of new colleagues to contact or new bibliographic databases to screen.

Your initial (and many subsequent) search iterations will each require completing the five steps explained in Goal 2, Appendix 3.1, Chapter 3. Later in this chapter, in Procedure C, as your team members become more skilled, they may find that their relevance judgments are sufficiently close (their precision, recall [if calculated], and Kappa rates remain appropriate) that they can reduce calibration sessions to one in every second or third iteration. Calibration sessions provide the necessary information for updating and clarifying the relevance criteria. It is very important to keep iterations small at this point, until the relevance criteria have been stabilized. Once stable, if additional criteria are added, it is necessary to redo all of the citations collected in the early iterations to make sure that relevance coding is consistent. It is very frustrating to have completed very large searches and selected articles for retrieval, only to realize that the relevance criteria need to be changed and the relevance coding redone.

At this point, you are ready to implement the search plan originated in Stage I, possibly with an augmented Task 1, Procedure A, processed in this chapter.

Products of Procedure B

The final products of your initial search iterations of locally available materials will be the following: (a) an initial database of relevance-coded citations, abstracts, and documents; (b) a stable set of relevance criteria; (c) the statistical results of calibration sessions; (d) updated documentation materials compiled and stored in specials files developed for that purpose; and (e) the most recent revision of your search plan from Step 5 of your last search iteration.

If you are successful, by the end of Procedure B, you should have compiled about a hundred citations and a collection of at least 10 to 25 relevant documents, including one or more "A+" relevance-coded reviews (if you are lucky) and "A" and "A-" relevance-coded research articles and other bibliographic leads.

Procedure C. Subsequent Iterations

TASKS FOR SUBSEQUENT ITERATIONS

1. Compile and relevance-code new citations; if rated "A" (A+, A, or A–), retrieve and code complete documents

2. Relevance-code references in documents retrieved; if rated "A" (A+, A, or A–), retrieve and code documents cited

3. Complete team calibration sessions when needed

4. Update documentation forms, calculate search statistics, and file all materials

5. Revise search plan, especially strategy and scope, as needed

Introduction

At this point, having a stable set of relevance criteria, you are ready to complete your definitive search to compile a final database for your synthesis. The resulting database will be semi-final because you may yet, while producing and reviewing your synthesis manuscript in Stage V, identify additional important references and documents to be added. However, at the end of Procedure C, your database and collection of materials should be nearly complete.

The material compiled by the end of Procedure C will determine the adequacy of your search effort, including how representative your resulting data may be of existing "invisible colleges." You will complete numerous iterations in this search effort. Consequently, in Procedure C, there is danger that you might "break the bank" if your fiscal and time resources are not managed properly.

Finally, you should note that your search in Procedure C differs from that of Procedure B in five aspects:

1. Whereas in Procedure B, you were restricted to local literature sources for practical reasons, in C you have no limitation regarding location of sources to screen.

2. In B, we suggested you take "small bites" in terms of the number of citations compiled in any one iteration (e.g., only 15 to 25 at a time), but in C you can compile as many as you can effectively manage in each iteration.

3. Whereas in B your relevance criteria were constantly being augmented or revised, in Procedure C they will remain the same, in contrast to your search scope and strategy which may continually change.

4. In B you need to have calibration sessions in every iteration to reach an acceptable level of agreement, but in C you may have to calibrate only occasionally (e.g., every second or third iteration).

5. In B all team members have to code the same citations, abstracts, and complete documents, but in C each rater usually works independently, coding different materials except for occasional calibration sessions. This latter difference assumes that team members continue to maintain acceptable interrater reliability, precision, and recall rates, the latter only being checked periodically.

The major tasks encompassed in Procedure C are listed below. Note that these are the same five steps of each search iteration explained above. Each is quite similar to those described above and thus will be augmented slightly, only as needed.

Task 1: Compile and Relevance-Code New Citations; If Rated "A" (A+, A, A–), Retrieve and Code Complete Documents

When you start this first task of Procedure C, you will be implementing the search plan from the final iteration of Procedure B. If there has been a long lull in your project since completing your last iteration, you may need to (a) think of several ways to "augment" your current search plan before starting its implementation and (b) review your "relevance cue logs" and your "relevance criteria list" to prepare for the iterations of the final search.

Task 2: Relevance-Code References in Documents Retrieved; If Rated "A" (A+, A, or A–), Retrieve and Code Documents Cited

For each iteration, you will compile a set of complete documents, whether they are notes from a consultant, articles, technical reports, or books. Within each you will identify their reference lists and relevance rate them. Again, you will retrieve and relevance-code these new materials for each of the A+, A, and A– references identified. Recall that the relevance ratings of these "references in references" check the context for each reference in the text as part of the coding process. This is one of the main factors that differentiate Task 1 from Task 2 in Procedures B and C.

Task 3: Complete Team Calibration Sessions When Needed

In the search iteration during Procedure C, you may or may not have to complete a calibration session for every iteration, as you did in Procedure B. If your interrater reliability, precision, and recall rates continue to remain high, it may be prudent to conduct calibration sessions only every second or third round (or iteration). You should use a minimum of 30 citations for calibration sessions. Obviously, if these rates drop to an unacceptable level, more frequent calibrations will be required. Otherwise, coders can conduct relevance coding independently. If the precision, recall (if calculated), and Kappa rates are adequate, it is likely your team is in agreement; if these rates are low, you may need to provide more training.

Task 4: Update Documentation Forms, Calculate Search Statistics, and File All Materials

For each iteration, the bibliographic documentation forms need to be updated. If this task is procrastinated, information may be lost as memories fade. Because relevance criteria now remain stable, augmentation of the relevance cue logs is not required. An exception might be the discovery of a new invisible college. In this case, if new relevance criteria are added, it probably will be necessary for you to recode all previous citations to maintain consistency and, possibly, find missed articles by members of that recently identified "college." Any new terms will also need to be included in your glossary, especially if they prove to be synonyms of terms already being used. However, if at all possible, the relevance criteria list should not be changed in Procedure C iterations. Most new documentation will be updating the master list of citations, as well as updating the fiscal and time ledgers. If you do not keep your master list up to date, you may retrieve and code the same article several times, wasting valuable time and resources.

In Procedure B, search statistics to be calculated were mentioned (precision, possibly recall, and Kappa rates). Remember that for each iteration, these statistics were calculated for that round only, with a final aggregation completed at the end of Stage II. The statistics will provide some of your best evidence as to how well you are doing in database development.

Task 5: Revise Search Plan, Especially Strategy and Scope, as Needed

In the many iterations of Procedure C, you will learn new information, particularly about missed bibliographic sources, new invisible colleges, or individual colleagues to contact. As such information is discovered, it might require revision of your search plan in this Task 5 of the iteration.

Products of Procedure C

The final products of Procedure C should be the cumulative harvest of materials from all iterations completed in this synthesis. Three categories of important items have been generated by Procedure C.

First are the final, A+, A, and A– relevance-coded books, book chapters, research reports (journal articles) from published medical literature, documents from unpublished sources, and information from consultants.

Second are filed search documentation forms, including (a) any updated relevance cue logs; (b) your standard set of relevance criteria; (c) completed calibration forms that document your interrater reliability statistical trends, as well as your citation and abstract precision rates (and occasionally recall rates); (d) your final master list of references, each with its unique relevance-coded citation and abstract; and (e) your set of sequential search plans from each iteration, documenting the evolution of your search scope and strategy.

Third is the actual data recorded for that iteration that should encompass your relevant database articles and documents, as well as your methods documentation. These statistics will be required to facilitate evaluation of this Stage II (in Chapter 7) and critical for data coding in Stage III (Chapter 8).

Procedure D. Search Termination

TASKS FOR SEARCH TERMINATION

1. Check master list for unprocessed "A" citation-abstracts
2. Analyze evidence for missed invisible colleges
3. Do a preliminary estimate of the file drawer problem
4. Verify "B" and "C" citation-abstract coding accuracy
5. Make your decision to stop or continue searching

Introduction

The most important issue in Procedure D is to decide when to terminate the Stage II search. This decision is determined by comparing the probability of subsequently finding critical new "colleges" and references, compared to the time and fiscal resources you still have available. Because it is nearly impossible to judge this probability for all references, it is important to take steps to avoid or minimize selection bias.

Several methods can be used to do this, most of which involve analyzing the pattern of resultant study effect sizes (usually in quantitative syntheses). These steps to reduce selection bias cannot really be taken until after the effect sizes have been recorded as described in Chapter 13. However, because the synthesis process is characterized by ongoing overlapping stages, likely the information required for this procedure (effect sizes) will already be in the process of being collected. If, based on what you know at that time, the probability of finding another important article is judged sufficiently low, you might consider ending your search.

Keep in mind that the termination of your search and retrieval efforts should consider many factors—for example, estimating the number of unretrieved studies with "null" or contradictory results needed to change your current conclusions (the file drawer statistic). Equally important is considering the degree to which you have actually retrieved existing relevant articles, the cost and effort of further screening, and your own project deadlines—all may be considered for this final decision to end Stage II.

In addition, you may have to address your publisher's final external review comments about your manuscript, which might require that several new documents be added to your database. In any event, it is helpful at this point to review five major tasks required for making this termination decision.

Task 1: Check Master List for Unprocessed "A" Citation-Abstracts

Screening the master list for inadvertently missed A+, A, and A– citations or abstracts is an important determinant of the adequacy of your search. It is also possible that you might identify an overlooked cue, such as finding an important author who was not contacted or whose own bibliography was not searched. Another cue would be a master file entry that was marked "article retrieved" with no relevance profile recorded, indicating the "references in references" may not have been coded. Such missed articles would have to be pulled from your files and their references properly relevance-coded and profiled.

Task 2: Analyze Evidence for Missed Invisible Colleges

If your database is to meet the requirement of being comprehensive and representative of current avenues of thought on your topic, you must complete an invisible college analysis at one or more times in your Stage II search.

This task might involve such subtasks as the following: (a) assemble all complete relevant studies for analysis; (b) analyze articles for clusters of documents that use similar theoretical frameworks, research designs, and jargon terms and phrases; (c) list the papers and investigators that each of these authors cites to determine where there are similarities and, especially, differences; and (d) check editorials or letters to the editor on several key articles in each cluster to identify critics of that article who might represent a competing "college" to explore. Similarly, new colleges may emerge when, for the same topic, different clinical disciplines have different approaches in their own bodies of literature. For example, research in nursing may be based on an entirely different conceptual area than research in clinical psychology, even though they are studying the same phenomena.

Task 3: Do a Preliminary Estimate of the File Drawer Problem

A file drawer problem estimate can be helpful in determining when to terminate a quantitative synthesis. This estimate consists of computing a preliminary estimate of the number of additional valid studies that have null results that might reverse your final conclusions. Such papers are often sound studies that were not published due to the author's finding of "null" results (i.e., a "negative" study accepting the null hypothesis). Table 6.1 can help you make this preliminary determination. One of the facts required for this estimate is the mean "effect size" for your set of studies. The final file drawer estimate cannot be computed until the end of Stage III, when nearly all effect sizes are recorded. However, because there is considerable chronological overlap between Stage II and Stage III, it is usually possible to make a preliminary estimate during the database compilation.

To use Table 6.1, you need three values: first, the number of articles you have retrieved thus far in your information search; second, selection of a significance level (alpha) for rejecting the null hypothesis when the results are combined across all studies (the traditional value is usually $\alpha < .05$, either one-tailed or two-tailed); and third, an estimated average, or typical standardized effect size, for all the retrieved studies in your current database. Typically, you will not know this final mean effect size at the time you would like to decide whether to continue or terminate your search process. However, you can pose a set of hypothetical conditions that can be evaluated, using the data in Table 6.1. For example, in your reasoning process, you assume (or guess) that you have relatively "small," "medium," or "large" effect size

TABLE 6.1 File Drawer Problem Management

Number of Currently Retrieved Studies	Estimated Typical Effect Sizes (Z, p) for Retrieved Studies									
	Z = 0.50 $p < 0.6$		Z = 1.00 $p < 0.3$		Z = 1.65 $p < 0.1$		Z = 1.96 $p < .05$		Z = 2.58 $p < .01$	
	Desired Alpha Level		Desired Alpha Level		Desired Alpha Level		Desired Alpha Level		Desired Alpha Level	
	.10	.05	.10	.05	.10	.05	.10	.05	.10	.05
1	NA	NA	NA	NA	NA	NA	NA	NA	1	1
2	NA	NA	NA	NA	2	1	4	2	8	5
3	NA	NA	NA	NA	6	3	10	6	19	13
4	NA	NA	2	NA	12	7	19	12	35	24
5	NA	NA	4	2	20	13	30	20	56	38
6	NA	NA	7	3	30	20	45	30	82	56
7	NA	NA	11	6	42	28	62	42	112	78
8	NA	NA	16	9	56	37	82	56	148	103
9	NA	NA	21	12	72	48	105	72	188	131
10	NA	NA	27	16	90	61	131	90	234	163
11	NA	NA	33	20	110	75	160	110	284	198
12	1	NA	41	25	132	90	191	132	339	237
13	3	NA	49	31	156	107	225	156	399	279
14	4	NA	58	37	182	125	263	182	464	325
15	6	NA	68	44	210	144	302	210	533	374
16	8	1	78	51	240	165	345	240	608	426
17	10	2	89	58	272	188	391	272	687	482
18	12	3	101	66	306	212	439	306	772	542
19	14	4	114	75	342	237	490	342	861	605
20	17	6	127	84	380	263	544	380	955	671
25	32	16	205	138	600	418	857	600	1498	1055
30	53	29	301	204	870	608	1240	870	1759	1525

NOTE: Estimating the number of negative file drawer studies (i.e., those that do not reject the null hypothesis) is required to overturn the conclusions from your currently retrieved studies. Numbers in each cell = number of file drawer negative (i.e., do not reject the null hypothesis) studies that would have to exist for the combined effect size to overturn your current results with a probability of chance less than the desired alpha threshold of .10 or .05. NA = not applicable; it literally means that less than 1 study could overturn the result. Z = effect size of current retrieved studies at the given *p* value. Desired alpha level = the selected probability that the difference between your present result and the result with the new combined number of studies is due to chance.

TABLE 6.2 Probability Values Associated With Various Z Statistics

Statistical Value (Z)	Probability Level
0.50	0.60
1.00	0.30
1.65	0.10
1.96	0.05
2.58	0.01

values for your test of significance. Consequently, this table contains a variety of different values you might encounter. If you have a substantial number of articles that have been validated and have had their effect size calculated, you can perform a preliminary estimate of the file drawer effect.

Note: The cell entries refer to the number of file drawer articles that must exist in order for the combined significance level to be below the desired threshold of $\alpha = .10$ or $\alpha = .05$.

The values in the first column of the table represent the current number of articles in your search (we report values ranging from 1 to 30 articles), and the remaining columns represent different hypothetical outcomes of research. The individual cell entries in the table represent the number of file drawer articles with null results that must exist to overturn your current conclusions. For purposes of estimating the file drawer effect, assume that you have converted your test statistic to a standardized score (Z) that is to be compared to a standard normal distribution, that is, a distribution with a mean = 0.00 and a standard deviation (variance) = 1.00.

Now return to the use of the file drawer in Table 6.1. To demonstrate its use, suppose you have obtained five studies in your search, all of which reject the null hypothesis (i.e., have significant results). You want to know how many file drawer studies (i.e., those with nonsignificant results) would have to exist for you to conclude that the null hypothesis is actually true. Suppose you anticipate that the typical study in your collection has a relatively small effect size so that the standardized test statistic would be of modest value (e.g., $Z = 0.5$, 1.00, or 1.65), as shown in Table 6.2.

If you have decided to accept the traditional, two-tailed threshold value for rejecting the null hypothesis as $\alpha < 0.05$, then you will reject the null hypothesis whenever the average $Z \geq 1.96$.

Table 6.1 is constructed so that you can determine the number of nonsignificant file drawer articles required to reduce the combined (i.e., published and unpublished articles) effect size to a nonsignificant value for your chosen threshold value (i.e., α = .05). To estimate the file drawer effect, look down the first column until you find the value 5 (the number of articles you have retrieved). Next, move across to the column headed by a Z value of 0.5 (the estimated average effect size of the studies). You will find a 0 or an "NA" in the columns headed by α = .05 and α = 0.10. This zero value indicates that you do not need to find any file drawer studies because the average Z value for the retrieved articles is not statistically significant from 0.00, so you cannot reject the null hypothesis by adding any number of negative studies.

Now examine the column where the anticipated Z score is 1.65. You will find a value of 13 under the column in which the threshold value is labeled as α = .05. If you had desired α = .10 as your minimum threshold value, then you would use the value of 20 as the file drawer number. As the table indicates, the number of required file drawer articles becomes quite large under two conditions: (a) when the number of currently retrieved studies is greater than 10 and (b) when the average Z score is greater than 1.00. The shaded areas indicate conditions in which the file draw phenomena should be of little concern because the number of required studies is prohibitively large. If your file drawer effect value falls in the shaded region of the table, you would be justified in terminating your information search without expending further effort to retrieve additional studies, given all other conditions are met.

Task 4: Verify "B" and "C" Citation-Abstract Coding Accuracy

There may be several B or C citations that were miscoded and should be rated at least A–. For example, you may discover that an early citation that initially appeared irrelevant (and was miscoded as C) was frequently cited later in other important articles on your topic. In this case, you would need to spot-check search recall (explained in Chapter 3). To do this, a sample of B and C citations should be selected and the complete documents retrieved for each. If an unacceptable proportion of these low-relevance citations yield high-relevance (A–, A, A+) articles, your recall rate would be too low and you would need to analyze why and, if possible, correct the problem. These coding errors are usually unavoidable, so you must make a final estimate of these false-negative documents that may have been missed. We have found it worthwhile to retrieve a random sample for relevance review of at least 25 C and 25 B articles (the more the better). You should retrieve and relevance-code the complete articles for each. If more than 2% to 5% of your C-coded citations or more than 10% of your B-coded citations were miscoded, then your relevance criteria, for example, might be reviewed and augmented for future searches. Because the above percentage thresholds are arbitrary, you may wish to adjust them to meet your individual requirements and values. If budgeted resources for the search are getting low, this task might be omitted, as it is likely to have a low yield for the expense.

Task 5: Make Your Decision to Stop or Continue Searching

Now comes the moment of truth when you must decide and then act on your decision. If the above tasks were completed adequately, you will likely make a sound decision as to whether to stop or proceed.

Products of Procedure D

The final products of Procedure D include (a) a final master list of citation-abstracts that have been screened to determine if any, inadvertently, were not processed; (b) a completed analysis to find clues of an invisible college of research colleagues interested in your topic; (c) an estimate of the file drawer problem effect for your information synthesis to confirm your decision to continue or terminate the search; and (d) a sample of B- and C-rated citations or abstracts that have been selected and reanalyzed to determine the proportion that might be false negative (i.e., A+, A, A–).

Summary

In Chapter 6, we presented and explained five overall procedures for any literature search (not to be confused with the five steps of a search iteration). These overall activities include the following:

Procedure A: Make final preparations for implementing your search, re-checking your plan and your team to be certain everything is ready and, in particular, checking your electronic and paper filing systems before the data and paper start piling up.

Procedure B: Stabilize your list of relevance criteria, finalize the goal of the initial search iterations, continue to enhance your team's search skills, and update your search strategy and scope.

Procedure C: Complete a semi-final database, including documentation files and results of calibration sessions, and compile search statistics.

Procedure D: Facilitate your search termination decision (e.g., repeat another file drawer problem analysis to check the need to continue searching). With all information at hand, in Chapter 7, you make your decision to stop the search and evaluate Stage II procedures or continue searching to build a more representative database. At this time, you might consider repeating another file drawer problem analysis or funnel plot check.

Remember that the key to a successful search is to recruit and calibrate a competent search team and provide detailed training as to the concepts, tasks, subtasks, and products of each procedure in Chapter 6. (In Appendix 3.1, Chapter 3, we suggest learning exercises to achieve the eight training goals listed there.) In all of the above procedures, we remind the reader to continually monitor both fiscal and time expenditures, to compare against your predetermined budget. Remember, in Stage II, you are most likely to have a cost overrun in terms of monetary or time resources. Next, we will move to Chapter 7 and discuss the procedures for estimating how thorough and accurate are the products of Stage II. At this point, you have retrieved and relevance-coded A+ and A documents and screened A– documents for leads to missed invisible colleges or other important references. If, in Stage III, these documents prove scientifically sound and homogeneous, they will provide the data for the Stage IV analysis and synthesis.

Evaluation and Improvement of Stage II

This chapter provides both strategic considerations and step-by-step procedures for evaluating Stage II methods and the resulting database.

STAGE II EVALUATION AND IMPROVEMENT PROCEDURES

Assess and enhance:
- A. Documentation adequacy
- B. Clinical significance
- C. Scientific soundness
- D. Cost-effectiveness
- Appendix 7.1   Screening for internal clues to missed studies
- Appendix 7.2   Screening for external clues to missed studies

Introduction

In coping with the evaluation of database development, there are a number of strategic factors that might be helpful.

Consideration 1: Mistakes and Omissions

One of the goals of Chapter 7, like all of the evaluation chapters in this book, is to identify and correct mistakes and omissions that might be found. Corrections may involve searching missed information sources and processing new citations, abstracts, or documents. However, the closer you get to the end of this data-gathering stage, the less likely you will have time or funds to correct serious problems. Even more important is the fact that the relevance criteria must be stabilized early in the search process. If you are approaching the end of Stage II, adding relevance criteria will require recoding all of your citations, abstracts, and complete documents to apply the new criteria. This is a serious problem that must be prevented rather than repaired at a time when your fiscal and time resources may be running short.

Consideration 2: Repeated Evaluations

The Stage II evaluation must be conducted early to midpoint in your database development and again, briefly, near the completion of your data gathering. The initial evaluation needs to be thorough and should be implemented after Chapter 6, Procedure B, search iterations are complete (i.e., when your relevance criteria have stabilized). At this point, you can still afford to correct serious problems, including revisions or additions to your relevance criteria and consequent recoding of previous documents and citations compiled. A final evaluation at the end of Stage II will be more cursory, looking mainly for errors that may not be correctable but that must be reported in the "limitations" section of your manuscript. For example, if at the end of Stage II you discover a missed college of investigators or new relevance criteria, it is usually too late to go back and repeat the search of every information source using these new clues and recoding your entire database.

Consideration 3: Author's Evaluation Role

The next strategic consideration is that Stage II evaluation should be conducted by the authors because they have the most to lose. This is especially true if the final database proves inadequate and threatens the scientific soundness of the final synthesis. Authors can rapidly spot-check for glaring errors or omissions. If these are found early, the staff can go back and do a more definitive assessment and correction of such flaws. If errors are found at the final evaluation as mentioned above, the authors must live with the consequences.

Consideration 4: Standard Evaluation Criteria

In Section E, Chapter 1, we listed four criteria by which you might evaluate your final information synthesis. At that time, you applied those criteria to assess your accomplishments in planning. In this chapter, you will apply those criteria to evaluate the accomplishments of Stage II, both in the middle and at the end of this stage.

Procedure A. Assess and Enhance Documentation Adequacy

The first important requirement in Stage II evaluation is to check how adequately your search methods are documented and your database is organized. If your documentation is thorough, it will be possible for an independent reviewer or editor to evaluate your database for adequacy to support your subsequent synthesis procedures. This same information will be included in your final synthesis manuscript in Stage V. If this documentation is sufficient, you or others can estimate how thorough your search was and how representative your resulting database might be of invisible colleges that exist on your subject. However, if your documentation is inadequate, further evaluation of Stage II will be difficult, if not impossible. If your methods recording and database files have been kept up-to-date as the search proceeded, it will likely require little augmentation. More important, it will support both an internal and external evaluation of your work and be critical to your final synthesis write-up.

TASKS TO ASSESS AND ENHANCE DOCUMENTATION ADEQUACY

1. Analyze search documentation forms and data
2. Review description of search plans
3. Check adequacy of relevance cue logs, relevance criteria, and master list
4. Review coded electronic citation printouts, photocopied reference lists, fiscal and time ledgers, and search statistics
5. Make additional revisions and augmentation as needed

Task 1: Analyze Search Documentation Forms and Data

Remember that most documentation is recorded on formatted forms suggested for Step 4 of each search iteration (as explained in Goal 2, Appendix 3.1, Chapter 3).

This material is organized and stored in its appropriate paper document file. Theoretically, by the end of Stage II, you should have a reasonably complete set of forms describing your search methods and statistical counts. If this was carefully done, this first compilation task should be rather simple.

Task 2: Review Description of Search Plans

Recall that the original search plan was completed in Chapter 3. In Stage II, this plan is continually revised as you complete Step 5 of each search iteration in Procedures B and C (Chapter 6). Consequently, you should now have a reasonably complete set of these plans documenting the evolution of your search scope and strategy that produced your current database.

We recommend you review these documents for adequacy. Check for any glaring omissions of search sources, especially prominent colleagues in your topic field who were not contacted, or any promising leads to the "fugitive literature" that were not followed. If, at some stage in this evolution, your team unintentionally "jumped the track" (e.g., were searching two different topics), and this was not corrected during calibration sessions, you may have some complex revisions that have to be accomplished at this late date.

Task 3: Check Adequacy of Relevance
Cue Logs, Relevance Criteria, and Master List

This task requires the authors to complete a cursory screening of the above documents, especially to determine whether they are up-to-date. Like business finance records, once you fall behind in doing your posting, it will be difficult to catch up and possibly be very expensive. In our case, you will be checking for serious omissions or redundancies, unreadable handwriting, and missing statistical counts for this documentation.

In addition, you will produce initial summary counts of relevant **parameters**. First, you will need to simply count all of the citations that fall into the relevance-coding categories. Then it is important to start checking for accuracy and completeness. For example, of the total number of citations in your electronic bibliographic printouts or photocopied reference lists, how many are relevance-coded? Of those coded citations and abstracts, were the relevance distributions in terms of A+, A, A−, B, and C meaningful? Of those A (A+, A, and A−) citations, how many were searched, and how many complete documents were retrieved? This latter count should correspond to the actual documents in your storage files.

Determine whether your electronic citation listings were accurately checked for duplications and the listings coded for relevance. Check the article retrieval status codes to establish if many A citations or abstracts were not followed up or are still being retrieved. You might want to ascertain whether the citations are in a similar recording style or if there are many glaring differences that must be corrected by your team. In Stage V, when you copyedit your final manuscript, you will again systematically check for such errors. Correcting such problems in Stage II will save much time later and will make your task much easier during manuscript preparation.

Task 4: Review Coded Electronic Citation Printouts, Photocopied Reference Lists, Fiscal and Time Ledgers, and Search Statistics

These paper hardcopy documents might prove valuable, especially if you experience a computer crash or accidentally wipe out some of your electronic files. These coded documents might also prove helpful for future copyediting and checking citation accuracy or if disputes arise about the actual relevance code given that citation or abstract. It is also helpful to spot-check the coding on the photocopied "references in references." (Remember that copies of these relevance-coded reference listings were given to your document retrieval staff to facilitate their library search activities.)

Your electronic master list of citation-abstracts is especially valuable. For example, the search statistics will facilitate assessing your documentation adequacy. You can find how many citations or reference lists were coded and profiled, how many A citation-abstracts were found, how many were searched, and how many documents were retrieved, coded, profiled, and readily available for data coding. Your master list of citations will provide many other clues to missed documents and possibly new invisible colleges.

Task 5: Make Additional Revisions and Augmentation as Needed

You might make some of the required revisions of your documentation at the time you discover errors. For example, while reviewing your citation printouts, you might find several citations that were not relevance-coded. At this point, you could send a note or talk to your coding team to assign a more careful recheck and relevance coding of these citation lists. However, many revisions can be delayed until later, when other tasks of this semi-final evaluation have been completed. (These tasks are "semi-final" because, when preparing your final manuscript of your synthesis, additional omissions or redundancies are likely to be discovered.) Your team should complete these tasks as soon as possible while recall of related factors is still fresh in their minds.

Procedure B. Assess and Enhance Clinical Significance

Remember that this Procedure B, "Clinical Significance," is discussed in detail in Procedure B, Chapter 4. Clinical significance is managed primarily by means of your relevance logs and your formal set of relevance criteria. Because these criteria evolve during the early phase of the literature search, it is necessary to ensure that they encompass the two elements of clinical significance—namely, importance (achievable population benefit) and maturity (readiness to be applied widely in the community).

At this point in your Stage II evaluation, you should reexamine your relevance criteria and skim through your final articles to be sure they meet this clinical relevance criterion. This should be done in your mid–Stage II evaluation, when you can still correct serious errors.

Procedure C. Assess and Enhance Scientific Soundness

To assess **scientific soundness**, we will not emphasize internal validity or statistical validity, which are primarily evaluated in Section C, Chapter 9. The measures of the scientific soundness of your database that are most important in applying Section C in this chapter are *construct* and *external* validity. As defined in Section E, Chapter 1, **construct validity** is the degree to which the content of your synthesis conforms to the assumptions and description of the conceptual model posed by your research question. Meeting this criterion is determined by the evolution of your relevance criteria. Equally important is **external validity**, which is the extent to which your database is representative (i.e., includes studies that cover the spectrum of different schools of thought on your topic). Meeting this criterion is determined by your search strategy. If the synthesis data gathering is haphazard, it is likely that neither the author nor the reader will be able to determine how representative or biased your data and conclusions might be.

As explained in Section E, Chapter 1, we conceptualize four tasks essential for assessing scientific soundness of a literature synthesis; at this point, only two will be covered:

TASKS TO ASSESS AND ENHANCE SCIENTIFIC SOUNDNESS

Assess and enhance:
1. Database construct validity
2. Database external validity

Task 1: Assess and Enhance Database Construct Validity

Again, as defined in Chapter 1, construct validity is the extent to which your database captures the key concept of your synthesis model or theoretical framework. We suggest four tasks to assess how well your database meets this requirement.

Review Original and Most Recent Project Plan. Reviewing your original, as well as your most recent, project plan should remind you of the specific synthesis purpose and goals you are trying to achieve. The information in these plans should indicate the theoretical construct guiding your research review. For example, your synthesis topic may be to determine, from the literature, whether routine use of the Short Form 36-Item Health Survey (SF-36) (Ware, 1998; Ware & Sherbourne, 1992), health outcome measurement instrument, and feedback of data to institutional staff is associated with better management action and improved **health** outcomes. In this construct, the key elements are routine SF-36 measurement of health status, feedback display of outcome data to the staff, development of quality management projects, and remeasurement of outcomes. These constructs should still be the focus of the project.

Assess Relevance Criteria. In assessing relevance criteria, your task is threefold: First, you must look for clarity, such as the need for rewording (e.g., being more general or specific as needed), also looking for redundancies; second, you must look for congruency between the constructs in the stated plan and the resultant relevance criteria; and third, look at potential missing criteria, especially exclusion criteria that could facilitate a more cost-effective future search.

This task is essential in the initial evaluation of Stage II, when it still might be possible to make improvements. Because your research construct sets the framework for establishing relevance criteria, you should examine these criteria carefully to determine whether they are directly related to your project's model.

Note that your exclusion criteria may be as meaningful as your inclusion criteria. Suppose you coded a citation titled "Importance of Quality of Life" as A–. On retrieving the complete article, you find that it is an abstract treatise with no mention of measurement, which is your central concern. The term *importance* might be added to your exclusion criteria to avoid retrieving what will likely be nonquantitative articles, thus improving the cost-effectiveness of your search.

Assess Random A+ or A Documents. To accomplish this task, you should establish a sampling plan, based on the prevalence of relevant documents you have collected thus far. If you have compiled less than 25 complete articles, use a universe sample and check them all. If you have found several hundred relevant documents, select a sampling method to yield at least 25 representative documents. (These sample sizes have somewhat arbitrary lower limits.)

With your synthesis construct fresh in mind, skim the articles in your sample to confirm that they are relevant. If this is your initial Stage II evaluation, and your articles are of peripheral relevance, assessment and revision of your search criteria would be indicated when you start a new iteration. If the profile of your articles was skewed to the right, having some As but many more Bs and Cs, you might still need to find out why and make subsequent plans accordingly.

Estimate and Improve Adequacy of Construct Validity. With the results of the above three tasks in hand, you and your team need to make a value judgment concerning adequacy of your construct validity. If your construct is clear, and the evidence indicates you have compiled a set of articles that match your assumptions and theoretical framework, you can instruct your team to continue completion of Stage II. On the other hand, if the team agrees that your documents poorly reflect your construct, you may have to rewrite your goals and relevance criteria and start over again.

However, as is often the case, if your construct validity is judged to be of questionable adequacy, a more in-depth analysis would be important to decide what steps are warranted for improving the relevance of your literature harvest.

Task 2: Assess and Enhance Database External Validity

EXTERNAL VALIDITY CONSIDERATIONS

External validity, defined in Section E, Chapter 1, is determined in Stage II by assessing how adequately your literature was sampled and how representative the results might be of existing schools of thought on your topic. Because a "universe sample" of all research ever written on your topic is usually impractical, if not impossible, you must compromise when making this assessment. This can be done using several methods; however, the one we suggest involves trying to represent the main invisible colleges of colleagues researching your subject.

CAUTION

The quicker and more haphazard your search, the higher will be the probability that you will miss important studies and possibly disseminate misleading information and conclusions.

To determine how adequately you have estimated external validity, we suggest the three tasks described below.

Identify Internal Clues to Missed Studies.   This approach again focuses on reanalysis of your search documentation. This task includes identifying overlooked studies to be retrieved or relevant clues to missed invisible colleges of colleagues to be contacted. For example, if you note that several A articles by the same author were in your master list but not followed up, your team would have to make a careful check for such omissions. Those that are found would have to be retrieved so the documents and their references could be relevance-coded. We assume these steps have been adequately accomplished during each iteration of your database search, so this check for internal clues, it is hoped, may not identify many serious problems.

In spot-checking for important missing documents or invisible colleges, we suggest the following six tasks (also described in detail in Appendix 7.1): analyze size of research database, analyze proportion of relevant citations, analyze scope of final search plan, check for citation-abstract and article miscoding, check for retrieval thoroughness, and review search team's interrater reliability and precision rates.

Identify External Clues to Missed Studies.   If resources allow additional searching for missed articles, you might consider the following five tasks (also detailed in Appendix 7.2): review or conduct a file drawer analysis, contact experts not previously consulted, complete a funnel plot analysis, search more intensively for fugitive literature, and briefly update database before finalizing Stage II.

Complete Our Checklist for Missed Generic Sources.   By the time you have completed this final review (Form 7.1, at the end of this chapter), it is possible that many new ideas will have occurred to your search team since the initiation of your project. As a "rule of thumb," if any of the sections of this form receive more than one no, an additional search effort might be considered in the area of that item.

At the completion of this task, you should have a rather thorough and representative database of relevant studies on your topic.

REMINDER

As with all of our checklists, the items shown are merely a starter set for you to alter, in any manner, for customizing these factors to your specific needs. Most likely, you will identify many more relevant factors for assessing the adequacy of your particular database.

Procedure D. Assess and Enhance Cost-Effectiveness

The purpose of this procedure is to determine how unnecessary and costly purchases or personnel time might, in the future, be avoided. The most important advantage of keeping such fiscal and time records is to manage this Stage II search effort efficiently. As mentioned before, it is during this stage that you might "break the bank" before completing your analysis and synthesis, let alone your manuscript preparation, which is the second most costly task in your project. If you plan to do many other syntheses, this information will also be valuable for planning subsequent work.

The documentation "files" of your budget should provide the needed data to estimate both direct purchases and personnel costs. As a caution, we recommend that only direct costs be considered. Indirect and opportunity costs should be left for a more erudite analysis, if that is ever warranted.

The cost-effectiveness criterion might be crudely estimated by completing the following five tasks:

TASKS TO ASSESS AND ENHANCE COST-EFFECTIVENESS

1. Calculate total direct (nonpersonnel) expenditures
2. Estimate personnel costs
3. Add any unbudgeted costs
4. Estimate likely contribution of your database
5. Judge whether your database seems worth the cost

Task 1: Calculate Total Direct (Nonpersonnel) Expenditures

Your budget files at the end of Stage II should provide a brief accounting of the direct dollar purchases of such items as books, computer equipment, software, online charges and licenses, copying, and other library charges. A major budget item you may not think of will be memberships and license fees for online services. One major essential cost is online access charges for use of their data files. One library, for example, charges close to U.S. $300 for a 1-year license to access its files. Multi-databank services provide access to numerous online information sources, libraries, journals, and books. For example, they may provide access to MEDLINE, EMBASE, the Cochrane Library, *ACP Journal Club* Evidence-Based Medicine, the *New England Journal of Medicine,* and many more valuable sites. However, they may charge more than $1,000 to $2,000 for use of their services. This may be high, but it would be even higher if you subscribed to each of the databanks encompassed by their service. We must face the reality that online information, in an informatics age, is going to be as expensive as it is essential. Thus, we must adjust to the fact that this will be another routine cost, just as travel and telephones are today.

For this purpose, you might use the same format as established in your original Stage I budget plan. One member of the team might be the bookkeeper assigned to maintain financial and personnel time records.

Task 2: Estimate Personnel Costs

Keeping personnel time records can be more complex. For the sake of practicality, we suggest that you *not* maintain meticulous time records. A more expedient method is to have each team member record an estimate of time expended during each iteration. Using a spreadsheet, or program evaluation and review technique (PERT) software, these estimates can be recorded and automatically multiplied by each person's salary rate to convert personnel hours to dollars. By this means, a crude total dollar estimate, in terms of both purchases and personnel costs, can be made for Stage II.

Task 3: Add Any Unbudgeted Costs

There can be many unexpected and unbudgeted expenses you might encounter. For example, if a new computer virus contaminates your software or documents, you will have to apply an updated virus detector that can identify and eradicate these malicious Internet messages. If you lose files and do not have an external backup disk, there may be substantial reworking that has to be done.

Another example might be the finding of an unexpectedly rich information source that would require direct dollar and personnel costs beyond your Stage II budget. The citation lists involved and the citation and abstract coding costs can be large, as can the costs of article retrieval, copying, and coding.

As with any project, there can be unexpected personnel turnover that will be very expensive. The disruption costs of having a team member leave, as well as the costs required in recruiting and training replacements, can be a financial burden. You must account for such unexpected costs in your projected budget.

Task 4: Estimate Likely Contribution of Your Database

Estimating, in Stage II, the likely value of your final product can be difficult. However, you will find many clues, such as the estimated size of your final compilation and/or the results of your preliminary file drawer problem analysis (based on effect sizes abstracted and coded thus far), that will suggest the value of the final product. There is always a possibility that little-known, unexpected excellent studies might be found that could make an immediate contribution to **healthcare outcome improvement**, or even to the state of the science in that topic area. Using team consensus judgement or seeking the judgment of respected colleagues, you might be surprised by the valuable information you have obtained.

To be more realistic, however, at this early date, there is usually a tendency to be overly optimistic about the contribution of your database and your final synthesis. Although such optimism might help motivate your work, do not be disappointed if the ultimate value of your effort is less than earlier anticipated. There is no way to avoid this other than being methodologically rigorous in each stage of your project.

Task 5: Judge Whether Your Database Seems Worth the Cost

In Stage II, this estimate will be rather crude. The same group that assisted you to estimate the likely value of your final product can also help make this final determination. This task requires a group value judgment that, in the Stage V overall manuscript review, could prove surprisingly sound. However, the importance of completing this preliminary estimate might be more in the methods training your team acquires at this point than in any realistic estimation of value.

Summary

The purpose of Chapter 7 is to facilitate your evaluating the product and process of Stage II database development. The product should be a compilation of relevant research or other documents related to your synthesis goal. This chapter is divided into four sections, providing both theoretical and procedural help in accomplishing a quality check of your data-gathering effort and product. In a brief introduction, we focus on some general considerations that might facilitate application of the four basic quality criteria you should consider.

The first procedure (documentation adequacy) helps you assess how well you documented your data-gathering procedures. The methods section of any scientific paper is the key to establishing how sound the conclusions might be. A poorly documented review, especially a quantitative synthesis, often produces "unusable numbers" that, if more thoroughly documented, might prove to an outside reviewer to be quite sound. This section helps you determine the thoroughness of your methods documentation, providing a number of tools that, if adequately applied, may increase the probability of your manuscript being accepted for publication.

The second procedure (clinical significance) is touched on only briefly because its major application was completed in Procedure B, Chapter 4.

The third procedure (scientific soundness) helps assess the soundness of the Stage II methods you applied and the resulting database you compiled. Here you focus on the structural validity of your work, which is based on how well-thought-out your synthesis model or theoretical framework is. This revolves around how well your database represents the spectrum of different research schools of thought, or "invisible colleges," related to your topic. This factor is often a major flaw of most reviews, even validated reviews. If your database represents only those investigators who have published in readily accessible journals or books, your conclusions might be seriously flawed. In a meta-analysis, a serious bias might be introduced by not being aware of the fugitive literature, which may include many unpublished quality studies that do not support or may even contradict your conclusions.

The fourth procedure (cost-effectiveness) outlines an admittedly simplistic approach to achieve a crude estimate of the likely contribution your database might make, in relation to the time and fiscal expenditures required. Remember that Stage II of your **synthesis project** probably will absorb nearly half of your resources. It is quite important to have a clear idea about the state of your budget at this point. If your results are not representative of the major research available or are poorly documented, your time and fiscal expenditures might have been for naught.

In Appendixes 7.1 and 7.2, we will go into more detail about evaluating and improving your database by checking for both internal and external clues regarding the adequacy of your search effort.

APPENDIX 7.1
Screening for Internal Clues to Missed Studies

When performing a particularly important health science information synthesis, where your database needs to be unusually comprehensive, screening for internal clues to missed studies might be considered. New, valid studies can be added to the database up to the finalization of the manuscript in Stage V, if they do not require changing the formal relevance criteria. However, such additions will require redoing the synthesis calculations. This reanalysis is especially important in quantitative syntheses or if the file drawer problem analysis indicates that very few null papers, or those having data in the opposite direction from yours, would be needed to reverse your current conclusions.

**PROCEDURES TO SCREEN FOR
INTERNAL CLUES TO MISSED STUDIES**

A.   Analyze size of database
B.   Analyze proportion of relevant citations
C.   Analyze scope of final search plan
D.   Check miscoding of B- and C-rated citation-abstracts
E.   Check retrieval thoroughness
F.   Review search team's precision and interrater reliability

---

Procedure A. Analyze Size of Database

TASKS TO ANALYZE SIZE OF DATABASE

1.   If low citation count
2.   If high citation count

If there is a paucity of research studies on your topic, you might have to cope with several unique problems and take actions for their solution. If you find a rich literature with numerous studies, you might have to cope with a different set of problems, also requiring some actions. Here we consider each possibility.

Task 1: If Low Citation Count

If your synthesis database consists of a small number of relevant citation-abstracts (say fewer than 50) and even fewer relevant complete articles (say less than 10), the probability of missed studies or invisible colleges may be high. In such a case, your search scope and focus will need to be adjusted. To accomplish this, you might concentrate on overlooked bibliographic data sources by contacting other authors listed in your database. These colleagues might suggest new key articles, electronic bibliographic databases and index descriptors, and especially referrals to other colleagues who might be helpful.

There is a possibility that your topic field is new, with little or no research or publications completed to date. This possibility can be affirmed if colleagues have spent considerable searching effort and have found very little on your topic. In this instance, you will have to consider selecting another subject for your synthesis. On the other hand, if other researchers have found an abundant literature, they might help you alter your search strategy. For example, you might reexamine old and new bibliographic printouts in MEDLINE citations and abstract listings. If you search PREMEDLINE, you can obtain recent references that have not yet been fully processed for the MEDLINE file. Currently, this file is included in MEDLINE for search purposes. For additional information, see the following Web address (last updated January 2001): www.nlm.nih.gov/databases/databases.html.

On the other hand, you can search OLDMEDLINE for references between 1960 and 1965. (Remember that the main MEDLINE database started in 1964 and was not fully operational until 1966.) These citations do not have abstracts and are quite limited in the indexing terms available for these older references. This Internet site goes to Grateful MED at the following address (last updated March 2001): igm.nlm.nih.gov/.

For earlier references, you can do a hand-search of the paper source "Cumulative Index Medicus" for articles before 1960. In this case, you might recheck for overlooked key words generated by the investigators themselves or official index descriptors (e.g., MeSH headings used by the National Library of Medicine [NLM]). These missed terms can provide valuable clues to overlooked concepts and ideas. A medical librarian should be consulted to help cope with this problem if you continue to have trouble. Clinical librarians can help you analyze MeSH **tree structures** and use truncation symbols and other such strategies. Before giving up on any bibliographic source, it is important to read its "HELP" and "Update" Web site material. For example, if you have been using HealthSTAR, you know it is a database that emphasizes evaluation of healthcare outcomes and is being continually updated (last updated March 2000): www.nlm.nih.gov/pubs/factsheets/healthstar. html.

If you read NLM's recent "News and Noteworthy," you would discover that, since 1999, CATLINE (former NLM book catalogue) entries are no longer listed in HealthSTAR. Consequently, if you need a book citation, you have to contact the LOCATOR*plus* Website, which can be reached by linking through "Library Services" (last updated April 2001) at www.nlm.nih.gov/libserv.html.

Likewise, you can locate relevant material from the National Information Center on Health Services Research and Health Care Technology (NICHSR) Web site (last updated March 2001): www.nlm.nih.gov/nichsr/nichsr.html.

This database became available in 1996; it provides comprehensive coverage of material of interest for synthesis development from such fields as health services research, technology assessment, and administration.

A broader approach is to search for a library that might have a more detailed catalogue of citations in your topic area. This strategy is getting to "the bottom of the barrel" and could be very time-consuming. NLM's library catalogWeb site is the following (last updated January 1999): www.nlm.nih.gov/libraries/libraries.html.

Using this site, you can search for a library in one of the following categories:

- National libraries
- Federal libraries
- Medical research libraries by state
- Consumer health libraries
- Libraries in the Washington, D.C. metro area

The national libraries' site includes both the United States and United Kingdom. (When we use the term *federal,* we refer only to U.S. government libraries.)

Task 2: If High Citation Count

If your master list contains several hundred or more relevant citations that have yielded numerous complete relevant articles, the likelihood of missing important clues in your current database may be high but for different reasons. With a rich literature harvest, it is likely that an adequate search of the reference lists in articles retrieved was not done or perhaps poorly done. To manage this problem, your search documentation will be essential. To illustrate, a careful reanalysis of the adequacy of your citation processing is indicated: There may be many "A+" or "A" references that were not retrieved, many "references in references" may have been missed, you have been too busy to conduct a science citation analysis on a few older A+ references, or, equally serious, you may have failed to screen the fugitive literature. Such omissions can result in overlooking important empirical studies and invisible colleges.

Next you must judge how well a given literature is processed. The number of reviews or bibliographies that have been developed on that topic indicates this dimension. If few or none are found, it might mean that you have hit a rich research vein of ore, where little has been refined. Obviously, this is an opportunity for developing syntheses, establishing new postulates or theories, and eventually obtaining new knowledge from this material. On the other hand, if there are numerous reviews, you must develop a search strategy to look for meta-validated or systematic synthesis information you may have missed to date. The Internet addresses in Table 2.1, as well as Section B, Chapter 2, and in the compendium of Internet sources at the back of the book, are good places to start such a search.

Procedure B. Analyze Proportion of Relevant Citations

Another way to estimate whether key literature may have been missed is to determine what proportion of initial citations in bibliographic printouts or reference lists proved relevant (A+ A, A–) to your synthesis topic. Another name for this term is *precision*. If this proportion is small, with more than two thirds of the initially identified citations being marginally relevant (Cs and Bs), it is likely that many important articles may have been missed. Remember, there is usually an inverse relationship between the proportion of relevant articles missed (false negatives) and the proportion of those found that proved to be irrelevant (false positives). Using the relevance ratings of the complete documents as a gold standard, it is possible to optimize (minimax) these errors. One way is to identify an appropriate point where the proportion of false-negative and false-positive articles is acceptable for your purposes. If resources allow, it is better to err on the side of too many false positives; however, the cost of doing this is lost time and dollars due to the effort required to retrieve and code much material that ultimately proves irrelevant.

On the other hand, minimizing the number of false-negative articles will be at a cost of missing important data that might reverse your current synthesis conclusions. This consequence might bring questions about the quality of your search and could be hazardous to patients whose care was based on your possibly erroneous conclusions. Overall, your primary intent should be to minimize the number of missed relevant articles providing clues to invisible colleges. The cost of processing false-positive documents should be taken into account when developing your original fiscal and time budget.

Procedure C. Analyze Scope of Final Search Plan

At this Stage II evaluation of your database, it is important to review your evolving search plans to determine whether they seem to be on track in relation to your goals and synthesis model. In view of the profile of your evolving database, did your search seem too broad or too narrow in scope? A review of the search documentation compiled in Stage II can provide this information. For example, you can recheck the limits of your search of data sources to be screened, language limitations, and calendar year restrictions applied, or you may have overlooked identifying and retrieving relevant books or book chapters. This omission could seriously bias how representative your database might be. At the following Web site, you can access references for books, monographs, and other hardcover materials in NLM's LOCATOR*plus* (last updated ??, as checked in September 2001): locatorplus.gov/.

This is NLM's major online catalogue of books, journals, and audiovisuals and provides access points to other medical research tools. LOCATOR*plus* covers all of the cataloged titles in the NLM collection from the 15th century to the present.

Analysis of the time limits of your search is also an element to check. If the literature screened extended back more than 10 years, it is likely that during that earlier time period, many current descriptors did not exist or had not been applied. If major descriptors were only recently added (e.g., the past 5 years) to the formal National Library of Medicine MeSH headings, a bias might be introduced. To cope with this problem in MEDLINE, for example, obtain the current volume the NLM publishes that provides the date in which "descriptors" and "tags" were added or dropped. To find these early citations included in MEDLINE but not indexed, a "free text" search of earlier literature might be required. This type of search will likely require consultation with a medical information specialist, such as a medical librarian.

Another approach is to find an older classic article whose content, though out of date, could facilitate a science citation search from the files of the Institute for Scientific Information (ISI). By this means, it is possible to identify more recent investigators who have cited this classic. This is an effective means of identifying missed articles, invisible colleges, or author networks. For instance, identifying those authors who have cited Dolcourt and Braude (1976) might identify much recent literature regarding the limitations and overlap of such bibliographic databases as Excepta Medica and Index Medicus.

Procedure D. Check Miscoding of B- and C-Rated Citation-Abstracts

You usually retrieve the complete documents for A+, A, or A– citation-abstracts so that false-positive relevance ratings are almost always detected. Because the complete articles for B- and C-rated citations and abstracts are not retrieved, you cannot measure relevance coding recall (false-negative coding rates). If B and C citations and abstracts have been miscoded, you might have lost important information. Thus, at some point, you might check the extent of this type of coding error.

One way to check is to randomly select a sample of B- and C-coded citation-abstracts and retrieve and relevance-code their complete documents. Your sample size of these B- and C-coded materials should be at least 30 to 50, although the more the better to narrow the confidence intervals about the false-negative rates you might find. Comparing the ratings of these complete articles with the initial ratings of the citation-abstracts lets you calculate false-negative rates. Assume that out of the 50 B- or C-rated citation-abstracts that you discover from reading their complete articles, you rate five as A. The 95% **confidence interval** (CI) for the proportion 5 in 50 would range from 2% to 22%. In other words, there is a 95% probability that the true proportion lies within the interval of 2% to 22%. Note that these CIs can either be looked up in a table or calculated (see Fleiss, 1981, pp. 14-15).

However, if you checked 100 citation-abstracts rated B or C and found 5 A-rated articles, your 95% CI would narrow down to 2% to 11%. You can see that identifying false-negative documents among B- or C-rated citation-abstracts can be very expensive in terms of the number of complete articles you must retrieve and relevance-code. It is up to you to decide whether the cost of retrieving a hundred extra articles is worth the 2 to 10 A documents you might obtain. Nevertheless, our suggestion is that, in a large project involving thousands of citations, you should estimate recall (i.e., check for false-negative coding) at least once or twice.

It is another issue to cope with the many other false-negative documents that never fell within the scope of your citation screening. Trying to identify invisible colleges is one strategy we have already suggested you try (see Task 2, Procedure D, Chapter 6).

Procedure E: Check Retrieval Thoroughness

Screening citation relevance ratings on the chronological master list might identify several important citations for which the complete articles have not been retrieved. Checking whether all promising A+, A, and A– citations or abstracts were actually obtained and processed is easily accomplished if the master list documentation has been kept up-to-date regarding reference retrieval status—for example, articles that were (a) retrieved and processed, (b) retrieved but not processed, (c) not yet retrieved, or (d) not accessible. There are so many tasks to complete in any search, and citations and documents pile up so rapidly that there is a frequent risk of important leads (coded A–, A, or A+) being overlooked. Reducing this risk is an essential task to ensure that your database will be representative. Identifying such overlooked leads can increase the number of relevant articles (and references within those articles) that could be added to your synthesis database and subsequently screened for new invisible colleges.

Procedure F. Review Search
Team's Precision and Interrater Reliability

Each iteration includes a relevance-coding precision rate and an interrater reliability computation. (Recall that the precision rate equals true positives divided by the sum of true positives and false negatives.) If these rates seem low, it is possible that relevance criteria are misleading, or that one or all of the literature retrieval team is incorrectly rating citations and articles for relevance. For example, if a Kappa rating is much below 0.60, it is important to determine the cause and whether this error has negatively biased the generalizability of your final conclusions. Another reason for low Kappas could be "topic drift," due to the team's failure to follow agreed-on relevance criteria. Or, it may be that earlier calibration sessions were not done, and early detectable "drift" was not noted or corrected until much later. Perhaps other factors can be identified to explain why an unacceptable level of agreement occurred among the search team members. At this point, you may still be able to correct some of these problems and enhance how well your synthesis meets the criterion of being representative of the total spectrum of invisible colleges, as we will discuss in Appendix 7.2.

APPENDIX 7.2
Screening for External Clues to Missed Studies

As with Appendix 7.1, when performing a particularly important health science synthesis where your database needs to be unusually comprehensive, the following tasks might be considered. New studies found can be added throughout the various stages of the synthesis development. If many relevant articles are added that seem to contradict your own conclusions at any given time, you will have to conduct a validation effort for these papers and repeat or revise your synthesis calculations in Stage IV. This reanalysis is especially important in quantitative syntheses or when the "file drawer problem" analysis indicates that very few null or contradictory studies would be needed to reverse your current conclusions.

PROCEDURES OF SCREENING FOR
EXTERNAL CLUES TO MISSED STUDIES

A. Review or repeat a file drawer analysis
B. Contact experts not previously consulted
C. Complete a funnel plot analysis
D. Search more intensively for fugitive literature
E. Briefly update database before finalizing Stage II

Procedure A. Review or Repeat a File Drawer Analysis

Recall that in Procedure D (search termination), Chapter 6, we defined and gave a brief historical note on the file drawer problem. We then discussed file drawer analysis as a method for coping with the decision as to when it is no longer cost-effective to continue your search.

Hunter and Schmidt (1990, pp. 510-513) provide further elaboration of Rosenthal's computational methods for making a file drawer estimate. However, we have developed a much simpler "look-up table" to help you quickly approximate this number without computation. In Table 6.1 (Procedure D, Chapter 6), we describe specific tasks on how to use this table.

NOTE

Again, it is important to understand that a final file drawer problem analysis cannot be computed until your research database effect sizes are determined, coded, and validated in Stage III. Because Stages II and III overlap considerably, you can at least make one or two preliminary file drawer estimates before the completion of Stage II.

If results of this analysis indicate that you require a large number of "missed" negative articles to reverse your conclusions, you might consider terminating your search. On the other hand, if very few missing articles would be needed to overturn your conclusions, you likely would want to continue your search.

Procedure B. Contact
Experts Not Previously Consulted

These "people" sources can provide one of the more efficient means for identifying missed relevant and valid articles, investigators, or invisible colleges. At this point near the end of Stage II, it is likely that new information has been generated in your field since you started your literature search. There might be recently identified new research missed in the initial search. This second survey of prominent colleagues might lead to new literature or especially to new investigators, key organizations, or professional groups that have not been contacted to date.

Procedure C. Complete a Funnel Plot Analysis

An effective method to estimate serious bias in your current database is to analyze Light and Pillemer's (1984, pp. 63-72) "Funnel Display." This concept was discussed in Section A, Chapter 5. Recall that this funnel display analysis might indicate, among other factors, such problems as publication bias or historical trends among statistical effects. Figures 5.1 and 5.2 provide a graphic illustration of a funnel display with and without nonpublished articles. When nonpublished studies are not plotted, you see the classic truncation pattern. This technique is a relatively simple visual approach to noting **heterogeneity** among the studies you have compiled thus far. If your database is not homogeneous, it might represent multiple research study populations that will not permit a valid quantitative analysis. If the quality of your studies varies, the funnel plot could be misleading (Petticrew et al., 1999). If discovered early in your Stage II evaluation, this serious bias can be corrected. On the other hand, if discovered in your final evaluation, unless time and resources allow, it is probably too late to make adjustments to compensate for such a heterogeneous population among the aggregate of your studies.

Procedure D. Search More Intensively for Fugitive Literature

One of the most neglected sources of valuable information encompassing clues to missing articles or invisible colleges is the "subterranean literature," "gray literature," or, as Marylou C. Rosenthal (1994) calls it, "fugitive literature." She provides detailed coverage on how to locate difficult-to-find unpublished or published sources of important information, such as (a) corporate technical reports; (b) government information files (especially information from the National Library of Medicine, the Agency for Healthcare Research and Quality, or the ongoing surveys by the National Center for Health Statistics); (c) studies in progress not ready for write-up; (d) university postgraduate student theses, dissertations, and reports; (e) proceedings of meetings and conferences; (f) final reports by blue-ribbon panels or commissions; (g) consensus reports; (h) little-known computer sources such as those on the Internet; and especially (i) contacting authors for their "negative" papers rejected or never submitted for publication. The U.S. Library of Congress can be surprisingly helpful in locating many of the above types of information. The index to this source is the following Internet address (last updated June 1998): lcweb.loc.gov/harvest/query-lc.html. Unpublished or published, sound material that you fail to identify is important for assessing the extent of publication bias. The "rejected" studies may represent a different point of view on the topic area, one that has not yet been widely circulated due to the bias against publishing null or "negative" findings or due to peer rejection of new innovative research approaches that are not understood or trusted. Valid published studies may have been missed because they were not within the scope of your search.

Procedure E. Briefly Update Database Before Finalizing Stage II

The length of time it takes to develop a quality manuscript for either journal or book publication is always far more than most authors anticipate. Consequently, scientific events in the field of your synthesis topic may have slipped by you since completing the Stage II database. There is usually very little you can do to cope with this reality except make a cursory last-minute effort to update your database and data set before completing your manuscript. Ideally, if you can find a literature historian in your field, he or she can be contacted to help you come up-to-date.

When writing your synthesis manuscript, you might also do a final PREMEDLINE, MEDLINE, or EMBASE computer search for the time period since you terminated your Stage II database search. A Science Citation Index (SCI) search on a favorite classic, limiting the time span to that covered since your last SCI search, can be done rather quickly. Finally, the most recent information in "Current Contents," online or published from the ISI, gives you a brief update from the table of contents in the most relevant serials you have used. Many of these same references can be found in PREMEDLINE as well. Again, remember that you cannot apply new relevance criteria at this point. You may add new highly relevant research studies to your reference list that meet your current relevance requirements. However, especially with quantitative syntheses, you must add the new data to your data set and recalculate your final results.

There is a possible exception that would negate the need for a final database updating. That exception would be if your final file drawer analysis indicates that a large number of new articles with null or contradictory results would be required to overturn your current conclusions. In such an instance, it may be unlikely that a last-minute search effort, or adding a couple of new papers, would make much difference.

FORM 7.1: DATABASE EVALUATION CHECKLIST
(Sorted by Generic Information Sources)

Iteration #_____

Date _____

Initials _____

Computer Sources

1. Have online "evidence-based" sources, especially in the United States and the United Kingdom, been screened for relevant "systematic reviews"? ___ Yes ___ No

2. Has a mini-synthesis of meta-validated reviews been done? ___ Yes ___ No

3. Have at least four online bibliographic databanks other than MEDLARS (e.g., BRS, Dialog, or EMBASE) been screened? ___ Yes ___ No

4. Have online electronic database descriptor lists been used (e.g., NIH Medical Subject Headings [MeSH] index?) ___ Yes ___ No

5. Have specific clearinghouses or continuing bibliographic search services been contacted for leads or updates? ___ Yes ___ No

People Sources

1. Have authors of relevant documents (i.e., systematic reviews, research articles) been contacted for references or leads? ___ Yes ___ No

2. Have groups that fund research or other activities (e.g., conferences) been contacted? ___ Yes ___ No

3. Have professional or lay organizations having a special interest in this topic been contacted? ___ Yes ___ No

4. Have reference librarians or information science specialists been contacted for advice on search strategies? ___ Yes ___ No

Published Paper Sources

1. Have indexes tabulating books and monographs, including book reviews, been searched? ___ Yes ___ No

2. Have "Current Contents" or other "Table of Contents" of recent journals or books been screened? ___ Yes ___ No

3. Has an SCI search of authors citing relevant early articles been conducted? ___ Yes ___ No

4. Have science writers for the lay press or leading newspaper   ___ Yes   ___ No
    or magazine files been contacted for references or leads?

5. Have letters to the editor been systematically screened for relevant   ___ Yes   ___ No
    publications or other leads?

Nonpublished Paper Sources

1. Were the investigators you contacted asked about unpublished   ___ Yes   ___ No
    research reports?

2. Have dissertation indexes been searched?   ___ Yes   ___ No

3. Have indexes to other nonpublished manuscripts, abstracts, or   ___ Yes   ___ No
    presented papers (e.g., Library of Congress) been searched?

4. Have deans or department chairpersons in relevant professional   ___ Yes   ___ No
    schools been contacted for leads regarding unpublished student
    papers or faculty research?

Document Retrieval Adequacy

1. Have all citation sources searched been recorded and the results   ___ Yes   ___ No
    tabulated?

2. Has there been an update search within 6 months of finalizing the   ___ Yes   ___ No
    manuscript of the synthesis?

3. Have all citation lists been checked against the master citation list   ___ Yes   ___No
    to identify new (as opposed to redundant) A or B references?

4. Has the percentage of "A" references, identified but not yet   ___ Yes   ___ No
    retrieved, been reduced to less than 5%?

DATABASE VALIDATION

CHAPTER 8

Data Extraction and Coding

Retrieving and coding of information and data from primary studies provide the foundation on which a synthesis is built. This process consists of distilling concepts to numbers in order for information to be compared across studies. In this chapter, both the theoretical issues in and practical steps for setting up accurate and efficient coding processes are presented.

SYNTHESIS DATA EXTRACTION AND CODING

    A. Theoretical issues in data extracting and coding
    B. Procedures for data extraction and coding

Section A. Theoretical Issues in Data Extracting and Coding

There are six general issues associated with the extraction and coding of data.

Issue 1: Coding Too Little or Too Much Data

If a synthesizer errs on the side of coding too much information or data, the biggest problem is wasted time, effort, and expense. The increased time may not be trivial. Adding only an extra five items that take an additional 3 minutes each, across 200 studies, may increase overall coding time as much as 10 hours per coder. Less likely, but just as important, is the possibility that data coded at too fine a granularity may result in findings that are not comparable from one study to the next. Also affecting comparability is the fact that constructs vary in the level of abstraction at which they are defined and measured. However, in the long run, it is much better to code too much data than too little, given equal resources; it is much more difficult and more time-consuming to go back and reread articles than to collect the information from the beginning.

If a researcher codes too little data or codes at too abstract a level, then there is an increased potential for error, lost information, and unreliability of data collection. To avoid such errors and at the same time minimize coding time, you should make every effort to explicitly define coding options and procedures before the coding begins. The original conceptual model of the information synthesis should guide decisions regarding what to code and how to define coding options. It is true, however, that the question and the definitions evolve over the synthesis process, so it is important that the model is addressed again at this stage (see Section D, Chapter 2, for a full discussion of this issue).

Issue 2: Missing Data

Data are rarely completely missing or completely present. The usual problem is that data are partially missing because they are unclear, incompletely specified, or available but undocumented. In addition, the consequences of missing data depend on how they are missing. If data are simply randomly missing, then there are different implications for the study than if the data are systematically missing. Understanding this problem involves the six factors discussed below:

Data Clarity. Data may not exactly be missing but may be quite unclear. For example, patients may be given presurgical instruction regarding deep breathing, but unless the study explicitly states that the patient was taught how to cough, it can only be assumed that such information was included. Hence, all data should be coded for clarity. One of the best ways to do this is to have coders report the degree of certainty in their ratings. For example, authors may report that research assistants were not informed of the group assignment of subjects, so we can infer that they were blinded, but we are not quite sure. However, if authors say that research assistants were blinded to the subjects' experimental condition by removing all identifying information from the chart, then coding of this item has more certainty. Using confidence or certainty ratings have many benefits, such as assisting the reviewer in identifying aspects of missing information, highlighting problems with the conceptual definitions of variables, and assisting the reader in interpreting the results of some sensitivity analyses. In their review comparing psychotherapy techniques, Glass et al. (1981)

found no relationship between therapist experience and effect size; however, as Orwin (1994) noted, therapist experience could only be extracted with confidence from 1 out of 10 reports. As a result, the strength of the conclusion regarding the relationship between experience and therapeutic outcomes is undermined.

Reasons for Missing Data. If data are totally missing, the reason must be specified. Missing data occur for several reasons, and some reasons will have more impact on the results of a synthesis than others; for example, data could be missing either because they were collected and not reported or because they were not collected. Understanding the source and cause of missing data is an essential first step in developing decision rules regarding coding the information.

Pigott (1994) and Light (1988) have analyzed the types and causes of missing data, with the underlying principle governing their categorization being the degree to which the missing variable is systematically associated with the results of the study. In other words, the important discriminations to make are whether the data are randomly missing, whether the pattern of missing data is associated with the value of the data, and/or whether they are associated with the results of the study. The type of missing data will determine the procedures for dealing with them later in the analysis. Table 8.1 displays the reasons for missing data and some possible solutions.

Missing Data Are Random. This type of missing data occurs when the information missing is a function of random error, author idiosyncrasies, or unavailability for reasons not associated with the value of the data or the results of the study. For example, information about a specific characteristic of the population may not be included because the author simply forgot to include it, because of research assistant error, or because of computer damage to databases. In these cases, there is no clear reason to associate the missing data with the value of the data (e.g., income data are only missing on elderly patients), the results of the study, or any other systematic characteristic of the study. In these cases, it is reasonable to use accepted methods of estimation to replace the missing values. Methods of estimation are discussed in Variation 5, Procedure B, Chapter 14.

Missing Data Are Systematic but Not Associated With Values of a Variable or Study Outcomes. This type of missing data is information missing for a reason associated with the study but not with the value of the variable. A major cause of this kind of missing data is different reporting practices in varied fields of study. For example, in medicine, it is often not customary to report the exact instructions given to subjects, whereas in psychology, this information is normally expected in the methods section. Similarly, data may be missing because the authors assume definitions are commonly agreed on, such as the exact methods for a medical procedure. In their meta-analysis on psychotherapy, Glass et al. (1981) found that the authors of primary studies

TABLE 8.1 Summary of How to Cope With Four Types of Missing Data

Type of Missing Data	Possible Solutions
Totally random: Reporting deficiencies not associated with any other variable, with the value of the variable itself, or with the results of the study.	1. Guessing conventions based on common practice. 2. Estimate missing data from known data from other studies.
Nonsystematic: Reporting deficiencies associated not with the value of the item missing or the results of the study but with variables already reported (e.g., assumed to be shared information).	1. Contact investigator. 2. Estimate missing data from known data in other studies. 3. Use expert judgment to estimate values.
Systematic: Reporting deficiencies systematically associated with the value of the item missing but not with the results of the study.	1. Contact investigator. 2. Use expert judgment to estimate values. 3. Estimate data statistically from other variables within the study itself.
Biased: Reporting deficiencies not only associated with the value of the item missing but also with the results of the study.	1. Contact investigator. 2. Avoid using that study, if possible.

NOTE: Right column entries refer to common solutions for managing missing data.

rarely described in full the type of psychotherapy. Groups of domain experts had to be used to make explicit the differing characteristics of each type of therapy. The result was that data were missing for a class of studies coming from a particular area. If there is no reason to suspect that a category of studies would have different findings than other categories of studies, then the values of the missing data may be estimated.

Missing Data Are Systematically Associated With Values of a Variable but Not Study Outcomes. This type of missing data presents more of a problem for reviewers. In this case, the information is missing in a specific pattern. One kind of pattern is due to the value of the information itself; for example, many authors do not publish nonsignificant results. Thus, the value of the variable determines whether or not it is missing. Or, the variable may be published only by certain specialties. For example, pharmacists may provide more thorough patient education on drug use than physicians. The result may be greater patient knowledge and compliance for those studies using pharmacists, but this information is missing. If the depth of patient education was not reported, and failure to report was associated with a dependent variable of interest (e.g., compliance), then you have a missing variable associated with the value of a variable.

If the value of the missing variable is not related to the outcome of interest (the quality of patient education may reasonably be thought not to relate to length of an incision), then the variable might be missing systematically but not bias the outcome. Some estimation procedures may be used here.

Missing Data Are Associated With Study Outcomes. If the outcome of a study (such as low infection rates) can be reasonably associated with the quality of patient health education, you have a variable whose missing data is systematically associated with the results of the study, and the outcome is therefore biased. Missing data of this type directly bias the size of the effect.

Because of the direct impact on effect sizes, this type of problem is difficult to deal with in meta-analyses. In some cases, it may be possible to infer the necessary information from other reported data or use complicated statistical procedures to predict the missing variable. For example, Glass et al. (1981), in their meta-analysis on psychotherapy, reported having to guess mortality rates from changes in the degrees of freedom from pretest to posttest.

Overall, decisions regarding how to deal with missing data depend on the underlying cause and the degree to which the missing data are systematically correlated with other aspects of the study, such as type of population examined, effect size, or author. If the data are missing as a result of a random process, quite accurate estimates can be generated statistically by using the available data. These procedures are outlined in detail in Variation 5, Procedure B, Chapter 14. When the data are missing for systematic (or nonrandom) reasons, then estimates based on the incomplete data set could be seriously biased.

Issue 3: Construct Coding

Construct coding includes how the variable was measured or manipulated and the conditions under which the manipulations and measurement occurred. In cases such as mortality, which is measured by death as determined by hospital records or the *International Classification of Diseases—9th Revision* (*ICD-9*) codes, the data are easy to code. However, other types of data may not have clear or exact methods of measurement for the dependent variables, nor may there be specific descriptions of manipulating the independent variables. In these cases, the coders must use their subjective judgments. Subjective judgments about construct definitions, even when made using explicit coding instructions, may be unreliable because of the difficulty accounting for all possible contingencies.

The issues of degree of treatment integrity and consistency with which the independent variable is operationalized in each study, as well as whether the specific operationalization matches the conceptual independent variable under consideration, are especially difficult. People implementing the independent variable (the treatment) may differ in their level of training, settings may differ in significant ways that are not expected, and only some aspects of the independent variable may be implemented consistently across all studies. For example, in one meta-analysis on the impact of a clinical pharmacokinetic system (CPS) for aminoglycoside drug monitoring, the definition of a CPS (the independent variable) varied from study to study. In some studies, the implementation of a CPS included education of the nurses and doctors, the writing of orders by pharmacists, and the implementation and use of specific formulas for assessing appropriate dosing. In other studies, the staff education component is not reported. In some studies, only physicians write all orders, but in other studies, pharmacists write everything. In other cases, only the type of dosing formula used and the collection of serum assays are the same for both control and experimental groups. It is essential that these differences in how the independent variable is conceptualized and operationalized are captured in the recording process.

Judgment, then, is required regarding how close each description of the independent variable is to the one under investigation by the reviewer. At the very least, the dimensions on which the independent variables differ from study to study need to be systematically identified and coded. Later, these dimensions can be used for systematic analyses assessing the impact of differences in the independent variable on study results.

The same level of subjective judgment is often involved in coding for dependent variables when the construct being measured is assessed in a variety of ways. Renal failure may be defined as the ratio of blood urinary nitrogen (BUN) to creatine in one study and only creatine levels in another, efficacy of treatment may be measured by blood or urine cultures, and depression may be assessed by different instruments. The result of this variation in measurement is decreased statistical power and increased probability of failing to find an effect that truly exists. Although these problems are pervasive, specific coding procedures can mitigate some of the problems. We will cover these procedures later in this chapter.

Issue 4: Selection and Calculation of Effect Sizes

Because "effect size" is defined as a mean difference between control group and treatment group interventions, it can be expressed in terms of raw numbers ($M_t - M_c$).

Effect sizes can also be standardized in terms of the error variance in the study. In that case, the mean difference is divided by a standard deviation $(M_t - M_c)/SD$. The particular standard deviation (SD) used is either that of the control group or the pooled SD of all groups. The advantage of using a standardized effect size is that results are comparable across studies. The only modification needed to pool the results is some weighting scheme to allow for different size samples.

Coding directly for effect sizes may be too global an approach. Rather, the specific items that comprise an effect size should be recorded and the actual effect size computed from the raw data. Glass et al. (1981) reported the effect sizes computed by two judges for six studies taken from the meta-analysis of the effects of psychotherapy. He showed that none of the six studies were coded identically, and the difference between coders ranged from 0.20 to 0.0.

It is not always clear which effect sizes to code. Multiple statistical tests may be conducted on the same data, making it difficult to determine which analysis to include, especially when the construct being assessed is broadly defined. For example, treatment efficacy may be measured by blood cultures, overall length of treatment, and length of stay. Which one to use and how many to use are complex questions. Answering the questions requires reviewing the conceptual model and specifying priorities.

Issue 5: Minimizing Coder Bias

In this subsection, we outline errors that can occur due to coder biases. Normal human information processing has limitations, and human perception is often a function of expectations and stereotypes. For example, the introduction of bias into the coding process occurs when certain authors of primary research are perceived as carrying more authority than others, results are more congruent with the coder's beliefs, or certain procedures are more favored. Coder bias in noting and recording information has significant effects on the resulting meta-analytic findings. Ample research in the psychological field has demonstrated the impact of investigator bias on research findings (R. Rosenthal, 1969, 1994). Potential sources of bias include tendencies to (a) rate famous authors as having better research methods, (b) rate findings inconsistent with previous work to be more valid, (c) find results consistent with our beliefs to be more valued or to be stronger, or (d) find results to be more significant that make our gender or our racial group look better. Sometimes, the effects are not trivial and may have significant policy implications (Wortman & Bryant, 1985).

Bias is a product of normal information processing. To minimize bias, its sources must be identified and systematic procedures established to deal with it. At least three sources of biases are (a) expectancy effects due to the source of the article (e.g., the journal, school, or author); (b) expectancy effects due to beliefs about the area of study, such as a theoretical position or educational background; or (c) self-serving biases, which include one's school, gender, racial group, or publications.

Fortunately, the procedures needed to minimize all of these sources overlap. **Blinding** coders to the authors, the school, the journal, and the results of the study will greatly minimize expectancy effects. Using coders who have some expertise in an area but who are not major experimenters removes some self-serving bias. Using at least two coders with different backgrounds maximizes initial differences that will later be helpful in refining coding criteria. Many of the protections used for primary research to eliminate research expectancy effects may be useful for coders; for example, if coders can remain blind to the purpose of the study or to the specific hypothesis, less bias would be expected. Evaluating the methods section independently of the results section prevents contamination of validity assessment due to knowing results of a study (Sacks, Berrier, Reitman, Ancova-Berk, & Chalmers, 1987).

Issue 6: Assessing Validation Team Coder Reliability

In this subsection, we discuss the concept of assessing coder reliability (agreement between validation coders), as well as the negative impact of poor consensus—an inherent part of the coding process. Not only does information about reliability provide feedback about the coding process to increase accuracy, but also reliability information helps clarify important conceptual and theoretical questions regarding the review itself. Assessing reliability also protects somewhat against coder bias (see above). Estimating reliability may not be clear-cut, and there are issues to consider regarding what items to include in a reliability assessment, as well as issues regarding how reliability is computed and the detail at which results should be reported.

Differences in coding between raters are extremely common. Sources of these differences vary, and their importance ranges from simple random variations to serious problems with the validity of definitions and codes. The impact on results may range from a minor attenuation of effect sizes (the relationship between independent and dependent variables is smaller when the reliability of the specific measures is low) to significant changes in results and conclusions. For example, Orwin and Cordray (1985) recoded a sample of studies from the meta-analysis on psychotherapy outcomes (Glass et al., 1981). They found that when the measures were adjusted for unreliability, the results of the analysis were significantly changed. Specifically, the reliability correction altered the ranking of predictors from the original regression analysis (Orwin, 1994). Given the potentially large impact of coding reliability on results, it is essential not only to assess interrater reliability but to report it as well.

Assessing interrater reliability can be complicated because it is not obvious how to group items for assessment or which interrater reliability index to use. Some authors simply compute agreement across all items for a total score. This procedure combines items that are not conceptually related (e.g., age of participants and year of publication) and those that would naturally be highly reliable (e.g., year of publication) with those requiring much more subjective judgment (e.g., presence of "blinding"). Orwin (1994) recommends a procedure developed by Yeaton and Wortman (1991) that first focuses on the lower levels of a category. For example, items that are included in the overall topic of experimenter blinding include the presence or absence of knowledge of the hypothesis, knowledge of group membership during data collection, and knowledge of the hypothesis during the analysis stage. These items could be combined and reliability assessed for the single concept of blinding. Then, in an additional step, validation reliability could be assessed across several other items.

In terms of what reliability indices to use, there continues to be some controversy among reviewers. In general, percentage agreement, Kappa, weighted Kappa, intercoder correlation, and interclass correlation are the indices most commonly used. Orwin (1994) presents an excellent discussion of this issue. We recommend using Kappa, either the weighted or unweighted forms, in order for you to best control for chance agreement (Cohen, 1968). Procedures for computing a Kappa are presented in Table 10.1, Chapter 10.

Section B. Procedures for Extracting and Coding Data

The coding process begins when articles are retrieved, numbered, and duplicated. Enough copies of each retrieved article should be made to supply all the coders. Coders are trained, pilot coding is done, and then actual data recording is performed. The process ends when all the validated data are in a computerized format, cleaned, and ready to analyze. The data extraction and coding process involves four tasks: develop coding criteria and manual, train team and calibrate its validation ratings, identify and manage missing data, and record data into data set.

Procedure 1: Develop Coding Criteria and Manual

This first procedure, development of coding criteria and procedural manuals, tends to be overlooked until problems become apparent. Careful attention to this phase early in the coding process will prevent significant loss of future time. The process starts with adoption of a generic coding list specific to the synthesis at hand. The conceptual model specifies the important questions associated with the review. Items to be coded should be chosen on both methodological and theoretical grounds and specifically tailored to every synthesis. Issues regarding the setting, the type of subjects, and the methodology identified in the conceptual model are now defined in detail through the coding criteria.

There are many taxonomies of codes. We have adopted Stock's (1994) coding categories here. The list in Table 8.2 is a template adaptable for future redesigns.

A template of initial items should be developed from the categories listed in Table 8.2. Once the items have been specified, the possible range for each variable is identified. For example, income could be coded into one of several categories (e.g., low, middle, or high), or the specific income could be coded (e.g., $37,500 per year). *Blinding* could be defined as having two qualities (yes or no) or consisting of many predefined levels that include no blinding, research assistants not aware of group membership, and research assistants not aware of the hypothesis of the study. Each variable should have a clear definition, criteria for coding, and examples developed for explanatory purposes. These definitions are entered into a coding manual to be used for training purposes. The coding manual is written simultaneously with the development of items and contains definitions, examples, and process instructions. At the same time, a coding sheet is prepared that matches the coding manual and is the actual place where data are recorded.

The coding manual should address several coding issues. First, items in the manual and on the coding sheet should be listed in the same order as they are found in the studies. Ordering is particularly important in coding studies for which there are multiple dependent measures, each with different effect sizes and characteristics, or when different information is provided about subgroups. Second, the categories in the manual and on the coding sheets should be described thoroughly. Third, items should be highlighted on the coding sheet in a readable and useful manner. Finally, all descriptions, issues, problems, and resolutions that arise should be included within the manual.

At this time the list of items to be coded should be sent to two or more persons familiar with the domain and with issues of methodology. Once their feedback has been incorporated into the coding definitions, a few pilot attempts with coders should be conducted to clarify any confusing items remaining.

Procedure 2: Train Team and Calibrate Its Validation Ratings

This second procedure, training a team and calibration of coder ratings, is essential to enhance efficiency and accuracy of the coding process.

Select and Train Coders. The coding team should be chosen for both its content knowledge and methodological expertise. At least two coders should be used to enhance reliability. When coders have been selected, they should be formally introduced to the project, the other players, and the procedures. It is not advisable to

TABLE 8.2 Generic Coding Categories

1. *Report identification* are items associated with the article or study itself, such as country where study occurred, author(s), and year of publication. Also included here is information about the authors' training, education, and theoretical orientation.

2. *Kind of design* refers to the process of categorizing the design into predetermined appropriate categories (e.g., information synthesis, randomized clinical trials, clinical trials, quasi-experimental, descriptive case study, descriptive population, or didactic).

3. *Setting/subjects* are items associated with the population being studied such as a sexually transmitted disease (STD) clinic, socioeconomic status (SES) of community, and specific issues associated with sampling. Also included here is sampling information (e.g., the diagnostic test used); description of the subjects' age, SES, and so on; and disease characteristics (e.g., severity).

4. *Independent variable manipulation* refers to the number of groups, characteristics of those groups, processes of handling the groups differently, and process of group assignment. Also included here are definitions of different variations in the independent variable.

5. *Study procedures* include any information regarding the procedures associated with the study across both groups—for example, how cultures were taken, what information was given to the subjects, the order of events (if important), and/or the training of the research assistants. Size of groups should be collected here.

6. *Methodology/research quality items* are presented and discussed under validation procedures in Chapter 6 and Chapter 7 but are usually collected at the same time as the other variables.

7. *Dependent variables* are those variables that were expected to be the "effect" of the experiment. Coding should include not only which variables were measured (a sort of checklist of all possible ones) but also a notation of how they were measured (requiring development of a list of all possible variations in measurement). Also included here is information about reliability, validity, and scaling.

8. *Statistical information* includes the results, means, standard deviations, reliability estimates of measures, proportions, confidence intervals, and significance for each dependent variable. Because articles often report data somewhat differently, every effort should be made to include sufficient statistical information, including whole tables of results, if possible. Also included here are all the codes for missing data.

9. *Coder information* includes the coder name, the time taken to code the article, certainty levels, and any open-ended comments.

10. *Theoretical background* involves the major theoretical justification of the research, either research paradigm, origin of hypothesis, or school of thought. Development of coding criteria for this class of items requires domain expertise.

inform them of the hypothesis, if possible. Except for early training sessions, we do not recommend that the author(s) take part in the validation procedures, due to his or her inherent bias. The author's responsibility is to be sure the validation team is on track and doing a good job, especially in terms of interrater reliability.

Pilot-Test Coding Manual. Coders must review the coding manual in a step-by-step manner, not only to educate themselves but to suggest any needed revisions as well. They should also set up procedures for communicating with the authors, with any outside experts willing to answer their questions, as well as with each other.

Once the initial training sessions are conducted, pilot sessions can begin. Each pilot session should include between two and five articles. Initial sessions should be conducted with the coders and one or more authors, so that discussions after each session can be incorporated into the manual and the coding sheet. Once several articles have been reviewed without requiring substantial discussion, coders can begin to work independently if resources do not allow dual coding of every article. If the latter is the case, this fact should be mentioned in the limitations section of the manuscript.

Practice Coding Reliability Assessment. At this point, formal reliability assessment of the validation team can be conducted. Sessions are kept deliberately small until reliability reaches a sufficiently high level to allow continuing with larger numbers of articles. We recommend that a Kappa greater than 0.80 be reached at this point, because reliability usually drops later, and should not go below 0.70 or, at worst, 0.65. To maintain interrater reliability, regular meetings should be held with coders and frequent reliability checks conducted. This process cannot be overemphasized because errors and unreliability in coding can change the conclusions and threaten the contribution of your synthesis.

There are several methods for assessing agreement or reliability, including intraclass correlations, percentage agreement, and Cohen's Kappa. Which one to use depends on the kind of data or ratings. For categorical data, we recommend using Cohen's Kappa because it is one of the few reliability indicators that control for chance agreement. However, Kappa results can be misleading when the base ratings are skewed. For example, it is possible to have a 97% agreement on items and still get only a moderate Kappa of about 0.50 when most items are in one category alone. For that reason, it is a good idea to report both percentage agreement and Kappa for indicating level of agreement.

For continuous data, such as ratings of quality and ratings of uncertainty, a Pearson correlation is recommended. Because most statistical packages can easily calculate a correlation, we are not going to provide specific computational instructions. We do recommend that data be kept in an electronic database management program to ensure easy conversion to statistical programs if needed (see the section below on database management programs).

Table 10.1 in Chapter 10 includes instructions for calculating a Cohen's Kappa (Castellan & Siegel, 1988). Conceptually, Kappa refers to the number of agreed items normalized by the number that could have been agreed on, minus chance agreement. In other words, Kappa is the proportion of agreement not due to chance. The easiest way to implement the above procedures is to use a spreadsheet, such as Microsoft Excel.

Procedure 3: Identify and Manage Missing Data

The third procedure is to develop strategies for handling missing data. These strategies will depend on the reasons or causes for why the data are missing. First, we recommend that all missing data be coded for the level of uncertainty involved in the missing data. We also recommend the following four categories be used as a descriptor field for each item:

1. No missing information about the item—item present in database.

2. No information available on the item at all—item classed as missing.

3. Incomplete information available on the item—item classed as missing.

4. Item content inferred from other data in article—item present in database.

Although using this field almost doubles the size of the database, it is possible to have defaults set in place so that the item is rated as fully present unless someone enters information in that field. A few additional text fields are essential for capturing explanations and clarifications by the coders. Decisions regarding whether or not authors have to be contacted will be made by the synthesis team as a function of the importance of the item to the analysis and the degree to which the missing data could bias the results.

Missing data that can be recovered independently of the author include the location of authors or information about the care setting. By using this code, the database can be sorted in terms of actions relevant to the recovery of missing data.

Data that cannot be recovered by contacting the author or by independent efforts must be estimated. There are three fundamental ways to estimate these data. The *first* is to use similar data from the published literature. Incident rates, procedural texts, and population averages are examples of data that can be estimated from other published literature. The *second* method is to use expert judgment. Appendix 2.1 in Chapter 2 contains detailed procedures for using structured group consensus for any number of purposes. In general, a group of experts (between three and seven) in a domain are selected to make systematic judgments regarding a decision. The *third* method is statistical and involves imputing the numbers systematically; these procedures are presented in more detail in Section C, Chapter 13.

Procedure 4: Record Data Into Data Set

We recommend that coders enter data directly into the database using prestructured forms (e.g., see Form 8.1 at the end of this chapter). However, such procedures may not be feasible, and coders may need to enter information onto a paper form first and then transfer it into the computer database. The order of the information input should be identical for both procedures to facilitate transfer between the two mediums. In addition, the persons entering data from coding sheets into the computer should not have to make any subjective judgments. The data should be in a form such that what they see on paper is what they record in the computer.

In addition, it is essential that all data entered be verified. A simple technique is to compare a printout of the current records, as they appear in the database, to the original coding forms. For some database software, simple quality checks can be constructed to check the length of the variable, the type of variable, and the expected values. Quality check and verification are often overlooked to gain time but are invaluable to prevent unnecessary data analyses later.

Summary

A. Theoretical Issues in Extracting and Coding Data

In any coding scheme, reviewers need to weigh the costs and benefits of coding too much information versus too little. We recommend erring on the side of too much, as long as it is possible to stay within the limits of your budget and timetable. In general, several issues need to be addressed.

First, deal systematically with missing data, (i.e., reporting deficiencies) within primary studies. Data need to be recorded in terms of whether they are missing and the likely reason for why they are missing. In addition, the degree of certainty to which variables are coded should also be captured.

Second, give careful attention to 'construct coding' for both the independent and dependent variables. Many variables are conceptually but not physically identical. Subjective judgment is then needed to discriminate between differing methods of measurement. Detailed decision rules need to be constructed to capture these variations in subjective judgment.

Third, choose which effect size to use, as it may be an issue in some domains where multiple dependent variables are examined within each study. Again, decision rules regarding this choice of effect sizes should be developed using both theoretical and practical considerations. The conceptual model of the synthesis will drive many of these decisions.

Fourth, deal with coder biases systematically. Such biases are a function of normal human information processing. Many of the accepted principles and procedures of research design are helpful in this area.

Fifth, regularly assess validation team coder reliability. Estimating reliability is not clear-cut, and there are issues regarding which items to include and how reliability is computed. Regular reliability checks ensure that your coders have not drifted from each other.

B. Procedures for Extracting and Coding Data

The process of extracting data from primary studies is complex and involved. The two opposite sources of tension that define this process are the need to code all data and the need to minimize labor. You should code as much information in as much detail as your timeline and budgetary considerations allow.

We divide the coding process into five procedures. The *first* is to develop coding criteria and a coding manual. We present a template of coding items that you can adapt for your use in future information syntheses. The *second* is to train the team and calibrate its ratings. This involves helping the coders become familiar with the coding protocol and conducting discussion and feedback sessions until reliability of the coders has reached an adequate level. In general, we recommend using the smallest unit possible and computing either a Kappa for categorical data or a Pearson correlation for interval data. The *third* procedure, routinely assessing *coder reliability*, is conducted throughout the remainder of the coding process. Regular reliability checks ensure that your coders have not drifted from each other. The *fourth* procedure is to identify and manage missing data. We detail ways that you can attempt to obtain missing data. In Section C, Chapter 13, we present statistical procedures for estimating missing data that cannot be obtained by any other means. The *fifth* procedure, recording data into the data set, involves entering the coding data into an electronic format for storage and later for data analysis.

FORM 8.1: VALIDATION DATA CODING FORM

Coder Initials: _____

Coding Date: _____

Reference

Citation #: _____   Country of Publication: _____

Authors: _____ Institution of Publication: _____

Document Year: _____

Study Designs

Please check one of the following study designs:

a. _____ Descriptive (case study, project description, product implementation)
b. _____ Didactic (review of pathophysiology, essays, textbook material)
c. _____ Time series (measures taken repeatedly more than twice, longitudinal)
d. _____ Quasi-experimental (missing either control group, random assignment, or experimental manipulation of independent variable)
e. _____ Experimental design (subjects randomly assigned, control group present, and manipulation of independent variable)

Setting

Please check which of the following settings and subject populations used were in the study:

a. _____ Public clinic
b. _____ University student
c. _____ Hospital inpatient
d. _____ Hospital outpatient
e. _____ Private clinic or office
f. _____ Home health

Samples

a. General population _____
b. Average age _____
c. Proportion female _____

    d.   Proportion with concurrent gonorrhea _____
    e.   Percentage attrition _____
    f.   Percentage diffused _____
    g.   SES information _____
    h.   Urban _____   Rural _____
    i.   Selection procedures _____
    j.   Type of validation of disease _____
    k.   Length of prior disease _____
    l.   Comorbidities _____
    m. Percent loss to follow-up _____

Practitioners

    a.   Physicians (include levels of specialty, education, location of practice)
    b.   Midlevel: nurse practitioner, physician's assistant, social work therapists, nurse midwives
    c.   Nurses
    d.   Pharmacists
    e.   Trained assistants

Groups

    a.   Selection process (random, matched, case control, case cohort)
    b.   Size of groups (initial and final)

Procedures

    a.   Procedures for data collection
    b.   Were subjects aware of the study?
    c.   Was data collection part of normal health care delivery?
    d.   Training of research assistants
    e.   Blinding of research assistants
    f.   Blinding of data analysts
    g.   Kinds of cultures
    h.   Kinds of labs
    i.   When was treatment given?
    j.   Length of time to follow-up
    k.   Method of measuring compliance

Theory

    a.   Specified (yes/no)
    b.   Inferred
    c.   Name of theory (develop coding scheme)

Publication Bias

a.   Retrieval from
        1 = computer database
        2 = invisible college (peers, experts)
        3 = reference from other study
b.   Review process
        1 = peer reviewed
        2 = not
        3 = not known

CHAPTER 9

Principles of Information Validation

In this chapter, we discuss several important principles related to the validation of individual studies you are considering for inclusion in your synthesis. These are described in five sections:

PRINCIPLES OF INFORMATION VALIDATION

A. Importance of validation of individual studies

B. Causes of poor scientific quality in published research

C. Analysis of quantitative validity

D. Analysis of qualitative validity

E. Use of validated information for synthesis

Appendix 9.1   Criteria sets for validating individual research studies (1977-2000)

Section A. Importance of Validation of Individual Studies

Unacceptable validity of scientific publications and other documents for disseminating information is a significant problem for the clinician and for the reviewer. We doubt most clinicians are aware of the fact that outcome studies may often produce unusable numbers and that the results of meta-analyses can differ significantly as a result of different validity assessments (Bailar, 1998). Consequently, we have devoted a major stage of this book to discussing this issue and options for its management.

Factors Related to Literature Validity Management

Most healthcare professionals do not have the time to read, let alone analyze, critical articles in their field. As a result, they turn to either experts or to formal literature reviews to assist them in their attempts to keep up with new scientific developments (Guyatt et al., 2000; Williamson et al., 1989). However, both of these approaches can have significant limitations. Experts are not always in consensus regarding the appropriate action to be taken in certain cases (Eddy, 1984); they are often slower to advocate a position than the literature (Antman, Lau, Kupelnick, Mosteller, & Chalmers, 1992), and they may be more susceptible to biases in decision making (K. J. Cook et al., 1992).

On the other hand, using formal literature reviews to assist decision making may also be a problem. Even two meta-analyses on the same question can produce differing results (Chalmers et al., 1987), leaving clinicians in search of a definitive answer empty-handed. Because few clinicians are familiar with the rapidly developing advances in the quantitative sciences of statistics and research methods, they are often poorly prepared to evaluate the scientific soundness of research publications or reports.

Importance of Validation in Syntheses and Reviews

In addition to the need by individual practitioners for validated information, many organizations are using systematic research summaries as part of guideline and protocol development. Both the Agency for Healthcare Research and Quality (AHRQ) and the National Library of Medicine (NLM) use systematic literature reviews extensively as part of their evidence development process. In this context, the issue of a critical validation becomes all the more important as information extracted from the literature is incorporated into national guidelines and recommendations.

In recent years, formal assessment of the validity of literature as part of the review process has become increasingly essential. One reason for the increased emphasis is the popularity of meta-analysis. One of the early complaints about meta-analyses as a review process was the indiscriminate inclusion of results from poorly conducted primary studies (Eysenck, 1978; Feinstein, 1995). Other authors noted that it was not until the advent of meta-analysis as an accepted synthesis method that the validity of primary articles became an issue (O'Rourke & Detsky, 1989). In other words, it may be that the popularity of meta-analysis has brought to light the inadequacy of much of the primary research and of methods flaws in meta-analysis itself.

Research Evidence of Literature Validation Problems

Evidence that there is a problem with the validity of many primary articles is substantial. In 1986, Williamson and his colleagues completed an analysis of 33 independently published validation analyses of sampled clinical literature published between 1970 and 1985. They found that more than 94% of over 2,000 reports in the most prestigious clinical journals were of questionable validity in terms of producing "usable numbers." That is, the reported findings could not, with confidence, be validly applied (Williamson et al., 1986). The Agency for Health Care Policy and Research (now the Agency for Healthcare Research and Quality) reported that the significant limitations regarding the quality and comprehensiveness of the medical literature severely hampered its ability to develop validated guidelines (Shekelle & Schriger, 1996). Similarly, other authors have found that the poor quality of the primary literature makes literature reviews difficult to conduct (Chalmers et al., 1987; Morris, 1983).

The effect of the quality of primary research studies on the conclusions of an information synthesis can be significant. Sacks, Chalmers, and Smith (1983) reviewed six therapies examined in both randomized clinical trials (RCTs) and historically controlled trials (HCTs). These authors found that for HCTs, 84% of the therapies were found to be effective, compared to only 11% for the RCTs. Khan, Daya, and Jadad (1996) found that poor-quality studies tended to report a positive effect with treatment, whereas high-quality studies more often accepted the null hypothesis. Chalmers et al. (1987) humorously described the inverse relationship between enthusiasm for findings and their methodological integrity, with the most enthusiasm given to new case studies having the poorest quality. As areas become more researched, findings often become less significant when better quality studies are conducted and reported.

In contrast, however, there may be no relationship between the quality of the primary research studies and the effects reported. Emerson, Burdick, Hoaglin, Mosteller, and Chalmers (1990) examined the relationship between quality scores and the size of the effect of seven meta-analyses (all using the same quality scoring method) and found no relationship between the two. They also found no relationship between quality scores and the variation in treatment differences. In other words, the results suggested that high-quality studies were just as likely to have large effects as low-quality studies. Because of the unknown relationship between the quality of the study and the strength of the findings, there is a strong consensus among researchers that the methodological soundness of any research being synthesized is a very important consideration.

Summary of Section A

Overall, assessing the validity of primary studies prior to the synthesis process is important for both the individual practitioner and for healthcare agencies. The individual clinician must be able to analyze the soundness of literature reviews to determine which report safe, efficacious, and cost-effective information to apply to his or her practice. Healthcare agencies are attempting to shape practice patterns based on scientific evidence and need to base their policy recommendations on solid data. When the quality of primary research is poor, the conclusions of a synthesis may be wrong and important clinical implications affected. Although the quality of medical research and corresponding literature reviews is improving, evidence suggests that there are still many problems, hence the need for validating systematic reviews.

Section B. Causes of Poor Scientific Quality in Published Research

There is mounting evidence that the editorial peer review process is not altogether sound. Several authors have reported serious problems related to current procedures (Bailer & Patterson, 1986; Berlin, Begg, & Louis, 1989). One of many contributions of George Lundberg, M.D., a recent editor of the *Journal of the American Medical Association,* was to originate and support a series of international conferences on the subject of editorial peer review. The purpose of this effort was to stimulate research on this topic and to improve the quality of the first assessment screen of medical literature (i.e., editorial peer review).

Editorial Policy Favoring Original Studies With Positive Findings

One of the many factors contributing to poor scientific quality of research papers is the editorial policy of publishers. We will discuss three examples.

Editorial Bias Against Negative Research Publications. One reason editorial peer review might result in publication of articles having poor methodological quality is the potential bias in editorial policy and its impact on the peer review process itself. These biases most often occur because of the tendency for editors to reject findings from negative studies (Dickersin, 1990; Mahoney, 1977). This is regrettable because negative studies may have a higher probability of being scientifically sound than those reporting "breakthroughs" (Williamson et al., 1986, pp. 380-381).

The outcome of having studies published with only positive results is a biased sampling of the universe of real results on a particular question. Just as in any other study with a sampling bias, the results of an aggregation of such research will, therefore, also be flawed. Editors also place much weight on an article being interesting to its readers. Unfortunately, negative studies are often not considered of interest. This notion that editors of journals selectively choose studies with positive results has received significant empirical support (Coursol & Wagner, 1986).

Editorial Bias Against Nonoriginal Research Reports. Some publishers adhere to an editorial review policy to accept only original articles. Consequently, such information is often premature for clinical practitioners. By not accepting replication studies, which may be many years from the time of the original publication, the finding that a given paper was dead wrong may occur after potential health damage or wasted care expense has taken place. It takes a substantial number of studies, after a so-called breakthrough report, to be able to assert efficacy, let alone cost-effectiveness and long-term safety. Thus, such editorial policy discourages researchers from conducting and submitting unoriginal studies that are so essential for evaluation by the scientific community.

Insufficient Reviewer Time for Adequate Manuscript Assessments. The reviewer panels for most journals have many notable researchers and clinicians, who, though qualified for the task, often do not have the time needed to do a thorough review. Editorial staff have a difficult time getting them to adhere to deadlines for returning their assessment reports. Not being up-to-date on many medical and statistical advances, these reviewers should put in the effort to contact colleagues or get on the Internet to figure out some puzzling research designs or procedures. However, it becomes very frustrating for them if they have a busy practice, or if students are waiting for their share of the reviewers' time. Under such circumstances, unless the reviewer is vitally interested in the subject matter, reviewing the manuscript may get low priority.

Inadequate Documentation of Study Methods. Another kind of publication bias is evidenced by the failure of authors to publish full details about their studies. Publishers often discourage large methods sections and do not provide sufficient space for authors to document research methods in detail. This space limitation creates problems for the synthesis validation process because it becomes necessary to directly contact authors to find out what procedures were actually performed. Many excellent studies are rejected because reviewers cannot judge whether the study is good or bad due to lack of critical methods documentation.

Inadequate Knowledge of Scientific Processes

Current assessments of the quality of primary studies support the general conclusion that clinical authors, especially, are still unaware of how to conduct good research (Shekelle & Schriger, 1996). It is almost impossible for physicians to keep up with their own subject matter, let alone achieve proficiency in the quantitative sciences. When primary practitioners and their opinion leaders were asked how they discern the scientific soundness of literature in medical journals, approximately 90% of each group claimed they compared study results with their own experience. Only 8% of practitioners, compared to 30% of opinion leaders, would check with a research methods specialist (Williamson et al., 1989, p. 157).

Authors' Contribution to Poor Scientific Quality

Authors themselves contribute to biased reporting. Authors working hard to advance their careers may give primary emphasis to original research and avoid time-consuming replication studies. Authors often decide not to submit studies with negative findings because experience tells them their papers will be rejected (Dickersin, Yuan, & Meinert, 1992). Also, authors may skimp on their methods sections to give more space for long, extensively detailed introductions or discussion sections that are far less important for evaluating the scientific validity of their investigations.

High Cost of Adequate Research Validation

With the flood of new manuscripts to the better known journals and the relatively small budgets editors are given, it is not cost-effective to assess these articles in terms of details of database development and, especially, to validate each article by means of research design-specific criteria. Many articles require time-consuming review by subspecialty research methodologists and statistical experts. Many editors are forced to "fill up the pages" to maintain their advertising revenue, so they do the best they can with the limited resources they have at hand.

Summary of Section B

Overall, the causes of poor-quality research are many and range from poor editorial review to lack of knowledge on the part of clinician researchers. Pressures to publish, and limitations on the amount of information that can be published, exacerbate the problem.

Section C. Analysis of Quantitative Validity

Assessing quantitative validity involves determining the degree of confidence we can have regarding the accuracy of the conclusions in any given article. There are at least four major approaches in use today for analyzing validity of this type. These approaches differ from each other in terms of relative emphasis on different validity threats, the type of summary provided regarding each study (e.g., an overall number vs. estimates of bias), and the manner in which biases and artifacts can be integrated into the results of an information synthesis. We cover the principles under each method but emphasize the "threats to validity" approach (Cook & Campbell, 1979).

"Threats to Validity" Method

Cook and Campbell (1979) developed a theoretical framework for research methodology. However, they did not develop their "threats to validity" approach as a system by which the validity of primary articles can be evaluated. Rather, they developed a theoretical framework for research methodology, and those who conduct literature validity assessments have used their conceptualizations and methods. The threats they present encompass four major categories and cover both experimental and quasi-experimental designs (Campbell & Stanley, 1963; Cook & Campbell, 1979).

Internal Validity. Internal validity refers to the strength of the inference regarding the causal connection between the independent and dependent variables. Internal validity is maximized when groups are comparable (e.g., when subjects are randomly assigned to groups), thereby minimizing systematic differences between them; when the independent variable is manipulated systematically; or when a control group is used for comparison purposes.

If groups are equal initially, then differences between the groups after application of that independent variable are thought to be "caused" by manipulations of the independent variable. For example, if patients are randomly assigned to groups that differ in the degree of behavioral specificity provided in their patient education materials, differences in how well they do those tasks after treatment can be attributed to the behavioral specificity of the instructions. However, many groups cannot be randomized. We cannot randomize individuals to gender, age groups, or disease severity. When these limitations are present, then "confounds" might be brought into the design. Confounds are alternative explanations for differences found between groups after an experiment.

CONFOUNDS

Confounds are variables that are associated with the independent variable and therefore could be an alternative cause of the effect of the independent variable.

For example, gender groups may differ not only on chromosomes but also on work experience, education levels, or average income. Males and females may differ in their response to a treatment, not because of the treatment but because of these other differences. Racial groups may differ not only on chromosomes but also on culture, income, and sociological influences. Groups that naturally differ because of race or gender may then show differences in effect, but not because of the treatment—rather, because of inherent differences between the groups. When studies have these kinds of confounds, our ability to attribute observed differences between groups as "causes," after an experiment, is weakened. In addition to **confounding** problems, groups may also differ because they have had different experiences, either before or during the experimental treatment. They may differ in terms of when they were brought into the study (historical controls). They may differ in terms of the rate at which they are changing (maturation or illness trajectory). Change comes about as a result of normal developmental processes (children are growing and adults are not) or as a function of disease staging (cancer stages) or even as a function of differential motivation (learning occurs faster with motivation). Different results of a treatment may then be a reflection of differences between groups in these variables and not because of the independent variable.

One of the most common problems in healthcare research, in terms of the comparability of groups, is that of "attrition" and "dilution." Often, patients in the control group who get very ill will be transferred (attrition) to the experimental group (dilution) in order to receive a treatment. The end result is that the control group is effectively less ill, and the treatment may appear to have less of an effect when contrasted with a more ill treatment group. Initial entry into a study should be standardized and results measured on an "intent to treat" basis.

Even randomized groups may be systematically different if randomization did not work. Randomizations will only "work" to produce equal groups if the population from which the selection occurs is sufficiently large and the sample size is also large. For example, randomizing a population of 12 into two groups does not ensure equality between the groups. Even with moderate-sized groups, it is important to verify that the groups are indeed not significantly different on other important variables.

Also, randomization will not be sufficient to equalize groups if the treatment was given differently in some subtle way for the different groups. For example, a study examining the effectiveness of different kinds of psychotherapy may try to have all groups have standardized treatment. However, if novices perform one kind of therapy and experts another, then the treatment does not differ on content alone. Rather, groups may differ as a function of a variable that is related to experience of the practitioner. Occasionally, differences such as these in treatment application are fairly subtle and difficult to detect. Nevertheless, they can have a large impact on study results.

Groups may also receive a different "treatment" when one of the groups tries harder or is given compensatory treatment of another kind. This may occur if a study of patient education provides control patients with most of the same material as the experimental patients in an effort to meet ethical standards. Or, in some cases, patients who know they are in the control group for a study on patient education may try extra hard (e.g., go to the library or talk more with friends). Biases introduced into data gathering as a function of beliefs held by the experimenter may also cause the experiences of two groups to differ. For example, data gathering and interpretation can be quite biased if the individuals involved know of the hypothesis. Interactions with subjects can be subtly altered. The result in all of these cases is a difference between how the experimental and control groups are treated, and hence the effects are spurious.

Internal validity is also determined by the degree to which the independent variable (the hypothesized cause) can be manipulated. Causation is strongly implied when the causative agent occurs before the expected effect. Hence, the expectation in research is that the independent variable is shown to precede the dependent variable (the effect), and this is generally demonstrated by direct manipulation.

However, it is often the case that some variables cannot be manipulated. They are simply observed to co-occur. In that case, the direction, or even the fact of causation, is unclear. For example, we may be studying the effect of good patient-provider communication on compliance with treatment. If we simply observe how they co-occur, we cannot say that good communication improved compliance. It could also be the case that those patients who are highly compliant may elicit good communication patterns from providers.

External Validity. External validity refers to the degree to which the results of a particular study can be generalized across persons, settings, independent variable, and time. Often, the constraints of time and money require that a researcher do a study on a single population and in only one setting. Only systematic random selection from the population of interest across all settings would ensure that the findings had sufficient external validity to be applied to the population at large. For this reason, many studies are limited in external validity.

Operationalization of the independent variable is also an aspect of external validity, as it refers to the extent the subjects in a study were exposed to an experience that conforms to what was intended. In other words, you can do an experiment evaluating the effect of running on mood. However, you cannot generalize those results to walking or weight lifting or even to a situation where the exercise was conducted under different conditions. For example, exercise involving groups can be much different than exercise alone. The conditions or procedures are a very important part of the independent variable. Some studies cause a great deal of subject "reactance" or changes in behavior as a function only of being in an experiment. In addition, many studies are quite constrained in how they operationalize the independent variable. The construct of interest may be provider communication style, but in some studies, it may be operationalized by only the time spent with the patient. Other aspects of the concept "communication" may be completely neglected, making comparisons between studies difficult.

Statistical Conclusion Validity. Statistical validity refers to the strength of the claim of a systematic relationship between the independent and dependent variable in a statistical sense. This means that the authors used the correct statistical test, such as a *t* test or a correlation coefficient, and that they did not violate the basic assumptions of that test. Statistical conclusion validity also refers to the degree that the measures used are reliable (they would measure the same if repeated). Unreliable measures can often obscure differences between groups because they add so much "noise." Another common threat to statistical validity is the tendency to perform too many statistical tests. If one is accepting an alpha of 0.05 as indicating significance, then 1 in 20 tests will be significant by chance alone. If too many tests are done, then the alpha needs to be made smaller to account for the higher chance of finding significant results.

Construct Validity. Construct validity is the degree to which the variables, as manipulated and measured, reflect the ideas being examined. Many studies may claim they are examining a construct, but when the specific methods used are examined, the operationalizations (how variables are manipulated and measured) of the construct are theoretical, incomplete, or just different from the ones you are interested in exploring.

For example, researchers may be examining the impact that quality of communication between the patient and the provider has on a patient's functional status. They may decide to measure communication quality in terms of time spent speaking to the patient. However, theories of communication may define quality of communication differently. These definitions could include the amount of information exchanged, the responsiveness of the provider to the effect of the patient, and other important components of the communication process. Some operationalizations may be more central to the construct and others less so. Authors may measure the number of lines in a progress note as a measure of the quality of communication—a construct a bit removed from the notion of communication quality. A low-quality construct in many ways invalidates the findings of a study or at least makes them less applicable.

These four categories reflect the "threats to validity" approach of Cook and Campbell (1979). They are broad and comprehensive, and there is little to help a reviewer determine how to weigh the different threats or biases. We recommend that review authors use these basic categories and construct specific validity criteria weighted according to the importance to validity in that domain of study. The method discussed next is a direct attempt to quantify the "amount" of validity in a systematic way. The hope is that a reviewer would be able to say that one study is more valid than another and that a threshold could be established for "valid" versus "nonvalid" articles.

Point Counting Method

T. C. Chalmers and his associates (Chalmers et al., 1981) developed a second system based on a point counting method for analyzing quantitative quality (validity). (Do not confuse this method with the synthesis design approach of "vote counting" by Light & Smith, 1971, or Glass et al., 1981, explained in Section C, Chapter 2.) This approach was developed to focus on RCTs. The end product of this system is an overall quality score. This score is based on many of the same principles outlined by Cook and Campbell (1979), but relatively more emphasis is placed on construct and statistical validity. In an article summarizing his approach, T. C. Chalmers (1991) proposed that the major issues to be assessed for validity are as follows:

POINT COUNTING METHOD: MAJOR VALIDATION ISSUES

1. Problems in patient selection
2. Biases in the randomization process
3. Ancillary treatments given along with the treatment of interest
4. Selective removal of patients before or after completion of study
5. Problems in the analytic process
6. Failure to "blind" patients and researchers to randomization process

SOURCE: Chalmers (1991, p. 973).

Although the method of T. C. Chalmers and associates has the limitation of not specifying a study's particular weakness, the procedure does provide an overall numerical assessment that can be used for summary descriptions of the research literature. The advantage of a single summary score is that it can then be used to make comparisons across articles. However, the use of such a global indicator has some-times been found to be unreliable (Wortman & Yeaton, 1987) and also to obscure systematic quality errors across all studies, making synthesis bias likely (Wortman, 1994). Finally, a single summary score fails to reflect the types of validity problems present in a group of studies.

Combination Method

Other authors have attempted the task of quantifying validity by doing what appears to be a combination of the above two approaches. Bryant and Wortman (1984) and Wortman (1994) propose performing a two-step decision strategy taken from an earlier work by Mansfield and Busse (1977).

Establish "Construct" and "External" Validity. The first step of the decision process is to establish construct and external validity. Assessing construct validity involves judging whether the procedures used to create levels of the independent and depend-ent variables are valid. A construct has high validity if the procedures used to create the treatment or condition are closely related to the theoretical ideas that are being examined in the research.

Assessing external validity involves estimating the degree to which the study reflects the setting, population, or time of the hypothesized question. If either con-struct fails to fit the definitions used in the review, then the study is omitted as not relevant. Wortman (1994) refers to this step as "acceptability," suggesting that if a study fails to meet minimum criteria in this area, then it is unacceptable and, there-fore, eliminated from further consideration.

Identify Measurement Bias. The remaining articles are then evaluated for specific measurement of bias, based on Cook and Campbell's (1979) "threats to validity" approach. The result is an assessment of the degree of bias in each domain rather than an overall score. Specific procedures for coping with measurement bias will be discussed in Section D, Chapter 13.

Bayesian Assessment

Eddy, Hasselblad, and Shachter (1992) introduced a Bayesian system of quanti-tative synthesis. This approach is quite similar to threats to validity strategy but emphasizes the various biases differently. Congruent with a threats to validity approach, Eddy et al. (1992) reason that all studies have some type of validity prob-lem. The goal of the validity assessment is to identify which particular type of problem characterizes a given study. In their meta-analytic procedures, Eddy et al. call for estimates of the following biases:

Patient Selection Bias. This bias occurs when different kinds of patients are studied in the treatment group versus the control or comparison group. Any differences between the groups may then be a function of those initial differences and not the treatment itself. One important clinical source of this bias is a function of disease progression. If nonrandomized groups differ in terms of where they are in the natural history of the disease, the result would be different treatment effects for each group. For example, patients might be chosen for treatment of hypertension from a screening clinic for one group. These patients might be fairly early into the disease process. Patients for the other group might have entered the healthcare system because of symptoms, suggesting that they might be further along in the disease process. Any comparison of the effects of a treatment would be biased as a result of these initial differences. Differences between groups may occur after selection, such as contamination, dilution, and differential loss to follow-up. This bias is one of the most serious threats to internal validity.

Population Biases. Population biases occur when the population involved in the initial investigation differs in important ways from the population to which generalizations are to be made. For example, experimental investigations frequently exclude patients with comorbid clinical conditions. However, actual patient populations often have multiple medical problems. Population bias is one kind of threat to external validity.

Confounding Factors. Confounding, or ambiguity, regarding the nature of the relationship between the independent and dependent variable occurs when the treatment and control conditions differ on some factor other than the variable of interest to the investigator. This concept was discussed earlier under internal validity. If alternative factors can affect the results of the study, then the investigator cannot determine whether the variable of interest or the alternative variable is responsible for the results.

Contamination and Dilution. These biases can occur in experimental investigations where random assignment is not maintained. Contamination occurs when the patients assigned to a control condition actually receive the procedure assigned to the experimental subjects. Dilution occurs when the patients in the treatment condition do not receive the procedures assigned to them. Contamination and dilution reduce the effectiveness of random assignment and are, therefore, a threat to internal validity.

Differences in the Intensity of the Independent Variable. This bias, as applied to the different experimental groups, may occur if the procedures or timing differ in some way between the groups. When this problem occurs, the results of the study may then be a function of the intensity or duration of the independent variable and not the variable itself. For example, in a psychotherapy experiment, some of the therapists may have only a moderate skill level, so they are unable to provide the same quality of therapeutic intervention as the other therapists in the group. If the therapists with the lower skill level are responsible for only the control group, then the two groups do not receive the same therapy. This bias is associated with threats to construct validity.

Errors in Measuring Outcomes. These errors may occur when the measures are not obtained accurately or reliably. They frequently occur when investigators use archival data (e.g., claims data, patient records, or death certificates) and the data themselves are poorly or inaccurately recorded. Error in measurement can also occur with unreliable instruments. This bias is one of the statistical threats to validity.

Errors in Ascertaining Exposure to an Intervention. These errors may occur when the investigator incorrectly determines the treatment received by a patient. This is also called a misclassification bias. This type of problem is especially likely in case-control studies in which the investigator must rely on archival data or provider and patient memories to ascertain the patient's treatment condition. For example, a study may be examining the impact of taking birth control pills on the likelihood of cerebral hemorrhage. If the researcher has to rely on the subject's memory regarding the type and strength of the birth control pills, there may be misclassification bias where some women are put in the wrong group. This bias is an internal validity bias.

Loss to Follow-Up. This bias occurs when the patients who are not followed differ on important characteristics from the patients who are followed. This problem can be especially important if different follow-up rates occur between cases and control patients, treatment and control patients, or interactions with the kind of treatment used. For example, it may be that at high dosage levels, unpleasant side effects may increase dropout rates, whereas at low dosages, patients may experience less unpleasant side effects and are, therefore, less likely to drop out of the study. This bias creates confounding differences in groups and so affects internal validity.

Length of Follow-Up. Because disease and illness is a progressive event that changes over time, any time groups are not measured at the same time, there is a significant risk of bias. Patients differ in terms of where they are in the disease process. For example, some patients who are in a study on hypertension may be asymptomatic and, as a result, are not as likely as those with symptoms to come back when requested. The result is that the follow-up time between groups is different, and some of them may be much more ill at the time of follow-up. The results, then, would not be comparable. Whenever there is a control group, whether randomly selected, matched, or historical, some effort must be made to ensure homogeneity of follow-up time periods.

Other Assessment Procedures

There are many other less systematic or less detailed proposed approaches to measuring validity, some of which are specific for the area of study. For example, Fowkes and Fulton (1991) outlined an overview of issues to consider in assessing the validity of epidemiological studies. Feinstein (1979) developed a checklist for assessing the quality of studies in the same area. Lichtenstein, Mulrow, and Elwood (1987) developed criteria specifically for case-control studies. T. D. Cook et al. (1992) organized fundamental quality attributes into higher categories, called "levels of evidence" in a format developed by the American College of Chest Physicians. Level I is randomized control trials with high power, Level II is randomized control trials with low power, Level III is studies of cohort comparisons, Level IV is nonrandomized historical cohort comparisons, and Level V is simply case series descriptions. Most of these systems focus on a small subset of designs or are overly broad in their assessments, making their usefulness minimal.

Summary of Section C

Although there are many methods in use to assess validity, the "threats to validity" approach is the most comprehensive. As no single study is without flaws, it is essential to approach the task of validity assessment with caution. The strength of inference from any single set of conclusions comes from many factors. Not only does the experimental design and lack of bias of any one study affect conclusions, but so does the overall size and maturity of the literature in which it is embedded. The value of validity assessment is that the results provide readers with some understanding of the reliability of the conclusions.

Section D. Analysis of Qualitative Validity

Qualitative validity concerns assessment of the soundness of the nonquantitative aspects of the study. Although these areas cannot be measured as quantitatively as scientific soundness, they may be of significant interest to some reviewers. In some cases, the purpose of the review is to examine the nature of research in a particular topic and to summarize not only effect sizes but also the field of inquiry itself. Qualitative validity, as we define it, involves three independent aspects of an article, shown as follows.

Theoretical Relevance

This construct refers to the degree to which a study is judged to advance **theoretical development** in an area. Most studies in medicine are not designed to test theory. However, because tests of theory are extremely important for the advancement of knowledge, noting and evaluating this dimension enhances the synthesis process. Theoretical advancements are particularly important in clarifying methodological and construct definition issues. Because of the specialized nature of theory development, evaluating this dimension requires a domain expert. This expert must be aware of current controversies in the field and understand the importance of any particular study.

Clinical Soundness

This area refers to the degree to which the study "makes sense" clinically. Are measures of effect congruent with levels of clinical decision making? Are the patients selected a reflection of patients usually seen by practitioners? Are the dependent measures related to clinical outcomes of importance? Are the results of the study reported in a format that can be used by clinicians? As in theoretical development, an expert is required to assess this dimension.

Heuristic Validity

Some articles may be important to consider in a synthesis because, despite serious quantitative flaws, they have a unique methodological approach, or they may make an especially important contribution to the field. This dimension is referred to as *heuristic validity,* and an adequate evaluation of this element would also require an expert who keeps up with a given field and can recognize a unique theoretical contribution.

Summary of Section D

Overall, assessing the qualitative validity of a study provides information about how the study "fits" into the literature in terms of theoretical relevance and heuristic value. Qualitative validity also covers clinical significance, a concept that is not often addressed in literature reviews.

Section E. Use of Validated Information for Synthesis

There are four basic approaches to using quality information from primary studies in an information synthesis. These approaches include (in order of desirability) the following: using quality scores in a **sensitivity analysis**, using quality information to weight the effect size, choosing criteria for selecting studies, and ignoring quality scores altogether (not recommended).

Using Quality Scores in a "Sensitivity Analysis"

The most general approach involves using quality scores to do a "sensitivity analysis" (i.e., to explore variations in results). Any overall judgment regarding inclusion in the synthesis is suspended, and the relationship between quality and effects receives the emphasis. We recommend this approach in that the sensitivity analysis can be done separately for the different threats to validity and for all levels of quality. When most of the studies are quasi-experimental, this approach is essential. For example, Detsky, Naylor, O'Rourke, McGeer, and L'Abbe (1992) sequentially combined trial results, starting with the study that had the highest validity score. At each combination, changes in the confidence intervals were examined. The width of the sequential confidence intervals reflected the added variability associated with poorer quality and bias. Similar activities appropriate for the area of interest can be devised. Quality scores can be correlated with effect sizes, or the studies can be divided into groups and the average scores compared across groups. For example, studies on the effectiveness of a coronary artery bypass graft (CABG) can be divided into those that are funded by insurance companies or health maintenance organizations (HMOs) and those that are conducted at research centers. The average quality score can then be compared between the two. It is also possible to simply report the results for both high- and low-quality studies as well. We recommend this approach because it provides the consumer with a much clearer idea about the state of the literature and the applicability of the findings.

Using Quality Information to Weight the Effect Size

Using quality information about primary studies to weight the effect size will result in a widening of the confidence interval as occurs with smaller sample sizes, which is an indication of less reliability (Eddy, Hasselblad, & Shachter, 1990). Although this method has several advantages, the exact amount of widening of the confidence interval that occurs with low-quality scores has little empirical support and is somewhat arbitrary (Detskyet al., 1992). However, an advantage of this method is that higher quality studies are given more weight in a meta-analysis.

Choosing Criteria for Selecting Studies

This approach sets criteria by which studies are to be included. The criteria can be as simple as an exclusion rule that eliminates all nonrandomized control trials. The actual procedures for establishing inclusion may vary from synthesis to synthesis. Perhaps only one aspect of quality will be used as inclusion criteria (e.g., randomization). Or an overall quality score can be computed as in the T. C. Chalmers method, and criteria are set for that number that determines inclusion. Deciding on criteria is, at best, subjective. However, some evidence is available regarding its efficacy in the literature. For example, Liberati, Himel, and Chalmers (1986) found an average score of 0.50 after a review of RCT trials of primary treatment of breast cancer. Although this number is relative, it can be used to compare against other averages to make a judgment regarding relative quality. Otherwise, criteria for inclusion may be based on a combination of factors judged to be important in the domain of study.

Ignoring Quality Scores Altogether (Not Recommended)

Finally, there is an approach that suggests, simply, that the quality attributes of primary studies be ignored in the synthesis process itself. Reporting them is considered sufficient. We do not recommend this approach.

Summary

In Chapter 9, we present the theoretical considerations regarding principles of science information validation. This chapter covers five sections.

In Section A, we discuss the importance of validation, including factors related to current literature validity management, the importance of validation in literature reviews and synthesis, and research evidence of the literature validation problem.

In Section B, we present causes of poor scientific quality and discuss the current inadequacy of editorial peer review, publication bias, and inadequate knowledge of scientific processes.

In Section C, we present a discussion on the nature of quantitative validity, including the "threats to validity" method as reported by Cook and Campbell (1979), the point counting method developed by Chalmers et al. (1981), the combination method developed by Bryant and Wortman (1984), the Bayesian assessment developed by Eddy et al. (1992), and other assessment procedures.

In Section D, we present another view of validity—qualitative validity, which includes three independent aspects of a scientific article: (a) the theoretical relevance of a study, (b) the clinical soundness of the content, and (c) the "heuristic" contribution of the study, or the degree to which the study makes a unique and innovative theoretical or methods contribution, independent of its quantitative aspects.

In Section E, we discuss the various ways that validated information is used in a synthesis, including using quality scores in a "sensitivity analysis," using quality information to weight the effect size, choosing criteria for selecting studies, and, least acceptable, ignoring quality scores altogether.

We suggest that understanding these principles will be essential to developing your quantitative synthesis on a sound scientific foundation. Actual procedures for putting these theoretical concepts into practical use are presented in the next chapter.

APPENDIX 9.1
Criteria Sets for Validating Individual Research Studies (1977-2000)

There are numerous sets of criteria in the literature for evaluating individual research articles for possible inclusion in a review. Although in no way comprehensive, the following are examples of such criteria that have evolved over the past 25 years of the senior author's experience. They are quoted directly from the various publications mentioned (with the possible exception of the numeration). Be aware of the U.S. and U.K. spelling differences. For example, *center* in the United States is spelled *centre* in the United Kingdom, and *maneuver* in the United States is spelled *manoeuvre* in the United Kingdom. Primarily, these criteria sets provide an overview of the evolution of these methods for analyzing individual studies. They also might provide ideas to help you establish your own criteria set for systematic review validation assessment.

CRITERIA SET A.
Criteria for Assessing Individual Research Articles

1. What is the source of the data or information upon which the article is based?

2. Has this work been replicated or is this an isolated report on the subject?

3. If the article encompasses an experimental study design:
   a. Was the health problem content specified in terms of criteria for inclusion and exclusion of the experimental subjects?
   b. Was a control group used in the design?
   c. Was there random allocation of the experimental treatment between [subjects to determine] control and experimental subjects?
   d. Are the experimental and control groups studied concurrently?
   e. Was a double blind design used in evaluating the results?
   f. Was the response rate adequate to justify generalization?

4. If a diagnostic validation study is described:
   a. How valid is the criterion [gold standard] against which the experimental procedure is to be tested?
   b. Are both false negative (e.g., missed diagnoses) and false positive (e.g., misdiagnosis) rates compared?
   c. Was the method for computing the false negative and false positive rates indicated?
   d. Was the practical standard indicating acceptable limits of the rate of false negatives and false positives stated?

5. If an epidemiologic study is described:
   a. Is the specific population to be sampled adequately described [including inclusions and exclusions]?
   b. Is the method of sampling described in some detail [if randomization used, what method was applied]?
   c. Were substitution methods used to replace those in the original sample who could not be contacted?
   d. Was the response rate high enough to support generalization?
   e. If a survey was based on the use of a questionnaire, was it pre-tested for communication effectiveness and were reliability-validity test coefficients determined?

6. For all research reports, was there adequate information to evaluate the statistical analysis utilized?

a. Was the statistical test used named or described?
b. Were assumptions related to the test applied mentioned in the study?
c. Was the level of statistical significance accepted made explicit?

SOURCE: Williamson (1977, pp. 6-8).

CRITERIA SET B.
Criteria for Judging Effectiveness of Treatment or Preventive Measures

The following set of criteria represents but one of three that the Canadian Task Force recommended for use to judge each potentially preventable condition. The other two were: criteria for judging the current burden of potentially ameliorable suffering [and] criteria for judging the manoeuvre undertaken in order to find or prevent the condition.

Three Levels of Effectiveness

I.   At least one acceptably designed randomized controlled trial has shown that treatment or prevention does more good than harm according to the following terms: survival; physical, social and emotional function; freedom from pain and anxiety.

II-1.   Well-designed cohort or case control analytic studies (preferably from more than one centre and by more than one research group) suggest that treatment or prevention does more good than harm.

II-2.   Comparisons between times or places with and without treatment or prevention suggest that treatment or prevention does more good than harm. Dramatic results in uncontrolled experiments (such as the results of the introduction of penicillin in the 1940's) could also be regarded as grade II evidence.

III.   Authoritative and respected experts in the field are convinced of the value or lack of value of treatment or prevention for the condition on the basis of descriptive studies, clinical experience or reports from expert committees or task forces.

Categories of Recommendation

A.   There is good evidence to support the recommendation that the condition be specifically considered in a periodic health examination.
B.   There is fair evidence to support the recommendation that the condition be specifically considered in a periodic health examination.
C.   There is poor evidence regarding the inclusion (or exclusion) of the condition in a periodic health examination, and recommendations may be on other grounds.

D. There is fair evidence to support the recommendation that the condition be excluded from consideration in a periodic health examination.

E. There is good evidence to support the recommendation that the condition be excluded from consideration in a periodic health examination.

SOURCE: Canadian Task Force on the Periodic Health Examination (1979, pp. 16-17).

CRITERIA SET C.
Critical Appraisal of Journal Articles

One of the better sets of criteria for evaluating individual research articles was published in the second edition of *Clinical Epidemiology: A Basic Science for Clinical Medicine* (Sackett, Haynes, Guyatt, & Tugwell, 1991, pp. 366-377). This set is a derivative of one developed for the Canadian Task Force on the Periodic Health Examination (1979). This reference is unique in that the authors present eight different sets of criteria, depending on the clinical subject matter of the article to be evaluated. These include therapy, diagnosis, screening, prognosis, causation, quality of care, economic analysis, and review articles. Due to the amount of material in this reference, we will only refer you to the above book that, it is hoped, can be found in any medical library. Most of these criteria have been published in the *JAMA* series "Users' Guide to the Medical Literature," published in the mid- to late 1990s. These exceptional references are as close as your nearest clinical library. These sets are also available in various editorials of the *APC Journal Club.* For access to the most recent edition of these "levels of evidence," see the following Web address (last updated November 1999): cebm.jr2.ox.ac.uk/docs/levels.html.

CRITERIA SET D.
Point Counting Method: Major Validation Issues (Meta-Analysis)

1. Problems in patient selection

2. Biases in the randomization process

3. Ancillary treatments given along with the treatment of interest

4. Selective removal of patients before or after completion of study

5. Problems in the analytic process

6. Failure to "blind" patients and researchers to randomization process

SOURCE: Chalmers (1991).

CRITERIA SET E.
Levels of Evidence for Treatment Efficacy

Level 1	The lower limit of the confidence interval for the effect of treatment from a systematic review of randomized controlled trials exceeded the clinically significant benefit.
Level 2	The lower limit of the confidence interval for the effect of treatment from a systematic review of randomized controlled trials fell below the clinically significant benefit (but the point estimate of its effect was at or above the clinically significant benefit).
Level 3	Non-randomized concurrent cohort studies
Level 4	Non-randomized historical cohort studies
Level 5	Case series

SOURCE: Cook, Guyatt, Laupacis, and Sackett (1992).

CRITERIA SET F.
Guidelines for Selecting Articles That
Are Most Likely to Provide Valid Results

Primary Studies

Therapy	Was the assignment of patients to treatments randomized?
	Were all of the patients who entered the trial properly accounted for at its conclusion?
Diagnosis	Was there an independent, blind comparison with a reference standard?
	Did the patient sample include an appropriate spectrum of the sort of patients to whom the diagnostic test will be applied in clinical practice?
Harm	Were there clearly identified comparison groups that were similar with respect to important determinants of outcome other than the one of interest?
	Were outcomes and exposures measured in the same way in the groups being compared?
Prognosis	Was there a representative patient sample at a well-defined point in the course of the disease?
	Was follow-up sufficiently long and complete?

Integrative Studies

Overview	Did the review address a clearly focused question? Were the criteria used to select articles for inclusion appropriate? Were the options and outcomes clearly specified?
Practice guidelines	Did the guidelines use an explicit process to identify, select, and combine evidence?
Decision analysis	Did the analysis faithfully model a clinically important decision? Was valid evidence used to develop the baseline probabilities and utilities?
Economic analysis	Were two or more clearly described alternatives compared? Were the expected consequences of each alternative based on valid evidence?[a]

SOURCE: Oxman, Sackett, and Guyatt (1993).

a. The validity criteria you might use in making this evaluation depend on the content area being addressed (e.g., therapy, diagnosis, prognosis, harm, or economics).

CRITERIA SET G.
Assessment of Trial Quality

1. Concealment of random allocation (protection against selection bias)
2. Completeness of follow-up
3. Blind outcome assessment
4. Reliable outcome, indicated by two or more raters with at least 90% agreement, or achievement of a Kappa value greater than 0.8
5. Baseline measurement of performance, or health outcomes measured before intervention
6. Assurance that contamination was unlikely (i.e., that the control group did not receive the experimental interventions)

SOURCE: Oxman, Thomson, Davis, and Haynes (1995, pp. 1423-1431)

CRITERIA SET H.
Abridged Checklist for Evaluating the
Quality of Study Methods for Various Study Designs

Therapy	Were patients randomly assigned to treatment?
	Was follow-up sufficiently thorough and were all of the patients accounted for?

            Were patients analyzed according to the groups to which they were randomly assigned?

Diagnosis   Was there an independent, blinded comparison with a reference (gold) standard?

            Did the patient sample include an appropriate spectrum of patients to whom the diagnostic test will be applied in clinical practice?

Harm   Were comparison groups clearly identified that were similar with respect to important determinants of outcome (other than the one of interest)?

            Were outcomes and exposures measured in the same way in the groups being compared?

Prognosis   Was there a representative patient sample at a well defined point in the course of the disease?

            Was follow-up sufficiently thorough?

SOURCE: Meade and Richardson (1998).

CRITERIA SET I.
ACP Journal Club Criteria for Review and Selection for Abstracting

To meet the basic criteria, all original research and review articles must be:
in English
about adult humans
about topics, other than descriptive studies of prevalence, that are important to the clinical practice of general internal medicine and its specialties
analyzed to assure that the data is consistent with the study question

Category-Specific Criteria

Studies of prevention or treatment must also include:
random allocation of participants to comparison groups
follow-up (end point assessment) of at least 80% of the participants entering the investigation
outcome measures of known or probable clinical importance
Studies of diagnosis must also include:
clearly identified comparison groups, at least one of which is free of the disorder or derangement of interest
interpretation of a diagnostic ("gold") standard without knowledge of the test result
interpretation of the test without knowledge of the diagnostic standard result

objective diagnostic standard, e.g., laboratory test not requiring interpretation of current clinical standard for diagnosis (e.g., venography for deep venous thrombosis), preferably with documentation of reproducible criteria for subjectively interpreted diagnostic standard (i.e., report of statistically significant measure of agreement beyond chance among observers)
Studies of prognosis must also include:
inception cohort of individuals, all initially free of the outcome of interest
follow-up of at least 80% of patients until a major study end point occurs or the study ends
Studies of etiology must also include:
a clearly identified comparison group for those at risk for, or having, the outcome of interest (i.e., randomized controlled trial, quasi-randomized controlled trial, non-randomized controlled trial, cohort analytic study with matching or statistical adjustment to create comparable groups, or case-control study)
blinding of observers of outcome to exposure (criterion assumed to be met if outcome is objective, i.e., all-cause mortality, objective test)
blinding of observers of exposure to outcomes for case-control studies or blinding of individuals in the study to exposure for all other study designs

SOURCE: American College of Physicians (1999, p. A-15).

CRITERIA SET J.
Levels of Evidence and Grades of Recommendations

This set of criteria for evaluating individual research articles has evolved from the earlier Canadian Task Force on the Periodic Health Examination prototype reported in 1979 (here labeled Criteria Set B). A later derivation is reported in a book by Sackett et al. (1991) (here labeled Criteria Set C). A more recent derivation is Criteria Set J, for which the URL address is (latest updated November 1999) as follows: cebm.jr2.ox.ac.uk/docs/levels.html.

CHAPTER 10

Procedures for Database Validation

The procedures we recommend for the quality assessment of primary articles have two major areas of emphasis. The first is the process of developing the validity criteria themselves. The second area of focus is the validation procedure itself. We will cover these topics within a framework of five procedures shown in the index box below.

PROCEDURES FOR DATABASE VALIDATION

    A.   Categorize studies by research design
    B.   Develop validation protocols
    C.   Select and train reviewers
    D.   Calibrate and standardize validity ratings
    E.   Validate literature for synthesis

Introduction

Experts need to be consulted and time devoted to ensuring that the criteria used are appropriate for the topic at hand. Simply adopting a ready-made set of criteria is not likely to be effective unless carefully adapted to your purpose and topic. We suggest using the conceptual framework of Bryant and Wortman (1984) that involves a judgment of relevance and then a judgment of validity. We extend this approach by including an evaluation of clinical and methods heuristic validity if resources are available. To accomplish this, we emphasize the importance of having expert input during this criteria development stage. Finally, we strongly support sensitivity analyses to determine the relationship between quality assessment criteria and the results of a meta-analysis.

As Meade and Richardson (1998) have noted, there are three purposes in assessing the validity of primary articles. The first is to understand the validity of the primary studies included in the review, which includes understanding the patterns and types of validity problems inherent in the literature. The second is to uncover differences among study results that are caused by reasons other than chance. (Differences in the quality of studies are one source of variability.) The third is to provide readers with sufficient information so they can judge for themselves the applicability of the systematic review in their clinical practice. Supporting this objective means that criteria are carefully developed and analyzed.

Procedure A. Categorize Studies by Research Design

We suggest that you first classify each article by its fundamental research design. This classification will determine the type and content of validation criteria that must be applied to estimate serious bias. Each design category will have different validity items. We classify articles into seven major design categories by their overall purpose: theory development, descriptive (nonexperimental), hypothesis testing, knowledge application, methods studies, qualitative research, and information reviews.

This research design categorization process is crucial for purposes of study validation. It will also be invaluable later when reporting results and clarifying the state of literature on a topic. This is especially true for certain applications, such as guideline development or management of a consensus conference. This classification is arbitrary and may be altered to meet your needs. Most current information syntheses focus only on articles whose purpose is to test hypotheses. However, there may be a real need to synthesize the state of the literature using publications that are not necessarily empirical. Note that this classification is based on the content of the author's purpose in writing the review.

Design 1: Theory Development

Theory development encompasses original theorization or research whose purpose is to develop or test theory. These articles report on the development of new constructs to explain current phenomena, usually through philosophic essays and theoretical writings. These suggest new pathways for research that likely have never been implemented. Most of the work in theory-based fields of inquiry, such as physics or basic psychology, is research designed to test theory. They also describe new ideas and constructs to explain other measured phenomena. Theory articles may include personal opinion critiques of other studies or projects, such as editorials or letters to the editor. There is a large body of such articles related to national or state healthcare reform; many represent the judgment and opinions of special interest groups, so it is important to discern the bias or slant of such publications.

Assessing the quality of articles in this field involves specifying the degree to which the article is comprehensive (covers the essential theoretical issues in the field), accurate (faithfully represents the positions and findings of other authors in the field), and creative (develops a new and important position in the area). If the work is empirical in nature (as you might find in the basic sciences), review criteria will be similar to quantitative research. However, because of the esoteric nature of the content, judging the quality of theory articles requires domain expertise. See White (1973) for a brilliant example of this design.

Design 2: Descriptive (Nonexperimental)

The purpose of these studies is to provide a simple description of a population, a case study, cohort, disease, program, project, or technology, without testing a hypothesis, trying to compile evidence of causality, or performing an evaluation. Such designs might include simple comparisons to describe similarities or differences among the subjects studied. Most simple epidemiological studies are of this type, with the exception of "epidemiological natural experiments." In this descriptive (nonexperimental) design category, we include studies that involve a time dimension—for example, natural history of disease, prognosis, and studies of "harm" (which describe such variables as functional disability, decreased quality of life, and death rates for a population as measured over time).

Design 3: Hypothesis Testing

The purpose of these studies is to test a hypothesis, either discerned from a theoretical model or derived from practical concerns. Often, they are used for establishing causal relationships. Almost all of the descriptions regarding validity issues in Chapter 9 refer to studies whose goal is hypothesis testing.

Also, there are natural epidemiological experiments in which evidence of causation is the purpose (e.g., measuring and comparing health status of a large group of individuals who avoid Western scientific medicine with a matched group who use such scientific healthcare).

Experimental. The use of a control group, random assignment, and manipulation of the independent variable characterizes experimental designs. This design has the power to provide the strongest evidence of causality between independent and dependent variables.

Quasi-Experimental. These designs are investigations that test a hypothesis but do not include all of the experimental controls present in an experimental design. However, the intention is to provide evidence from which inferences can be made. Often, one of the independent variables is being systematically manipulated, but the other is simply measured, as when issues such as race, gender, socioeconomic status (SES), or disease categories are being examined (Cook & Campbell, 1979). In other words, there is not random assignment to all groups. Examples of this kind of work include regression analyses, personality investigations, pre-post studies, case-control, and longitudinal cohort studies. Causal implications are compromised by the lack of experimental control so that the validation assessment must give some estimate of the degree of bias. Evaluating this research takes more expertise, as issues of group size, applications of measurement, and statistics become more important. The researcher must identify all threats explicitly and rule them out, one by one. Typically, researchers use statistical control (e.g., through regression techniques) rather than experimental control in an attempt to select among plausible competing hypotheses. Quasi-experimental studies also include "natural" epidemiological experiments, and there are many that can be conducted. For example, suppose a religious group does not believe in Western medicine and refused antibiotics for bacterial infections sensitive to these drugs. An epidemiological outcome study can be completed for this population and compared to a matched group who receives antibiotics for the same infections. Other studies might be generated to explain why no differences are found. Just as in the quasi-experimental studies, statistical control is often used to select among plausible competing hypotheses.

Descriptive Experimental. These are investigations that are not only missing random assignment to groups but also missing a control group and manipulation of the independent variable, as with "natural" epidemiological experiments. No intention to make inferences to a large population group is intended. Natural epidemiological experiments usually attempt to gather evidence regarding causation and thus go beyond simple descriptive designs.

Design 4: Knowledge Application

Knowledge application studies include formal program evaluation, quality improvement studies, and technology assessments. In this category, the purpose is not to test a hypothesis but rather to examine the factors associated with successful implementation of a program, activity, or technology. For example, knowledge applications in healthcare guidelines, practice parameters, protocols, and computerized expert systems would be included in this design. Educational program evaluation studies to determine the extent of learning are also included here. These usually examine the degree to which a program or instrument reaches its goals, achieves reliability and validity, and is applicable to practice. In many ways, these evaluation studies are similar to descriptive studies, differing by the fact that a criterion measure is compared to a standard that is based on a value judgment.

Design 5: Methods Studies

The fifth major design category of research literature is **methods studies**. These studies include the development and assessment of new methods, tools, or instruments. A study that reports the development of an instrument to measure severity of illness, or to compare its validity against others, is an example of a methodological study. Another example is diagnostic instrument validation studies in which a measurement made by the instrument being tested is compared to a gold-standard measurement. In technology assessment studies, explicit standards are used wherein researchers or regulators may set the criteria for performance themselves.

Validation of methods studies focuses on the relationship between the concepts or constructs being measured and their respective operationalizations. The validation process emphasizes a detailed examination of construct, convergent, discriminate, and predictive validity. For example, an assessment of the predictive (or criterion-related) validity of an instrument would measure the extent to which the measurement methods compare with a gold-standard measurement method. In contrast, discriminate validity would be tested by assessing the degree to which the measure is associated with other measures that are conceptually not related. In addition, measures of interitem reliability, test-retest reliability, and split-half reliability should all be performed on instruments being developed. Nunnally's (1978) *Psychometric Theory* is an excellent sourcebook to guide this kind of assessment.

Design 6: Qualitative Research

In contrast to experimental designs, **qualitative research studies** are based on ethnographic research techniques. In qualitative research, the purpose is less to predict and control and more to provide an "interpretive explanation," an elaboration of meaning, and a mechanism to enrich human discourse (Glasser & Strauss, 1967; Noblit & Hare, 1988; Popper, 1968). As a result, validation procedures for qualitative investigations involve a different approach than studies in which the focus of validation is on data.

Few authors discuss assessing the validity of qualitative studies. Here we present three authors who use slightly different approaches. Noblit and Hare (1988) suggest that a central aspect of quality assessment is the evaluation of the core metaphors used in the study. They suggest that the quality of metaphors can be judged on the following five dimensions:

CRITERIA FOR JUDGING QUALITY OF METAPHORS

1. *Economy,* or the ability of the metaphor to express a large amount of information
2. *Cogency,* referring to "elegantly efficient integration"
3. *Range,* referring to the capacity of the metaphor to cross other symbolic domains
4. *Apparency,* the ability of the metaphor to evoke understanding versus describing facts
5. *Credibility,* the degree to which the metaphor is understood and accepted by the intended audience

SOURCE: Noblit and Hare (1988).

Altheide and Johnson (1994) provide a thorough discussion of the general issue of "qualitative confirmation." Their discussion indirectly provides a method by which to assess the validity of a qualitative investigation. In their description of the "rules of evidence" for qualitative reviews, these authors describe possible criteria to be used for validating a reviewer's conclusion. Finally, Leininger (1994) has suggested that evaluating qualitative literature should be done using six criteria:

QUALITATIVE LITERATURE EVALUATION CRITERIA

1. *Credibility,* or the "believability" of the findings
2. *Confirmability,* or the degree to which the conclusions are congruent across respondents or relevant settings
3. *Meaning in context,* or the degree to which data are explained in their context
4. *Recurrent patterning,* or degree to which repeated instances of an event appear across experiences or life-ways
5. *Saturation,* or the degree to which the researchers are able to demonstrate full immersion into the phenomena
6. *Transferability,* or the degree to which particular findings from a qualitative study can be transferred to another similar context or situation

SOURCE: Leininger (1994).

Regardless of which taxonomy is used, researchers validating qualitative work have to systemize the judgment task to communicate their findings. We advocate the use of multiple judges and systematic analyses. Although numerical responses may not be possible, analyses that relate the quality of the study to the conclusions can still be performed as part of a sensitivity analysis.

Design 7: Information Reviews

The final category of research design is the review article. These articles are designed to compile and synthesize previous research on any topic. This category includes traditional reviews; systematic reviews, including quantitative (such as meta-analyses) and qualitative reviews; and consensus conference reports.

Oxman and Guyatt (1991) provide an illustrative list of specific validation criteria for assessing review articles or information syntheses. These are listed in the following box. This criteria set is but one of many shown in Appendix 18.3. Cochrane Collaboration evaluation forms used by its experts to validate systematic reviews are especially helpful for these procedures. You can link to its abstract index of Cochrane Synthesis Reviews at the following Web site (last updated ?? after January 2000): hiru.mcmaster.ca/cochrane/cochrane/cdsr.htm.

CRITERIA FOR ASSESSING REVIEW ARTICLES

1. What is the precise purpose of the review?
2. How were studies selected?
3. Is there publication bias?
4. Are treatments similar enough to combine?
5. Are control groups similar enough to combine?
6. What is the distribution of study outcomes?
7. Are outcomes related to research design?
8. Are outcomes related to characteristics of programs, participants, and settings?
9. Is the unit of analysis similar across studies?
10. What are the guidelines for future research?

SOURCE: Oxman and Guyatt (1991).

These criteria are really documentation criteria as they ask to what degree these issues are presented in the review. As a list of possible items to address, they also lend themselves as criteria to assess the quality of an information synthesis.

Procedure B. Develop Validation Protocols

This procedure calls for establishing validation criteria applicable to each type of research design used. The first step involves developing the criteria list. In general, we recommend beginning with the validity assessment instrument in Form 10.1 at the end of this chapter. Items can be added to this list as a function of the type of primary articles involved. Once a sample criteria list has been developed, it should be approved by a group of experts. The members you select to be in the expert group depend, of course, on the topic; however, in general we recommend a clinical expert, a research methodologist or statistician, and a domain expert as a minimal set. These experts will evaluate quality criteria items for relevance and decide which ones to leave in and which ones to remove.

Once the task of inclusion is finished, the same group will rate the importance of items in terms of how the criteria affect the validity and usefulness of the results of any study in this area. We recommend this judgment be made using a scale of 1 through 7, with 1 being *no impact* and 7 being *substantial impact,* for each item. The experts should make this judgment twice, both times anonymously (first before discussion and the second time after discussion). Items that receive an average score of less than 3 after the second vote could be eliminated entirely.

Once the protocol has been constructed, specific instructions and examples for each item should be written in a codebook. In addition, the validation protocol should be included as an appendix to your final synthesis report to document this critical and often neglected function. Form 10.1 provides an illustrative instrument for validating individual research reports in your database. It encompasses 20 criteria. We judge the categories of these criteria to be essential, but the individual criteria within each category must be customized to your particular topic and purpose.

Procedure C. Select and Train Reviewers

Training reviewers is an important but often overlooked aspect of good validations. Reviewers can vary a great deal, even when they have scientific and research training (Orwin, 1994; Oxman et al., 1991). Typically, we select at least three raters, two of whom have completed a minimum of six quarters of coursework in research methods and statistical analysis. The third rater should have clinical experience. A fourth domain expert is also desirable. One of the reviewers should be very familiar with multivariate statistical procedures such as multiple regression analysis, multivariate analysis of variance (MANOVA), discriminant analysis, factor analysis, and other multivariate procedures covered in the research literature. The actual level of reviewer sophistication depends, in part, on whether articles to be reviewed report advanced statistical procedures to analyze the research.

Training the reviewers consists of selecting a set of articles similar to the content of the articles to be reviewed. Raters are first trained to identify methodological problems of the type included in the rating criteria. They are then trained using the protocols and the protocol instruction book for at least three articles. Once they have learned the process, an initial pilot run of about 12 articles is conducted, with each rater working independently. At the completion, reliability between raters is computed using Cohen's Kappa.

Procedure D: Calibrate and Standardize Validity Ratings

Periodic calibration sessions are conducted to determine interrater reliability of the validation ratings. The Kappa statistic is the method we suggest for this purpose. Exact procedures for performing a Kappa are shown in Table 10.1.

A Kappa of greater than 0.75 reflects good agreement, values below 0.40 indicate poor agreement beyond chance, and values between 0.40 and 0.75 represent fair to good agreement (Fleiss, 1981, p. 218; Landis & Koch, 1977). Kappas lower than 0.40 indicate that raters should meet, discuss their differences, and repeat the process on a new set of items. When the Kappas are high (above 0.75 team agreement), you can infer that the team is doing well.

For purposes of training, Kappas should be conducted on an item-by-item basis to discover meaningful differences. Reporting the mean and the range of Kappas in your manuscript is an indication of thorough documentation. Calculating the Kappa statistic can be done by hand or, preferably, by a spreadsheet having the formulas programmed in prior to data analysis.

Procedure E. Validate Literature for Synthesis

The overall purpose of this procedure is to ensure that the synthesis bibliographic database is valid, correct, and complete. This procedure consists of checking for document duplication, numbering the documents for reviewer assignment, and ensuring that each document contains a level of detail consistent with the planned review. In addition, we recommend that every effort be made to minimize bias in the rating process. "Blinding" raters to the results of the study while they are rating the methods is important, as is "blinding" the raters to the authors and to the journal title.

Reliability among the raters is assessed initially and at various intervals. Retraining is conducted periodically to protect against rater drift. The final result of the validation effort is a brief report indicating the major biases identified in terms of quantitative validity (and qualitative validity if resources allow). Some authors suggest that interrater reliabilities be examined for the coding sheets (i.e., the sheets

TABLE 10.1 Procedures for Computing a Kappa Using Multiple Judges

Step 1. *Set up spreadsheet*—For the purposes of the original spreadsheet, the citations are arranged on the vertical axis, and the raters are arranged on the horizontal axis.

Step 2. *Compute parameters*—The following parameters must be set initially.

N = #citations (2)
m = # categories (5)
k = # raters (3)

Step 3. *Record data*—Use the following format.

			Columns			
A	B	C	D	E	F	G
						Sum of Squares
Citation	# of A+s	# of As	# of A–s	# of Bs	# of Cs	(SS)
No. 1	2	1	0	0	0	5
No. 2	0	1	1	1	1	4
Sum	2	2	1	1	1	9
(p_j)	2/Nk	2/Nk	1/Nk	1/Nk	1/Nk	
	2/6	2/6	1/6	1/6	1/6	
(p_j)^2	(2/6)^2	(2/6)^2	(1/6)^2	(1/6)^2	(1/6)^2	

Step 4. *Calculate the Kappa*—Use the following nine computational procedures:

a. Sum up the number in each category by summing down columns (A+, A, A–, B, C).
b. Divide each column sum by Nk to get the proportion (p_j) for that category.
c. Compute the square of (p_j) for each column.
d. Compute $P(E)$ (the expected proportion by chance by summing across columns: $P(E) = (2/6)^2 + (2/6)^2 + (1/6)^2 + (1/6)^2 + (1/6)^2$
e. Then sum the cell's frequencies squared $(2^2 + 1^2 + 0^2 + 0^2 + 0^2)$ across rows. ($S = 5$)
f. Sum down this column to compute I.
g. Compute $P(A)$: Multiply this sum (I) by $(1/Nk(k − 1))$
h. Subtract $(1/k − 1) = P(A) = (I)*(1/12) − 1/2$
I. $K = P(A) − (P(E) / (1 − (P(E))$

SOURCE: Castellan and Siegel (1988).

NOTE: The parameters for K that vary and need to be specified somewhere up front, each time, are as follows: N (# of citations), k (# of raters), and m (# of categories).

involved in summarizing the specifics of a study) for future meta-analysis (Hunter & Schmidt, 1990).

Summary

The procedures we recommend for conducting an information validation involve four steps. (a) Articles are categorized by type of research design. (b) Validation protocols are developed that combine a basic template of validity criteria, with the criteria needed for the unique types of studies being synthesized. Experts are used for this process to maximize validity. At this point, the criteria are also rated in terms of the degree of relevance to the area of study. (c) Once the protocols have been developed and coding books written, the raters can be trained. Training involves an iterative process with piloting materials, calibrating agreement, and then retraining. Once raters are trained and are reliable, actual coding can begin. (d) We recommend minimizing bias by separating the parts of each manuscript so that raters analyze the methods section, without having the results section available. Once they understand and rate the study methods, they are then given the results to evaluate.

Once the validity ratings have been done, a decision needs to be made regarding how the results of the validity analysis will be included in the overall review. Currently, no consensus exists among authors in the field as to the best method to deal with invalid results. One compromise is to use methodological rigor as a control and test it directly (Glass, 1977; Wortman, 1994). If the literature has a large amount of experimentally sound research, then there is an opportunity to assess the affect of rigor on effect size directly, and, consequently, all articles should be included. If, however, there were only a few rigorous studies on a given question and many where there is considerable methods weakness, then it would be preferable to include only those with the most scientific rigor (Wortman & Yeaton, 1987). Another compromise is to use only the most rigorous studies as "best evidence," even if the number is very small (Slavin, 1986). This issue will be explored in more depth in the succeeding chapters on methods of synthesis.

FORM 10.1: AN ILLUSTRATIVE DATABASE VALIDATION INSTRUMENT

Instructions

Step 1. Develop Database Validation Criteria

The first step in a database validation is to develop design-specific criteria for assessing individual studies. The criteria are established in terms of how important each area is to the validity of studies in the review. The final product should be a readily understandable list of specific criteria that are easy to apply. Each of our illustrative list of 20 criteria is represented by a number in the first column of the score sheet. You may elect to have more or less than this number of validation criteria.

Step 2. Establish Weights for Each Criterion

On the score sheet, distribute 100 points across each of your criteria to represent your judgment as to the importance of that criterion to the validity of your conclusions. Record these weights in column A of the score sheet such that all weights add up to 100.

Step 3. Apply Criteria

(a) Reviewers should evaluate only what is stated in the individual research reports. If information required for validation is not explicit, do not make assumptions of what may have or should have been considered. Judge each article only on what has been stated directly in the report. In other words, if a procedure is not stated, assume it was not done.

(b) Use the following rating scale (0.0 to 1.0) in assessing an article on each criterion and record that rating in column B of the score sheet:

        0.0 = inadequate
        0.25 = somewhat adequate
        0.5 = partially adequate
        0.75 = mostly adequate
        1.0 = fully adequate
        NA   = not applicable

(c) Each item is also rated on a certainty scale (0.0 to 1.0) to be recorded in column C of the score sheet:

        0.0 = completely uncertain as to rating (used for missing information)
        0.25 = somewhat certain (some information missing; suggestive, not clear)
        0.5 = partially adequate (reasonable judgment but still not clear)
        0.75 = mostly adequate (fairly certain regarding rating)
        1.0 = fully adequate (completely certain; item is very clear)
        NA   = not applicable

Step 4. Compute Final Validity Scores

Multiply the validity weight in column A by the validity rating in column B for each criterion and record the result in column D.

Step 5. Decide on an Overall Validity Rating

At the bottom of the score sheet, make an independent judgment of the overall validity of the article, not an average of ratings in column B.

Note: Disregard columns E, F, and G of the score sheet until the consensus meeting.

A. Internal Validity Criteria

1. Initial differences between groups regarding either subjects or settings as they relate to the items below; assess pretreatment comparability on all relevant demographic and outcome variables.

   - Stage of illness—early, late, or terminal
   - Timing of treatment—in relation to stage of illness
   - History—groups compared against differing time periods
   - Extreme scores—on the first test, the nontreatment groups with extremely low scores (very ill or very low performance) are likely to improve the second time around by chance alone
   - Testing—different kinds of tests used to put subjects into different groups

2. Threats to validity by confounding variables or covariates effectively managed by one of four options: (a) random assignment, (b) statistical control, (c) matching, or (d) none.

3. Procedural standardization across comparison groups or times either for treatments or for measurement is appropriately standardized (e.g., pre–post) for the following:

   - Independent variable—treatment regimen, adjunct or ancillary regimes, follow-up periods are consistently applied.
   - Measurement—measures/instruments, data collection methods are the same across groups.
   - Experimenters and personnel between groups are equal as to education and behavior.
   - Diffusion or sharing of information (about the independent variable) is minimized or identified.
   - Reactance or motivation to act differently, as a function of being in an experiment, is the same across groups (e.g., one group is paid to participate and the other is not, or one group knows more about the experiment than the other).

4. Observers and subjects kept blind as much as possible, such that researchers are blind to subjects' status on the independent variable (unless impossible, e.g., male vs. female) and, if relevant, to ongoing results; researchers or data collectors are blind to the hypotheses; researchers are blind to individual subject data.

B. Statistical Validity Criteria

5. Appropriate instrumentation in that standard instruments with previously reported validity and reliability, or new instruments with accompanying documentation of validity and reliability, are used; there is no evidence of ceiling or floor effects.
6. Assumptions of statistical tests are not violated.
7. Error rate is minimized by not applying too many tests on the same data, thereby decreasing significant results by chance.
8. Reporting is sufficient, especially in terms of methods documentation.
9. Inaccuracies are not evident or, if present, are acknowledged.

C. Construct Validity Criteria

10. Sample frame has sufficient coverage of the range of possible values in the application of the independent variable. Is the independent variable sufficiently congruent with other manipulations of the same construct?
11. Treatment adequacy—independent variable was sufficiently intense to produce a meaningful effect (e.g., treatment quantity, quality, follow-up period).
12. Evidence of possible confounds—the construct being manipulated is really the one intended, and other variables are not being manipulated inadvertently.
13. Reactance—degree to which the experimental situation causes other effects for participants (e.g., increased patient education may also cause increased evaluation apprehension).

D. External Validity Criteria

14. Sampling denominator population clearly explained, including criteria of inclusion and exclusion.
15. Sampling method (subject selection) and results clearly explained, especially how the final subjects used in the experiment were "like" the population to which they are being generalized.
16. Setting in which the experiment took place is "like" the settings to which the results are being inferred.
17. Time in which this experiment was conducted is "like" the time to which the results are being inferred.
18. Healthcare providers encompassed were comparable to those who would usually provide care to the population being studied.

E. Heuristic Validity

19. Research theory or methods contribution of the study has sufficient heuristic value in terms of research theory or method, for the purposes of this review, to justify its inclusion, apart from its external and internal validity.
20. Clinical theory or methods contribution in this study has sufficient heuristic value in terms of clinical theory or methods that, for the purposes of this review, its inclusion is justified, apart from its external and internal validity.

F. Overall Validity Judgment

In view of the above ratings and any other factors, what is your overall validity judgment (0.1 to 1.0 [1.0 high]) for including this study in your synthesis?

Synthesis # _____			Reviewer_____					
Topic_____			Date of Review_____ Date of Consensus Meeting _____					

ARTICLE VALIDATION SCORING SHEET

Criterion #	A Importance Weight	B Validity Rating	C Certainty Scale	D Validity Score (A × B)	E Mean Group Validity Rating	F Mean Group Certainty Scale	G Group Validity Score (A × E)	H
1								
2								
3								
4								
5								
6								
7								
8								
9								
10								
11								
12								
13								
14								
15								
16								
17								
18								
19								
20								
Sum of Importance Weights	100							
Overall Validity Estimate				Individual Reviewer		Group Mean		

CHAPTER 11

Evaluation and Improvement of Stage III

F our evaluation criteria were proposed in the Introduction (Section E, Chapter 1) as being important for evaluating any information synthesis. In Chapter 7, we assessed how well these criteria were applied in validating the individual research studies in the synthesis database. In this chapter, we assess how well these validations, as a whole, were conducted. The importance of this procedure is based on the following assumption:

DATABASE VALIDATION REQUIRES ASSESSMENT

We assume that the probability for bias is inversely related to the stringency of the research methods validation effort. The more formal and systematic the validation, the less biased and more sound the final synthesis evidence might be and the more value this synthesis might achieve. Based on this assumption, we deem that the effort required to verify the validation methods and products is well worth the cost.

The following index outlines the four standard validation criteria, the application of which will be the focus of the four procedures of this chapter.

PROCEDURES FOR STAGE III EVALUATION AND IMPROVEMENT

Assess and enhance:
   A.   Documentation of validation procedures
   B.   Validation of database clinical significance
   C.   Validation of database scientific soundness
   D.   Validation of database cost-effectiveness

Procedure A. Assess and Enhance
Documentation of Validation Procedures

The main purpose of assessing the adequacy of the validation documentation effort is to determine whether you can be confidant of the results of subsequent validations, which depend on the soundness of this documentation. If your documentation is inadequate to assess how well you validated the individual studies in your database, applying the other three criteria (B, C, D) above may be questionable. Coping with the problem of inadequate validation documentation might require that you reconvene your search team to fill in as much missing information as possible while it is still fresh in everyone's mind.

   If all of the relevant information required to evaluate Stage III were recorded, you could proceed to evaluate how well the application of the remaining three criteria are validated, giving major emphasis to "scientific soundness." The checklist in Form 11.1, presented at the end of this chapter, can be used as a rough guide to estimate the adequacy of your validation documentation. If most of the items on Form 11.1 are checked "Yes," you are ready to complete an assessment of the validation methods applied in Stage III. If many of the items are not completed, additional effort will be required to fill in the missing information.

Procedure B. Assess and Enhance
Validation of Database Clinical Significance

In Stage III, there is only minor emphasis on evaluating the validation of a research study's clinical significance because this procedure was conducted in Stage I (Chapter 4) and Stage II (Chapter 7). Recall that we conceptualize clinical significance in terms of population net benefit for the subject content of any of the eight cells of the healthcare outcomes cluster matrix illustrated in Figure 2.4, Chapter 2. (For more details, see Section F, Chapter 2.) The most desirable end result would be substantial health improvement or health risk reduction for a specified population. In other words, you could estimate an average net benefit (improvement achieved minus harm) per person, times the number in the population who might thus be helped. The content of the net benefit could also be economic, satisfaction, or other outcomes such as reduction of medical-legal risks for either the consumer or **provider** of care.

We also assume that only those articles that prove relevant in content that is reasonably mature can be judged to be clinically significant. Note that the discovery of the gene for colon cancer is highly relevant but is premature for immediate application by healthcare practitioners in the community. The articles passing this clinical significance filter are candidates for Stage III scientific methods validation of Procedure C in this chapter.

Procedure C. Assess and Enhance Validation of Database Scientific Soundness

The output from Stage III is a validation rating on each database article indicating its scientific soundness. Making this assessment of your validation procedures is somewhat similar to the technology assessment of any scientific measure. Evaluation of such an instrument includes assessing specific validity factors, such as construct validity, predictive validity, criterion validity, and discriminant validity. Instrument evaluation also involves investigation into its reliability or internal cohesiveness.

Besides the kind of validity that is reflected in an instrument assessment, measuring scientific soundness depends on the degree to which the validation process was adequately planned and implemented. A starter set of validation questions to assess soundness follows and provides a list of basic tasks to be conducted.

TASKS TO ASSESS AND ENHANCE VALIDATION OF DATABASE SCIENTIFIC SOUNDNESS

1. Evaluate outcomes of validation instrument
2. Determine reliability of validation instrument
3. Assess integrity of data set
4. Assess adequacy of validation procedures

Task 1: Evaluate Outcomes of Validation Instrument

Two questions must be asked to evaluate the outcome of your validation of each relevant article in your database: (a) Will experts, independently evaluating each article, agree that the overall validation ratings you applied are sound? (b) Will expert ratings of the four evaluation dimensions (internal, external, statistical, and construct validity) compare favorably with those of your team?

We consider a "structured group judgment" method to be the most rigorous assessment of your Stage III database validation task. However, later we will mention some alternatives you might consider. The listed subtasks here assume you select a group judgment approach, using the "estimate, talk, reestimate" format or some modification of these subtasks (see Chapter 2, Appendix 2.1, for a more detailed explanation of this approach).

Overview of Article Validity Assessment. For this approach, compare the results of your team's validation assessment for each article with an acceptable "gold standard." Such a standard could be expert team consensus validation ratings of each relevant database article. Experts include research methodologists or statisticians in the health field. In addition, two clinical researchers who are expert on your synthesis topic should be included to evaluate the clinical and **heuristic validity** of the article. Using a 2 × 2 contingency table, determine your team's percentage of false negatives (i.e., where the experts rated an article valid that you rejected as unsound) or your team's percentage of false positives (i.e., where an article your team rated as valid was rejected by the experts) (see Figure 11.1). Compare these results to your team's previously agreed-on threshold of maximum acceptable percentages of false-negative and false-positive validity ratings of the articles in your database. Remember we calculate a false positive rate as (1 − **positive predictive value * 100**) **to transform this value to a percentage.**

The main advantage of this approach is that it can be completed rather rapidly, and the results have acknowledged credibility. The main disadvantage of this method is the expense in consultation dollars and the work required to recruit these experts and elicit their validation ratings for each article.

Agree to Number of Experts and Articles Needed. If you have more than 50 to 100 articles to validate, database sampling methods might be considered. The number of experts you recruit should be sufficiently large so that no one consultant has to read and validate more than 10 articles. If a face-to-face meeting is considered, 7 to 11 members are good in terms of group dynamics and efficiency of operations. Try not to have fewer than 5 or more than 13 members.

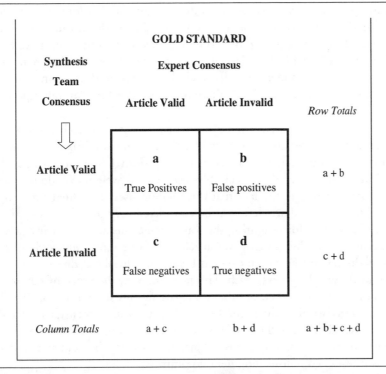

Figure 11.1. 2 × 2 Matrix for Literature Validation Coding Accuracy

Recruit and Train Your Research Methods Experts. Recruitment of an expert in research methods and statistics can be difficult and expensive. If you are near a university medical center, you can readily identify several who might be willing to assist in this task for evaluation of validation methods. If you are connected to the university, they may provide a couple of hours as a courtesy. If not, you will have to pay their consulting rates.

You should prepare an instrument to elicit expert judgments regarding five validation dimensions (listed below) for each article or document being rated.

VALIDATION RATINGS FOR EACH ARTICLE

1. Internal validity
2. External validity
3. Statistical validity
4. Construct validity
5. Overall article validity (optional)

The experts are instructed to take into account the first four ratings and then make a fifth independent judgment of overall validity, with the caution not to average the preceding four ratings. A brief training session of about 10 minutes will facilitate their familiarity with the project and application of your validation instrument. (See Form 18.2 for a model form that includes validation dimensions 1 through 4 shown above. If desired, a similar fifth item can be added for "overall validity.")

Elicit and Aggregate Individual Experts Validation Ratings. For each of the four validity dimensions and the article as a whole, request your experts to complete your questionnaire, giving each item a weight ranging from 1 (low) to 5 (high). By this scale, all of the articles could conceivably receive a "5" weight. We do not suggest a ranking approach due to the fact that this method uses an ordinal scale, in which even the highest ranked article might be considered very poor by a weighted measure. Another reason for weighting the four dimensions and the article as a whole might be that the highest one or two articles might be scored above the threshold, but all of the remaining articles scored below the threshold due to poor quality reflected by the weight given to each. This fact cannot be discerned by ranking methods. It is important to remember that aggregate ratings should be done (preferably using a team statistical median score) for each of the four dimensions of validity, as well as for the weighting of the article as a whole. For example, the experts' consensus judgment on external validity across all articles provides the gold standard against which your team's consensus judgment is compared.

Complete a Validation Analysis and Critique the Approach. The final analysis is quite simple because it involves a value judgment of your team as to what proportion of false negatives and false positives is acceptable. In this analysis, either false negatives or false positives can seriously bias your synthesis conclusions, depending on your topic. The implications of an unacceptably high proportion of either or both would indicate immediate reanalysis to determine if these proportions can be improved. If the experts cannot come to a consensus (i.e., they achieve rather low Kappas), then a face-to-face meeting or a conference call should be done to allow them to discuss their differences.

If the above approach is not desirable, feasible, or affordable, then a series of compromises can be considered. For example, a smaller number of articles could be sampled for evaluating validation accuracy. A smaller team might be more affordable (the lowest limit being three).

If neither of these actions is reasonable, then it might be helpful to have at least one outside methodological expert rate each article on the five dimensions (i.e., internal, external, statistical, construct validity, and the overall article rating) using implicit judgment. If there are more than 25 to 50 articles, you could select a representative sample. Finally, you would compare the experts' responses with those of your team.

Task 2: Determine Reliability of Validation Instrument

Reliability in this case refers to the degree to which the items in an assessment instrument (see Form 10.1 for an example) correlate together. The usual statistic for this analysis is **Cronbach's alpha**, and most statistical programs have a reliability analysis that gives you the overall alpha plus additional statistics. Cronbach's alpha is the average of each item's correlation with every other item. An alpha of 0.80 is considered acceptable.

Task 3: Assess Integrity of Data Set

The data set is the compilation of coded values, including the validity assessments, demographic variables, and publication information retrieved from each article in your database. Before these data can be analyzed, they need to be evaluated for completeness and accuracy. Several techniques can be used to accomplish this task.

The first and most common technique is to run an analysis called **frequencies** or **frequency distribution** on the data. Any statistical program can do this easily. Spreadsheets can also produce counts of each variable value. Frequencies can tell you how many items have each value; what the mean, mode, and median are; and the range and standard deviation. Examination of the results of this analysis can reveal variables that have an unusual or impossible value. For example, a given site (location) may have one of the following codes: 1 = hospital, 2 = sexually transmitted disease (STD) clinic, and 3 = fertility clinic. If the frequency distribution reveals one study with a code of 30, the study would have to be reexamined and the correct value determined.

A second technique to ensure data set completeness is to make sure that each study has the same types of data. This is essential for statistical analysis but can easily be overlooked if this kind of analysis is not planned.

A third technique is to carefully examine the team's interrater reliability (Kappa) for each variable. Those with low interrater reliability could easily be a function of error.

A fourth approach is to check the data themselves for accuracy by randomly sampling four or five articles and coding them to see if there are differences between these ratings and those that your team established previously.

Task 4: Assess Adequacy of Validation Procedures

One component of scientific soundness is the degree to which procedures have been followed to preserve scientific integrity. As stated previously, Form 11.1 is a checklist you can use to assess whether or not the validation procedures were completed.

Procedure D. Assess and Enhance
Validation of Database Cost-Effectiveness

Cost-effectiveness refers to the degree to which your literature database is worth the direct fiscal and time expenditure required for its development. Three tasks are suggested for this process:

TASKS TO ASSESS AND ENHANCE
VALIDATION OF DATABASE COST-EFFECTIVENESS

1. Determine fiscal and time costs of database validation
2. Assess contribution of database validation results
3. Was value of the database validation effort worth the cost?

Task 1: Determine Fiscal and Time Costs of Database Validation

Quantifying the costs for conducting Stage III involves analysis of the fiscal and time ledgers where direct expenditures, personnel time, and "salary codes" are recorded. The salary code is the median of a range of salaries at five different levels, so that the specific salary for each staff member is kept somewhat confidential.

Your first concern is to determine whether the fiscal and time data seem reasonable. For example, are there receipts to document direct fiscal expenditures? As mentioned in Stage II (Procedure D, Chapter 7), the time spent by each team member, as well as by specialty consultants, is multiplied by their "wage code" and then added to approximate personnel costs (Form 3.3 in Stage I might be helpful). Even if members of the team are not being paid directly, their time and salary code should be recorded. Your final crude cost-effectiveness estimate will be more complete and allow comparison with future information synthesis projects you may want to implement. In addition, your fiscal ledgers should include all direct costs such as Internet, books, hardware, software, travel, postage, and copying costs. The final sum will be the total cost of your database validation effort.

Task 2: Assess Contribution of Database Validation Results

The rationale for validation analysis is that you will most likely have many research papers to process, which requires considerable time and, with statistical consultation, may be expensive. Assessment of the validation of the contributions may be very rigorous using experts, or (in certain syntheses) the database need not be so rigorously analyzed. This decision depends on the consequences to your final conclusions of seriously inadequate article validation. To make this determination, you must ask how serious the consequences might be if you rejected the **null hypothesis** of your meta-analysis based on invalid research data input. We suggest that the required rigor, expense, and quality of your database validation may depend on the purpose and likely impact of your synthesis.

Having calculated your total Stage III validation time and fiscal expense, your next step is to determine what value you achieve for this expenditure. We suggest that one approach would be for you to assess the value of Stage III database validation as follows.

Estimate Validation Stringency Required. What is a *stringency analysis*? We conceptualize this term as shown below:

STRINGENCY ANALYSIS

We define the jargon term **stringency analysis** as a procedure to assess how rigorously a validation task was planned, implemented, and evaluated as compared to what was required. In the context of validating individual database articles, this analysis estimates the extent to which validation tasks and results meet previously agreed-on stringency standards for your topic. This analysis applies to both processes and outcomes of Stage III validation.

Your team should briefly estimate the level of stringency required for the validation of articles in your synthesis. Later you will judge what level of stringency was actually accomplished for each article. Comparing the two values might give you a rough estimate of how well your validation task was done.

Using an **estimate-talk-estimate** procedure, your team can establish the probability of the worst consequence that might result if your validation is inadequate or seriously wrong. In other words, what is the probability that serious negative consequences might occur if your synthesis reader assumes your inferences are valid when in fact they are not? Table 11.1 presents a starter list of possible negative consequences to be considered.

Your team might augment this list to meet your specific circumstances. For example, if your topic is related to the care of a patient with a spinal cord injury, more detailed specification might be made as to potential negative consequences of invalid treatment information (e.g., loss of mobility, serious depression). For such a topic, a neurosurgeon and an orthopedic surgeon specializing in spinal injuries should provide input to your team.

TABLE 11.1 Potential Negative Consequences of Inadequate Synthesis Validation	
Loss of life years	Substantial loss of money
Serious disability	Substantial loss of time
Pain and suffering	Minor loss of money
False hope/expectations	Minor loss of time
Threat to principal investigator's reputation	Increased legal risk

Grade Validation Stringency Achieved. In terms of the Stage III effort, what level of validation stringency is, in fact, achieved? This requires examination of your Stage III documentation. With this material, you can reanalyze the extent to which your validation stringency goals meet your requirements. Another approach is to examine specific process elements closely to answer questions such as the following: (a) Were all articles validity coded? (b) What interrater reliability (Kappas) trend was achieved during the calibration sessions? (c) What policy was applied if, after two calibration rounds, the Kappa for a given article remained below 0.4 to 0.6? (d) Did you obtain advice from an independent research methods expert to help you improve your validation effort? (e) Did you contact the authors of articles having insufficient data to accomplish a validation? (f) If you validated articles applying a gold standard for diagnosis, methods, or instrument assessment, did you evaluate how sound that standard might be? (g) Were there any obvious redundant steps or unnecessary expenditures that reduced your Stage III efficiency?

In any event, at this point, the validation team and/or authors must make a judgment as to whether validation stringency meets or surpasses agreed-on standards. If an adequate validation effort was not done, and resources do not allow correction of this serious flaw, readers must be made aware of this omission. This will alert them to the fact that they must now judge for themselves whether your product is sufficiently trustworthy for a specified use.

For each synthesis, you must develop your own Stage III validation protocol for methods assessment. The items listed above provide a few examples of the types of questions you might ask to estimate the quality of the Stage III validation process and product.

Estimate Stringency Using a Simple Ordinal Scale. A simple subjective approach to this Stage III evaluation of validation quality is to make an overall judgment as to which level (1-7, 1 being best) on the ordinal scale in Table 11.2 you most likely achieved.

TABLE 11.2 Levels of Validation Stringency Achieved for Database

1. Definitive evaluation: Both a quantitative validation by research methodologists/statisticians and a qualitative review by subject matter experts were conducted using explicit criteria protocols for evaluating each A+ or A document included in the synthesis database.

2. Less than definitive, but systematic validation: A formal evaluation either by external quantitative specialists or by external qualitative specialists was completed. This validation applied explicit criteria based on research design.

3. Formal evaluation by authors: For this level of validation, explicit criteria protocols are applied by the authors, evaluating all A+ and A articles used in the final synthesis.

4. Informal evaluation by independent reviewers: At this level, only implicit criteria are used, with no formal protocol or research design-specific criteria.

5. Informal evaluation by authors: This level relies heavily on trusting traditional editorial peer review of the journal articles included and applies validation criteria implicit in the minds of the authors.

6. No formal validation of database was done: This would infer that the information included, as well as inferences and conclusions, did not undergo any specific, formal validation for scientific soundness.

Admittedly, this scale only gives a "ballpark" estimate, again based on the quality of your **validation process**. If this Stage III evaluation effort achieved a high level on Form 11.2, you can subjectively estimate that your data input to Stage IV of the synthesis is adequate. Furthermore, an overall validation assessment at Stage IV might well facilitate a later validation of your final synthesis conclusions.

Task 3: Was Value of the Database Validation Effort Worth the Cost?

Once Tasks 1 and 2 are accomplished, your final task will be to formulate a judgment comparing the value of your Stage III validation product (a compilation of validated articles) with the direct costs involved. Perhaps a brief nominal group technique could be applied or other consensus approach to elicit the validation team's judgment of the extent to which your database validation was worth the total expenditures of time and money. Whatever your results, having thought through these concepts should help you determine how you might improve these procedures.

Summary

This chapter outlines a brief method for validating your Stage III database of research reports. This approach emphasizes two of the four overall synthesis evaluation procedures—namely, establishing adequacy of documentation and scientific soundness. However, some mention is made of validating clinical significance and cost-effectiveness of the Stage III database validation process.

Procedure A. Assessing adequacy of validation documentation is briefly discussed because this factor is needed to establish scientific soundness, which is covered under Procedure C. Again, we assume that it is important to assess your validation documentation process as soon as it is feasible so that you do not lose valuable information that might grow dim in your mind later on when it might be needed. Form 11.1 provides a starter set of items to consider.

Procedure B. Assessing validation of the database's clinical significance was conducted in Stage I (planning) and also in Stage II (database development). However, in this chapter, two factors are explained to help you identify measures and evidence related to this criterion—namely, "net benefit" and "information maturity."

Procedure C. Assessing validation of database scientific soundness applies directly to this stage. Its purpose is to ensure that individual research reports and articles are of sufficient scientific validity to be included in Stage IV of the synthesis. We can safely assume that all research has flaws to some extent. The challenge, in light of your goals, is to determine whether or not the article flaws are of little consequence and/or can be adjusted so as not to threaten the validity of your synthesis conclusions. Form 11.2, presented at the end of this chapter, is provided as a suggested set of criteria for evaluating your Stage III validation procedures.

Procedure D. Assessing validation of database cost-effectiveness is briefly discussed. Were your final validation ratings (the main product of Stage III), with whatever flaws may have been included, worth the expenditures of time and fiscal resources required to validate these articles? This is an important question and is worth some effort to judge, if for no other reason than to help you improve your next synthesis. We suggest several admittedly simplistic tasks for you to apply to obtain a rough estimate of the cost-effectiveness of your Stage III product and process. If you were not able to achieve a minimally sound validation of the articles synthesized, this information must be reported to your readers. Then, whatever the negative consequences of invalid information, this places the responsibility in the readers' hands to decide whether or not to apply your conclusions to their own needs.

With Stage III adequately completed, it is likely that in your Stage V evaluation (Chapter 18), little or no revision will be required. On the other hand, if at that time, serious deficiencies are noted, it might be too late to correct them, and the overall quality of your synthesis might be compromised.

At this point, you should have a relevant and valid database required to accomplish the procedures of your formal data synthesis in Stage IV.

FORM 11.1: DATABASE VALIDATION METHODS DOCUMENTATION

Date: _____

Coder: _____

Instructions: Have members of the search team independently check the following items and then come to some consensus as to a yes or no answer.

Team members (names and credentials on file) _____ Yes _____ No

Validity assessment instrument (produced and used) _____ Yes _____ No

Validation protocol (recorded and on file) _____ Yes ___ No

Validation coding manual (produced and on file) _____ Yes _____ No

Training manual (produced and used) _____ Yes _____ No

Interrater reliabilities (recorded and on file) _____ Yes _____ No

Missing data (recorded and on file) _____ Yes _____ No

    If yes, is cause reported? _____ Yes _____ No

    If yes, are data now available (e.g., author contacted)? _____ Yes _____ No

    If not found, is management method stated? _____ Yes _____ No

Research methods expert (consulted at least twice) _____ Yes _____ No

Completion rate (articles validated/total to be validated) _____%

FORM 11.2: CHECKLIST FOR ASSESSING DATABASE VALIDATION

Date: _____

Coder: _____

1. Were the validation procedures sufficiently documented to facilitate a formal evaluation? ____ Yes ____ No

2. Were the validation goals clear? ____ Yes ____ No

3. Was your database double-checked for errors? ____ Yes ____ No

4. Were research methods experts or statistics experts consulted? ____ Yes ____ No

5. Were outside clinical research experts on the synthesis topic used? ____ Yes ____ No

6. Were explicit "design-specific" validity criteria applied? ____ Yes ____ No

7. Were respective validation criteria agreed on by your team and

 quantitative reviewers? ____ Yes ____ No

 qualitative reviewers? ____ Yes ____ No

8. Was a qualitative or heuristic validation completed? ____ Yes ____ No

9. Were the raters assessing qualitative and heuristic validity:

 up-to-date on clinical advances on your topic? ____ Yes ____ No

 able to recognize important conceptual contributions? ____ Yes ____ No

10. Were two coders used for at least a third of the articles? ____ Yes ____ No

11. Was interrater reliability calculated for each item early in the coding process and then repeated as needed? ____ Yes ____ No

12. Was interrater reliability for each item at least .70 (kappa)? ____ Yes ____ No

13. Were rater certainty assessments measured for each item? ____ Yes ____ No

14. Were coding conventions explicit? ____ Yes ____ No

15. Were validity coders "blinded" to author, journal, and results? ____ Yes ____ No

16. Were most sources and causes for missing data explored? ____ Yes ____ No

INFORMATION ANALYSIS AND SYNTHESIS

CHAPTER 12

Basic Statistics for Quantitative Synthesis

T he purpose of Stage IV is to accomplish the final synthesis of the information compiled in your database. At this point, we assume you want to complete a **quantitative synthesis** and have compiled a relevant and scientifically sound database for this purpose. Although, potentially, a meta-analysis is the most rigorous and meaningful method of integrating quantitative data, it is also an approach most fraught with hazards of statistical errors that, perhaps, only the most sophisticated can recognize and properly manage. However, Chapter 14 provides careful coaching through each of the nine steps of seven possible variations of a meta-analysis. Following these procedures and tasks can help you be more confident that your results will be sound.

This chapter provides a briefing on the fundamental quantitative concepts that might prepare you to learn the concepts (Chapter 13) and procedures (Chapter 14) of a meta-analysis. (For those of you who are already sophisticated in these basic statistical concepts, we suggest you move on to Chapter 13.) We also recommend that you read other recent publications on this subject such as Fleiss (1994), Lau et al. (1997), and Egger et al. (1997).

BASIC STATISTICS FOR QUANTITATIVE SYNTHESIS
(Sections of Chapter 12)

A. Basic statistical concepts
B. Effect sizes: Calculation and use
C. Hypothesis testing in meta-analysis
Appendix 12.1. Contingency table statistics

A quantitative synthesis is the statistical analysis of the pooled data from many individual studies. The goal is to provide a more effective integration of these results to answer a research question better than can be accomplished in a traditional narrative review (Glass, 1976). To conduct such a synthesis, a formal, *quantitative* representation of the meta-analytic model is needed. Constructing this quantitative model requires an understanding of the basic principles of statistical analysis and hypothesis testing. The purpose of this chapter is to review the basic statistical concepts required to perform a quantitative health science information synthesis, or meta-analysis. This chapter is for relative beginners who have a basic understanding of **statistics** at the first-year graduate study level but are inexperienced in their use for developing a quantitative synthesis. You should already know how to calculate basic statistical indices (e.g., means, proportions, correlation coefficients, standard deviations, and variances) and be familiar with hypothesis-testing procedures, *t* tests, analysis of variance, and chi-square procedures. Readers who are more experienced in statistical theory and practice as applied to quantitative syntheses might skip this chapter and move on to Chapter 13 for more in-depth coverage of meta-analytic theory. Three general areas are covered:

Section A covers basic statistical concepts such as samples, statistics, populations, and **sampling distributions** and is meant for a brief review only. Section B discusses effect sizes and their history, calculation, and use. In this section, we provide a detailed description of methods for computing the most common effect sizes. Section C presents inferential statistics in meta-analysis, including a discussion on the sampling distribution of effect sizes, and provides a brief overview of methods to obtain parameter estimates such as the average or mean of the sampling distribution of effect sizes.

Section A. Basic Statistical Concepts

Four fundamental conceptual areas will be reviewed. For each one, we present the basic definition, summarize how the concept is related to other statistical concepts, and emphasize the similarities between meta-analysis and traditional statistical analysis methods.

Samples and Populations

In both traditional and meta-analytic procedures, an investigator formulates questions about *samples* to make generalized statements about *populations*. In traditional studies, statistical procedures are used to make these guesses about the population based on a single sample. An important feature of meta-analytic procedures is that the results from many samples (studies) are used to make guesses or estimates about the population. The results achieved by combining these studies together can produce a more rich and accurate source of information than can be achieved from any of the individual studies alone. Thus, an investigator can be more confident making generalizations about population estimates based on meta-analysis results from many studies rather than estimates based on a single study (Cooper & Hedges, 1994).

One of the most important issues in meta-analysis is proper specification of the population to be studied for the synthesis. The definition of the population influences the types of generalizations to be made from the data. Although the process of defining the population in a meta-analysis is similar to defining the population for a single study, an important distinction exists—the definition must be broad enough to include all study samples in your synthesis database. In meta-analysis, a population is the complete set of all possible studies that *might* be conducted for a particular research hypothesis. The population is defined initially as part of the relevance criteria (e.g., acute myocardial infarction [MI] patients or premature infants with hydrocephalus). After coding the studies for relevance, an investigator will have selected several (possibly many) studies to include in the database and will have excluded many others for failing to meet the relevance criteria. This process of establishing the relevance criteria will define the population.

Many of the failures in meta-analysis can be explained by inadequate definition of the population to which the analysis will be applied. In the interest of creating the largest sample size possible, investigators may be tempted to find a way to include studies that do not strictly meet the relevance criteria; it is important to avoid this temptation (Feinstein, 1995). The result is a nonmeaningful mix of studies.

For example, suppose a meta-analysis on a new treatment for serum glucose regulation in diabetic patients is planned. These patients may have a variety of coexisting medical conditions (e.g., kidney failure, heart disease, visual problems, skin infections, or neurological problems) in addition to their diabetes. Depending on the level of disease progression, these patients may be receiving several types of medical or rehabilitation treatments.

Thus, any given subgroup of patients will most likely have different combinations of medical conditions and clinical interventions in addition to the specific problem that is the focus of the meta-analysis. Furthermore, each of the individual studies in the database will have different subsets of these patients. The results that are reported for this diverse set of studies would have a high degree of variability. This variability cannot be explained easily by the independent variable (the treatment) and moderator variables. As a consequence of this unexplained variability, the researcher usually cannot determine the population to which the research findings can be generalized.

In addition, the treatment itself may actually differ substantially from study to study. Using the above example, a patient education program may consist of handing out reading material for an interactive computer simulation. Pooling studies using this intervention may provide little real information on the general impact of patient education on compliance for diabetic patients.

To effectively manage this diversity, it is essential to fine-tune the model to answer specific questions of variability. If several carefully defined populations are included in a meta-analysis, generalizations across these specified populations are possible.

For example, suppose that the conceptual model postulates that a particular medical treatment has different effects on diabetic patients, depending on whether or not they have kidney failure. Suppose that none of the individual studies in the database include *both* patients with and patients without kidney failure but instead only focus on one type of patient. By combining both populations (i.e., sets of patients with and without renal disease) in the same meta-analysis, it is possible to determine whether the findings regarding the medical treatment generalize across the two populations (Hunter & Schmidt, 1990, pp. 36, 292-303, 415-419).

In general, the problem of defining the population of interest can be described as the "apples and oranges" problem. On one hand, we are concerned that quite different constructs (apples vs. oranges) are being combined. On the other hand, apples and oranges may both be examples of a higher order common construct that is of interest (fruit). If the studies are actually studying a common concept (i.e., fruit), then combining these studies will be meaningful. However, if the studies examine different processes and constructs (i.e., different populations), then any statistical combination of results will be misleading.

Statistics and Parameters

A *statistic* is any measurement taken on a sample. A *parameter* is the same measure taken on the population. Conceptually, parameters are similar to statistics in that parameters define some aspect of the population and statistics define that same aspect in the sample. For example, the mean of a sample is a statistic, while the symbol μ (pronounced "mu") represents that mean or "parameter" of the population. Both indicate the same measure of central tendency. We are familiar with the mean or average as the most common statistic used in data analysis. However, results of primary studies are reported using a variety of statistics, especially in the health field. In this section, we assume that the reader is familiar with the calculation of means, proportions, and correlation coefficients. Hence, we will not cover these definitions and calculations here. Readers are referred to a good beginning statistics text if they would like to review these calculations.

Statistics calculated on samples can be used for both descriptive and inferential purposes. Descriptive statistics may be used to *characterize* the average size of the treatment effect of a given drug or surgical procedure. Alternatively, statistics can be used to *infer* population parameters through inferential statistics. In the case of descriptive statistics, the goal is to *describe* the sample; in the case of inferential statistics, the goal is to use the sample statistics to *estimate* the population parameter.

Continuous Measures. Continuous variables are those where the measure is at least on the level of an **interval scale** (assume equal distance between measures), such as a temperature scale or a Likert scale measuring attitudes. These statistics are called *parametric* because it is assumed that their underlying natural distribution is that of a normal curve. Means and correlations are the most common parametric statistics. For more complex multivariate designs, the statistical results could be expressed as regression weights, discriminant function coefficients, canonical correlation coefficients, or factor loadings. If the reader is interested in further instruction on the computation of multivariate statistics, we recommend the book *Using Multivariate Statistics* (3rd ed.) by Tabachnick and Fidell (1996).

Categorical Measures. Many research studies in the health field report their results not in the form of parametric statistics but rather by use of non parametric statistics and frequency table indices. These are statistics not based on assumptions of a normal distribution. They are usually dichotomous variables where the information of interest is the number or frequency of cojoint events. Some of these indices include sensitivity, specificity, relative risk ratios, or odds ratios.

Contingency tables combine the independent and dependent variables in a 2 × 2 matrix such as Figure 12.1.

In this contingency table, the independent variable Y is presented on the left side and the dependent variable Z is represented at the top of the table. The data collected in these studies are the number of individuals who appear in each of the four cells of the table, labeled a, b, c, d, respectively. Many statistical indices have been developed to characterize the relationship of the independent to the dependent variable for these fourfold tables. (Appendix 12.1 contains detailed description on the computation of some of these statistics—specifically, odds ratios, sensitivity, specificity and receiver operating characteristic [ROC] curves.)

Sampling Distributions

To perform a meta-analysis, you will need to be familiar with the statistical principles of *sampling distributions*. This concept is sometimes confusing to those who are initially learning about inferential statistics. A *sampling distribution* is a distribu-

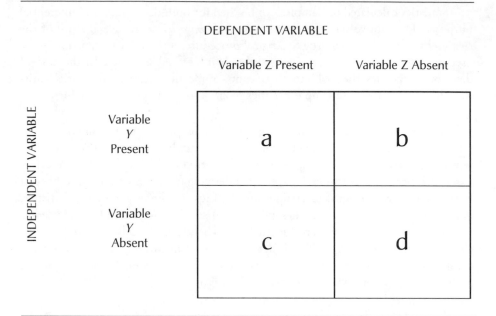

Figure 12.1. Illustrative 2 × 2 Contingency Table Where Two Variables Are Measured in a Population

NOTE: Z = the dependent variable; Y = the independent variable. The results are recorded in each of the four cells (a, b, c, d) of the matrix.

tion of the statistical values (i.e., means, proportions) that would be obtained if all possible samples of a given size were drawn from a population, the statistic measured for each sample, and the resultant list of statistics graphed in a frequency distribution. For example, the sampling distribution of the mean can be constructed by taking samples from a specific population (say 40 each), computing the mean of those 40 items, redrawing another sample of 40, computing the mean, and so on. Each mean will be somewhat different, but the graph of those means will be a normal distribution, and the mean of that distribution will be very close to the mean of the population. This distribution of means is called a sampling distribution.

We are very interested in the shape and characteristics of sampling distributions because we want to compare the measurements of our one sample against a theoretical population of possible samples. When the size of each sample is large (greater than 30 is the rule of thumb) and the samples are drawn randomly, the sampling distribution of many different statistical indices approximates the normal distribution. Because the statistical characteristics of a normal distribution are well known and easy to compute, the tendency for sampling distributions to take the normal form is fundamental to how statistical analyses are performed. The average or *expected value* of the sampling distribution is the average of the population. This fact is the heart of the central limit theorem, the basis of inferential statistics. This theorem is reflected in Formula 12.1:

$$\mu_{\bar{x}} = \mu_x.$$ (12.1)

The *variance* of the sampling distribution, however, is less than the variance of the population by a factor related to the size of the samples from which the statistic is drawn. The variance of a sampling distribution ($\sigma_{\bar{x}}^2$) of the mean is a function of the population variance (s^2) and the size of each sample (n) (Formula 12.2). In other words, as the size of the sample gets larger, the variance of the sampling distribution of the means gets smaller. The consequence of drawing large samples, then, is that the error around our estimate is quite small. When the sample size reaches the size of the population itself, there is *no* error as the mean of that very large sample is the mean of the population. The variance of the sampling distribution of means is sometimes called the *conditional variance* of the mean (Shadish & Haddock, 1994). The square root of this value is the standard deviation of the sampling distribution of the mean and is called the standard error of the mean.

$$\sqrt{\sigma_{\bar{x}}^2} = \sqrt{\frac{\sigma^2}{n}}$$ (12.2)

The value of the central limit theorem is that we can use this new distribution to make judgments about the relative probability of getting our sample mean if we were sampling from the population. We can make this judgment because the distribution is normal and we know the standard deviation (standard error) and the mean, so that we can compute any area under the curve.

The central limit theorem is relatively immune to the distribution of the original population. You could be sampling from a very skewed population (not normal), but the sampling distribution of the mean would still be normal. The consequence is that inferential statistics can be used to examine the likelihood of samples from a wide variety of original populations with little difficulty.

Statistical Power

One of the major benefits of a meta-analysis is that it greatly increases the **statistical power** for testing the null hypothesis (Hunter & Schmidt, 1990). Many research investigations are performed with inadequate statistical power because the sample size is too small. It is important, therefore, to understand the basic principles related to this power concept.

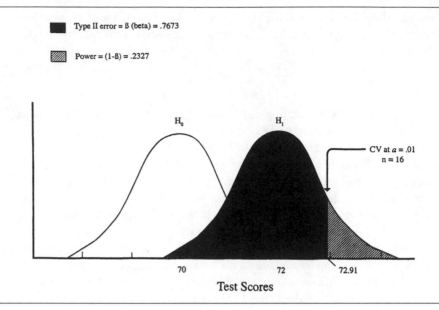

Figure 12.2. Sampling Distribution of Differences: Sample Size of 16

Statistical power is defined as the ability to detect an effect when one exists. In research, there are two kinds of errors. The first, called a *Type I error,* is the probability of rejecting the null hypothesis when in fact it should be accepted. That is, we make a Type I error when we say that we have a significant effect when, in reality, the treatment of interest really has no effect. Scientists usually focus their efforts on avoiding Type I errors. They are conservative and do not want to say there is an effect when in reality there is not an effect. The usual alpha chosen ($\alpha = .05$) in statistical analysis reflects this emphasis.

The second type of error is called a Type II error. A *Type II error* is defined as the probability of *accepting* the null hypothesis when, in fact, it should be rejected. In other words, with an agreed-on threshold of $\alpha = 0.05$ and a measured *p* value of 0.07, we would reject our alternative hypothesis of a treatment effect and accept the null hypothesis of no difference between groups. But we could be wrong if there actually were an effect. In other words, our sample of 16, drawn by chance, showed no difference when a difference might have been found in other samples. The probability of being wrong in accepting the null hypothesis is defined as ß (beta). Beta can *only* be determined by looking at the sampling distribution of the alternative hypothesis. We plot our findings on that distribution and compute the area (probability) under that curve. Power is defined mathematically as $1 - ß$ (1 – Type II error).

Figure 12.2 illustrates the two sampling distributions and the relative areas (probabilities) for a particular experimental example. In this example, an occupational health nurse is responsible for giving quality-of-life assessments to all incoming employees. She has two forms of the test: one with a normed mean score of 70 (Form A) and another with a normed mean of score 72 (Form B). Both have a known standard deviation of 5. She inadvertently failed to record which form she was using for 16 employees and she wants to make a guess. She would like to know first what her power would be if the tests were Form B (as compared to a null hypothesis that they were Form A).

In Figure 12.2, the sampling distribution of the null hypotheses (H_o) is represented on the left with a mean score of 70. The sampling distribution of the alternative hypothesis (H_1) is reflected on the right in the curve with a mean score of 72.0. The point of the abscissa, labeled critical value (CV) under the null hypothesis curve (H_o), is the value for which we would say that it differs statistically from 70.0.

The first step in calculating power is to calculate the standard error of the sampling distributions. In this case, we know the standard deviation of the population ($\sigma_x = 0.5$) and the size of our sample ($n = 16$). The standard error is calculated with Formula 12.3:

$$\sigma_{\bar{x}} = \frac{\sigma_x}{\sqrt{n}} \tag{12.3}$$

In this example the standard error is: (s/square root of n) = 5/4 = 1.25. Furthermore, because we know the population parameters, we can use the Z distribution. The critical value (CV) on this sample using a Z test is 2.33 at a = .01 (one-tailed). Translating this critical value of Z into actual numbers is done by multiplying the Z value by the standard error and adding the mean of the null sampling distribution, as shown in Formula 12.4:

$$CV_o = (Z_K)(\sigma_{\bar{x}}) + \mu_o \tag{12.4}$$

$(2.33)(1.25) + 70 = 72.91$. We next determine the probability of finding this value under the alternative sampling distribution (H_1) (see Formula 12.4).

$$72.91 = (Z_{H1})(1.25) + 72$$

In this distribution, CV_o is 72.91, so we subtract 72 from the CV_o (72.91) and divide by the standard error (1.25) to get the corresponding Z score (Z_{H1}) for the alternative distribution: $(72.91 - 72)/1.25 = 0.73 = Z_{H1}$. Checking tables of Z score probabilities, we find that a $Z = 0.73$ has a probability of 0.7673 (i.e., 76.7%). Figure 12.2 presents the probability of making a Type II error or of having a result that is really drawn from the population with a mean of 72. It is the shaded area under the H_1

curve. The power of correctly rejecting the null hypothesis is defined as shown in Formula 12.5.

$$Power = 1 - \beta$$
$$Power = (1 - 0.7673) = .2327 \text{ (i.e., 23.27\%).} \qquad (12.5)$$

In other words, with a sample of 16 (see Figure 12.2), we could only correctly determine where this sample came from 23% of the time. This is considered low power.

The most acceptable method of increasing power is to increase the sample size. Because the standard error of the mean is inversely related to the square root of the sample size (n), a large sample produces a small standard error. When the standard error is smaller, the critical value is smaller and closer to the mean of the null sampling distribution. The following example illustrates this principle.

Taking the same example as above but increasing the sample size to 25 (see Figure 12.3), we determine that the standard error of both sampling distributions is 1.00. Given that standard error, the CV_0 under the null sampling distribution would be $(2.33)(1.00) + 70 = 72.33$. This CV_0 has a Z score under the alternative sampling distribution of

$$72.33 = (Z_{H1})(1.00) + 72$$

Solving for $Z_{H1} = (72.33 - 72.00)/1 = 0.33$. From a table of Z score probabilities, a Z of 0.33 has a probability of 0.6293 (i.e., 72%). This value is β, or the probability of a Type II error (accepting the null hypothesis when, in reality, it should have been rejected). The corresponding number for power would be $(1 - \beta) = 0.3707$ (i.e., 28%). Thus, as you can see, we have increased the power by increasing the sample size. Figure 12.3 illustrates this example. The shaded area reflects the power associated with a sample size of 25.

Other factors can increase the power of a study as well. Increasing alpha will also increase the power. Because the CV of interest is associated with the corresponding Z score at the alpha level, a larger alpha would create a lower required Z score. In other words, with a larger alpha, we are more likely to reject the null hypotheses, making a Type II error less likely. In clinical practice, setting the alpha is a matter of determining the costs and benefits of the two kinds of errors. Sometimes, we want to make sure that if there is an effect, we detect it. Patients are more likely to want an intervention, even if the odds are low that it actually has an effect. In scientific circles, it is sometimes permissible to set the alpha as high as 0.10. The result will be an increased ability to detect an effect of the independent or treatment variable if there is one.

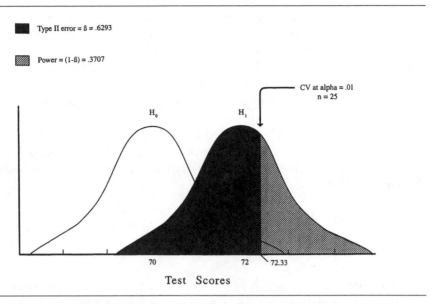

Figure 12.3. Sampling Distribution of Differences: Sample Size of 25

Section B. Effect Sizes: Calculation and Use

Definition and History

Typically, the meta-analysis parameter of interest is a numeric index that represents the *effect size* for the population, which reflects the size of the impact of an independent variable on a dependent variable. We adopted the notation introduced in Cooper and Hedges (1994) and use the symbol d_i to represent the population effect size.

Historically, two general approaches have been used to create effect size indices, called the *d* and *r* approaches (R. Rosenthal, 1994). In the *d* approach, an effect size is expressed as the *difference* between the means of two conditions (hence the *d* notation). Alternatively, in the *r* approach, the effect size is expressed as the strength of the relationship between an independent and a dependent variable; this index is usually measured as a correlation coefficient (hence the *r* notation).

Suppose that a researcher has studied the effects of a particular drug versus a placebo (these two conditions represent the two levels of the independent variable) on a patient's kidney functioning as measured by serum creatinine (the dependent variable). The population is defined as all patients who might be treated for diabetes.

The *d* effect size parameter for this example would be the average improvement effect (e.g., lowered serum creatinine level or *mean difference*) of the drug over the placebo condition for all possible patients. The *r* effect size index would be the correlation of the dichotomous independent variable with a continuous dependent variable (e.g., using a point biserial correlation) or the correlation of the dichotomous independent variable with a dichotomous dependent variable (e.g., using a phi, Φ, correlation coefficient).

A mean difference can be expressed as a correlation coefficient and vice versa, so an investigator can convert back and forth between the two approaches depending on which is most appropriate for the particular problem being addressed (R. Rosenthal, 1994).

Effect Size Calculations

Traditionally, a meta-analysis on mean differences involves the creation of a **standardized mean difference** (d_i), which serves as the effect size estimate for a single study, *i*. The effect size based on mean differences for study *j* can be represented by the differences between the experimental and control conditions, as in Formula 12.6:

$$d_i = \frac{(\bar{X}_i^t - \bar{X}_i^c)}{S_i}.$$

(12.6)

In this formula, $\bar{X}_i^t$ is the mean for the experimental condition, $\bar{X}_i^c$ is the mean for the control condition, and S_i is a pooled estimate of the within-group (i.e., within-study) standard deviation.

Formula 12.6 represents a typical *d* effect size that compares the means of an experimental and a control condition. Commonly, this difference is divided by an estimate of the within-condition standard deviation. As you will see later, one of the major problems to solve in a meta-analysis is to determine which estimate of the standard deviation should be used in the denominator of this expression. Some authors suggest that the combined standard deviation from both the experimental and control groups should be used, but others suggest that only the standard deviation from the control group be used. We recommend the former, using the pooled standard deviation; we will discuss this issue more in the next chapter.

As an estimator of the population effect size δ_j, shown in Formula 12.7, the statistic d_j is unbiased. Bryk and Raudenbush (1992) note that the accuracy of d_j as an estimate of δ_j depends on the actual sample sizes in the study.

$$\delta_j = \frac{(\mu_{E_j} - \mu_{c_j})}{\sigma_j}. \tag{12.7}$$

Note that δ_j has a conditional variance V_j in Formula 12.8:

$$V_j = \frac{(n_{E_j} + n_{C_j})}{(n_{E_j} * n_{C_j})} + \frac{d_j^2}{[2(n_{E_j} + n_{C_j})]}. \tag{12.8}$$

By substituting dj in this formula, we can assume that V_j has a known value. This value (V_j) is the conditional variance of the sampling distribution of effect sizes. The standard error is the square root of this value.

An investigator also may decide to estimate an r index for each study, and a typical computational formula is represented in Formula 12.9. The r statistic is itself an effect size measure. However, it is a somewhat biased estimator of the population effect size, δ_j, and must be standardized by conversion to a Z statistic.

$$r_{xy} = \sum_{i=1}^{N} \frac{Z_x Z_y}{N} = \sum_{i=1}^{N} \frac{\dfrac{(X - \bar{X})}{S_X} \dfrac{(Y - \bar{Y})}{S_y}}{N}. \tag{12.9}$$

In Procedure B, Chapter 14, we demonstrate the use of four effect size indices that are used most frequently in health-related research: (a) mean differences (the d approach), (b) the size of a correlation between an independent and a dependent variable (the r approach), (c) the difference in proportions between two conditions (e.g., the proportion of patients who died in a treatment minus the number of patients who died in the control group), and (d) an **odds ratio** that measures the ratio of the proportions in two conditions (e.g., a ratio of the proportion of people who die in a treatment condition to the proportion who die in a control condition). (For a more complete description of effect sizes and their computation, see R. Rosenthal, 1994, p. 233.)

In the research literature, there are references to small, medium, and large effect sizes (Cohen, 1988; Lipsey, 1990). These terms are used to describe the effect sizes (measured as standardized indices) that have been reported by other investigators in a particular research domain, and these values can be a useful reference point for investigators to judge the effect sizes of their syntheses. Cohen has referred to effect sizes of 0.20 as small effect sizes. An effect size of 0.20 indicates that the difference between treatment and control conditions is 0.20 standard deviation units. Cohen describes 0.50 as a medium effect size and 0.80 as a large effect size. The power of a statistical test indicates the probability of rejecting the null hypothesis given that the hypothesis is false (i.e., the treatment and control groups are different). However, the likelihood of rejecting the null hypothesis depends both on the effect size and the sample size.

Lipsey (1990, p. 23) has documented that most published research in medicine has rather low levels of statistical power. He has compiled an estimate of the statistical power for rejecting the null hypothesis (the hypothesis of no difference) in a number of research domains. He reports the statistical power of small effect size studies as being 0.37 in occupational therapy, 0.37 in gerontology, and 0.14 in medicine. For medium effect size studies, the power was 0.65 in occupational therapy, 0.88 in gerontology, and 0.39 in medicine. For large effect sizes, the published research had statistical power of 0.93 in occupational therapy, 0.96 in gerontology, and 0.61 in medicine. Thus, we would expect 86% of studies (100% − 14% = 86%) in medicine to fail to reject the null hypothesis, even though a small effect size was present. Similarly, 61% of medical studies would fail to detect a medium effect, and 39% of studies would fail to detect a large effect size.

In addition to the indices for effect size calculated on the individual samples, an investigator also calculates summary statistics *across* all the samples. These summary statistics typically are measures of the central tendency and the variability of the effect size indices obtained from the individual studies. In meta-analysis, the usual index of central tendency is a *weighted average* calculated across all the effect sizes from the individual studies. To produce this average, studies may be given different weights depending on values of the variances or samples sizes for each study. Weighting is usually done by multiplying the average effect size by a factor that is related to the sample size. Calculation of study variances and weighting factors is also presented in Chapter 14.

Section C. Hypothesis Testing in Meta-Analysis

Hypothesis Testing

One of the major goals of meta-analysis is to determine whether the existing evidence supports the premise that the independent variable is related to the dependent variable. The process of defining hypotheses in meta-analysis is quite similar to the method taught in introductory statistics classes. Typically, an investigator postulates two competing hypotheses about the value for δ_j, the population effect size parameter. The first is called the null hypothesis, and it postulates that the independent variable is *not* related to the dependent variable ($\delta j = 0.00$). The other hypothesis (the alternative or experimental hypothesis) asserts that a relationship *does exist* between the independent and dependent variable so that the absolute value of the population effect size $|\delta_j|$ is greater than 0.00.

As with other types of statistical analysis, the hypothesis testing process begins by assuming that both the null hypothesis and the alternative hypothesis are plausible. Each hypothesis predicts the mean of a particular sampling distribution from separate populations (each representing one of the hypotheses). Next, the statistical analysis determines whether the null hypothesis is plausible given the results from the various investigations. If an investigator fails to reject the null hypothesis, then only the alternative hypothesis is retained. An investigator retains only the hypothesis stating that some relationship does exist between the independent and dependent variable. (A more comfortable wording might be to "accept the null hypothesis" except that from a scientific perspective, one has only the choice of rejecting or not rejecting the null hypothesis, not accepting the null over the alternative. In other words, one cannot prove the null hypothesis.) The assumption at this point is that the sampling distribution with the alternative hypothesis mean value is the population from which the sample is selected. If the null hypothesis is rejected, an investigator usually will estimate the actual value of the effect size parameter and create a confidence interval around this estimate.

The methods of inferential statistics provide decision tools to help evaluate generalizations about the populations from which the samples were selected. In their hypothesis testing procedures, research investigators usually propose several competing hypotheses, and each hypothesis represents different hypothetical populations with different parameter values.

One hypothetical population is the *null distribution* in which the population parameter for the effect size is assumed to be 0.00. A zero effect size indicates no difference between the control group and the experimental group or no relationship between the independent and the dependent variable. The alternative population hypothesis specifies that the population parameter values are *not* equal to 0.00 (i.e., either greater than 0.00 or less than 0.00). Using the same type of strategy employed in traditional hypothesis testing, the observed statistical values of the averaged effect size across studies ($T\bullet$), as obtained from the sample of studies, can be compared to the values that would be expected if the null hypothesis were true. Calculation of the distribution to which the value of $T\bullet$ is compared is the *sampling distribution of effect sizes,* and comparing the $T\bullet$ with that distribution involves calculation of the variance of each study, then using those variances to estimate the variance of the sampling distribution. These calculations are covered in Chapter 14.

Parameter Estimation in Meta-Analysis

One goal of inferential statistics is to *estimate* the population parameter from the sample of studies that has been identified. For example, an investigator can use an index of effect size central tendency, such as a median, mode, or mean, that is calculated across all studies to estimate the population parameter (e.g., μ). The average effect size across studies will be used to estimate the "real" size of the effect. Not only can the size of the effect be an estimate, but also the degree of certainty regarding the estimate can be estimated. An investigator can then calculate measures of the variability or uncertainty associated with the specific parameter estimates.

A convenient and commonly used estimate of uncertainty is the *confidence interval* calculated on the samples. The confidence interval is calculated by estimating the range of values within which the parameter value is likely to be found. This interval defines the upper and lower limits for this range of values. Basically, it involves adding 2x the standard error (standard deviation of the sampling distribution) to the estimated average effect size for the upper limit and subtracting 2x the standard error from the average for the lower limit. The formula for calculating the confidence interval is also presented in Chapter 14.

When investigators use estimation strategies in meta-analysis, they are trying to find the best possible estimate of the population parameter and obtain some idea about the likely range of values for this particular parameter estimate. The estimation strategy is particularly useful when cost-effective **decision analyses** are performed. Suppose that two different drugs (A and B) are used in a clinical setting. Clinicians know that Drug A is statistically significantly better than Drug B in reducing the number of days of stay in the hospital. However, Drug A is much more expensive than Drug B. In order to choose between the two drug treatments, an investigator needs to know whether the reduction in costs associated with shorter hospital stays is sufficient to offset the higher cost of treatment for Drug A.

Meta-analysis procedures can be used to estimate the population parameters associated with drug costs and hospital length of stay. The goal in this analysis is not to test statistical significance. Rather, the goal in the estimation procedure is to obtain effect size estimates. By knowing the costs and the treatment effects for both drugs, an investigator can estimate the benefit that would be expected relative to the cost for each drug. An investigator can also obtain an estimate of the variability that occurs across studies. If high variability (i.e., wide confidence intervals) in the estimate of hospital length of stay is found, then the estimates of the cost savings associated with one drug would be uncertain. With low variability in estimates across studies, an investigator would be much more confident about the estimates.

Sampling Distributions for Hypothesis Testing

In the sections that follow, we provide detailed information about the sampling distributions for specific effect size statistics that you might want to test. Included are descriptions about d and r. Each of the sampling distributions is described in detail, including how the averages and variances are computed. Again, actual procedures for combining the effect sizes and doing hypothesis testing are reserved for Chapter 14.

A very important feature of these procedures is that the data entering into the analysis are statistically independent. Statistical dependence often arises when several comparisons are made within the same study (Condition 1 vs. Condition 2 and Condition 2 vs. Condition 3). It can also arise when both an initial and a follow-up study are reported in which a subset of subjects appears in both studies. Whenever data dependencies exist among the study samples, the properties of the sampling distribution change and estimates must be modified to accommodate these changes. In these cases, the procedures reported in this chapter cannot be used unless a multivariate approach is adopted. Under these circumstances, a valuable resource for you to use is available in Gleser and Olkin (1994).

The Sampling Distribution of the Composite Mean Effect Sizes. In the formulas we present in this section, $T\bullet$ is used to represent the average effect size. The variable t_i is the effect size calculated for each study, and w_i is a weighting factor that represents the variance for each study in Formula 12.10. k is the number of studies to be averaged. The actual effect size index value used for t_i can be calculated from a number of effect size indices, including correlation coefficients, mean difference in proportions, mean differences, odds ratios, or other effect size indices. Depending on your selection of an effect size index, you will need to choose an appropriate formula for calculating the *variance estimates* (v_i) of each study that is to be used (Shadish & Haddock, 1994). The weighting factor (w_i) is always calculated as the inverse of the variance.

In Chapter 14, we present the calculations for both a quality-unweighted and a quality-weighted approach. You would use the following formula to calculate a combined effect size if you wanted to weight the results by the study variances but not by measures of research quality. We refer to this approach as an unweighted solution. In Formula 12.10, you are calculating the average effect size or your estimate of the mean of the sampling distribution of effect sizes:

$$\overline{T\bullet} = \frac{\sum_{i=1}^{k} w_i t_i}{\sum_{i=1}^{k} w_i}. \tag{12.10}$$

With this formula, you multiply the effect size for each study by the reciprocal of the variance for that study. With this procedure, you will give greater weight to the studies that have smaller error variances.

The weighting factors (w_i) are derived from the actual variance within each study. These estimates are needed to calculate confidence intervals for the overall (average) effect size. You will also use these values if you decide to test the average effect size for statistical significance. There are several solutions to the problem of estimating variances. The most direct solution is to "average" the variances obtained in the individual studies. However, this procedure is not recommended. Because we actually use the value of 1/variance (symbolized as $1/v_i$) in our calculations of (w_i), we need to compute the averages from ($1/v_i$) instead of v_i, as shown in Formula 12.11. The value of v_i is the variance estimate obtained from each of the individual studies (i). These variances are computed individually for each study and differ depending on the statistic used. In almost all cases, v_i is usually based on the sample size and varies inversely with the sample size. In other words, the larger the sample size, the smaller the variance. We use the notation w_i to describe this inverse value for each study. $V\bullet$ is the conditional variance (standard error squared) of the sampling distribution.

$$w_i = \frac{1}{v_i}. \qquad (12.11)$$

Formula 12.12 provides an estimate for the conditional variance of the sampling distribution. This formula is based on the variances within each study, and they provide an estimated variance of the sampling distribution of effect sizes. This formula is needed for calculating confidence intervals and for performing hypothesis tests.

$$V_\bullet = \frac{1}{\sum\limits_{i=1}^{k}(w_i)} = \frac{1}{\sum\limits_{i=1}^{k}(1/v_i)}. \qquad (12.12)$$

At first glance, this formula may seem to be a bit unusual. If you want to calculate an average variance, you might expect to add up the variances and divide by the number of variances. To understand why we use the formula above, you need to recall that we are actually using the value of ($1/v_i$) in our calculations so that we need to calculate the average value of ($1/v_i$). You can easily show that the value generated by Formula 12.12 does not agree with the value you would obtain if you simply averaged the variances from each of the studies.

The Sampling Distribution for Combined Correlation Coefficients.   The following section addresses issues of combining correlation coefficients when an investigator does not have access to the original data (i.e., only has access to published correlation or covariance coefficients). Two different approaches have been introduced for combining correlation coefficient effect sizes. The first approach is based on traditional methods of combining correlation coefficients following Fisher's (1925) recommendations, as cited in Runyon and Haber (1991). The second approach is based on a method recommended by Hunter and Schmidt (1990, 1994).

The sampling distribution of combined correlation coefficient effect sizes is an approximately normal distribution when the sample size is sufficiently large and the null hypothesis value for ρ_{xy} is close to 0.00. However, when the population value of ρ_{xy} is not 0.00, then the sampling distribution for r_{xy} can be highly skewed. Fisher (1925) identified a transformation of the sample correlation coefficient whose sampling distribution is approximately normally distributed for any value of ρ_{xy}. The r to Z transformation is presented in Formula 12.13; this expression can be used in meta-analysis to generate combined effect size estimates (Shadish & Haddock, 1994). Tables for r to Z transformations are located in most basic statistics texts.

$$z_i = \frac{1}{2}\ln\left[\frac{(1+r_i)}{(1-r_i)}\right].$$
(12.13)

The expected value (mean of the sampling distribution) of Z_j is represented by ζ_j (Greek letter zeta) in Formula 12.14:

$$\zeta_i = E(Z_j) = \frac{1}{2}\ln\left[\frac{(1+\rho_i)}{(1-\rho_i)}\right].$$
(12.14)

The variance estimate for the sampling distribution of Z_j is presented in Formula 12.15. This formula is valid when the underlying distribution of X and Y is bivariate normal. The value of n_i in this formula is the sample size of the ith study to be combined in the meta-analysis.

$$v_i = \frac{1}{(n_i - 3)}.$$
(12.15)

Shadish and Haddock (1994) recommend that the obtained values of the average effect size be converted back to the original metric of correlation coefficients. These authors note that the following transformation, Formula 12.16, can be used to convert r back to these original values.

$$p(z_i) = \frac{(e^{2z} - 1)}{(e^{2z} + 1)}.$$
(12.16)

Hunter and Schmidt (1990) recommend an alternative approach to combining correlation coefficients. These authors suggest that the untransformed values of r be averaged together. Next, the variance of these effect sizes is estimated from Formula 12.17:

$$v_i = \frac{(1 - r_i^2)}{(n_i - 1)}.$$

(12.17)

Shadish and Haddock (1994) note that the values calculated using Formulas 12.15 and 12.17 will be very close for large sample sizes and for circumstances in which r is close to 0.00. However, when values of r are substantially different from 0.00, then the values in Formula 12.13 will be quite different from the untransformed values, and the variance estimate in Formula 12.15 will be substantially larger than the estimate from Formula 12.17. We agree with Shadish and Haddock's recommendation that Formulas 12.13 and 12.15 should be used for averaging correlation coefficients.

Summary

This chapter assumes you have a reasonably sound database of empirical studies that are homogeneous and have specific data (e.g., effect sizes) for synthesis. We review several basic statistical concepts important to help you implement the meta-analysis variation most appropriate to your needs.

The first section (A) reviews fundamental concepts such as populations, statistics, power, and sampling distributions. Specific descriptions are given for some of the more common statistics used in the healthcare field, such as odds ratios and relative risk ratios. Readers are assumed to have had exposure to means, correlations, and proportions.

The second section (B) presents a generic overview of effect sizes, including two different historical perspectives, the d and r effect size. The basic calculation for an effect size based on mean differences is presented as well as the variance calculations for that statistic.

The third section (C) reviews hypothesis testing in meta-analysis. We again review the concept of sampling distribution and how that concept applies to a meta-analysis. The process of hypothesis testing using a sampling distribution is reviewed with emphasis on its use in meta-analysis. Parameter estimation is also described and defined. This section ends with a short description of the sampling distribution of several important statistics, most particularly odds ratios, means, and correlations.

APPENDIX 12.1
Contingency Table Statistics

NOTE

For those of you unfamiliar with 2×2 contingency tables, it is important to understand the following labeling convention as used throughout this book.

The general nomenclature of a 2×2 contingency table labels the four cells using four alphabetic letters: a, b, c, and d, usually in lower case. The upper left cell is a, the upper right cell is b, the lower left cell is c, and the lower right cell is d.

For validation purposes, for example (see Figure 11.1), the vertical columns represent the gold-standard measures shown as marginal totals at the bottom of the columns. Thus, a + c equals the total gold-standard positive, whereas b + d equals the gold-standard negative results.

The horizontal rows represent the results of the test being validated, shown as the marginal totals to the right of the table. Thus, a + b equals the positive test results, and b + d equals the negative test results.

With this configuration, the upper left cell "a" indicates the "true positives," the upper right cell "b" the "false positives," the lower left cell "c" the "false negatives," and the lower right cell "d" the "true negatives."

Table 12.1 shows a different configuration of a 2×2 contingency table in which the independent variable represents the columns and the dependent variable the rows, which will now be discussed in the following example.

In a typical study, individuals either have or have not been exposed to some risk factor (say asbestos), which is the independent variable, and each individual is classified as having or not having a specific disease (say lung cancer), which is the dependent variable. Suppose an investigator hypothesizes that asbestos is a causal agent (independent variable) in producing lung cancer (dependent variable). If asbestos causes lung cancer, then a research study should find that a higher proportion of individuals exposed to asbestos, as opposed to those not exposed, have lung cancer. This relationship is easy to see in a contingency table such as Figure 12.1.

The demonstration of an association between asbestos exposure and lung cancer does not *prove* that asbestos exposure causes cancer. However, two variables that share a causal mechanism *should* be associated with each other. If an investigator is unable to establish evidence of a statistical association between two variables, then there is no evidence to support the plausibility of a causal relationship between them.

TABLE 12.1 Summary of Hypothesis Testing in Meta-Analysis Procedures

Hypothesis to Be Tested	Sampling Distribution	Central Tendency	Variability
Null hypothesis	Approximately normal	$\delta_j = 0.00$	Standard error of estimate $(V)^{1/2}$
Alternative hypothesis	Approximately normal	$\delta_j \neq 0.00$	Standard error of estimate $(V)^{1/2}$

NOTE: Cell entries refer to the elements of statistical decision making in meta-analysis.

Suppose an investigator has two groups of individuals who are hypothesized to represent two different populations (risk factor present or not present). For this presentation, we have adopted the notation of Fleiss (1994) and Shadish and Haddock (1994). Within each group, individuals are classified into dichotomous categories as being diseased or not diseased. The *probabilities of disease* in these two populations are represented as Π_1 (risk factor present) and Π_2 (risk factor absent). The proportion of diseased individuals in single samples from these populations is represented as p_{i1} for the risk factor present and p_{i2} for the risk factor absent.

We will now present four different types of hypothesized relationships between the population parameters Π_1 and Π_2. These descriptions of population differences will be followed by descriptive statistics often computed using contingency tables.

STATISTICS ON CONTINGENCY TABLES
(Sections of Appendix 12.1)

A. Difference in proportions
B. Relative risk ratio
C. Proportional reduction
D. Odds ratio
E. Sensitivity and specificity
F. Receiver operator characteristic curves
G. Precision and recall in literature searching

A. Difference in Proportions

Differences in proportions are the simplest type of effect to be tested with a contingency table. This test is based on the premise that the two populations are the same (the null hypothesis) so that the difference (Δ) between the two population parameters would be 0.00 (Formula 12.18).

$$\Delta = (\Pi_1 - \Pi_2) = 0.00. \qquad (12.18)$$

B. Relative Risk Ratio

Relative risk ratio is another test that can be done using a 2×2 table. The *relative risk ratio* is defined as the ratio of the two population proportions. Again, it is assumed that the parameters do not differ, so the null hypothesis is that the ratio of the parameters is equal to 1.00. If the exposure group is indeed more at risk, then the numerator will be larger (higher probability of disease) than the denominator, and the relative risk (RR) ratio will be greater than 1.00 (Formula 12.19). The relative risk ratio (RR ratio) is not to be confused with relative risk reduction (RRR), which will be explained later.

$$Relative\ Risk = \frac{\Pi_1}{\Pi_2} = 1.00. \qquad (12.19)$$

C. Proportional Reduction

Proportional reduction is the relative decrease in the likelihood of an adverse outcome when individuals are not exposed to a risk factor. The investigator can compare the rate of disease in a control condition to an exposed or experimental condition. For example, an investigator may want to estimate the reduced likelihood of lung cancer in individuals who are not exposed to asbestos. A third way to express the null hypothesis is through proportional reduction (PR). The null hypothesis is that PR = 0.00, as shown in Formula 12.20. In this formula, the added amount of risk, or rate of disease associated with being in the exposed group, is divided by the amount of disease in the nonexposed group.

$$Proportional\ Reduction = \frac{(\Pi_2 - \Pi_1)}{\Pi_2} = (1 - RR). \qquad (12.20)$$

D. Odds Ratios

Odds ratio is the fourth type of null hypotheses generated from 2 × 2 contingency tables. Odds ratio is a widely used statistical index for research purposes, especially for prospective, retrospective, and cross-sectional studies that have categorical independent variables (Fleiss, 1994). The odds ratio contrasts two different ratios: the odds of disease for groups when a risk factor is present versus the odds of disease for groups when the risk factor is absent. In our example of asbestos and lung cancer, the odds ratio would be the probability of disease for a group exposed to asbestos as compared to the probability of disease in the group not exposed to asbestos. However, Douglas, Deeks, and Sackett (1998) point out that there are times when odds ratios should be avoided.

To understand odds ratios, you need to understand the concept of odds. For example, an investigator might ask what the odds are of contracting lung cancer within one of the populations (i.e., the one given exposure to asbestos). If three fourths of that population had lung cancer, then the odds of having lung cancer would be expressed as the following ratio (Formula 12.21):

$$Odds\ of\ disease = \frac{(\Pi_1)}{(1-\Pi_1)} = \frac{3/4}{1/4} = \frac{3}{1}. \tag{12.21}$$

An odds ratio (Formula 12.22) is the ratio that compares the odds in one population to the odds in the other population. Hence, the null hypothesis for a test of the odds ratio is that they are equal, producing a ratio of 1.0.

$$\omega = \frac{\frac{(\Pi_1)}{(1-\Pi_1)}}{\frac{(\Pi_2)}{(1-\Pi_2)}}. \tag{12.22}$$

The null hypothesis states that the odds are the same in the two populations. Hence, the odds ratio would equal 1.00 if the null hypothesis were correct. A typical alternative hypothesis is that the odds ratio is not equal to 1.00. In the example cited above, suppose that 1 out of 20 people in the *asbestos nonexposed* group had lung cancer. Then the odds ratio would be (3/1)/(1/19) or a value of 57.

Formula 12.22 can be simplified based on the cell frequencies in the four-cell (2 × 2) table (see Figure 12.1) with the letters "a" through "d" representing the individual cell frequencies (Formula 12.23).

$$\omega_i = \frac{ad}{bc}. \tag{12.23}$$

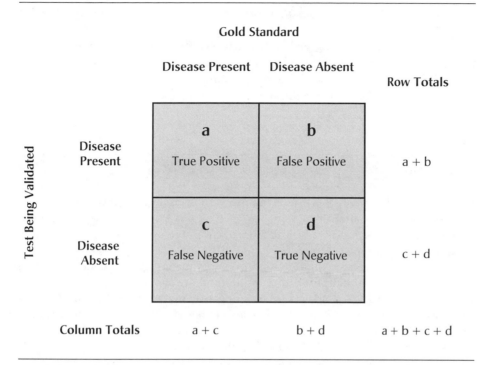

Gold Standard

Figure 12.4. Population Measured by Gold-Standard Test and by Test Being Validated
NOTE: Cell entries refer to the frequency of occurrence.

E. Sensitivity and Specificity

Sensitivity and **specificity** are another set of common statistics in healthcare using a
2 × 2 contingency table, when validation is the goal. In these cases, the tables reflect
slightly different questions than the relationship of a risk factor to a disease. More
commonly, they are used to assess the accuracy of a test as compared to a gold standard. The table is usually constructed the same way, but on the top along the horizontal dimension is the gold standard, and on the left side along the vertical dimension is
the test (see Figure 12.4 for an illustration).

Sensitivity and specificity are related and are essentially rates or simple proportions. Using Figure 12.4, *sensitivity* is defined as the proportion of true-positive
patients (cell a), where the gold-standard test and the test being checked agree the
patients have the disease, divided by the total patients that the gold standard indicates have the condition (cell a + cell c). Formula 12.24 illustrates this computation.

$$Sensitivity = a/_{a+c} \qquad\qquad (12.24)$$

Similarly, *specificity* is defined as the proportion of true-negative patients (cell d) where the test and the gold standard agree that patients do *not* have the disease, divided the gold-standard total that indicates those who do *not* have the condition (cell b + cell d). Formula 12.25 illustrates this computation.

$$Specificity = d/_{b+d} \qquad\qquad (12.25)$$

NOTE: FALSE-NEGATIVE AND FALSE-POSITIVE RATES

False-negative rate: This represents the proportion of total positive findings by a gold-standard assessment that a new, or routine, test finds negative. In literature searching, it is the same as (1 – recall rate); in clinical research, it is (1 – sensitivity), or beta value or a Type II error.

False-positive rate: We judge that it is most meaningful to conceptualize a false-positive rate as that proportion of the total positive findings of a test being validated that the gold-standard test finds negative. In literature searching, it is the same as (1 – precision rate); in clinical research, it is (1 – positive predictive value), or alpha value or a Type I error.

By this convention, both the false-negative and false-positive rates are usually whole integers that range from 0 to 100 (in percentage terms) and are immune to the effects of prevalence levels that fall below 1%. Figure 12.6 illustrates this latter effect of prevalence.

F. Receiver Operator Characteristic Curves

The *receiver operator characteristic* (ROC) curve is a graphical display of the relationship between sensitivity and specificity. See Figure 12.5 for an illustration.

ROC curves are used to evaluate the performance of decision processes across a range of possible cutoff points. The curve plots the true-positive rate (sensitivity) against the false-positive rate (1 – specificity). When these two numbers are graphed together for each value of a test, they capture the performance of the test across that range of values. The area under the curve reflects overall performance. The greater the area, the fewer false positives and the more true positives.

For example, you could have a test of myocardial damage that could take on a value of 1 (not at all severe) to 5 (very severe). When you graph the proportion of correctly identified patients with myocardial infarctions (MIs) at each level of the test, with the proportion of those where an MI is falsely identified, you will produce a curve. If the curve has a steep slope at first (when the false-positive rate is low while

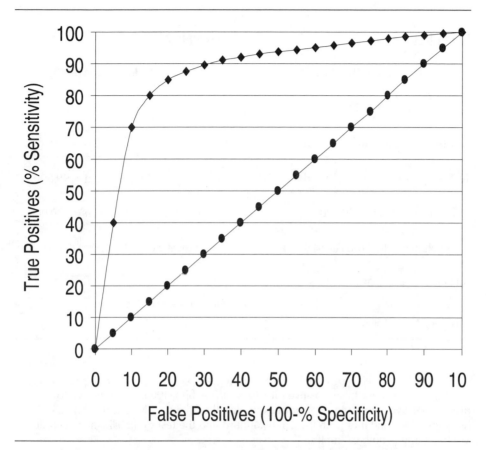

Figure 12.5. Receiver Operator Characteristic (ROC) Curve

the true-positive rate is high), then the test is a good one. When the test has about equal true-positive and false-positive rates across all conditions, then the line is a straight diagonal and the test performs no better than chance. It is the difference in the area under the curve between a straight diagonal and the higher curve that is the measure of the quality of the test.

These curves, however, can be misleading if the prevalence of the condition being studied is much lower than 1.0%. See Figure 12.6, where the prevalence calculation is depicted as ([a + c]/[a + b + c + d] × 100). When the prevalence is low, the false-positive rate of the ROC curve rapidly drops to small fractions, whereas the false-negative rate remains constant.

Readers interested in using ROC curves, sensitivities, and specificities in a synthesis should review their characteristics by reading a text on the issue, such as Sackett et al. (1991) or Moses, Shapiro, and Littenberg (1993).

Example 1

Gold Standard

	(+)	(−)
Test (+)	a = 60	b = 100
Test (−)	c = 40	d = 9,800

a + c = 100   n = 10,000

Prevalence = 1 in 100 (1.0%)

False (−)	=	40.00%
False (+)*	=	1.01%
False (+)**	=	2.50%

Example 2

Gold Standard

	(+)	(−)
	a = 60	b = 100
	c = 40	d = 99,800

a + c = 100   n = 100,000

Prevalence = 1 in 1,000 (0.1%)

False (−)	=	40.00%
False (+)*	=	0.10%
False (+)*	=	62.50%

* The traditional false-positive rate, $fp = (b/[b + d]) \times 100$ is sensitive to prevalence.
** Our formula for a false-positive rate, $fp = (b/[a + b]) \times 100$ is not sensitive to prevalence. We assume that for both examples, the total positive population (a + c) is homogeneous and that both the gold standard and the test's reliability and accuracy are the same in both examples.

Figure 12.6. Effect of Prevalence on Traditional False-Positive Rate (i.e., [1 - specificity])

G. Precision and Recall in Literature Searching

Closely related to sensitivity and specificity are the concepts of **precision** and **recall**. These concepts, as applied in assessing literature search results, use a 2 × 2 contingency table. In this case, *precision* indicates the proportion of all positive documents retrieved that are also found positive by the gold standard. In other words, this is the lack of false positives. On the other hand, *recall* indicates the proportion of gold-standard positive documents that actually exist (within a defined universe of literature) that the search actually retrieves. In other words, this is the lack of false negatives.

Another way that precision is used is in asking how narrowly defined a measurement or estimate might be. The most frequent way of expressing these terms is by means of a confidence interval (CI) about the given measure or estimate. The CI defines the range that represents the limits of accuracy of a measurement. Furthermore, the range is set at a specified probability, usually 95%. This means that, with a 95% probability, the true measure lies somewhere within that range (i.e., between the upper and lower limits of the CI). An estimate is precise if it is sharply defined (i.e., has a narrow CI). (Note that *recall* does not have meaning in terms of measurement or estimation outside of searching.)

In terms of the 2 × 2 contingency table nomenclature, *precision* would be cell a divided by the sum of cell a and cell b (multiplied by 100 if percentage results are preferred). Similarly, *recall* would be cell a divided by the sum of cell a and cell c (also times 100 if percentage values are preferred). Note that recall is calculated the same as sensitivity, and precision is calculated the same as positive predictive value.

Conceptual Aspects of Meta-Analysis

A quantitative research synthesis, or meta-analysis, is a formal approach for identifying the consistencies and inconsistencies in studies that examine the same research hypothesis (Cooper & Hedges, 1994; Egger et al., 1997). We have stated that, in our judgment, meta-analysis is one of the most sound methods of synthesizing quantitative data. Although many investigators agree (Egger & Smith, 1997), this assumption is not shared universally (Hasselblad et al., 1995). For example, recently the question has been raised as to whether a large-sample randomized clinical trial (RCT) produces more valid results than meta-analysis of many small sample trials (Cappelleri et al., 1996). In a *New England Journal of Medicine* editorial, Bailar (1998) addresses this issue and is quite critical of meta-analyses as they are conducted today. If you are to avoid the hazards that these experts point out, it is important that you understand the theoretical aspects of this form of systematic review.

Chapter 13 is organized around seven major issues that are central to the theory of the design and performance of a meta-analysis. A brief synopsis is provided at the end of each section, as well as a complete chapter summary at the end of the chapter.

We will focus on studies that produce randomized data. However, it is possible to develop meta-analyses of diagnostic tests (Irwig et al., 1994; Moses et al., 1993) or even nonrandomized, uncontrolled data such as synthesis of dose-response studies (Lau et al., 1997; Tweedie & Mengersen, 1995).

CONCEPTUAL ASPECTS OF META-ANALYSIS

    A.   Designing multivariate models
    B.   Selecting effect size index
    C.   Managing missing data
    D.   Managing artifacts and biases
    E.   Heterogeneity of effect sizes among studies
    F.   Combining effect sizes
    G.   Sensitivity analysis

Each of the above issues is briefly described in Table 13.1. Many are somewhat controversial, and there is no exact right or wrong way to deal with them. Understanding the complexity and implications of each is the most effective method for making a correct decision. As but one example of the effect of RCT quality on the final efficacy of meta-analysis results, see Moher (1998).

Section A. Designing Multivariate Models

A formal quantitative model is essential to conducting a quantitative synthesis. The conceptual model developed during the planning stage provides the best foundation for the construction of a quantitative model in the synthesis stage. As much as possible, a multivariate quantitative model is needed to address the multiple independent and dependent variables that are contained in the conceptual model (Becker & Schram, 1994). A quantitative restructuring is the first issue in the synthesis process itself. All hypotheses must be specified in measurable terms to be tested. However, there are several problems commonly associated with turning a multidimensional conceptual question to a quantitative multivariate testable model. A multivariate model contains one or more independent variables and more than one dependent variable. The following section will elucidate these problems and their management in more detail.

Because of the necessity of quantifying the model prior to the actual synthesis, many authors of meta-analyses severely limit their model to a simple question of cause and effect between two variables. This tendency in meta-analyses to oversimplify the question is one of the major complaints about it (Feinstein, 1995; Guzzo, Jackson, & Katzell, 1986). In the past, a meta-analysis made limited use of multivariate approaches to examine mediating or interactive effects on research outcomes.

TABLE 13.1 Description of Issues to Be Addressed in Performing a
Meta-Analysis

Issue Name	*Description*
A. Multivariate models	Converting the conceptual framework to a quantitative, multivariate synthesis model
B. Effect size index selection	Determining which effect size to use
C. Missing data management	Identifying sources and reasons for missing data and managing solutions
D. Management of biases and artifacts	Estimating degree of impact of artifacts and biases and correcting them if possible
E. Heterogeneity of effect sizes	Testing for significant differences in effect sizes and adjusting plan based on results
F. Combining effect sizes	Determining which combination strategy is suited to the data and to the question
G. Sensitivity analyses	Recombining data in different ways to test how robust the results are

This overemphasis on univariate strategies resulted from two common problems that authors of meta-analyses still face.

The first problem is that original investigators do not report all the data that might be required for a multivariate approach. For example, most multivariate analyses require a variance-covariance matrix; this statistical matrix measures the strength and direction of relationships among all of the measures; frequently, this matrix is not available in published reports. This problem might be solved by contacting the original investigators and soliciting the data from individual research participants (i.e., the raw data) rather than from the aggregated data reported in publications. With these original data, it might be possible to perform multivariate analyses for the studies in a data set. Lau et al. (1997) state that "meta-analysis of individual patient data may represent the highest step in the hierarchy of evidence" (p. 825). In support of this statement, they reference Olkin (1995).

The second problem is a function of the theory construction process itself. Univariate theories are relatively weak in providing explanatory principles. In contrast, multivariate models are more desirable because they are conceptually more complete (see Becker, 1992; Becker & Schram, 1994). The actual models researchers develop typically postulate interactive effects among several variables. Moderators are identified that affect either the direction or amount of effect that the independent variables have on the dependent variables. Mediators are variables that are postulated to cause the relationship between the independent variables and the dependent variables. In satisfactory theoretical models, both the cause and the context are identified. The result is a better "explanation" of the phenomena.

Although it is desirable to test a multivariate model, most often it is not possible. Many reviewers find that most primary studies test only one part of a model (sometimes a few more); rarely does a study test all of the relevant components. Thus, you may not be able to locate enough studies to test a specific interaction or multivariate hypotheses, and alternatives need to be used. Below we discuss three approaches to expanding the quantitative model to include multivariate questions. In all cases, questions should be set up á priori to minimize the likelihood that conclusions are inappropriately biased by chance or random sampling processes.

Testing Moderator and Mediator Variable Hypotheses

Under some circumstances, you can adopt one relatively simple reformulation solution to address complex theoretical interactions in your meta-analysis. That is, you can identify a specific variable that may moderate the relationship of the independent variable to the dependent variable. For example, you may hypothesize that the relationship depends on whether you are studying patients treated in public versus private clinics (location of treatment would be the **moderator variable**), or you might hypothesize that the results are moderated by the patient's age, gender, or severity of illness.

You might perform the meta-analysis separately for studies reporting results within specific populations or within levels of other interacting independent variables. That is, you might perform separate meta-analysis for male and female subjects if there appears to be an interaction between the primary independent variable and the gender of research participants. Or, you might be able to perform separate analyses for studies in which the patients are severely ill versus those studies in which the patients are not very ill.

If you have a sufficiently large set of studies in your data set, you might classify the studies by two different moderator variables and look for possible interactive effects between them. Hunter and Schmidt (1990, pp. 524-527) provide an example of this approach using hypothetical data. In their example (see Figure 13.1), each of two variables apparently moderated the meta-analysis results.

Moderator Variable B \ Moderator Variable A	Present	Absent	Average for Moderator B
Present	0.40	0.20	0.30
Absent	0.20	0.20	0.20
Average for Moderator A	0.30	0.20	0.25

Figure 13.1. Example of the Interactive Effects of Two Moderator Variables

NOTE: Cell entries are (hypothetical) mean effect sizes for studies that have the presence or absence either of moderator variable A or moderator variable B. The average row and column represent mean effect sizes calculated across the presence or absence of a moderator variable. These data are adapted from an example described in Hunter and Schmidt (1990, pp. 524-527).

In this hypothetical example, we assume that the independent variable has produced a mean effect size of 0.30 when Moderator A (e.g., a comorbid condition) is present but an effect size of 0.20 when the moderator is absent. Similarly, the mean effect size is 0.30 when Moderator B (e.g., a second comorbid condition) is present but 0.20 when Moderator B is absent.

As the results in Figure 13.1 indicate, the two moderator variables actually produce an interactive effect on the meta-analysis results. When both moderators are present, the effect size is 0.4. When either or both of the moderators are absent, the effect sizes are 0.20. In this example, the researchers are able to examine the interactive effects of three variables (the two moderator variables plus the primary independent variable). You may find this approach to be a valuable tool to examine some of the multivariate assumptions in your model when the available data do not permit a direct test of some hypothesized interactive effects.

Subgroup Analyses Applied to Incomplete Designs

Another useful strategy for conducting a multivariate analysis, when none or few of the primary studies address the entire theoretical model, is to identify subgroups of studies based on the control group. Control groups can vary depending on the question. For example, the control group for a study examining effectiveness of a drug could be a group that receives no drug or a group that receives a different drug. Because the control group subjects have not been influenced by the experimental treatment, these individuals can provide an assessment of how the various study samples differ prior to the introduction of the treatment conditions. This approach can be used for circumstances in which the available studies in the data set do not provide sufficient data to test all of the planned hypotheses. Berlin and Antman (1994) suggest subgroup analysis should only be used as a means to generate hypotheses. Michels and Rosner (1996), on the other hand, claim this approach can provide important insights.

Eddy et al. (1992, pp. 241-250) describe a variation of the subgroup analysis technique. This example describes the synthesis of research on two different thrombolytic agents for patients who had experienced a myocardial infarction. One drug was called tissue-type plasminogen activator (t-PA), and the other drug was called streptokinase (SK). Thrombolytic agents are designed to dissolve blood clots that prevent perfusion of blood to heart tissue. If either drug is administered quickly enough after the formation of a blood clot in the coronary arteries, the medication can reduce damage to heart tissue that results from the lack of blood flow to these tissues. Both of the medications are designed to produce rapid reperfusion of the heart tissue (an intermediate outcome) as well as reduce mortality during the first year after the infarction (the long-term outcome).

REPERFUSION RATE

After coronary artery occlusion by a thrombus (clot), early administration of thrombolytic drugs usually dissolves the clot (at least partially) and allows reperfusion of blood through the coronary arteries. A "reperfusion rate" is the proportion of patients who are diagnosed as having an acute myocardial infarction (MI) who receive thrombolytic agents (i.e., reperfusion therapy) within a few hours of the onset of symptoms. For example, if a patient receives these drugs within 1 hour of onset, mortality can be lowered more than 40% to 50%, and the extent of cardiac damage and subsequent disability is substantially reduced (National Institutes of Health [NIH], 1993). There is a clear time relationship between the onset of pain and administration of thrombolytics to mortality in percentage terms: If treated within 1 hour, mortality is 3.2%; within 2 hours, 3.7%; within 3 hours, 5.2%; and within 4 hours, 6.2%.

TABLE 13.2 Summary of Evidence Examining the Effectiveness of Two Thrombolytic Agents on Coronary Artery Reperfusion Following a Myocardial Infarction

| | Research Conditions | | | |
Individual Study	*t-PA*	*SK*	*Usual Care*	*Placebo*
TIMI	0.66 (118)	0.36 (122)	(0)	(0)
Collen	0.76 (33)	(0)	(0)	0.071 (14)
Kennedy	(0)	0.69 (134)	0.12 (116)	(0)
20 trials	(0)	(0)	(0)	(0)
Combined	0.68 (151)	0.54 (256)	0.12 (116)	0.071 (14)

NOTE: Numbers in parentheses are sample sizes. The other cell entries are the proportion of patients successfully perfused. The proportions in the combined row are the weighted average of the nonempty cells above.

In this example on thrombolytics, we describe three studies that evaluated these drugs using different types of control conditions (Eddy et al., 1992, p. 242). The first study was conducted by the NIH Blood Thrombolysis in Myocardial Infarction trials, called TIMI; the second was labeled Collen; and the third was labeled Kennedy, as shown in Table 13.2.

Researchers in these studies measured reperfusion rates and used various combinations of t-PA and SK in treatment conditions and "usual care" or "placebo" for the control condition. We have summarized the results from these studies in Table 13.2 to illustrate how combined rates can be used when there are missing data cells.

In the last row of this table, we illustrate combined results for all of the studies that report data on this condition. The combined reperfusion rates were as follows:

t-PA = 68%

Streptokinase = 54%

Usual treatment = 12%

Placebo treatment = 7%

SOURCE: National Institutes of Health (1993).

Even though none of the studies actually compared t-PA with usual care, we can use the data from the last row in Table 13.2 to make this comparison. The data in the combined row suggest that t-PA raises perfusion to 68% as compared to the usual care rate of 12%. In a similar manner, the data provide evidence that SK raises perfusion to 54% as compared to the placebo rate of 7.1%. That is, the combined results permit tests of hypotheses that did not occur in any of the individual studies.

We recognize that these types of comparisons should be made very cautiously. For example, you may suspect that the various studies represent different populations of patients or treatments. A common problem in health research is that patients have coexisting medical conditions that contrast to the illness that is the focus of treatment. Some of the patients may be receiving treatment for these conditions. As a consequence, the patients in one study could be quite different from the patients in another study.

You would have reason to suspect a problem of this sort in the present example because the two studies of streptokinase produced substantially different rates of perfusion (36% vs. 69%). A number of explanations are possible for these different rates. For example, the patients might represent different populations (say, differing in age, comorbidity, or other treatment characteristics). The studies may also differ on other characteristics such as the actual measurement procedures for assessing reperfusion or differences in other treatment variables (e.g., the experience level of clinicians treating patients). Regardless of these limitations, the synthesis process can provide approximate evidence about what might be expected if an experiment were to be performed comparing t-PA with conventional care.

Structural Equation Modeling

Other approaches that can be used to examine multivariate conceptual models include the use of various **path analyses**, structural equations modeling, or regression models (Becker, 1992; Bryk & Raudenbush, 1992; Shadish, 1992). These techniques are more sophisticated and involve significantly more statistical expertise. However, their use may be very rewarding in complex meta-analyses. As we indicated earlier, the essential data for these types of analyses often are not reported in published accounts, and you might have to contact original investigators to obtain it. The current availability of such informatics resources as the Internet and e-mail makes the transfer of data sets much easier and more direct than was possible in the past.

Structural equations modeling is a multivariate statistical technique that permits examination of complex patterns of relationships among a set of variables. Using this technique, a researcher can simultaneously create a measurement and a causal model. The process basically involves two steps.

The first step is to create more accurate measures of the theoretical constructs being examined in the multivariate model. An important assumption in this approach is that many of our concepts can only be measured indirectly. For example, we do not have a direct measure of depression. However, the investigator can use one or more of several indirect measures (e.g., irritability, loss of appetite) that might support an inference about this health problem. Some researchers might use a subjective sense of the patient's affect and appearance, some might infer depression from a careful history, others might use psychometric tests, and still others might check the medications the patient is taking. These approaches assess somewhat different aspects of the same underlying concept, depression. However, they vary in their validity and reliability. The abstract construct that they are all trying to measure is termed the "latent" concept. Presumably, some combination of these various measures can provide a more accurate assessment of the latent concept than any one type of evidence alone. The goal of the first step, then, is to create a composite of the various measures so as to permit a more accurate inference or assessment of the latent concept.

The second step in a structural equation approach is to examine hypothesized relationships among a set of latent variables. Typically, these relationships are expressed in path-analytic terms. In other words, the causal latent variables are shown on the far left of the model, the next step in the causal pathway might be in the middle, and the outcome of interest would be on the far right. A line indicating the strength of their relationship would connect each variable. They are sometimes referred to as hypothesized causal relationships.

The study begins with analysis of the "baseline model." This model is intended to be a simple and parsimonious explanation of the results (i.e., correlations among the measures). In this step, we attempt to determine whether all of the measures appear to reflect a single empirical construct. If this hypothesis is correct, then only a single latent variable is needed to account for all of the correlations among the measures. Typically, we would be disappointed if the findings supported this reasoning. We usually want to examine a multicomponent model in which we are trying to estimate relationships between all of the components. If we need only a single construct to represent all of these relationships, we will have developed a very parsimonious but possibly a too simple representation of our multicomponent theory. The next step is to test our more elaborate and complex hypothesized model against a simple baseline model. A **chi-square test** for improvement of fit can be calculated to determine whether the more complex model provides a better explanation than the baseline model in accounting for all of the observed relationships among our measures.

Using a model of this type in a meta-analysis can be complicated because there will rarely be a study that includes all aspects of the model and its paths in one study. However, it may be possible to break down different aspects of the model to more focused individually relevant questions (Becker, 1994, has several examples).

Synopsis of Section A

One of the first issues in the synthesis process is to quantify a model. Often reviewers reduce their model to a simple question of the relationship between one independent variable and one dependent variable. This model often fails to include explicit discussion of the factors that might moderate that relationship (e.g., setting, disease type, experience of the clinician, or an analysis of other causal or mediating factors). As a result, findings from these meta-analyses often are either too broad to be applicable to real-life settings and/or too simplistic to extend knowledge. If at all possible, we recommend that a multivariate design be chosen. However, actual implementation of a multivariate analysis is often difficult because the necessary primary studies are not available.

If a multivariate design is chosen, then there are several options available. Simple extension of the model to include moderator variables is a common approach that has the advantage of being able to generalize the results. The subgroup analysis techniques can be very effective for examining interactive relations of the independent and dependent variables. Although useful, these approaches cannot be used under some circumstances. As Hunter and Schmidt (1990, pp. 292-303) indicate, subgroup strategies can lead to a substantial reduction in the total sample of studies or subjects for each subgroup analysis, resulting in low statistical power. Furthermore, you should carefully plan these subgroup analyses so that they do not turn into "fishing expeditions." That is, you can perform so many subgroup analyses that you substantially increase the number of possible chance findings (Hunter & Schmidt, 1990, p. 88). Finally, you can develop a full structural equation model using and estimating the data from primary studies.

Section B. Selecting Effect Size Index

The second issue, Section B, is the selection of an effect size index. Most meta-analyses involve the synthesis of research findings that examine the relationship between an independent and a dependent variable. That relationship is usually expressed by the calculation of an effect size. In Chapter 12, we defined effect sizes and described how they are computed. In this section, we discuss the issues surrounding the selection of the particular effect size calculation. Factors that influence effect size use include decision rules regarding selection, standardization, small sample sizes, and the impact of different research designs.

Decision Rules for Selection of Effect Sizes

Many problems in selecting the proper statistic as a measure of an intervention effect precede their computation. Attention to several decision rules is an essential component of the task of defining an explicit model.

The first rule is to ensure that measures of effects are independent from each other. In other words, two or more measures of the same effect should not be included in the same overall average effect size. Determining which effect size to use from a study that reports many effects may be difficult. For example, doctor-patient communication may be measured in one study as both the amount of information given to the patient and the reports of patient satisfaction with the information given. If both were used independently in the overall list of effect sizes, the same sample would unduly influence the findings.

Studies from the same set of researchers may also not be independent because they often could involve some of the same subjects or geographic regions and the same intervention techniques. For example, researchers may report follow-up data on the same patients across several successive publications. A study may report separate findings on different samples as well. Although there may be no overlap between the subjects' in-groups, there is significant overlap between the population from which each is drawn and the procedures by which they are measured.

The only solution to lack of independence is to decide beforehand what the **unit of analysis** will be or to build a model that directly tests for nonindependence. If there are clearly groups of researchers, each of which publish many articles on the same topic (and the correlation between their findings is quite high compared to the correlation across researchers), then an average of all of their findings might be appropriate. On the other hand, this approach is quite conservative and may unnecessarily limit your findings. If there is evidence of significant heterogeneity, the initial solution suggested or a post hoc analysis may be warranted.

Most solutions to this problem center on using studies as the unit of analysis and developing a set of rules that will determine which effect size index to use to analyze data from each study. One possibility is simply to average them, another is to choose one on theoretical grounds, or the median can be used (Cooper, 1998, p. 98). In any case, an explicit criteria index must be developed and used for selecting an effect size index for each of the data sources in your analysis.

A second rule is to decide the level of abstraction at which the effect size will be calculated. For example, a researcher can be looking at the degree to which antidepressant drugs affect patient outcomes. Because outcomes are so variously measured from study to study, it is sometimes difficult to justifiably combine them all as being the same. However, a researcher can make the case that all of them reflect a general construct of overall functioning. Or the researcher can select a set of categories to which each type of outcome can be assigned. Effect sizes would then be aggregated within categories.

A third rule is to determine issues of timing in selecting and defining the appropriate effect size. *Timing* refers to when measures of the dependent variable are taken. Usually, measures will vary in terms of time since treatment. For example, some studies may measure exercise tolerance 1 month after treatment, whereas others may measure 6 months after treatment. In healthcare studies, timing issues may be more subtle. Measurements may be taken at the same length of time since treatment, across all studies, but on populations who vary in how far along they are in their disease process. Or populations may vary in terms of when, in their disease progression, they were selected for treatment. Some patients may be diagnosed on routine screening events and thus be asymptomatic. Others may have entered the study population because they were sick enough to have had symptoms. Finally, there is the familiar problem of patients lost to follow-up, which produces a different population and hence a different effect measure than those studies that lost very few to follow-up. In all cases, the issue of timing, as the precise measure of effect, needs to be expressly defined.

A fourth rule is to take into account appropriate study characteristics when defining effect size. Even though each study purports to examine the effect of an antidepressant on depressive mood, the conditions under which the medication is given may actually constitute a different independent variable. For example, in some studies, antidepressant medications are always given with psychotherapy; in other studies, patients are given medications with a variety of other types of treatment. The author must decide as part of model development exactly which effect(s) are associated with the variable of interest. Sometimes guessing criteria must be developed as well.

Standardization of Effect Sizes

Many of the early models for meta-analysis advocated the use of standardized effect size indices. In this approach, the mean difference between treatment and control conditions is divided by the standard deviation, usually of the control group, but the investigator might instead pool the standard deviations of treatment and control groups.

One important reason for using a standardized effect size is that an investigator can compare his or her results to those of other meta-analyses. Suppose that a meta-analysis examines the effect of one type of family therapy intervention on a clinical outcome measure (e.g., depression). Investigators may wish to compare their results to other meta-analyses on the same topic, such as other family therapy models, or meta-analyses that involve different types of treatment (e.g., drug therapy or individual psychotherapy). Standardized effect sizes make these comparisons possible.

The most common issue in the standardization process is to choose an appropriate denominator. This problem often arises when the two conditions being compared within a single study have different variances. In this case, the calculation of a standardized score is made difficult because it is not clear which of the two standard deviations to use as the divisor. Differences in variances of the conditions within a study are likely to occur when a **restriction of range** exists for the dependent variable, such as a **floor effect** or **ceiling effect**. A floor effect occurs when most of the individuals have scores on the low end of the continuum. A floor effect would occur if a very difficult test were administered to a group of untrained individuals. A ceiling effect occurs when the possible scores are limited on the high end of the continuum. A ceiling effect would occur if a very easy test were administered to a group of highly trained individuals. The range restriction issue becomes especially problematic when only one of the two conditions has a restriction of range. For example, imagine an investigation of an experimental drug on coronary artery disease. The untreated patients in the control condition who receive a placebo could have a wide variability in health outcomes. When patients receive an experimental treatment (the drug under investigation), they may experience a substantial improvement in their health status. As a consequence, the patients in the treatment condition may be quite healthy and have little variability in health outcomes. In this case, the variance in the experimental condition would be much smaller than the variance in the control condition. The difference in the variances between the two conditions is a contraindication for simply combining them.

When large differences in variances between the treatment and control condition occur, the most appropriate variance estimate for standardizing effect size estimates must be carefully selected. The major question regarding the variance estimate is whether the average of the within-condition variances (i.e., the pooled variances) or a variance estimate from only one of the conditions should be used (see Glass et al., 1981; Hedges & Olkin, 1985). In most cases, you should choose the control condition variance when estimating effect sizes for each study (Glass et al., 1981; R. Rosenthal, 1984, 1994). That is, standardize the condition differences based on the variability in the control group rather than on the pooled variance effects. By choosing the variance of the control condition for the standardization process, an investigator compares the size of the mean difference between the experimental treatment and control condition to the natural variability that would occur without the introduction of the experimental treatment (i.e., to the variability in the control condition).

Under some circumstances, an investigator might want to standardize differences using only the variance of the experimental (treatment) group, but these circumstances are much less common. For example, only some of the patients in an experimental treatment condition may benefit from the treatment, resulting in much greater variability in this condition than in the control condition. In this circumstance, an investigator would compare the size of the difference between the treatment and control conditions to the variability produced within the treatment condition.

Even when the issue of the appropriate denominator has been solved, the standardization approach has significant limitations and should not be used in all cases. For example, comparisons across studies cannot always be achieved through a simple conversion to a standardized index. A relatively common problem arises when original researchers use different types of measurement instruments, such as different questionnaires or a questionnaire and an interview for the same construct (e.g., functional status). Often, these many versions of the same variable have different means, standard deviations, and ranges. As a consequence, the scores obtained from these instruments are not directly comparable. Therefore, you cannot use an approach in which you add a known constant, or divide by a constant value, to convert one measure into another.

The standardization approach also may have some negative consequences in a meta-analysis. An implicit assumption in the standardization approach is that the variation among studies is noise or random error. The standardization procedure removes this source of error from the calculation of average effect sizes. However, this standardization procedure actually discards a potentially important source of data about the studies—namely, the between-study differences in means and variances. Cooper and Hedges (1994) propose that one of the major challenges in meta-analysis is to account for apparent consistencies and inconsistencies on a research topic. The between-study variation can sometimes point to an important hypothesis that may explain the different kinds of treatment effects found in a research domain and can only be seen when the raw mean differences or unstandardized effect sizes are used. Some of the newer methods in meta-analysis attempt to model all of the sources of variance to better explain them and, as a result, to better explain the findings (Becker & Schram, 1994; Bryk & Raudenbush, 1992, chap. 14).

As an example, suppose that a research synthesis project involves a number of studies examining the effects of a new anti-cancer drug. In this hypothetical example, suppose that different types of cancer were not differentiated in the various investigations. That is, one investigator might have used patients with gastrointestinal (GI) neoplasms, whereas another used patients with a variety of non-GI neoplasms. Suppose that in the first study, the experimental cancer treatment had a small overall improvement as compared with the control group (actual mean difference), but because the variability within the group was small, the standardized effect size would be relatively large. In contrast, the overall mean difference in the study using patients with a variety of non-GI neoplasms was quite large, but because the variability within that study was also quite large, the computed standardized effect size would be the same or smaller than in the first study. If an investigator standardizes the results in all the studies before combining the results, the differences in the effect sizes between GI cancer patients and those with non-GI cancer would be inappropriately eliminated.

An investigator may conclude that between-study variation is an important source of information to be modeled in the meta-analysis. Between-studies variation can be modeled as a setting, author, or population type variance. These between-study sources of variance can be modeled using unstandardized effect size indices such as differences in means, proportions, rates, or covariances rather than correlations as measures of association (Fleiss, 1994; Hasselblad et al., 1995; Shadish & Haddock, 1994). This kind of modeling, however, involves a multivariate meta-analytic strategy such as hierarchical linear modeling (Bryk & Raudenbush, 1992, chap. 14) or structural equation modeling (Becker & Schram, 1994; Byrne, 1998).

Adjusting for Small Sample Sizes

The sample size is another important factor in estimating effect sizes. To test whether or not our computed averaged effect size differs significantly from zero, we need to be able to describe the sampling distribution that would be expected if the null distribution is correct. For this purpose, we need to know three things about the distribution—namely, the shape (or form), the central tendency (or mean), and the variability of the sampling distribution of effect sizes. You can usually solve the shape and central tendency quite easily when the studies have large sample sizes (say, greater than 30) and all of the studies have approximately equal sample sizes. That is, you will often be able to assume that the shape of the sampling distribution is approximately normal. The central tendency of the sampling distribution can be estimated from the grand mean calculated across all of the studies.

However, estimates of the shape, central tendency, and variability of the sampling distribution can become quite complex when some of the studies have small sample sizes. Small and large sample size studies can produce substantially different estimates for the standard deviation (i.e., standard error) of the sampling distribution. Consider a circumstance in which some of the studies have 9 subjects per condition, whereas other studies have 81 subjects per condition. The standard error is calculated by using the square root of the sample size in the denominator of the expression. Thus, the standard error for the small studies has $(9)^{1/2} = 3$ in the denominator, whereas the larger studies have $(81)^{1/2} = 9$ in the denominator. In other words, the standard error for the small studies will be three times the size of the larger studies (Lilford, Thornton, & Braunholtz, 1995). Because the sampling distribution for the studies with large sample sizes has a smaller standard error and a more restricted range of sampling variability, we can view these estimates as being more precise (Bryk

& Raudenbush, 1992; chap. 4). As a consequence, we may want to give greater weight to the studies with small standard errors.

The effect sizes from the various studies are sometimes given different weights in calculating the average, as well as the overall variance estimate (Bryk & Raudenbush, 1992, p. 159). This adjustment to the mean effect sizes and variance estimates is particularly important when the sample sizes vary substantially across the studies. The calculation procedures in Chapter 14 permit differential weighting by sample size.

Synopsis of Section B

In this section, we discuss some of the problems to be addressed in choosing and calculating an effect size index. It is important to consider the type of research design, the type of statistics used, and whether or not you want to standardize the effect size. When the different studies use different summary statistics, you might have to adjust the effect sizes to a common effect size index, such as an r or a d. You also should consider whether the parameter and statistic effect size indices should be standardized or unstandardized. Standardization may be warranted if you want to assume no between-study effects or, in other words, if you want to assume a fixed effects model with no independent contribution of variation by the studies. You may lose overall mean differences, but you gain in having comparable numbers. On the other hand, using unstandardized effect sizes allows you to model as much between-study variation as possible. More complex models will contribute greatly to your understanding of events.

Section C. Managing Missing Data

Types of Missing Data

During the synthesis process, you will likely discover many areas in which data are missing. We conceptualize four broad types of missing data:

Unpublished investigations

Unretrievable investigations

Incomplete reports on individual variables

Uncollected data on individual variables

You will have managed the first and second types of missing data problems during your search procedures, discussed in Section E, Chapter 5 and in Section D,

Chapter 6, Stage II. You will have managed some of the third and fourth types during the data coding process in Section B, Chapter 8. Your focus now involves the process of quantitatively estimating missing data on the variables to be included in the meta-analysis. An important consideration in the replacement of missing values is whether they are missing due to random or systematic processes. Below we discuss the traditional approaches, such as assigning a zero or the mean, as well as newer multivariate approaches.

Traditional Approaches

Many mechanisms have been proposed for handling missing data. The traditional suggestions are still often used but have considerable potential for bias and error. We review these mechanisms, describe their shortcomings and their benefits, and let the readers decide which would work best for them.

Assigning Zeros. One traditional approach has been for the analyst to assume that the null hypothesis is true for unknown data and then assign an effect size of zero for any unknown (missing) values. This approach might be considered appropriate under some circumstances. Suppose that you need to adopt a conservative approach concerning some topic. You may decide that the evidence has to be very compelling before you will reject the null hypothesis. In this case, you might be willing to assume that all missing data were sampled from a population distribution in which the null hypothesis is true. However, this approach can produce biases in the means, variances, and covariances of the resulting data set (i.e., where missing values have been estimated and replaced) (Little & Rubin, 1987). Most of the time, you will probably be more interested in finding the best possible estimate of the population effect size, as well as the variance of these estimates. Under these circumstances, you should not adopt an approach that may introduce biases into the estimation procedure. We do not endorse this solution for managing missing data.

Guessing Conventions. Guessing conventions are a second traditional approach that you can develop to help coders standardize their responses to missing data. For example, if the method for collecting a culture is not specified, then one can assume by default that the method applied was accepted practice and code it as such. Another possibility is to outline the distribution of types of cultures done across studies that report them and then "guess" in those studies not reporting the data, using similar proportions to the distribution of those that do report the data. By delineating the content of the "guess," the review process is more replicable. The danger of a guessing convention is that systematic bias may be introduced in place of random error, possibly distorting parameter estimates and diminishing variance

(Orwin, 1994). Counts, therefore, need to be kept on both the content of what data are present and absent and, if absent, whether or not a guessing convention was used to fill in the missing information.

Mean Replacement. A third traditional approach is to replace the missing values with the mean obtained from all known data. As stated previously, this practice can produce biases in the means, variances, and covariances of the resulting data set (i.e., where missing values have been estimated and replaced) (Little & Rubin, 1987). If the null hypothesis were true (i.e., all of the studies were sampled from a population in which the true effect size was 0.00), and values were missing for random reasons, this approach would provide an unbiased estimate of the expected (mean) effect size. However, the systematic strategy of replacing missing data with the mean of a distribution produces a bias in the estimates of any variances and covariances that are calculated using these values. In general, substituting the mean decreases the variance because all of the substituted values have no variability about the mean; these estimates increase the number of items that cluster at the mean of the distribution. In most circumstances, we would expect the randomly missing values to have the same variances and covariances as the nonmissing values. This being the case, substituting the mean for the missing values leads to an underestimate of the variance and the covariances of the population values.

Newer Approaches

Recently, there has been considerable progress in developing newer methods to manage missing data. We will discuss two of these.

Multiple Regressions. A newer approach researchers sometime use is to estimate the missing values by use of multiple regression procedures. In this approach, you perform a regression analysis to identify the variable with missing values from other measures in the studies. Using the regression equation that is generated, you can estimate the missing values for those variables used as dependent variables in the regression equation. Suppose that you have 25 studies in your database. Furthermore, suppose that one of these studies is missing data on an important measure. Also, suppose that this study does have observed values on three other measures, and these measures are highly correlated with the variable that has missing data. You can create a multiple regression equation in which the dependent variable is the one with missing data, and the other three measures serve as independent variables in the regression equation. The mean scores for each study on each of these measures serve as the observed values in the regression equation (i.e., the study is the unit of analysis). You

TABLE 13.3 Sample Values to Demonstrate the Multiple Regression Approach to Estimate Missing Values

	Variable 1	Variable 2	Variable 3
b_i weight	0.70	0.60	0.45
Variable value	65.0	72.0	86.0
$b_i \cdot X_i$	45.5	43.2	38.7
a intercept (when $X_i = 0$)	45.2	45.2	45.2
Y	90.7	88.4	83.9

NOTE: Cell entries are hypothetical values to be used in estimating missing data.

then calculate the regression equation generating the nonstandardized regression coefficients (i.e., the *b* weights and the intercept *a*, as in Formula 13.1):

$$\hat{Y} = a + b_1 X_1 + b_2 X_2 + b_3 X_3 \tag{13.1}$$

Next, we focus attention on the study with missing data. You can obtain the *b* weights from the regression equation for each independent variable, as reported in Table 13.3. In our hypothetical example, the observed values in the study with missing data on your three independent variables are also as presented in the table. In this example, the value of the intercept is 45.2.

The predicted value to be used for replacing the missing data would be calculated as follows:

$$\hat{Y} = 45.2 + (0.70*65) + (0.60*72) + (0.45*86) = 172.6$$

This estimation approach is quite useful when you have several measures that have reasonably high correlations among each other (say, correlations greater than 0.5) and you have a small number of missing scores. One possible problem with this approach is that it leads to an underestimation of the variance among the predicted scores that are used to estimate the missing values. This bias occurs because the variance of the estimated scores is proportional to $R^2 \bullet s^2$, but the variance of the true scores is s^2. Because R^2 usually is < 1.00, then $(R^2) \bullet (s^2)$ is typically less than s^2. In other words, the estimated scores have a smaller variance than the true scores, and these estimated scores are closer to the mean (on average) than the actual scores.

However, this decrease in the variance is less than occurs when performing the mean imputation strategy.

Imputation Strategies. One solution to this problem of decreased and biased variance due to imputation of data is to use a multiple imputation strategy (Little & Rubin, 1987; Pigott, 1994, pp. 170-174). Although this procedure is rather complex, we can provide an approximate idea for the approach. With this approach, you would initially use regression procedures to determine that one or more variables (say, X_1 and X_2) can be used to estimate missing values for another variable (say, X_3). Next, you would identify a study K_i with missing data. Suppose that study had data present on variables X_1 and X_2 but not on X_3. In the third step, you would identify all the remaining studies that have the same (or nearly the same values) as study K_i on variables X_1 and X_2. Next, you would randomly sample one of the X_3 values from these "matched" studies and substitute the value into K_i. If none of the other variables can be used to predict X_3, then we randomly sample from all the X_3 values and substitute this random value into the missing value for study K_i. This imputation strategy minimizes the likelihood of biasing the mean, the variance, or covariances of the augmented data set (i.e., where missing values have been estimated and replaced).

The procedures for performing multiple imputations are quite tedious if you have very much missing data. Fortunately, you can obtain "shareware" software to perform this task. Recent releases (after 2000) of more general software packages such as SPSS and SAS contain procedures for performing multiple imputation. This shareware can be found through the Pennsylvania State University Methodology Center Web site (last updated July 1999) at www.stat.psu.edu/~jls/misoftwa.html.

Several different software programs are available at this Web site, and the statistical programs can be downloaded directly to your computer. The software can be used in a graphics user interface format. The software NORM can be used for multivariate continuous data using a normal distribution model. CAT can be used for multivariate categorical data for use in log-linear analyses. MIX can be used when you have mixed continuous as well as categorical variables; this program may be the most generally useful for health care researchers who have mixed types of data. A final program called PAN is useful for panel data or other types of clustered data when the researcher plans to use a multivariate linear mixed effects model.

Synopsis of Section C

In this review, we focus on the process of estimating missing data for variables needed in a meta-analysis. As we indicate, you should be careful about using the mean of known data on a variable to serve as an estimate of missing data. When you substitute the mean for missing values, you may be underestimating the variance on that variable. That is, the variance calculated after substituting the mean will be smaller than the variance before the substitution. Because you will use the sample variance in the denominator of many of your tests of significance, you will be creating a larger test statistic when you have reduced the sample variance. If you use estimates of the missing scores applying multiple regression procedures, you will not produce such a strong bias in your estimate of the sample variance. The best procedure for minimizing the bias of means, variances, and covariances is to use the multiple imputation strategy.

Section D. Managing Artifacts and Biases

The fourth issue to address is the management of artifacts and biases. Both artifacts and biases can alter the results significantly. In this chapter, we will use the two concepts interchangeably, but the major focus will be on biases.

ARTIFACTS AND BIASES

Artifacts are nonsystematic or random errors in measurement or design that change results. If the study were to be repeated, these artifacts would not be there, resulting in a nonreliable system.

Biases are systematic alterations or nonrandom errors in the data as a result of design or measurement. If the study were to be repeated, it would likely have the same distorted results.

The validation process described in Stage III is designed to assess for most of the important artifacts and biases. There is no easy or agreed-upon procedure to correct for either artifacts or biases. However, potential biases can be identified and managed to some degree. We discuss some of these management procedures below.

Flawed Early Approaches

In earlier approaches to meta-analysis, two common strategies were used to manage the effects of bias. Because of their limitations, we do not recommend either of these approaches; however, you might encounter them in your reading.

Discard Invalid Studies. One of these flawed strategies involved simply discarding studies containing significant sources of bias in the data. A fundamental assumption of this approach is that only high-quality studies can provide the best estimates of effect sizes. The major problem with this approach is that all studies are likely to contain some type of artifact or bias because any investigation involves a set of compromises among different types of potential problems. Thus, if only "high-quality" studies (those without biases) were to be used in a meta-analysis, the researcher might find that there were none to combine. There is, however, one approach that does involve limiting the synthesis to only the very high-quality studies. That approach is called "best evidence synthesis" and has been proposed by Slavin (1986). For the interested reader, Section C in Chapter 2 discusses this approach.

Ignore Sources of Bias.   A second early approach was to ignore the various sources of bias and perform the analysis on all existing data. The fundamental assumption in this approach is that biases reflect random variation in the implementation of research on the topic of interest. Presumably, by averaging across all these supposedly random errors, the biasing effects will cancel each other out. The result would be an unbiased estimate of the true effect size. Furthermore, it is presumed that calculations of the average effect size and confidence intervals describe the actual central tendency and variability of effect sizes for the currently existing research findings on a given topic. This approach is reasonable if you simply want to describe what already has been published rather than make significant inferences. In other words, this approach to meta-analysis provides an accurate appraisal of the types of data you might find when you examine currently available research on a topic, but that data would not necessarily be accurate.

A first major problem with this latter approach as a tool for managing research biases is that it does not control for variability across studies. You will often note that the existing findings on a topic are likely to be highly variable. When there is a wide range of quality in the set of studies used for the synthesis, the variability is likely to be even higher. This high variability creates two types of problems. First, you will have trouble rejecting the null hypothesis (i.e., the effect size comparing conditions is statistically different from 0) because of the high variability among studies. Detecting a statistically significant effect size averaged across studies requires that a large enough difference must be found relevant to the overall "scatter" of findings across all groups. When there is a lot of "noise" or variation among studies, it is very difficult to detect the mean difference.

A second major problem is that you cannot justify much confidence in the mean effect size you calculate (i.e., the confidence intervals are likely to be very wide). Because you may want to have a more precise estimate of the average effect size so that you have narrower confidence intervals for your effect size estimates, you are likely to seek some method of accounting for the between-study variation in these estimates. Often it is possible to explain some of the variability across studies by examining the specific types of research biases or artifacts that occur within the studies of your database.

A third major problem with the "ignoring biases" approach is that you cannot assume the biases in the research literature are strictly random processes. Suppose you are examining the effects of prevention programs on drug abuse among adolescents who are at high risk of using drugs. Also suppose that the activities planned for the youths are much more interesting in the treatment condition than in the comparison condition. Due to the interesting nature of the intervention conditions, more of the high-risk youths might remain in the treatment than the comparison group. As a consequence, the average level of risk in the treatment condition may be higher than the control condition. The differential retention rate for treatment and comparison groups can introduce a bias that could either increase or decrease the average effect size that would be expected if similar retention rates occurred in both conditions.

Consider another circumstance in which errors in a research area actually were random. In this circumstance, the random errors should balance out so that the mean effect sizes would provide the best possible estimate of the overall effect of an independent variable. The random variation in errors would cause the error variance to be increased with an associated increase in the width of the confidence intervals calculated among the reported results. Thus, the presence of biases would influence our estimates of variance across studies but would not influence our estimates of the mean values for the effect size parameters. In other words, randomly generated errors would probably have a greater influence on our estimates of the variance of parameters (i.e., the width of the confidence interval) than the specific expected value for the parameter. Nonrandom bias can influence both the variance as well as the average effect size across studies.

Improved Recent Approaches

Numerous papers have been written to demonstrate that research biases are not likely to be random and that we can expect these errors to influence the expected value (i.e., the mean) as well as the variance of the effect size parameter. More recently, meta-analysis procedures have been developed to estimate the influence of these biases and to adjust for their directional influence on parameter estimates. We will describe, briefly, three general approaches to solving this problem: (a) the psychometric approach (Hunter & Schmidt, 1990), (b) the Bayesian approach (Eddy et al., 1992), and (c) the multivariate modeling approaches, including hierarchical linear modeling (Bryk & Raudenbush, 1992) and structural equation modeling. Depending on the particular type of problem you are studying, you may decide to use any one (or a combination) of these approaches. Each tends to emphasize slightly different sources of bias.

Psychometric Approach. The **psychometric approach** (Hunter & Schmidt, 1990) is the oldest of the three newer approaches. This strategy is based on psychometric theory, which provides statistical procedures for estimating the effects of bias, such as restriction of range, sampling errors, and unreliability of measurement, on the predictive and construct validity of psychological tests. The psychometric approach to meta-analysis assumes that once you have corrected the variables for sources of error (such as sampling, measurement, unreliability, or restriction of range), the heterogeneity between studies will be effectively eliminated. Using the psychometric approach, effect sizes are adjusted for factors such as sampling bias, unreliability of measurement, or attenuation due to restriction of range of measurements. In this way, the results are "corrected" for sources of invalidity. Below we present the four major sources of random error that the psychometric approach was designed to address. The actual procedures for addressing these sources of error can be found in the work of Hunter and Schmidt (1990, 1994).

(1) *Error and unreliability in measurement.* The use of unreliable instruments can have a significant impact on a study's findings. Suppose that you had a way of knowing the "true" correlation between an independent variable and a dependent variable (i.e., the true correlation in the population, ρ). In addition, you would have an "expected" observed correlation (ρ_o). Following Hunter and Schmidt's (1994) notation, we use the symbol a_i to represent the level or amount of imprecision in each study, and these values range from 0 to 1.0. When dealing with measurement bias, a_i is the square root of the instrument's reliability. The true correlation will be decreased by the imprecision of measurement to produce the "expected" (observed) correlation. The relationship of the "true" correlation and the observed correlation can be expressed as follows:

$$\rho_o = a_i \rho \qquad\qquad (13.2)$$

Suppose that the true correlation of an independent variable and dependent variable is $\rho = 0.80$. Also, suppose that you have several studies that have used one of two different versions of the same instrument to measure the dependent variable. For example, some of the investigators used an abbreviated version, which has a reliability of $r_{yy} = 0.49$, whereas other investigators used a more expensive and time-consuming version, which has a reliability of $r_{yy} = 0.81$. The level of imprecision (a_i) in the latter study would be $(0.81)^{1/2}$.

The expected observed correlation (ρ_o) with the more reliable measure would then be (a_i) times the true correlation (0.80):

$$\rho_o = (.81)^{1/2} * (0.80) = (0.90 * 0.80) = 0.72$$

For the less reliable instrument, we would expect to observe smaller correlations of approximately

$$\rho_o = (.49)^{1/2} * (0.80) = (0.70 * 0.80) = 0.56$$

As this example shows, unreliability of measurements can have substantial effect on study results. You might be able to account for the variation in your data set by considering whether the various studies have different levels of unreliability in their measurements. Procedures for actually "correcting" the observed correlation as a function of unreliable instruments can be found in Hunter and Schmidt (1994).

(2) *Artificial dichotomization of a variable.* Artificially dichotomizing a variable, or taking a continuous variable and dividing it into two types of results, limits the size of observed correlations between that variable and another. Original investigators may split their sample into groups as an outcome, but others will have maintained a continuous measure of the same outcome variable. For example, the original index may contain a continuous measure of level of illness. This measure might be dichotomized into an index of mild illness or severe illness. Correlations between that variable and another will be attenuated and perhaps not comparable across studies. The problem becomes even more difficult when investigators have used different cut points in their dichotomization procedure.

Hunter and Schmidt (1994) have shown that using a cut point at the median can lead to a 20% reduction of the observed correlation, below what would be expected from correlations based on continuous measures. A cut point yielding a 90/10 split in the sample can produce a 40% reduction in the size of the observed correlation. In summary, you might expect substantial variations in study results depending on the strategies used by original investigators in producing dichotomous outcomes.

(3) *Low construct validity.* Another potential source of imperfection in study results may be created by low construct validity of either the independent or dependent variables. Construct validity refers to the degree to which the variable being measured is actually assessing the concept of interest versus some concept not quite related. *Construct validity* can be defined as the correlation between the observed variable and another variable thought to be somewhat more accurate for assessing that variable (Hunter & Schmidt, 1994). Suppose that one study used a measure with a construct validity of 0.75, whereas another study had a construct validity of 0.90. The first study would produce approximately a 25% reduction in the observed correlations of independent and dependent variables as compared to the values expected if the measures had perfect construct validity. The second study would produce approximately a 10% reduction. If there is any reason to suspect that construct validity varies between studies, it is a good idea to find some mechanism by which this can be estimated, by comparing to a gold standard, using expert judgment, or by comparing across different measures.

(4) *Restriction of range.* Restriction of range refers to situations where values on a measured variable have a narrow spread. Scores could either cluster around the top of

a scale, as occurs when experts are responding, or values could be all at the bottom, as might occur when patients are very ill before treatment. This problem occurs quite frequently in clinical research. Range restriction might occur because of selection procedures that include only the very healthy or the very sick in a study (for an example, see Miller, Turner, Tindale, Posavac, & Dugoni, 1991).

There are two important signs of range restriction. The first sign is a highly skewed distribution in which a large number of individuals have the most extreme score possible. The second indication of restriction is the finding that there are substantially different variances in the treatment and the comparison groups.

Assessment for the impact of range restriction is somewhat more complicated than other procedures. Hunter and Schmidt (1994) provide the following formulas for assessing the potential impact of range restriction on your study results. For the first step, the standard deviations of the study samples are compared against the standard deviation of a reference population; this ratio of standard deviations is expressed as μ.

$$\mu = \frac{S_x \text{ of study sample}}{\sigma_x \text{ of reference population}} \qquad (13.3)$$

The resulting value provides an estimate of the degree of range restriction. In general, we would expect that the standard deviation of the population would be larger than that of a sample. The smaller the sample variance is, compared to the population variance, the smaller the fraction that is μ. The relationship of this value to the multiplier a_i (which is the component of the correlation due to random error) is expressed as follows:

$$\alpha_i = \sqrt{(\mu^2 + \rho^2 - \mu^2\rho^2)} \qquad (13.4)$$

Suppose that the range restriction on your study population is 75% of the reference population, and the true correlation of the independent and dependent variable is 0.30. Then the value of a_i is the following:

$$\alpha_i = [(0.75)^2 + (0.30)^2 - (0.75)^2 * (0.30)^2]^{1/2} =$$
$$[(0.5625 + 0.09) - (0.5625 * 0.09)]^{1/2} = [(0.6525) - (0.0506)]^{1/2} = 0.775$$

In other words, we would expect a 22.5% reduction in the size of observed correlations with these particular values of range restriction and population parameters. As with artifacts and biases, each study should be examined carefully for restriction in range to assess the need for further evaluation.

We have presented these examples of the psychometric approach for two reasons. First, you might want to make the kinds of adjustments that we have described for the imperfections that might exist in the studies in your data set. However, actually making these adjustments might be difficult. As other authors have noted, you frequently do not have the exact numbers to make the Hunter and Schmidt (1990, 1994) adjustments. Second, and more important, these adjustments or analyses may provide plausible explanations for heterogeneity of effect sizes. Under these circumstances, you can use the ideas presented here to explore the possible role of imprecision in measurement as an explanation for the observed variation in study results.

Bayesian Approach. In the Bayesian approach to managing artifacts and biases, parameter estimates are adjusted subjectively, that is, they are adjusted based on what the author's perceived judgment is regarding their effects. An important feature of this approach is that it provides adjustments to expected values (e.g., means) and variance estimates. The primary goal of this adjustment is to have weights given to the studies, based on your "subjective" judgments about the quality of a study on a certain dimension, and the importance of that dimension to the conclusions of the meta-analysis (see Gelman, Carlin, Stern, & Rubin, 1995).

When you first read about Bayesian analysis where prior and posterior distributions are used, you may be a little confused about the concept of prior and posterior probabilities. However, most of us implicitly think in a Bayesian fashion using these principles. That is, we develop initial expectations about the likelihood of something happening, and then we subsequently adjust these expectations following some experience with the event.

For example, suppose that you decide to submit a grant proposal to a federal agency. In making this decision, you learn that the agency funds about one in four of the applications. Without any additional information, you could reasonably expect to have a 0.25 probability of having your grant funded. In Bayesian terms, this probability is called the **á priori probability** (i.e., it occurs prior to the outcome of the test, which is to be applied to your experience). If you have some additional evidence (e.g., you are either more or less skilled than other applicants), then you might adjust your initial estimate upwards or downwards given this additional information.

When you submit the grant application and receive feedback, you will know the outcome (i.e., the outcome that you either receive funding or you do not). Suppose now you decide to submit another grant application. What is the perceived likelihood that you will have this new grant application funded? If you rely solely on the outcome of the first grant application, your á priori probability (i.e., the subjective estimate prior to the outcome of the event) would be either 0.00 if the initial grant was not funded or 1.00 if the initial grant was funded. In other words, if your current expectation is based solely on the outcome of the one instance, you would have an expectation of certainty that the new application would be funded or would not be funded.

In fact, most of us would temper our conclusion based on the outcome of the first application as well as our prior expectation. Again, suppose the grant was actually funded. You started with the expectation that only 25% of grants are funded. You might believe that you have a better chance than the average person does in submitting grants (after all, you did get the grant), but you also know that you could have been lucky. So your final estimate may be a combination of your initial expectation and your actual experience with your first test. This combined estimate is called your **á posteriori estimate** (i.e., your judgment is conditional on your actual experience with the first application). This example of a Bayesian approach has been adapted from a description by Louis and Zelterman (1994).

You can now apply these Bayesian principles to your meta-analysis examples. With the Bayesian strategy, you would establish á priori likelihoods in your confidence about a study's results. For example, you might use your validity ratings on each article in the data set to provide different á priori weights to the various studies. Studies with high validity scores would be given high á priori confidence, whereas low validity studies would receive much lower á priori weight.

One valuable feature of the Bayesian approach is that it provides a multivariate approach to your meta-analysis. That is, you can simultaneously incorporate several sources of validity ratings together in one analysis to search for interactive effects of the various validity factors. When you perform a meta-analysis, you may discover that different types of bias occur within various experimental conditions. In Table 13.4, we assume some individuals were offered an experimental treatment, whereas others were assigned to a control condition and not offered this treatment.

Contrary to the planned interventions, some of the individuals actually received the treatment that was assigned to them, whereas others in the intervention group were not treated. This latter group represents a dilution of the experimental condition.

Furthermore, some patients assigned to the control condition actually received the conditions as assigned (i.e., not treated), whereas others received the treatment. This latter group represents a contamination of the control condition. Furthermore, suppose that the original investigator intended to follow up the patients at a later point in time but was unable to locate or obtain cooperation from some of these patients. Losing subjects to follow-up can create a sampling bias because the "lost" patients may differ in some way from the "followed" patients. You can estimate or "guess" the degree to which each of those biases affected the direction of the results for each of the studies in your data set. Your estimate (presented as a probability) can be used directly to compute adjustments. If you decide to pursue a Bayesian weighted approach, you can read Louis and Zelterman (1994) or Eddy et al. (1992).

TABLE 13.4 Possible Sources of Bias and Their Effects on Outcomes

Follow-Up Status	Research Condition			
	Offered Treatment		Not Offered Treatment	
	Treated	Not Treated	Treated	Not Treated
Followed	Intended data	Dilution	Contamination	Intended data
Not followed	Sampling bias	Dilution	Contamination	Sampling bias

NOTE: Adapted from an example presented in Eddy et al. (1992, pp. 143-158).

The actual computations are rather complicated, but the FAST*PRO software program provides a convenient method for making these adjustments.

Multivariate modeling. In this section, we present a short overview of some latent variable approaches. These types of analyses include path analysis, structural equation analysis, multidimensional scaling, hierarchical linear modeling, and others. Although it is not in the scope of this book to present the details of these approaches, we provide a general overview. The reader may consider pursuing these approaches because they can be extremely useful for modeling all aspects of a proposed model, including the effects of biases and artifacts (Bentler, 1995; Byrne, 1998).

Structural equation and hierarchical modeling estimate the independent effects of many variables simultaneously, including measurement error, the interaction between variables, and their separate effects on the dependent variable. An important assumption is that many concepts can be measured only indirectly. For example, we do not have a direct measure of depression, but several indirect measures have been created to assess this concept. Each approach assesses somewhat different aspects of the same underlying concept, although all have limited validity and reliability. Presumably, some combination of these various measures can provide a more accurate assessment of the latent concept than can be achieved by any one of the instruments. In structural equation modeling, the variables measuring the same concept are "combined," and the resultant "latent" estimates are the variables used in the analysis.

A second assumption of most multivariate modeling is that the relationship between variables is linear. In other words, changes in one variable result in straightforward (linear) changes in the predicted variable. In actual practice, a regression analysis is used to estimate the strength of the relationship between the "latent" predictor variables and the "latent" predicted variables.

In general, all latent variable analyses perform the same tasks. A proposed model is tested against a "baseline model" using a chi-square test as a test of goodness of fit. In practice, the "test" is a comparison of covariance matrices (i.e., the nonstandardized correlation between any two variables). If the two models are not significantly different, then we can judge that the data are a good fit for the proposed model. Values of goodness-of-fit indices below 0.85 usually indicate that the proposed model does not adequately explain the covariance relationships between the measures. In addition, all parameter estimates should be statistically significant (i.e., loading on the factors must be statistically significant). Finally, all modification indices must be less than 10.0 for an observed variable to be retained as an indicator.

In meta-analysis, the investigator is looking for equivalent model structures across studies. The first step is to develop good-fitting models in separate runs for each study. Then, a baseline model across studies is created on one run with none of the individual parameters (variances, factor loadings, regression weights) constrained to be equal. In the baseline model, there are no assumptions that the same variable (e.g., patient-doctor communication) is the same in every study, nor do we assume that the populations are the same or that the relationships between the variables (e.g., patient-doctor communication and patient compliance) are the same.

The model is tested, then, in three ways by creating a series of increasingly restricted models (by setting some parameters as having to be equal between studies) and testing each against the previous less restricted model. Specifying that certain parameters are equal, in this context, is the same as saying that we are theoretically sampling from the same population, and we only expect as much variance between studies as you would obtain from random samples from the same population. The steps are further explained below.

The first test is for equivalence of factor structures across studies (tested against the baseline model). In other words, the question examined is whether the measured variables are "hanging together" the same way across studies. This model is tested against the baseline model. If the result is nonsignificant, then we can reliably say that the factor structures of the variables from the various studies all appear to be sampled from the same population (i.e., these structures are the same). If not, then there is no reason to continue. The studies must be divided into subgroups for further analysis.

The second test is for equivalence of variances and covariances across studies. A model is created that specifies that the variances of each variable should be equal between studies. This restriction is the same as asking if the variables were measured on the same population in every study. This model is tested against the model created in the previous test. If the difference is nonsignificant (meaning that setting them equal did not change the structure of the model), then we can assume that the studies involved similar populations.

Finally, the third test asks if the relationships between the variables (the strength of the effects) are the same in all studies. This model is created by specifying that the regression weights between each set of variables are the same for each study. If this model is not significantly different from the previous model, then we can assume we have successfully and reliably modeled the relationship between variables across all the studies. The resultant estimated partial correlations (beta weights) between each pair of variables in the statistical model can then be assumed to reflect a synthesis of the relationship across the studies in question. Estimates can be calculated in EQS (Bentler, 1995), AMOS in SPSS, SAS CALIS, or in LISREL (Joreskog & Sorbom, 1988).

Synopsis of Section D

The issue of addressing artifacts and biases of the original studies continues to be controversial, and many methods are used in meta-analysis. The methods range from ignoring quality aspects of the original studies, eliminating all studies with quality problems, to various methods of incorporating the quality ratings into the synthesis process (Chalmers et al., 1981; Detsky et al., 1992; Moher et al., 1995; Mulrow, Linn, Gaul, & Pugh, 1989). Lau et al. (1997), in their section on quality, state that "to date, no scale has been proven to correlate consistently with treatment efficacy" (p. 825).

Keeping the Lau et al. (1997) statement in mind, which methods you choose depends on the type of synthesis, the purposes of the synthesis, and skills of the reviewer. If you choose to use quality ratings, we suggest using those (quality ratings) of the original studies in the synthesis process itself. Quality ratings can be incorporated into the synthesis by simply testing for the impact of quality on outcomes. Or quality ratings can be used to systematically adjust the outcomes, as advocated by some authors such as Eddy et al. (1992) and Shadish and Haddock (1994). Finally, quality ratings and even specific biases and confounds can be incorporated into the model using structural equation analysis or hierarchical linear modeling. The result should be statistical estimates of their impact on the outcomes of interest.

Section E. Heterogeneity of Effect Sizes Among Studies

A fifth issue central to conducting a meta-analysis is the decision authors make regarding heterogeneity of effect sizes across studies. This issue can be complicated, but the underlying problem is quite straightforward. We present a short explanation of the issue first, followed by a description of how heterogeneity might be managed.

Understanding Heterogeneity in Meta-Analysis

Significant heterogeneity across studies implies that the effect sizes do not come from the same population and, therefore, are not answering the same question. Accepted practice is that then they must not be combined, unless you can account for the source of heterogeneity. This problem is ubiquitous and controversial. When possible, you should include anticipated heterogeneity into your problem formulation and a statistical hypothesis-testing model in the beginning. Even if you carefully plan for heterogeneity, however, you may find unexpected sources of this problem in your synthesis. It is the author's responsibility to make an attempt to explain these differences. Most researchers use a chi-square heterogeneity of variance test to determine whether the parameter estimates are consistent for all the studies. Interpreting the meaning of evidence of heterogeneity is not straightforward. The following discussion on "fruit" illustrates several of the issues.

Suppose that you plan a meta-analysis examining the effects of a particular fertilizer on the weight of fruit and you have located a number of studies on this topic. Consider the following metaphor in thinking about these diverse studies. Imagine that the collection of investigations is similar to a bowl of fruit composed of apples, oranges, bananas, grapefruit, and pears. (Each piece of fruit represents a single research "participant.") If the focus of your effort is on the growth of fruit (regardless of the specific type), then the diverse fruit all can be viewed as members of the same population. The diversity among the types of fruit simply reflects the diversity within the population. We can express this total diversity as the sum of the within-fruit and the between-fruit diversity in the following formula:

$$\sigma^2_{Total} = \sigma^2_{between-fruit} + \sigma^2_{within-fruit}. \tag{13.5}$$

If the between-fruit and within-fruit variances are the same, then you do not have evidence of heterogeneity. In other words, whatever measure you are taking on the fruit (weight, circumference, length), the accumulated results "clump" together in one pile. The proportion of increase expected for the fertilizer experiment in each kind of fruit would be more or less the same. You could use either the within-fruit or the between-fruit variance as an estimate of the population variability in your formulas for inference testing.

Suppose that the between-fruit variance is larger than the within-fruit variance. This would occur if you were measuring some dimension where the types of fruit differed a great deal on some measure, such as in moisture content. Then you would find that instead of clumping together, you would have two clumps or groups of fruit. This situation occurs when the between-fruit variance is larger than the within-fruit variance. This finding raises a number of concerns about how to proceed. First, you have evidence that the individual pieces of fruit do not appear to be sampled from the same population. That is, the variability within the sample of each type of fruit is smaller than the variability between the types of fruit. When the variability among types of fruit is substantially greater than the variability within fruit, then you do not know which standard deviation to use. If you use the within-fruit standard deviation, then you will underestimate the amount of random variation that will occur due to sampling across all the fruit. The amount of random variation to be expected in your research synthesis would be influenced by the between-fruit differences. Hence, your estimates must account for this between-fruit variability as well as the within-fruit variability. In an analogous way, your meta-analytic results must consider both the within-study sources of variability and the between-study sources of variability.

Either you can define the between-fruit variability as a second independent variable, or you can define the various types of fruit as all belonging to different populations. In this latter case, you need an estimate of the between-fruit variability to determine how much variability in random sampling will be expected in the various individual types of fruit.

If we apply this analogy to meta-analysis, the individual studies are analogous to types of fruit. As you examine the various studies in your database, you are likely to find different types of research participants within each study. Some of the studies will sample only a single type of research participant, such as the elderly; others will include all ages. When you calculate variance estimates within each study, your estimate will only reflect the variability within that group. As you combine the results from all of the studies in your database, the differences among types of patients will appear as differences associated with the age of subjects among the various studies.

An additional problem that can arise is that there might be an interaction between the treatment and a specific subpopulation. Suppose you find an anxiolytic drug that reduces the stress of all patients having mood disorders, but the impact varies both within and between patients having different kinds of such conditions. For example, suppose the drug has a greater impact on the anxiety of patients with bipolar disorder (manic-depressive illness) than it does on patients with unipolar disorder (e.g., depression alone). Depending on your choice of definitions, you might have either two different populations (bipolar and unipolar disorder) or a single population (all forms of mood disorders). If you determine that you have two populations, then you might proceed with separate analyses within each population; under this circumstance, you would not attempt to combine the results from the two different populations.

You will encounter similar problems within your studies. Consider another example in the health area. Suppose that your synthesis compares the treatment effects of two different antibiotics on the management of gram-negative infections. As you examine the various studies on these different antibiotics, you might find that the patients in these studies have a wide variety of gram-negative infections (e.g., *Escherichia coli, Pseudomonas aeruginosa,* and *Haemophilus influenzae*). You must then decide whether your synthesis is designed to make generalizations to a single population that includes all types of these infections or whether you are going to make different generalizations to multiple populations, each of which has a different type of bacteria (see Bailey, 1987).

The kind of explorations and analyses described above will need to be conducted on all meta-analyses. The source of heterogeneity is always idiosyncratic to the particular study. Following is a review of some of the issues involved in managing heterogeneity once you know that it exists.

Managing Variation in Meta-Analysis

Importance of This Factor. One important decision to be made in meta-analysis is whether to perform a fixed or a random effects analysis (Borzak & Ridker, 1995; Raudenbush, 1994). This decision is really one of specifying the universe to which the researcher wants to generalize the results. One perspective, the most common, is the fixed effects approach. The second perspective is the random effects approach, and although it has been less common, it is now being used more frequently (Berlin, Begg, & Louis, 1989; Borzak & Ridker, 1995).

Your plan for dealing with the variation in research outcomes will be a function of which approach you choose. We always expect some variation in the results across studies because of the impact of random sampling of individuals. However, we need to decide whether the various levels of the independent variable are also the result of random sampling effects. In other words, we need to decide if the kinds of treatment used in the studies (and the ways that those treatments vary) are also random selections from a universe of treatments that randomly vary. In medicine, there are times when either case could be true.

We need to make this decision because our primary goals are to estimate the strength of the relationship between the independent and dependent variables and the uncertainty associated with these estimates. Random sampling effects will influence the strength of the observed relationship between these two variables.

Fixed Effects Model. In the fixed effects approach, the universe to which generalizations are made consists of a set of identically conducted studies. The independent variable differences are not presumed to be from different populations. When we conduct the research, we imagine that we are sampling from a population of individuals. Some of these individuals appear in the treatment condition, whereas other individuals appear in the control condition. For a fixed effect model, any differences between treatment and comparison groups are presumed to be attributable to one of two sources: Either differences are due to the treatments or the coincidental assignment of some individuals to the treatment and others to the comparison groups. If the size of the difference between treatment and comparison group is greater than we would expect from random assignment of individuals to conditions, then we reject random assignment of individuals as a plausible explanation for the differences between treatment and comparison groups.

In other words, we are trying to choose between an explanation of group differences, based on either random assignment of individuals or the impact of the treatment intervention, as the two plausible explanations for the differences between treatment and comparison groups. In the fixed effects analysis, the only random process that we consider is the assignment of individuals to groups. The specific levels of the independent variable are considered to be fixed (they do not represent randomly varying effects).

Suppose you conduct two different studies that are designed to replicate each other exactly, and you randomly sample your research subjects from the same population. Because of the effects of random sampling from the population, you would ordinarily not expect the results to be identical. When you use a fixed effects statistical model, you are assuming that the effects of random sampling of the population can explain all of the variation among the studies. None of the between-study variance is seen as due to differences in the studies themselves. This approach is very similar to the reasoning strategy of fixed effects analysis of variance.

The criteria for using the results are to determine how similar other studies are to the studies being used in your meta-analysis. The more alike the studies are, the more confident you can be that the results of your meta-analysis will be generalizable. The difficulty, of course, is determining exactly how alike the studies really are.

Random Effects Model. In this approach, the various study results in your database are expected to vary from each other as a function of additional sources of random variation. Not only do you have to consider the uncertainty produced by random sampling of individuals from within the population, but you also have to consider other sources of random sampling. One potentially important source of variation among the studies is the selection of levels of the independent variable. Imagine that the independent variable has many levels. Suppose that various investigators arbitrarily pick different values of this independent variable when they conduct their research. The different studies, then, do not have the same level of the independent variable. Instead, we can view all of these replications as random samples from the possible levels of the independent variable. We now have two sources of random variation to address. The first source is the variation due to random sampling of individuals, and the second is variation due to random sampling for levels of the independent variables. The level of variation among studies can then be explained by random sampling principles. That is, any single study can be viewed as a random sample from a population of studies, each somewhat different from each other. Thus, the size of the differences between treatment and comparison groups may be influenced both by the random effects due to assignment of people to conditions and the random selection of levels of the independent variable.

Other sources of random variation can occur in our database. Suppose you plan a meta-analysis to examine the effectiveness of a hospital-based treatment. Furthermore, suppose that each of the studies to be synthesized is conducted within a single hospitals. These hospitals might differ on a number of characteristics such as size, level of professional training, of staff, staff budget, age of hospital facilities, or distance to other facilities. These between-hospital sources of variability can be viewed as an additional source of random variation that can influence the study outcomes. That is, these additional sources of random variation can influence the size of the difference between treatment and comparison groups that can be expected from random sampling. Now, we have to include the random effects due to sampling of people, sampling for the level of the independent variable, and sampling for attributes of the hospital. In a fixed effects analysis, we ignore all sources of random variation except the effects attributable to the sampling of people.

In our meta-analysis of inferential statistical procedures, we attempt to determine whether the effect size (difference between treatment and comparison groups) is greater than the size of the effects that would be expected based on random sampling processes. When the investigator inappropriately ignores important sources of random variation, then he or she may underestimate the degree of sampling error that can occur. This underestimation can lead to an increased likelihood of falsely rejecting the null hypothesis. The random effects meta-analysis provides an approach to address these between-study sources of variability (Raudenbush, 1994).

Although using a random effects model seems straightforward, the reviewer will have significant difficulties determining the universe from which the studies are assumed to have been randomly sampled. Because studies are not random designed or conducted, careful attention has to be made in the problem formulation stage to identify the population accurately.

Quantitative Estimates of Heterogeneity

We can use sampling distribution principles to address the apples and oranges heterogeneity problem. First, we will examine this problem as a single sample problem, and then we will reexamine the problem as a two-sample case. Suppose that the various studies are not random samples from a common population but represent samples from various populations (say, apples, oranges, bananas, pears) with different means.

$$\mu_{x_1} \neq \mu_{x_2} \neq \mu_{x_3} \ldots$$

The variability among studies would reflect both the true differences among the population means as well as the fluctuation expected from normal random sampling within each population. As a consequence, we would expect the variance among studies to be greater than the variability within studies:

$$\sigma_{\bar{x}}^2 = \frac{\sigma_x^2}{n} \tag{13.6}$$

We can determine whether this between-population effect is statistically significant by using the F distribution with $(k - 1)$ and $n * (k - 1)$ degrees of freedom:

$$F = \frac{\sigma_{\bar{x}}^2}{\sigma_x^2/n} = \frac{n * \sigma_{\bar{x}}^2}{\sigma_x^2} \tag{13.7}$$

Because we usually do not know the population variances, these values can be estimated from sample variances:

$$F = \frac{n * S_{\bar{x}}^2}{S_x^2} \tag{13.8}$$

The procedure that we are describing is the same as performing a one-way analysis of variance with the individual studies serving as the k levels of the independent variable. A significant F statistic indicates that the variability between studies is significantly greater than would be assumed based on the values expected from the random effects represented in the sampling distribution. We would conclude that all of the study samples do not appear to be coming from the same population.

In other words, you reason that the samples may or may not come from the same population. With this evidence, the information reviewer needs to find an explanation for this significant heterogeneity. We will address this issue in greater detail after we have examined a meta-analysis of the two-sample problems.

You also should be careful about another possible inference error. Failure to reject the null hypothesis is no assurance that all of the studies come from the same sample. You need to consider the level of statistical power associated with your hypothesis test. That is, you cannot conclude that all of the samples come from the same population even though you have failed to reject the null hypothesis. This point is the same one made in traditional statistical hypothesis testing. When you fail to reject the null hypothesis, then you retain both the null and the alternative hypotheses; you do not accept the null hypothesis.

The formulas above are useful for understanding heterogeneity when you are sampling one mean at a time. However, in most meta-analytic problems, you will want to determine the heterogeneity of effect sizes, not the difference among single means sampled from each study. Thus, you will also need to calculate heterogeneity effects for a two-sample problem (i.e., when you are comparing the difference between two conditions). Formula 13.9 provides these estimates for assessing the heterogeneity of effect sizes across k studies. The value of q for each study is the quality rating for the study. If you are not going to use a quality-adjusted approach, then you would set the value of $q = 1.0$ for each study. The value of T is the effect size for each study, and the value of w is the variance estimate.

$$Q = \sum_{i=1}^{k} q_i w_i T_i^2 - \frac{(\sum_{i=1}^{k} w_i q_i T_i)^2}{\sum_{i=1}^{k} q_i w_i} \tag{13.9}$$

This Q statistic is distributed as a χ^2 statistic with $k - 1$ degrees of freedom. If the statistic is significant, then the data provide evidence that the between-study variance in effect sizes is larger than the within-study variance (see Formula 13.10; also see Formula 13.5).

$$\sigma^2_{between-study} > \sigma^2_{within-study} \tag{13.10}$$

As a consequence, the within-study variance does not provide an appropriate estimate of the amount of sampling variability to be expected for the various investigations. The presence of significant heterogeneity suggests that a random rather than a fixed effects model should be used to test effects. Efforts should be made to identify the sources of the variance as well. For additional insight into this topic, see Oxman (1994).

Synopsis of Section E

In summary, an important issue to address is creating a meta-analysis model that is an adequate balance between being too simple and being too complex. Your model must be complex enough to account for the research domain but also simple enough so that you can find a sufficient number of studies to test the hypothesized relationships in the model. Addressing the issue of heterogeneity, then, becomes central to problem formulation and meta-analytic model construction.

Writers must decide prior to performing statistical tests whether they are going to assume a fixed effects model or a random effects model and how they expect to translate their assumptions to the problem definition and model. A fixed effects model assumes that studies and treatments are not random samples from a larger group. Rather, results are expected to generalize to studies that are assumed to be nearly identical. A random effects model assumes that studies are randomly sampled from a universe of studies and that the studies themselves bring to the equation some variance in predicting the population effect size.

Testing for heterogeneity is straightforward in a statistical sense, but the results may not be definitive. A positive test for heterogeneity just says that it is likely that the studies do not come from the same population. It does not offer any more detailed explanations. One common solution to this problem is to formulate a series of meta-analytic models to determine the source of heterogeneity. In any case, dealing with heterogeneity is a significant problem.

Section F. Combining Effect Sizes

In this sixth section, we need to address methods for combining effect sizes. This concerns the differences between nonparametric (e.g., vote counting) and parametric combination strategies (e.g., weighted effect sizes).

In this section, you will learn about some of the different problems that must be addressed in selecting a combination model. These problems include choosing a software program, using a nonparametric versus a parametric combination strategy, weighting for biases, using a random versus a fixed effect model, and adjusting for variances and sample sizes across studies.

Nonparametric Methods for Combining Effect Sizes

Vote-Counting Methods. You might find any of three types of evidence from original articles that you are going to include in your analysis. These indices of evidence are the following: Type 1 data that can be used to calculate effect sizes, Type 2 data concerning the statistical significance of the hypotheses being tested (e.g., *t* tests with levels of significance), and Type 3 data concerning the direction of the statistically significant outcomes (Bushman, 1994). When available, the first type of data provides a more compelling basis for synthesizing results across studies. However, you may have access only to data of the second or third type, so that you cannot calculate effect sizes.

Vote counting is a procedure for determining whether the majority of studies in a domain provide evidence to support, contradict, or provide no evidence concerning a research hypothesis (Glass et al., 1981; Light & Smith, 1971). In the synthesis process, you would count how many articles report data that are consistent with each of these three outcomes. That is, you would treat each study as if it provided a vote in favor or against the hypothesis. You decide which of the three outcomes is most plausible depending on the number of articles that fall into each of the three categories (i.e., support, contradict, or are neutral). Often you can see this approach used informally in many narrative synthesis when the authors conclude that "most" of the evidence is consistent with (or contradicts) the hypothesis. Explicit procedures for conducting a vote-counting synthesis using the sign test and other methods are described in detail by Bushman (1994, p. 193).

Three major problems occur in vote counting (Bushman, 1994). *First,* the procedure ignores sample size (the likelihood of a statistically significant effect is greater with larger sample sizes). The reason for concern is that the small sample size studies may have too little power to reject the null hypothesis. The vote-counting procedure may give too much weight to the small sample size studies as compared to the large sample size studies (Light & Smith, 1971). A *second* problem is that vote counting ignores the differences in the sizes of the effects obtained in each study. Hence, a very small negative effect is given the same weight as a very large positive effect (Glass et al., 1981). *Third,* the vote-counting procedure has relatively low statistical power for detecting effects (Bushman, 1994; Hedges & Olkin, 1985).

However, you may discover that some of the research articles in your data set do not report enough data to calculate effect sizes, and you may be forced to use some type of vote-counting procedure. Bushman (1994) describes a useful approach for performing a vote-counting method, and we recommend that you read his chapter if you confront this problem.

Combining Significance Levels. You may be able to use another technique when you do not have sufficient data to calculate effect sizes for some of the studies in your data set. For example, suppose some of the original authors did not report enough within-condition information such as standard deviations, sample sizes, or statistical test values for significance. However, the authors of the studies in your data set might have reported the significance levels (probabilities or p values) associated with tests of significance. These p values represent the probability of observing a specific test statistic given that the null hypothesis is true (i.e., these values are the probability of a Type I error).

You may be able to combine these probability values from the studies of your database to test the overall significance level (Becker, 1994). If you decide to pursue this approach, we recommend that you examine a chapter by Becker (1994), who presents several useful techniques in combining significance levels.

In this approach, you decide which type of sampling distribution is appropriate for your data; typically, you would use the standard normal distribution. Next, you determine the exact Z score value on a standard normal distribution that would be associated with a given p value. Suppose that a two-tailed test of significance for a study in your database has a p value of 0.05. The standard normal Z value for this p value is 1.96. You can use tables of the standard normal distribution to estimate a Z score for most p values. You would obtain the Z score for every study and then combine the results using Formula 13.11. The value of k in the formula is the number of studies to be combined:

$$\overline{Z} = \sum_{i=1}^{k} Z_i / \sqrt{k} \tag{13.11}$$

We can determine whether this value is statistically significant by comparing the obtained value with that required to reject the null hypothesis at a particular significance level, typically $\alpha = .05$. If you find that the absolute value of the observed mean Z is greater than the threshold value of $Z_{(1 - \alpha)/2}$, then you would reject the null hypothesis.

Becker (1994) also presents a method for combining studies using the logs of the significance levels. You perform this procedure by computing the natural log of the probability values associated with each study. If you sum these values and multiply by (-2), you obtain a χ^2 value with $2k$ degrees of freedom, where k is the number of studies being combined. You multiply by the minus sign because the log of a decimal is a negative number, and the multiplication converts the result to a positive number:

$$\chi^2 = -2 \sum_{i=1}^{k} \ln(p_i) \tag{13.12}$$

These procedures are relatively easy to compute. Because these combination procedures represent nonparametric analyses, they can be more appropriate than effect size approaches when your database studies do not satisfy the stricter assumptions of parametric analyses (Becker, 1994). Whenever the studies satisfy the assumptions of parametric analyses, the methods for combining significance levels, rather than effect sizes, are relatively unsatisfactory. That is, effect size methods provide all of the information that can be obtained from the significance level approach.

In addition, the effect size approach also provides information about the size and the strength of effects (Becker, 1994).

Parametric Models for Combining Effect Sizes

You may select among a number of models for actually combining the results of the various studies to produce parameter estimates (e.g., means and variances) of the treatment effects. We will discuss briefly six such models: Bayesian, hierarchical linear modeling, variance weighted, **Mantel-Haenszel**, **Peto**, and **DerSimonian and Laird**.

Bayesian. This approach is called an *equal effects model*, and it assumes that all the studies to be combined are estimating the same parameter (or effect size). This approach is becoming more popular, and because of its flexibility, we expect it to become one of the leading standards for performing meta-analyses. This approach is quite similar to the process of weighting studies by sample size (e.g., usually you will give more weight to studies with larger sample sizes or greater validity).

The Bayesian approach will help you solve the problem of combining data from nonnormal distributions. A common problem in meta-analysis is to assume, incorrectly, that the data are sampled from a normal distribution. However, you will find in the health fields that data often cannot be viewed as being normally distributed. For example, healthcare researchers frequently sample from skewed population distributions that can best be described as either a Poisson or Bernoulli distribution.

These distributions occur when your measurement procedure involves proportions of events or counts.

Suppose that you are studying a treatment program that is designed to improve medication compliance among asthma patients. One of your dependent variables is the number of times a patient visits the emergency room for care. A patient cannot have a negative number of visits, so the range of possible values is restricted to 0.00 or above. You might find that most patients never visit the emergency room, but some patients visit many times. This pattern of results will appear as a positively skewed distribution that can be best described either as a Poisson or a Bernoulli distribution.

As you attempt to combine results across the studies, you need to be able to adjust the findings according to the type of underlying population from which the values were sampled. The Bayesian approach is very flexible for these purposes. This approach also permits the creation of findings from subjective judgments made about each study, such as estimating the between-study variance in a random effects model (Dumouchel, 1995). Even though you can model a variety of population types, all study samples within a single meta-analysis must have the same distribution type.

Hierarchical Linear Modeling. This model is a *random effects model,* and it assumes that all investigations are estimating the same parameter. However, the model allows for some unidentifiable random differences between the "true values" estimated by each experiment (Raudenbush, 1994). One goal of this approach is to estimate the mean effect size of the parent distribution. This estimation process includes both the uncertainty associated with the inherent within-study variation due to sampling problems and the variation arising from the random differences in the "true values" that influence different experiments. The consequence is that the hierarchical model approach has a wider range of uncertainty about the parameter of interest compared to the Bayesian approach (Eddy et al., 1992, pp. 405-414). Future work in meta-analysis will increasingly use hierarchical linear modeling as the questions become more complex.

Variance Weighted. This approach is based on an *equal effects model.* The combination procedure operates on the mean and variance of the profiles (Shadish & Haddock, 1994). Because this approach is not a Bayesian model, the analyst cannot calculate á posteriori probability distribution. Instead, the analyst must generate an estimate of a parameter and the variance of this estimate (Eddy et al., 1992, pp. 405-414).

Mantel-Haenszel. This approach would be used to calculate a combined odds ratio from source experiments whose results can be reported as odds ratios. In Variation 7, Procedure B, Chapter 14, we present a detailed computational example of this method. The procedure uses an *equal effects model,* and it assumes studies are to be taken at face value (i.e., no adjustments are made for internal or external validity biases). The method can be used to combine odds ratios calculated directly from two-arm experiments involving dichotomous outcomes and 2×2 **case-control studies**. The results include parameter estimates and a 95% confidence limit for the combined odds ratio.

Peto. This approach is similar to the Mantel-Haenszel method, and it has the same restrictions. The procedure does not provide a method to adjust individual observed study results for the effects of biases (Eddy et al., 1992, pp. 405-414). However, Berlin, Laird, Sacks, and Chalmers (1989) and Lau et al. (1997) point out that this approach may introduce large biases if the data are unbalanced.

DerSimonian and Laird. You can use this approach if you decide that you need to use a *random effects* rather than a *fixed effects* model (DerSimonian & Laird, 1986). The procedure can be used with any distribution except the generalized *F.* One important feature of this approach is that you can incorporate estimates of biases to adjust parameter values, and the parameters can be created from subjective estimates about each study. One possible limitation of the approach is that all sample distributions must have the same distribution type. The primary difference between this approach and other random effects approaches, such as the hierarchical model, is the role of Bayesian modeling. The approach uses information about the "prior distribution" for the mean and variance as a part of the process of estimating posteriori probability distributions for the parameters (Eddy et al., 1992).

Synopsis of Section F

This section discusses the issue of quantitative integration strategies. We describe how you might choose among nonparametric (e.g., vote counting) and parametric combination strategies (e.g., weighted effect sizes). In addition, we discuss issues that may influence your decision to adjust effect sizes by the research biases of the studies. These decisions permit you to give more weight to studies with few biases rather than to those with many biases. We also discuss differences between fixed and random effects models. Finally, we summarize some of the principles that might determine whether you would use a Bayesian or a non-Bayesian approach for combining these bias-adjusted effect sizes. We present a brief review of the major conceptual issues you need to understand to make these choices.

Section G. Sensitivity Analysis

This section addresses sensitivity analysis. After the initial results of the meta-analysis have been obtained, the researcher can examine the robustness of the solution by use of this method. This concept will be explained in the three subsections shown below.

A large number of decisions are made throughout the meta-analysis process. Sensitivity analysis is a method for exploring the impact of some of these decisions on the conclusions, uncertainties, assumptions, and judgments (Greenhouse & Iyengar, 1994). A major goal of sensitivity analysis is to demonstrate that the findings are robust when evaluated by a broad range of methods. Greenhouse and Iyengar (1994) note that sensitivity should address issues such as possible biases in the search and retrieval database development. They also address possible impacts of outliers in the synthesis process. As in other forms of data analysis, a few studies with extreme values on the measures may have an undue effect on the results. Another major concern is the method of estimating effect sizes (e.g., random versus fixed effects). Eddy et al. (1992, p. 310) describe three basic approaches to sensitivity analysis: (a) modifying distributions, (b) modifying data in the model, and (c) using analysis of covariance.

Modifying Distributions

The first approach involves varying the types of distributions assumed for the process being studied. For example, the investigator might examine the effects of assuming an underlying Poisson rather than a normal distribution. This particular approach typically requires access to a software program that permits these types of transformations. For example, the FAST*PRO and HLM programs described in Resource 5, Procedure C, Chapter 3 can be used to test assumptions about a variety of competing distributions (e.g., Bernoulli, Poisson).

Modifying Data in the Model

A second approach (Eddy et al., 1992, p. 311) involves repeating the analysis using different assumptions about independent and dependent variables. This approach is widely used to assess the stability of the final conclusions by adding or dropping studies that may not be equivalent to other studies in your database. The procedure involves exploratory analyses in which many competing explanations about the findings can be examined to determine whether the study conclusions are unduly influenced by a small number of potentially flawed studies.

First, the investigator may successively include or exclude particular pieces of evidence. For example, the analyst might successively include studies in which the independent or dependent variables deviate from the prototypic study. One strategy is to examine results from small samples versus large samples to see if the results differ. Other approaches include the successive inclusion or exclusion of studies that have particular types of research artifacts or research biases. Some have termed this approach as **cumulative meta-analysis** to assess the impact of each study (Lau et al., 1992; Lau, Schmid, & Chalmers, 1995). Some researchers may include and then exclude unpublished studies from their computations.

Second, the analyst might include or exclude adjustments for various combinations of biases (e.g., contamination and dilution with or without sampling bias estimates).

Third, the analyst might select different approaches to incorporate adjustments for biases, weighting strategies versus psychometric methods versus Bayesian approaches.

Fourth, the analyst can assume a fixed value for the magnitude of the bias but incorporate estimates of the degree of uncertainty about the presence or absence of the bias. In other words, a study might be coded as possibly having a 25% dilution rate in the treatment condition. There can be uncertainty about whether this dilution actually occurred. Thus, the possibility of this dilution might be considered to be of very low, moderate, or high likelihood.

Fifth, the problem might be reanalyzed with the judgment of experts used as a source of data. Expert consensus judgment can provide subjective estimates of parameters in the problem. If the experts substantially disagree about any of the parameter values, the meta-analysis can be conducted under the competing sets of estimates.

Analysis of Covariance

Another widely used approach in meta-analysis is to use an analysis of covariance approach to evaluate the stability of the observed effects. This approach is particularly useful when a test for heterogeneity of effect sizes is significant. In this approach, the investigator performs an analysis of covariance in which the effect size index for the individual studies is used as the dependent variable, and a possible source of variation among studies is used as a covariate. For example, the reviewer might use the year of publication, the size of a clinic in which the study was conducted, the proportion of patients with comorbid conditions, the experience of clinicians, or other variables as possible covariates (Bryk & Raudenbush, 1992; Eddy et al., 1992; Greenhouse & Iyengar, 1994). Another approach is meta-regression to assess the impact of each study (Berlin & Antman, 1994). However, caution must be used here because aggregate values may not represent important minorities (Greenland & Robins, 1994; Langbein & Lichtman, 1978; Morgenstern, 1982). Lau et al. (1997) point out that a variety of methods, including weighted least squares, logistic regression, and hierarchical models, can be used for meta-regression analysis. They reference Berlin and Antman (1994), McIntosh (1996), Morris and Normand (1992), and Smith, Spiegelhalter, and Thomas (1995).

Synopsis of Section G

In this section, we describe some of the problems to be addressed in performing a sensitivity analysis, which is used to evaluate the robustness of your results. You might switch from one effect size index to another (e.g., from mean difference to correlation coefficients). Alternatively, you might determine how the results would differ if you assumed a nonnormal distribution. You might decide to delete some of the studies that have specific types of research biases to determine whether the overall findings remain stable. You also might perform various subgroup analyses to determine whether interactive effects occur among **moderator** or **mediator variables**. You will find the graphical procedures described in Chapter 12 an important resource for planning sensitivity analysis.

Summary

This chapter presents some of the theoretical issues involved in designing a systematic review using meta-analysis. As with any research endeavor, your efforts require careful planning and execution. The planning must begin with converting a conceptual model of the problem under investigation to a concrete quantitative meta-analytic model. If a careful analysis of the problem is done, many other issues will not confound your effort.

Section A. The first consideration is the use of a multivariate model. Although difficult to specify and manage, a multivariate model is more desirable than a univariate model statistically, theoretically, and clinically. Different approaches to identifying a multivariate model are presented.

Section B. Next, we discuss the selection of an effect size index. Often overlooked, solving the complexities of this issue can make or break your meta-analysis. In general, we advise that you give careful attention to defining the exact effects you are going to examine, plan for dependence between data points, and use a nonstandardized effect size if possible.

Section C. We explain how to manage missing data. There are four broad types of missing data that should be understood because each requires a somewhat different strategy. We discuss both traditional and more recent approaches to manage this problem. Each of the traditional methods has rather serious disadvantages compared to the newer methods. Overall, we suggest the use of imputation procedures as being the least biased approach when coping with missing data.

Section D. We next discuss management of artifacts and biases. This issue is complex and controversial because currently there is no agreement about the best way to proceed. Authors are advised to consider their specific area carefully and to think through how the quality of the primary studies might affect their findings. Specific approaches are described, but no single method will be able to solve all problems.

Section E. We then discuss dealing with the issue of heterogeneity of findings. One of the fundamental criticisms of meta-analysis is the tendency to combine studies that do not belong together. The results then cannot be interpreted. Because study results are bound to vary, how much is too much? We suggest how to test this and how to interpret heterogeneity when it is found.

Section F. In this section, we discuss the issues involved in combining effect sizes. Several methods exist today, and each has its advantages and disadvantages. Selecting the best method will depend on assumptions about distributions, models, and the availability of software.

Section G. Finally, we explain the importance of completing a sensitivity analysis. This procedure is a way for authors to test the robustness of their findings. By selectively altering different aspects of the question, the number of studies, and the assumptions underlying the synthesis, a clearer understanding of the findings can be achieved. Sensitivity analysis increasingly is becoming used by authors of information syntheses and should be considered a fundamental component of the meta-analytic processes.

CHAPTER 14

Step-by-Step Procedures for Meta-Analyses

I n Chapters 12 and 13, we provided a description of basic meta-analytic statistical principles and discussed some of the issues that need to be addressed as
you plan a meta-analysis. This chapter consists of three parts and demonstrates step-
by-step procedures to be implemented in performing a quantitative synthesis. In the
first procedure, we outline the specific tasks required to develop your synthesis plan.
In the second procedure, we provide a step-by-step guide to develop any of seven
variations of meta-analyses. Only one of these examples is likely to be used in any
one meta-analysis. Finally, in the third procedure, we explain steps for doing a sensitivity analysis to explore the impact of uncertainties, assumptions, and judgments
that might affect your final product.

Before starting, however, you should be familiar with other manuals, software,
and simplified step-by-step articles on meta-analyses and systematic reviews. These
materials can provide a useful adjunct to the procedures we describe below. *The
Reviewers' Handbook* by the Cochrane Collaboration is likely the most detailed manual on conducting systematic reviews of which we are aware. Details can be found at
the following Web site: www.cochrane.org/cochrane/hbook.htm.

Software packages available that provide detailed instructions include RevMan
from the Cochrane Collaboration and Metaxis, both being available from Update
Software (London and San Diego, CA).

Several other articles provide a more simplified overview of the basic procedures
involved. A few examples are the following: Normand (1999); Egger, Smith, and
Phillips (1997); and Lau et al. (1997).

> ## STEP-BY-STEP PROCEDURES FOR META-ANALYSES
>
> A. Develop a strategic plan
> B. Implement one of seven variations of a meta-analysis
> C. Conduct a sensitivity analysis

Each of these procedures encompasses an independent part of this chapter. You should read Procedures A and C in preparation for conducting any meta-analysis. In Procedure B, we explain the specific tasks for each of seven variations that have different assumptions and different statistical methods for calculating effect size. Consequently, you need only read those meta-analysis variations that are of immediate interest or relevance for planning purposes. Although each of these variations uses the same nine procedural tasks, each is based on a different type of effect size measure and thus requires a somewhat different approach.

Procedure A. Develop a Strategic Plan

Procedures for strategic planning of the synthesis process involve completion of six tasks. These tasks are usually required before implementing your meta-analysis project plan, and they help authors maximize resources and time. The box below lists the six suggested tasks. Each will be described in detail.

> ## TASKS TO DEVELOP A STRATEGIC PLAN
>
> 1. Develop a quantitative model
> 2. Review project resources
> 3. Select software for calculating effect sizes
> 4. Select method for calculating effect sizes
> 5. Develop plan for managing artifacts and biases
> 6. Select model for combining effect sizes

Task 1: Develop a Quantitative Model

If, at this point, you decide to perform a meta-analysis rather than a qualitative or narrative review of the topics contained in your original plan, you will have to reformulate and quantify the causal model developed at the beginning of the synthesis. A quantitative model must be explicit and quantitative. Every question within the model should be listed and addressed separately. When the question is listed, the author should state whether it is multivariate or univariate. Within each question, each of the variables to be included in the analysis should be precisely and quantitatively defined. Specific emphasis should be on quantitative definitions so that variables are defined in the same form of measurement that they are found in the original studies. Assumptions regarding random versus fixed distribution of these variables also should be specified for each at this time. Finally, those variables or analyses that will be adjusted for quality should also be specified ahead of time. If both quality-weighted and non-quality-weighted analyses are to be performed, then those plans should be specifically identified at this point.

The result of this plan will be a meta-analytic model derived from the conceptual model you developed in Section D, Chapter 2. Because your goal at this stage is to estimate the parameters for some of the essential components in your hypothesized model, the meta-analysis model will be more restricted in scope than the causal model.

Task 2: Review Project Resources

At this point, it is important to revisit your overall project plan, as the project is now about midway, and many aspects of the plan may have changed during Stages I, II, and III (the first part of the review process). Issues to be resolved include the availability of adequate skills for the remaining tasks as well as current budget limitations and time constraints. Most of the fiscal resources will have been spent for securing articles. If consultant fees are necessary for a quantitative synthesis, it is important to ensure that funds are still available. We recommend that you obtain needed meta-analysis software if they are not now among your resources. You may be able to obtain publicly available software for this purpose. We recommend that you conduct a search on the Internet using the search terms "meta-analysis" and "software." Some of the software is available for public use. If you cannot locate public software, then you might have to purchase this software. The work required for the quantitative synthesis itself can be very time-consuming. At this point, an estimate should be made regarding your ability to make your time deadlines; adjustments may have to be made to the model to ensure that you can meet those deadlines.

Task 3: Select Software for Calculating Effect Sizes

If you do not have access to any of the formal meta-analytic software programs, you can achieve most analyses using widely available spreadsheets and data management programs such as EXCEL, FOXPRO, Lotus, ACCESS, or Dbase. You can also use any of a variety of statistical software programs such as SPSS, SAS, BMDP, or S-PLUS. Although these programs enable you to perform most meta-analyses, they are not specifically designed for this purpose; as a result, you have to create many of your own specific command files and diagnostic procedures. You will need to create effect size and variance estimates for each of the studies in your data set. If the research designs are at all complicated, then you may need to use special software to assist you in these calculations. We describe in Chapter 3 many programs available to help you perform a meta-analysis.

Task 4: Select a Method for Calculating Effect Sizes

Select an Effect Size Measure. The particular effect size measure selected depends on the type of research design and level of measurement in the dependent variable. These issues were detailed in Section B, Chapter 12, and we refer the reader to that section.

It is important to be cautious about combining too many different types of effect sizes together in the same meta-analysis. You will be tempted to include effect sizes that come from different patient populations, different types of research settings, or different methods of implementing the independent or dependent variables. For example, you might have effect sizes for a construct using similar, but not identical, versions of the same test instrument. Alternatively, you have located studies in which various researchers have used similar, but not identical, manipulations of the independent variables. You will often find that researchers have different inclusion or exclusion criteria for the acceptance of patients with comorbid medical conditions.

At times, you may decide to pool these various types of studies together because you are trying to assess the generalizability of the findings across diverse groups of measures, manipulations, and patient populations. However, a common outcome of this strategy is that these diverse studies are not adequately focused on specific research questions. The pooling of these diverse effect sizes can produce such heterogeneity in effect sizes that it is difficult to detect a systematic pattern of effects.

Check for Independence of Effect Sizes. Be certain to check for data dependencies across the various effect size indices available to you. Your effect size indices often involve comparisons between two groups of study participants. If the original study from which you have obtained data actually contained more than two groups, then the pairwise comparisons among all of the groups are not independent. For example, suppose that you found a study with three groups (we will call them Groups A, B, and C). When you examine all possible comparisons between any two groups, you obtain the comparisons A to B, B to C, and A to C. In these comparisons, the data within each group are used twice to make a comparison to other groups. In other words, the three sets of comparisons are not based on independent data, and the three effect size estimates are not independent. If you plan to use more than one effect size index from each study, then you must select a method to adjust for the nonindependence of the effect sizes.

Decide on Standardized or Nonstandardized Indices. Standardized indices are valuable when the scales of measurement of the various studies are not equivalent. These approaches are also useful when you want to compare your effect sizes to results from other meta-analyses. You can use standardized indices when you consider the between-study variations to be unimportant for the purposes of your research.

Nonstandardized indices are chosen when you need to understand and explain the variation among the studies. This situation most often occurs when you have found heterogeneity of effect sizes. Typically, you will need to know whether the variation among studies is due to differences in the means (numerators) or the variances (denominators) of the effect size measure.

Task 5: Develop a Plan for Managing Artifacts and Biases

You will need a strategy to manage the artifacts and biases identified in the data validation stage. Each flaw, or configuration of flaws, must usually be managed differently. Your main purpose is to minimize the effect of these factors on the soundness of your final conclusions. There are three general procedures used. These are all discussed in Chapter 13 and include the following: (a) the psychometric approach (Hunter & Schmidt, 1990) (see Section D), (b) the Bayesian approach (Eddy et al., 1992) (see Section F), and (c) the hierarchical linear model approach (Bryk & Raudenbush, 1992) (see Section F). If you decide to use one or more of these, you should consult the relevant text. Depending on the particular type of problem that you are studying, you may decide to use any one (or a combination) of these approaches.

Task 6: Select a Model for Combining Effect Sizes

You must select among a number of procedures for actually combining the results of the various studies to produce parameter estimates (e.g., means and variances) of the treatment effects. The various solutions involve different types of assumptions about the underlying distributions from which the data were sampled. You also need to decide whether to use a Bayesian or a non-Bayesian method for combining effect sizes. You should review the discussion in Section F, Chapter 13 to choose among these alternatives.

Procedure B. Implement One of Seven Variations of a Meta-Analysis

In this section, we present computational procedures for implementing a quantitative analysis. We demonstrate the methods using a variety of different types of statistics, such as correlation coefficients, differences in means, proportions, and odds ratios. There are nine steps in each of seven variations that we will explain in detail below.

SEVEN VARIATIONS OF A META-ANALYSIS

1. Combining study effect size differences in correlation coefficients
2. Combining study effect size differences in means
3. Combining study effect size differences in proportions
4. Combining study effect sizes using a quality weighted approach
5. Perform random rather than fixed effects meta-analyses
6. Combining study effect size differences in odds ratios
7. Combining study effect size differences in odds ratios with small sample sizes (e.g., Mantel-Haenszel)

As an extension of the differences in proportions, we demonstrate the use of quality-weighted procedures that give higher quality studies greater weight in the analysis. We also demonstrate the use of fixed and random effects models. Our approach is based on the work of Shadish and Haddock (1994).

For each of the variations, we describe a basic list of nine tasks for implementing a meta-analysis; these tasks are generic in that they apply to all of the variations in this chapter. However, exceptions to the tasks exist for some of the variations, and these exceptions are noted when relevant.

NINE META-ANALYSIS TASKS

1. Calculate an effect size index within each study (t_i)
2. Calculate a variance estimate within each study (v_i)
3. Calculate the weighting factor (w_i) for each study
4. Adjust each study effect size by the weighting factor ($t_i * w_i$)
5. Calculate the average effect size $T\bullet$
6. Calculate a conditional variance ($V\bullet$) and standard error of estimate across all studies
7. Calculate a confidence interval for $T\bullet$
8. Calculate the heterogeneity of effect size statistic, Q
9. Perform a test of significance on the average effect size

In the formulas we present in this section, $T\bullet$ is used to represent the average effect size. Formula 14.1 illustrates the basic computation of $T\bullet$ regardless of what kind of statistic is used in the effect size calculation. This is a generic formula in that each of the variables might be calculated differently, but the final combination step is the same for all examples:

$$\overline{T\bullet} = \frac{\sum\limits_{i=1}^{k} w_i t_i}{\sum\limits_{i=1}^{k} w_i} \tag{14.1}$$

The variable t_i is the effect size calculated for each study. The actual computation of this variable will depend on the type of statistic used for effect size estimates. The symbol v_i is the variance of that effect size and is also calculated within each study (its calculations also vary as a function of the type of effect size). Depending on your selection of an effect size index, you will need to choose an appropriate formula for calculating the variance estimates (v_i) that are to be used in your calculations (Shadish & Haddock, 1994). Each type of effect size index has its own unique formula for computing the variance.

The symbol w_i refers to a weighting factor that is used to represent the variance of each study in most of the studies (see Formula 14.2):

$$w_i = \frac{1}{v_i} \tag{14.2}$$

The weighting factor (w_i) is always equal to the inverse of the individual study variance (i.e., $1/v_i$), and hence Formula 14.2 is a generic formula across most types of statistics. The weighting factor allows for the effect size of each study to be modified by the sample size. With this procedure, you will give greater weight to the studies that have smaller error variances.

The conditional variance ($V\bullet$) is the variance of the sampling distribution of effect sizes. The square root of that number is the standard error of the sampling distribution. In the process of performing a meta-analysis, you need to have an estimate of the variability in the effect sizes reported in each of the original studies. These estimates are needed to calculate confidence intervals for the overall (average) effect size ($T\bullet$). You will also use these values if you decide to test the average effect size for statistical significance. As you read through these examples, be sure to distinguish between formulas using the within-study variances (v_i) versus the between-study variances ($V\bullet$).

You will discover that there are several solutions to the problem of estimating the conditional variance ($V\bullet$) of the sampling distribution of effect sizes. The most direct solution is to average the variances obtained in the individual studies (i.e., v_i). However, this procedure is not recommended. Because we actually use the value of 1/variance (symbolized as $1/v_i$) in our calculations, we need to compute the averages from $1/v_i$ instead of v_i. The value of v_i is the variance estimate obtained from each of the individual studies.

The following formula provides an estimate for the conditional variance of the sampling distribution of effect sizes across all studies and is calculated from Formula 14.3. (Recall that the square root of the conditional variance is the standard error.) This formula is needed for calculating confidence intervals and for performing hypothesis tests:

$$V\bullet = \frac{1}{\sum_{i=1}^{k}(w_i)} = \frac{1}{\sum_{i=1}^{k}(1/v_i)} \tag{14.3}$$

At first glance, this formula may seem somewhat puzzling. If your goal is to calculate an average variance, you might expect to add up the variances and divide by the number of variances. To understand why we use the formula above, you need to recall that we are actually using the value of $1/v_i$ in our calculations, so that we need to calculate the average value of $1/v_i$. You can easily show that the value generated by Formula 14.3 does not agree with the value that you would obtain if you simply averaged the variances from each of the studies.

We now present seven variations with examples of the nine computational steps involved in performing a meta-analysis. The formulas for this approach come from Shadish and Haddock (1994). Each of the seven variations can be performed using widely available spreadsheet programs such as Excel, Quatro, or Lotus.

Variation 1: Combining Study Effect Size Differences in Correlation Coefficients

The following example demonstrates the calculation of combined effect sizes for correlation coefficients. We have used the notation system in Shadish and Haddock (1994) to present our computational approach. The data set for this example is presented in Appendix A of Cooper and Hedges (1994, pp. 543-544).

In this variation, the studies, from which this data set was extracted, are designed to evaluate the validity of student ratings of instructor performance. In each of the original studies, the investigators correlated student ratings of instructor performance with student achievement. For each study, the class or section is the unit of analysis. The number of classes or sections in these studies ranges from 10 to 75. The investigators first calculate means across each section for the student ratings of the instructor and the student's achievement scores in the class. In the original studies, a correlation coefficient was computed across all sections between the mean student rating of the instructor and the mean achievement score for the students in the class. In some of the studies, students had been randomly assigned to instructors, and in other studies, a control variable measuring student ability was used as a covariate to control for differences in student ability. The measure of effect size was a product moment correlation or a partial correlation coefficient. We present the actual study results and effect size calculations in Table 14.1.

As illustrated in Table 14.1 and in all subsequent tables, we summarize the calculations to be used in Tasks 1 through 9 of each variation of a meta-analysis. In Table 14.1, we denote the column headed by "Study #" as the first column, which indicates the specific study number. The second column, labeled "Topic," specifies the type of study sample. The third column, labeled "Sample," identifies the total sample size (*n*) for each study, and the fourth column, labeled "*r*," reports the size of the correlation for each.

Task 1 (Variation 1):
Calculate an Effect Size Index Within Each Study (t_i)

In Table 14.1, the data reported in the columns headed by *r* and *Z* are used to calculate effect sizes for each of the studies. Because the correlation coefficient is a standardized effect size, the combined correlation effect sizes are also standardized effect size indices. Extensive research and statistical theory have demonstrated that the value of r tends to be biased (e.g., see Hays, 1973, 1997). A more appropriate index is called the *r* to Z_i transformation. Because the sampling distribution for the value of *r* is not normally distributed, we use the Z_i transformation to generate an estimate that is approximately normally distributed. Although it is easier to use a table to determine the transformations (available in almost any statistical textbook), Formula 14.4 for the r_i to Z_i transformation is as follows:

$$Z_i = .5\{\ln[(1 + r_i) / (1 - r_i)]\} \tag{14.4}$$

The initial effect size measure in each study is the correlation coefficient (column headed by r_i). The actual values of the coefficients range from −0.11 to 0.68. The mean value calculated across the studies (ignoring differences in sample size) is 0.378. The values for the *r* to *Z* transformation are presented in Table 14.1 under the column labeled Z_i. (Note that this index is not a traditional standard score.) These values can be easily calculated in a spreadsheet program such as Excel or Quatro. The value of the *r* to *Z* transformation calculated for the first study is 0.829. The values of *Z* range from −0.110 to 0.829. The absolute value of *Z* can be larger than 1.00. The mean value for *Z* in this data set is 0.417. Thus, the mean value is quite close to the number obtained for the average value of the r_s, which is 0.3782. You would expect

TABLE 14.1 Data for Meta–Analysis Variation 1 on Correlation Coefficients

Author	Study #	Topic	Sample (n)	r_i	Z_i	v_i	$w_i = (1/v_i)$	$t_i * w_i$	$t_i * t_i * w_i$
Bolton	1	psych	10	0.680	0.829	0.143	7.000	5.804	4.811
Brysoin	2	algebra	20	0.560	0.633	0.059	17.000	10.758	6.812
Centra	3	psych	22	0.640	0.758	0.053	19.000	14.405	10.917
Centra	4	biology	13	0.230	0.234	0.100	10.000	2.342	0.548
Crooks	5	physics	28	0.490	0.536	0.040	25.000	13.402	7.182
Elliot	6	chemistry	36	0.330	0.343	0.030	33.000	11.313	3.882
Ellis	7	psych	19	0.580	0.662	0.063	16.000	10.599	7.012
Frey	8	calculus	12	0.180	0.182	0.111	9.000	1.638	0.298
Greenwood	9	geometry	36	-0.110	-0.110	0.030	33.000	-3.645	0.399
Hoffman	10	math	75	0.270	0.277	0.014	72.000	19.934	5.524
McKeachie	11	psych	33	0.260	0.266	0.033	30.000	7.983	2.123
Remmer	12	chemistry	37	0.490	0.536	0.029	34.000	18.226	9.768
Sullivan-1	13	science	14	0.510	0.563	0.091	11.000	6.190	3.487
Sullivan-2	14	psych	40	0.400	0.424	0.027	37.000	15.675	6.652
Sullivan-3	15	math	16	0.340	0.354	0.077	13.000	4.603	1.629
Sullivan-4	16	biology	14	0.420	0.448	0.091	11.000	4.925	2.208
Wherry	17	psych	20	0.160	0.161	0.059	17.000	2.744	0.441
Sum			445	6.430	7.096	1.050	394.000	146.896	73.692
Mean			63.57	0.378	0.417	0.062	23.176	8.641	4.335

bigger differences between an average r and an average Z when the values of r are greater than 0.60.

Task 2 (Variation 1): Calculate a Variance Estimate Within Each Study (v_i)

The next value to be computed is the variance (v_i) for each of the studies. Each study will be weighted by an estimate of the study variance; this procedure creates a standardized effect size index weighted by the sample size. Formula 14.5 for the variance of the transformed Zs is:

$$v_i = \frac{1}{(n_i - 3)} \qquad (14.5)$$

For the first study in the table (Bolton), the value of $v_i = [1/(n-3)] = [1/(10-3)] = [1/7] = 0.143$. A similar approach is used for calculating v_i in each of the other studies. The sum of these numbers is 1.050.

Task 3 (Variation 1): Calculate the Weighting Factor (w_i) for Each Study

The next value to be calculated is w_i, which is $1/v_i$ (Formula 14.2). For the Bolton study, this value is $(1/0.143) = 7$. The values of v_i and w_i for the remaining studies are also presented in Table 14.1.

Task 4 (Variation 1): Adjust Each Study Effect Size by the Weighting Factor ($t_i * w_i$)

Now, the effect size for each study can be adjusted by the variance to construct a standardized weighted effect size. This adjustment is done computationally by multiplying each effect size by the weighting factor ($t_i * w_i$). Thus, in the Bolton study we would calculate $0.829 * 7 = 5.804$. Examples of this computation can be seen in Table 14.1. The values in Table 14.1 for this example range from -3.645 to 19.934 across the studies. The sum of those numbers (146.896) in the column headed by $t_i * w_i$ will form the numerator of the formula required to compute the overall average.

Task 5 (Variation 1): Calculate the Average Effect Size $T\bullet$

We have now calculated all of the data necessary to determine the average effect size across the studies. To compute this average, use Formula 14.1* below. Formula numbers presented with asterisks (*) indicate that they were previously presented in this chapter. Remember that the Z transformations are the computed (t) effect sizes in this formula.

$$\overline{T \bullet} = \frac{\sum\limits_{i=1}^{k} w_i t_i}{\sum\limits_{i=1}^{k} w_i} = \frac{146.896}{394} = 0.373 \tag{14.1*}$$

First multiplying the weight by the effect size for each study and then adding those results determine the numerator. These numbers range in size from –3.645 to 19.944. The sum of these values is 146.896. Finally, you divide the sum of the adjusted effect size by the sum of the weights. The sum of the weights in this example is 394, that is, the sum of the column labeled w_i. This value is the denominator term of Formula 14.1*.

The resulting value 0.373 is the average effect size for all the studies in the data set. Note that this value is quite close to the value obtained simply by averaging the individual correlations. When the individual correlations are less than 0.60 and the samples are similar in size, then you would expect to obtain similar results from the r effect size index and the Z effect size index.

Task 6 (Variation 1): Calculate a Conditional Variance (V•) and a Standard Error of Estimate Across All Studies

The average effect size has a conditional variance ($V\bullet$), which is the average variance across samples, or the estimate of the variance of the sampling distribution. For this example, this value is the inverse of the sum of the w_i. For meta-analyses other than the correlation coefficient, these values can be rather complex. The sum of the column labeled w_i yields a total of 394. To convert this number to a conditional variance, we divide it into 1, which yields a value of 0.003 (Formula 14.3*).

$$\overline{V \bullet} = \frac{1}{\sum\limits_{i=1}^{k}(w_i)} = \frac{1}{\sum\limits_{i=1}^{k}(1/v_i)} = \frac{1}{394} = 0.003 \tag{14.3*}$$

To generate a standard error of estimate, we calculate the square root of this value to yield 0.0504.

Task 7 (Variation 1): Calculate a Confidence Interval for T•

We represent the population effect size by the symbol δ. To calculate the confidence interval for our estimate of δ, you need an estimate of the standard error of estimate. The standard error of estimate is another way of saying the standard deviation of the sampling distribution of effect sizes. We calculated this value 0.0504 in

Task 6 above. Formula 14.6 provides the calculations for the confidence interval of the average effect size. The value of C_α in this formula is the critical value in the sampling distribution, after which you would decide that the results were significant. Another way of saying this is that the critical value is the value of Z in a normal distribution in which we decide the effect has a probability of alpha. (The value of alpha is usually set at 0.05.) For a two-tailed test for the normal distribution with an alpha = 0.05, the value of C_α = 1.96.

$$[\overline{T \bullet} - C_\alpha (V\bullet)^{\frac{1}{2}}] \le \delta \le [T \bullet + C_\alpha (V\bullet)^{\frac{1}{2}}] =$$
$$[0.373 - (1.96)(.003)^{\frac{1}{2}}] \le \delta \le [0.373 + (1.96)(.003)^{\frac{1}{2}}] =$$
$$[0.274] \le \delta \le [0.472] \tag{14.6}$$

When we complete these calculations, we have 95% confidence that the population value for the effect size parameter lies between 0.274 and 0.472.

Task 8 (Variation 1): Calculate the Heterogeneity of Effect Size Statistic (Q)

Our next task is to perform a test to determine whether the various effect sizes are heterogeneous. Use the Q statistic to estimate the heterogeneity of effect sizes from Formula 14.7:

$$Q = \sum_{i=1}^{k} w_i t_i^2 - \frac{\left(\sum_{i=1}^{k} w_i t_i\right)^2}{\sum_{i=1}^{k} w_i} = \left(73.690 - \frac{(146.896)^2}{394}\right) = 18.924 \tag{14.7}$$

This value (Q) = 18.924 is distributed as a χ_2 (chi-squared) statistic with k −1 degrees of freedom (the number of studies in the data set minus 1) and can be evaluated using a standard χ_2 table. These tables are usually found in any introductory statistic book. This value of the Q statistic with 16 degrees of freedom is not statistically significant. To be statistically significant with an alpha = 0.05, the observed value would have to be greater than 26.3 with 16 degrees of freedom. The implication of nonsignificance is that the effect sizes are derived from the same population and can be combined.

Suppose that the heterogeneity statistic had been statistically significant. Under this circumstance, you would consider the possibility that the various studies were sampled from different populations. Typically, the next step would be to identify the source of the heterogeneity. Going back to the example of student ratings of instructor performance from which the data in Table 14.1 were derived (see example used at the beginning of Variation 1), you might consider that some of the studies had students who came from private schools, whereas other studies had students who came from publicly supported schools. If you controlled for the type of school, then the variability might disappear. However, if you were unable to identify the source of variability, then you might proceed with a random effects analysis instead of a fixed effects analysis. We will examine this procedure in more detail in the following sections.

Task 9 (Variation 1): Perform a Test of Significance on the Average Effect Size

The formula to be used for testing the statistical significance is similar to a traditional Z or t test. (Note that this value of Z is different than the "r to Z" concept.) In the traditional Z test (Formula 14.8), the numerator contains the absolute value of the mean effect size (Formula 14.1), and the denominator is the square root of the pooled variance estimate ($V \bullet$), calculated in Formula 14.3.

$$Z = \frac{\left| \overline{T} \bullet \right|}{(V \bullet)^{1/2}} = \frac{\left| 0.373 \right|}{(0.003)^{1/2}} = 7.40: p < .001 \qquad (14.8)$$

For the example described in Table 14.1, the value for Z is equal to 7.40, which is statistically significant (a Z greater than 1.96 would be statistically significant at the 0.05 level). The data set provides evidence that the null hypothesis is false for this set of research participants. The average effect size is significantly different from zero. The results for each study are the correlations between student ratings of the performance of their instructors and the students' grades in the class. The average effect size calculated across all of the studies provides evidence that the null hypothesis (stating that the correlation is 0.00) is not supported by the combined study results. The findings are consistent with the premise that all of the studies are sampled from a comparable population because the heterogeneity of variance test does not provide evidence that the studies differ in effect size.

Variation 2: Combining Study Effect Size Differences in Means

The most commonly used descriptive statistic in research is the mean. As a result, mean differences are the prototypical effect measure for many researchers, both inside and outside the health field. Variation 2 demonstrates the method for performing a meta-analysis on differences in means. This example uses Table 14.2 as the source data for computations. This table contains hypothetical scores on a functional status instrument that was normalized to have a mean of 50 and a standard deviation of 5.0. The treatment was a specialized exercise program, and 12 hypothetical studies were created to form the basis of the meta-analyses. We will use the same conceptual steps identified in the overview.

In Table 14.2, we have summarized the calculations to be used in Tasks 1 through 9 in performing a meta-analysis of mean differences. The first column, labeled "Study #," identifies the specific studies; the next three columns are labeled *n*, *M*, and *SD* for the control groups (the sample size, mean, and standard deviation). The next three columns represent the same variables for the treatment group.

Task 1 (Variation 2):
Calculate an Effect Size Index Within Each Study (t_i)

The data reported in columns for the control and treatment groups are used to calculate effect sizes for each of the studies. To compute the effect size for a mean difference, you should use Formulas 14.9 and 14.10.

$$S_i^2 = \frac{(n_{t_i} - 1) * S_{t_i}^2 + (n_{c_i} - 1) * S_{c_i}^2}{(n_{t_i} + n_{c_i} - 2)} \tag{14.9}$$

$$d_i = \frac{(\overline{X}_i^t - \overline{X}_i^c)}{S_i} \tag{14.10}$$

In Formula 14.9, the mean of the control group for the ith study is subtracted from the mean of the treatment group. That difference is presented in the column labeled "DIFF" for each study. The pooled standard deviation (the combination of the standard deviation for the control group and the treatment group) is computed in the column labeled S_i. The column labeled t_i contains the computation of the effect size d_i. For Study 1, the value of t_i (i.e., *d*) is (71-42)/5.756 = 5.038. Similar calculations are made for the other studies.

Task 2 (Variation 2):
Calculate a Variance Estimate Within Each Study (v_i)

The next step is to calculate the variance estimates for each study. Each of the studies will be weighted by an estimate of the study variance; this procedure creates a standardized effect size index. Formula 14.11 indicates the variables needed for these calculations.

TABLE 14.2 Data for Meta–Analysis Variation 2 on Mean Differences

| Study # | Control | | | Treatment | | | Diff | S_i | $t_i(d_i)$ | v_i | w_i | $t_i * w_i$ | $t_i * t_i * w_i$ |
	n	M	SD	n	M	SD							
1	122	42	6.23	120	71	5.23	29	5.75592	5.0383	0.06898	14.4976	73.0430	368.0115
2	16	56	8.48	16	64	6.55	8	7.5767	1.0559	0.14242	7.0215	7.4138	7.8280
3	80	48	5.54	82	44	5.25	−4	5.39514	−0.7414	0.02639	37.8907	−28.0925	20.8280
4	42	40	3.22	42	32	4.48	−8	3.9012	−2.0506	0.07265	13.7647	−28.2265	57.8826
5	219	52	6.94	220	68	7.92	16	7.44726	2.1484	0.01437	69.5950	149.5209	321.2368
6	54	49	4.31	48	53	4.22	4	4.26794	0.9372	0.04366	22.9055	21.4675	20.1198
7	26	38	6.46	23	44	5.55	6	6.0511	0.9916	0.09197	10.8728	10.7810	10.6900
8	11	37	7.66	12	59	8.67	22	8.20457	2.6814	0.33055	3.0253	8.1121	21.7520
9	14	66	6.63	14	58	5.4	−8	6.04636	−1.3231	0.17412	5.7432	−7.5989	10.0542
10	66	44	2.38	70	66	5.78	22	4.4666	4.9254	0.11863	8.4297	41.5199	204.5043
11	44	40	3.49	44	48	4.33	8	3.93249	2.0343	0.06897	14.4993	29.4964	60.0055
12	54	54	7.72	50	56	5.69	2	6.82063	0.2932	0.03893	25.6859	7.5318	2.2085
Sum	748	566	69.06	741	663	69.07	97	69.065	419	366.033	233.931	284.9684	1105.12124
Mean	62.33	47.167	5.755	61.75	55.25	5.7558	8.0833	5.7554	34.9167	30.5027	19.4943	23.7474	92.0934

$$v_i = \frac{(n_{t_i} + n_{c_i})}{(n_{t_i} * n_{c_i})} + \frac{d_i^2}{[2(n_{t_i} + n_{c_i})]} \qquad (14.11)$$

For Study 1 in Table 14.2, Formula 14.11 is calculated as follows:

$$v_i = \frac{(122 + 120)}{(122 * 120)} + \frac{(5.0383 * 5.0383)}{2(122 + 120)} = 0.06898.$$

This value is reported in Table 14.2 under the column labeled v_i.

Task 3 (Variation 2): Calculate the Weighting Factor (w_i) for Each Study

You will also need to calculate the value of $w_i = 1/v_i$. For the first study, this value is (1/0.06898) = 14.4976. The values of v_i and w_i for the remaining studies are also presented in Table 14.2, in columns with those same labels.

Task 4 (Variation 2): Adjust Each Study Effect Size by the Weighting Factor ($t_i * w_i$)

Next we create an "adjusted effect size" by multiplying the nonstandardized effect sizes (t_i) by the weighting factor (w_i). This procedure produces a value of 73.0430 for Study 1, and this value is reported in the column with the $t_i * w_i$ label. Appropriate values for the remaining studies are also presented under the column labeled $t_i * w_i$.

Task 5 (Variation 2): Calculate the Average Effect Size T•

To compute the average effect size, use Formula 14.1*:

$$\overline{T\bullet} = \frac{\sum\limits_{i=1}^{k} w_i t_i}{\sum\limits_{i=1}^{k} w_i} = \frac{284.968}{233.9312} = 1.21817 \qquad (14.1^*)$$

To compute the average adjusted effect size, first multiply the weighting factor and the effect size for each study. Then, sum those figures across all of the studies. In our example for Table 14.2, this sum equals 284.968. Taking this sum, you divide by the sum of the variance estimates (the sum of the column labeled w_i = 233.9312).

The resultant number = 1.21817. This value is the average effect size combined across all of the studies in our data set.

Task 6 (Variation 2):
Calculate a Conditional Variance (V•)
and Standard Error of Estimate Across All Studies

The next step in conducting a meta-analysis is to test the significance of the average adjusted effect size. To do this test, it is necessary to compute the estimated variance of the sampling distribution of effect sizes. Formula 14.3* for computing this variance is as follows:

$$V\bullet = \frac{1}{\sum\limits_{i=1}^{k}(w_i)} = \frac{1}{\sum\limits_{i=1}^{k}(1/v_i)} = \frac{1}{233.9312} = .00427 \qquad (14.3^*)$$

Using Table 14.2 to perform the calculations, we get the following numbers: $V\bullet = 1/233.9311 = 0.00427$. The square root of this figure is the standard error, which, for the set of studies in Table 14.2, would be 0.0654.

Task 7 (Variation 2): Calculate a Confidence Interval for T•

Creating a confidence interval involves calculating upper and lower limits of the average effect size (as in Formula 14.6*). The value of C_α in this formula is the critical value in the sampling distribution that includes alpha proportion of the sampling distribution. For a two-tailed test for the normal distribution with an alpha = 0.05, the value of C_α = 1.96.

$$[T\bullet - C_\alpha(V\bullet)^{\frac{1}{2}}] \le \delta \le [T\bullet + C_\alpha(V\bullet)^{\frac{1}{2}}] =$$
$$[1.21817 - (1.96)(.00427)^{\frac{1}{2}}] \le \delta \le [1.21817 + (1.96)(.00427)^{\frac{1}{2}}] =$$
$$[1.09002] \le \delta \le [1.34632] \qquad (14.6^*)$$

Thus, we have 95% confidence that the population value for the effect size parameter lies between 1.09002 and 1.34632.

Task 8 (Variation 2):
Calculate the Heterogeneity of the Effect Size Statistic (Q)

Use this statistic to determine whether all the studies in your data set appear to come from the same population. The following Formula 14.7* is used to compute an estimate of the degree of heterogeneity among the effect sizes. The numbers used to compute Q are already computed in your spreadsheet, except for the $w_i * t_i * t_i$. In our example, this computation is performed in the column labeled $w_i * t_i * t_i$ of Table 14.2:

$$Q = \sum_{i=1}^{k} w_i t_i^2 - \frac{\left(\sum_{i=1}^{k} w_i t_i\right)^2}{\sum_{i=1}^{k} w_i} = \tag{14.7*}$$

$$\left(1105.1212 - \frac{(284.968)^2}{233.931}\right) = 757.981$$

This value (Q) is distributed as a χ^2 (chi-squared) statistic with $k - 1$ degrees of freedom and can be evaluated using a standard (chi-squared) χ^2 table. For the example in Table 14.2, the value for the $Q_{(11)}$ statistic is 757.981, which is statistically significant, $p < .001$. This value of the Q statistic with 11 degrees of freedom (the number of studies in the data set minus 1) is statistically significant, suggesting that the studies do not come from a common population. As a consequence, we need to explore the potential source of variability among the studies. A first possibility is to try using one of the other coded variables from the data extraction phase. You could implement one of the subgroup analysis procedures described in Chapter 13. For example, you might split the sample of studies in your data set into subgroups based on setting characteristics, research design characteristics, or research participant characteristics such as age, severity of illness, and comorbid conditions. A second possible solution is to use a random rather than a fixed effect model for testing hypotheses about these data. You would resort to the random effects approach only if you were unable to identify the source of heterogeneity among studies.

Task 9 (Variation 2):
Perform a Test of Significance on the Average Effect Size

The formula to be used for testing the statistical significance of the average effect size is similar to a traditional Z or t test. The numerator contains the absolute value of the mean effect size, and the denominator is the square root of the pooled variance estimate calculated in Formula 14.8*.

$$Z = \frac{|T \bullet|}{(V \bullet)^{1/2}} = \frac{|1.218|}{(0.00427)^{\frac{1}{2}}} = 18.6317; \, p < .001. \qquad (14.8^*)$$

The resultant Z is significant, or in other words, for the example described in Table 14.2, the combined results provide evidence that the null hypothesis is false. The average effect size of 1.218 is unlikely to have been sampled from a population with a mean effect size of 0.00.

To summarize, the meta-analysis procedures that you have followed permit you to address a number of issues about the studies in your data set. You can determine whether the average effect size is significantly different from 0.00. Thus, the pattern of findings across all studies is consistent with the premise that differences between treatment and comparison groups are significant across all of the studies. You will also have developed an estimate of the average effect size across all studies, and you will have developed a confidence interval for this average estimate. Finally, you will have performed a test to determine whether significant heterogeneity exists across the various studies. The heterogeneity test does not have much statistical power. As a consequence, you may fail to reject the null hypothesis, and there still could be important sources of variability among the study samples.

Variation 3: Combining Study Effect Size Differences in Proportions

A commonly used descriptive statistic in health research is the proportion. A number of studies report differences in proportions between treatment and control conditions as a measure of the treatment effect. Hasselblad et al. (1995) and Fleiss (1994) both discuss the advantages and disadvantages of the use of proportions. Variation 3 demonstrates the method for performing a meta-analysis on differences in proportions. We will use the same nine tasks identified in the introduction to Procedure B.

The following calculations are based on a meta-analysis that the authors previously performed. This meta-analysis compares the effects of two different treatments on patient outcomes. Some of the studies are experimental designs, and others are quasi-experimental designs. Each of the 17 studies compares the rates of successful aminoglycoside therapy for gram-negative infections. In the "treatment" condition, a coordinated team of pharmacists, physicians, nurses, and other clinical support staff work together to make sure that the drug therapy is administered at an appropriate time with an appropriate dose. In the control conditions, usual clinical practice serves as the research intervention. The studies, then, were designed to determine whether the clinical team approach produced more successful outcomes than the control condition.

In Table 14.3, we have summarized the calculations to be used in Tasks 1 through 9 in performing a meta-analysis on proportions. The first column identifies the specific study number, and the column headed "Total (n)" identifies the sample size for each study. These values do not enter into any calculations for effect size. The procedures for comparing differences in proportions is similar to the method for comparing differences in means. You can conceive of a proportion as a sample mean. First, assign each observation a value of 0 or 1. If you calculate a mean for these observations, you sum the values of all observations and divide by the total number of observations. This value is the same value you would obtain by calculating the proportion of 1s. The major difference between variations 2 and 3 is the method for estimating the variances of the individual studies.

NOTE

In the last three columns of Table 14.3, you may find our numbers after the decimal different from those you calculate. This is often due to our using more decimal places than are commonly used in such calculations.

Task 1 (Variation 3):
Calculate an Effect Size Index Within Each Study (t$_i$)

The data reported in the columns headed "Treatment Success" through to the column headed "Control (p_2)" are used to calculate effect sizes for each of the studies. The columns headed "Treatment Success," "Treatment Failure," "Control Success," and "Control Failure" report the frequency of success and failure in the treatment and control conditions. For example, in the first study (Table 14.3), 22 patients had successful outcomes and 58 had failed outcomes in the treatment condition. For the control condition, 2 patients had successful outcomes and 71 had failed outcomes. We use these numbers to determine the proportion of individuals with successful outcomes in the treatment (p_1) and the control (p_2) conditions.

To estimate an average effect size using Formula 14.1, we need to calculate the different proportion of success patients for the treatment condition versus the control conditions. The column headed by p_1 reports the calculated proportions of successes for the treatment condition, whereas the column headed by p_2 reports the proportion of successes in the control condition. The proportion of success in the treatment condition is obtained by dividing the number of success cases by the total number of patients (p_1 = Treatment Success/Total Treatment). For Study 1 in

TABLE 14.3 Data for Meta-Analysis Variation 3 on Differences in Proportions

Study #	Total (n)	Treatment Success	Treatment Failure	Control Success	Control Failure	Treatment (p_1)	Control (p_2)	$t_i(p_1-p_2)$	v_i	$w_i = 1/v_i$	$t_i * w_i$	$t_i * t_i * w_i$
1	153	22	58	2	71	0.27500	0.02740	0.24760	0.00286	349.99176	86.65892	21.45699
2	41	8	10	5	18	0.44444	0.21739	0.22705	0.02111	47.36087	10.75343	2.44160
3	148	21	40	12	75	0.34426	0.13793	0.20633	0.00507	197.33648	40.71669	8.40113
4	41	17	5	10	9	0.77273	0.52632	0.24641	0.02110	47.38401	11.67596	2.87709
5	143	58	12	44	29	0.82857	0.60274	0.22583	0.00531	188.35170	42.53578	9.60593
6	110	49	26	8	27	0.65333	0.22857	0.42476	0.00806	124.10408	52.71469	22.39119
7	50	9	15	2	24	0.37500	0.07692	0.29808	0.01250	80.02163	23.85260	7.10991
8	145	49	26	11	59	0.65333	0.15714	0.49619	0.00491	203.58389	101.01639	50.12337
9	262	97	4	52	109	0.96040	0.32298	0.63741	0.00173	576.45095	367.43829	234.21056
10	60	14	16	3	27	0.46667	0.10000	0.36667	0.01130	88.52459	32.45902	11.90164
11	46	10	13	6	17	0.43478	0.26087	0.17391	0.01907	52.44397	9.12069	1.58621
12	54	20	7	12	15	0.74074	0.44444	0.29630	0.01626	61.50938	18.22500	5.40000
13	2,011	1,098	429	189	295	0.71906	0.39050	0.32856	0.00062	1602.43946	526.49928	172.98719
14	217	108	60	10	39	0.64286	0.20408	0.43878	0.00468	213.60386	93.72414	41.12386
15	89	33	33	11	12	0.50000	0.47826	0.02174	0.01464	68.32049	1.48523	0.03229
16	435	125	78	137	95	0.61576	0.59052	0.02525	0.00221	452.94342	11.43515	0.28870
17	77	45	7	17	8	0.86538	0.68000	0.18538	0.01094	91.37201	16.93896	3.14022
Sum	4,082	1,783	839	531	929	10.29232	5.44606	4.84626	0.16237	4445.74253	1447.25022	595.07786
Mean	240.118	104.882	49.353	31.235	54.647	0.60543	0.32036	0.28507	0.00955	261.51427	85.13237	35.00458

Table 14.3, the proportion of successes in the treatment condition is 0.275 = (22/[22 + 58]). A similar approach is used to obtain the proportion of successes for the control condition (p_2 = Control Success/Total Controls). For Study 1, the proportion of successes in the control condition is 0.027 = (2/[2 + 71]).

With these values, we can calculate the effect size for each study (symbolized as t_i). The effect size is calculated as the difference in the proportion of successes for the treatment versus the control condition ($t_i = [P_{i1} - P_{i2}]$). For Study 1, the value of t_i is 0.248 = (0.275 − 0.027). Similar calculations are made for the other studies.

Task 2 (Variation 3):
Calculate a Variance Estimate Within Each Study (v_i)

The next step is to calculate the variance estimates for each study. Each of the studies will be weighted by an estimate of the study variance; this procedure creates a standardized effect size index. Formula 14.12 indicates the variables needed for these calculations.

$$v_i = \frac{[p_{i1} * (1 - p_{i1})]}{(n_{i1})} + \frac{[p_{i2} * (1 - p_{i2})]}{(n_{i2})} \qquad (14.12)$$

The two numerators are the variance estimates, respectively, for the treatment condition and for the control condition. For Study 1, Formula 14.12 is calculated as follows:

$$v_i = \frac{[0.275 * (1 - 0.275)]}{(80)} + \frac{[0.027 * (1 - .027)]}{(80)} = 0.00286.$$

This value is reported in the column labeled as (v_i).

Task 3 (Variation 3): Calculate the Weighting Factor (w_i) for Each Study

You will also need to calculate the weighting factor, $w_i = (1/v_i)$ (Formula 14.2). For the first study, this value is 1/0.00286 = 349.992. The values of v_i and w_i for the remaining studies are also presented in Table 14.3.

Task 4 (Variation 3):
Adjust Each Study Effect Size by the Weighting Factor

Next we create an "adjusted effect size" by multiplying the unstandardized effect sizes (t_i) by the weighting factor (w_i). This procedure produces a value of 86.659 for Study 1, and this value is reported in the column with the $t_i * w_i$ label. The values of $t_i * w_i$ for the remaining studies are also presented in Table 14.3.

Task 5 (Variation 3): Calculate the Average Effect Size T•

To compute the average effect size, you use Formula 14.1*. First, you sum all of the $t_i * w_i$ calculated for each study. (The sum across all of the studies = 1447.250.) You divide this sum by the sum of the average variance estimates (the sum of the column labeled w_i = 4445.742). (Note: your own calculations may be slightly different from that which we show in Table 14.3, unless you use at least eight decimal places in your calculations.)

$$\overline{T•} = \frac{\sum_{i=1}^{k} w_i t_i}{\sum_{i=1}^{k} w_i} = \frac{(1447.250)}{(4445.742)} = 0.325 \qquad (14.1^*)$$

The resulting value (0.325) is the average effect size combined across all of the studies in our data set.

Task 6 (Variation 3):
Calculate a Conditional Variance (V) and
Standard Error of Estimate Across All Studies

The first step in computing a standard error and then testing for significance is to compute the variance of the sampling distribution of effect sizes. The formula for computing this variance is

$$V• = \frac{1}{\sum_{i=1}^{k} (w_i)} = \frac{1}{\sum_{i=1}^{k} (1/v_i)} \qquad (14.3^*)$$

Using Table 14.3, the conditional variance would be 0.0002. The square root of this figure is the standard error, which would be 0.015 for the set of studies in Table 14.3.

Task 7 (Variation 3):
Calculate a Confidence Interval for T•

Calculating the confidence interval involves calculating upper and lower limits of the average effect size (as in Formula 14.6*). The value of C_α in this formula is the critical value in the sampling distribution that includes (1- alpha) proportion of the sampling distribution (usually 95% of the sampling distribution). The mean effect size (0.325) was obtained in Task 5. For a two-tailed test for the normal distribution with an alpha = 0.05, the value of C_α = 1.96.

$$[T • - C_\alpha (V•)^{\frac{1}{2}}] \leq \delta \leq [T • + C_\alpha (V•)^{\frac{1}{2}}] =$$
$$[0.325 - (1.96)(.0002)^{\frac{1}{2}}] \leq \delta \leq [0.325 + (1.96)(.0002)^{\frac{1}{2}}] = \quad (14.6*)$$
$$[0.296] \leq \delta \leq [0.355]$$

Thus, we have 95% confidence that the population value for the effect size parameter lies between 0.296 and 0.355.

Task 8 (Variation 3):
Calculate the Heterogeneity of the Effect Size Statistic (Q)

You use this statistic to determine whether all the studies in your data set appear to come from the same population. Formula 14.7* is used to calculate the heterogeneity of effect sizes:

$$Q = \sum_{i=1}^{k} w_i t_i^2 - \frac{\left(\sum_{i=1}^{k} w_i t_i\right)^2}{\sum_{i=1}^{k} w_i} =$$

$$\left(595.078 - \frac{(1447.250)^2}{4445.742}\right) = 123.945 \quad (14.7*)$$

Using the numbers from Table 14.3, the value of 595.078 was obtained by summing the column headed by $w_i * t_i * t_i$, and the value of 1447.250 was obtained by summing the column headed by $w_i * t_i$. The value of 4445.7425 was obtained by summing the column headed by w_i.

This value (Q) is distributed as a χ_2 statistic with k-1 degrees of freedom and can be evaluated using a standard χ_2 table. For the example in Table 14.3, the value for the $Q_{(16)}$ statistic is 124.430, which is statistically significant, $p < .001$. These results suggest that the variability among the studies is greater than what would be expected based on the "average" variability observed within studies from the same population.

This value of the Q statistic with 16 degrees of freedom (the number of studies in the data set minus 1) is statistically significant, suggesting that the studies do not come from a common population. As a consequence, we are led to some approach to understand the potential source of variability among the studies. A first possibility is to try using one of the other coded variables from the data extraction phase. A second possible solution is to use a random rather than a fixed effect model for testing hypotheses about these data.

Task 9 (Variation 3):
Perform a Test of Significance on the Average Effect Size

The formula to be used for testing the statistical significance of the average effect size is similar to a traditional Z or t test. The numerator contains the absolute value of the mean effect size (0.325), and the denominator is the pooled variance estimate (0.0002) calculated in Formula 14.8*.

$$Z = \frac{\left|\overline{T} \bullet\right|}{(V\bullet)^{1/2}} = \frac{|0.325|}{(0.0002)^{1/2}} = 21.7056: p < .001 \qquad (14.8^*)$$

For the example described in Table 14.3, the combined results ($Z = 22.981$) provide evidence that the null hypothesis is false for this set of research participants. The average effect size of 0.325 is unlikely to have been sampled from a population with a mean effect size of 0.00.

Variation 4: Combining Study Effect Sizes Using a Quality-Weighted Approach

In this variation, each study has been rated according to its research quality. The index used to conduct the rating can be based on any number of models. In this case, the quality rating is an overall number ranging from 0 to 1.0, which is a combination of internal and external validity criteria. In this chapter, we demonstrate the methods for adjusting each effect size by the quality index and for combining these quality-weighted effects sizes into an average effect size. The numbers used for this example are derived from Table 14.3 (in the previous variation) and are re-created in Table 14.4 with the addition of the quality-weighted information. The basic tasks are the same as in the previous variation; the specific computations differ. The reader is advised to review Variation 3 prior to using this one.

Task 1 (Variation 4):
Calculate an Effect Size Index Within Each Study (t_i)

The data that are reported in the three columns headed by "Treatment Success," "Treatment Failure," and "Control Success" of Table 14.3 from Variation 3 provide the first step in calculating a quality-weighted solution. The effect size (t_i) along with the columns headed by v_i and w_i are listed again in Table 14.4. That is, these values are the proportion of successful outcomes in the treatment ($P1$) and the control ($P2$) conditions, and the column headed by t_i reports the differences in the proportion of success patients for the treatment versus the control conditions. The difference in proportions is the effect size. The effect size for Study 1 is 0.2476.

Task 2 (Variation 4):
Calculate a Variance Estimate Within Each Study (v_i)

The next step is to calculate the variance estimates for each study. This task is identical to the quality-unweighted solution, and the values for each study are reported in column v_i of Table 14.4. Formula 14.12* for calculating the within-study variance is

$$v_i = \frac{[P_{i_1} * (1 - P_{i_1})]}{(n_{i_1})} + \frac{[P_{i_2} * (1 - P_{i_2})]}{(n_{i_2})} \qquad (14.12^*)$$

Task 3 (Variation 4):
Calculate the Weighting Factor (w_i) for Each Study

We will also need to have the values of $w_i = (1/v_i)$, and these values are reported in the column labeled w_i of Table 14.4.

TABLE 14.4 Data for Meta–Analysis Variation 4 on Quality–Adjusted Approach

Study #	Study Size (n)	Quality q_i	t_i (P1 – P2)	v_i	$w_i = 1/v_i$	$w_i * q_i$	$w_i * q_i * t_i$	$w_i * q_i * q_i$
1	153	0.80300	0.24760	0.00286	349.99176	281.04338	69.58711	225.67784
2	41	0.66800	0.22705	0.02111	47.36087	31.63706	7.18329	21.13356
3	148	0.66800	0.20633	0.00507	197.33648	131.82077	27.19875	88.05628
4	41	0.70700	0.24641	0.02110	47.38401	33.50049	8.25491	23.68485
5	143	0.71200	0.22583	0.00531	188.35170	134.10641	30.28548	95.48376
6	110	0.57200	0.42476	0.00806	124.10408	70.98753	30.15280	40.60487
7	50	0.76000	0.29808	0.01250	80.02163	60.81644	18.12798	46.22049
8	145	0.38900	0.49619	0.00491	203.58389	79.19413	39.29537	30.80652
9	262	0.33600	0.63741	0.00173	576.45095	193.68752	123.45927	65.07901
10	60	0.26900	0.36667	0.01130	88.52459	23.81311	8.73148	6.40573
11	46	0.47600	0.17391	0.01907	52.44397	24.96333	4.34145	11.88254
12	54	0.44200	0.29630	0.01626	61.50938	27.18714	8.05545	12.01672
13	2011	0.72100	0.32856	0.00062	1602.43946	1155.35885	379.60598	833.01373
14	217	0.41300	0.43878	0.00468	213.60386	88.21839	38.70807	36.43420
15	89	0.41300	0.02174	0.01464	68.32049	28.21636	0.61340	11.65336
16	435	0.57700	0.02525	0.00221	452.94342	261.34835	6.59808	150.79800
17	77	0.55800	0.18538	0.01094	91.37201	50.98558	9.45194	28.44995
Sum			4.84626	0.16237	4445.74253	2676.88487	809.65080	1727.40140
Mean			0.28507	0.00955	261.51427	157.46382	47.62652	101.61185

Task 4 (Variation 4): Adjust Each Study Effect Size by the Quality Index and Weighting Factor ($t_i * w_i * q_i$)

The quality index is based on 0.00 to 1.0 for each study, with higher scores indicating higher quality. The quality index for each study is reported in the column labeled "Quality (q_i)" of Table 14.4. For example, the index for Study 1 is 0.803. To use this quality score, we create a quality-weighted inverse variance ($w_i * q_i$) by multiplying the weighting factor by the quality index. For Study 1 of Table 14.4, this value is (349.9918) * (0.803) = 281.0434 and is reported in the column labeled $w_i * q_i$.

The next step is to use this modified weighting factor to adjust the effect size. The weighting factor adjusts the effect size by the study variance. By multiplying all three $w_i * q_i * t_i$, you have modified the effect size for both the weighting factor (adjusted for variance) and the quality score. This value is reported in the column labeled by $w_i * q_i * t_i$. For Study 1 in Table 14.4, this value is (0.2476) * (281.0434) * 69.5871.

Task 5 (Variation 4): Calculate the Average Effect Size T•

We create the numerator value for our average effect size (Formula 14.1*, weighted here for quality) by summing the column labeled by $q_i * w_i * t_i$ in Table 14.4 to yield a value of 809.6508. We obtain the denominator value for this equation by adding the values in the column headed by $w_i * q_i$, the sum of which is 2676.8849. Our quality-and variance-weighted average effect size is now calculated in Formula 14.1* (here weighted for quality) as (809.6508/2676.8849) = 0.3025.

$$\overline{T\bullet} = \frac{\sum_{i=1}^{k} q_i w_i t_i}{\sum_{i=1}^{k} q_i w_i} = \frac{(809.6508)}{(2676.8849)} = (0.3025) \qquad (14.1^*)$$

Task 6 (Variation 4): Calculate a Conditional Variance (V•) and Standard Error of Estimate Across All Studies

In the next step, we calculate the conditional variance with Formula 14.13. The numerator value of the conditional variance includes the quality weight as well as the usual weighting factor. This requires that we first calculate $q_i^2 * w_i$ for each study by multiplying values in the column labeled $w_i * q_i$ by the column labeled q_i, and these values are reported in the column labeled $w_i * q_i * q_i$. For Study 1 of Variation 4, this value is 225.6778.

$$V\bullet = \frac{\left(\sum_{i=1}^{k} q_i^{\,2} w_i\right)}{\left(\sum_{i=1}^{k} q_i w_i\right)^2} = \left(\frac{(1727.4014)}{(2676.8849)^2}\right) = .0002 \qquad (14.13)$$

The sum of the numbers in this column yields a value of 1727.4014. We calculate the denominator value of the conditional variance by adding the values of the column labeled $w_i * q_i$, which yields a value of 2676.8849, and then we square this value. We divide this into the numerator value, which yields a value of 0.0002, the conditional variance. We also calculate the square root to yield a value of 0.0155, which is our standard error of estimate.

Task 7 (Variation 4): Calculate Confidence Interval for $T\bullet$

We again use Formula 14.6* to provide the calculations for the confidence interval of the average effect size. The value of C_α in this formula is the critical value in the sampling distribution that includes alpha proportion of the sampling distribution. For a two-tailed test for the normal distribution with an alpha = 0.05, the value of $C_\alpha = 1.96$.

$$[T \bullet -C_\alpha (V\bullet)^{\frac{1}{2}}] \le \delta \le [T \bullet +C_\alpha (V\bullet)^{\frac{1}{2}}] =$$
$$[0.3025 - (1.96)(.0002)^{\frac{1}{2}}] \le \delta \le [0.3025 + (1.96)(.0002)^{\frac{1}{2}}] =$$
$$0.2720 \le \delta \le 0.3329 \qquad (14.6^*)$$

Thus, we have 95% confidence that the population value for the effect size parameter lies between 0.272 and 0.333. Remember that the quality-unadjusted confidence interval in Variation 3 ranged from 0.296 to 0.355. Thus, the quality-adjusted confidence interval is just slightly larger than the unadjusted confidence interval.

Task 8 (Variation 4):
Calculate the Heterogeneity of Effect Size Statistic (Q)

As we stated in the previous section, you need to determine whether all the studies in your data set come from the same population. Formula 14.14 is almost identical to Formula 14.7, with the exception of the inclusion of the quality-weighted information as noted.

$$Q = \sum_{i=1}^{k} w_i q_i t_i^2 - \frac{\left(\sum_{i=1}^{k} q_i w_i t_i \right)^2}{\sum_{i=1}^{k} q_i w_i} \qquad (14.14)$$

$$= 299.734 - [(809.6508)2 \,/\, 2676.8849] = 54.8468.$$

This χ^2 with 16 degrees of freedom is statistically significant, suggesting that the studies do not come from a common population. As a consequence, we are led to consider some other approach to understand the potential source of variability among the studies. A first possibility is to try explain the variation among the studies using the measures of research quality or one of the other coded variables from the data extraction phase. A second possible solution is to use a random rather than fixed effects model for testing hypotheses about these data.

Task 9 (Variation 4):
Perform a Test of Significance on the Average Effect Size

The formula to be used for testing the statistical significance is similar to a traditional Z or t test. The numerator contains the absolute value of the mean effect size, and the denominator is the square root of the pooled variance estimate shown in Formula 14.10*.

$$Z = \frac{|\overline{T} \bullet|}{(V \bullet)^{1/2}} = \frac{|0.3025|}{(0.0002)^{1/2}} = 19.4805: p < .001 \qquad (14.10^*)$$

The results (19.4805), based on the quality-weighted statistics, are also statistically significant. The weighted effect size (0.3025) is smaller in absolute value than the unweighted value (0.3254), and the conditional variance estimate is about the same (0.00022 vs. 0.00024).

Variation 5: Perform Random Rather Than Fixed Effects Meta-Analysis

One of the subtle but important considerations in meta-analysis is the use of random rather than fixed effects procedures. This distinction has both theoretical and practical implications. The usual assumption of a fixed effects model is that all of your studies were sampled from a single population. This population is assumed to have a mean parameter value for the effect size, and this value is often represented by the symbol "theta." However, you may be actually randomly sampling from multiple populations simultaneously. For example, some of the studies in your meta-analysis could be sampling from a treatment population that is elderly, and others could be from a treatment population that is young. Each of these populations will have an effect due to the treatment and an effect due to the age of the patient. To model effectively the variation due to the treatment and to different populations, it is useful to use a random effects model.

In developing the random effects model, we need to estimate the combined effects of both the treatment and other parameters. In practice, this means estimating the between- and within-study variances. We demonstrate the random effects approach using our example from the fixed effects model (Variation 3) presented again in Table 14.5.

Task 1 (Variation 5):
Calculate an Effect Size Index Within Each Study (t_i)

This procedure is the same as the procedure to be used with the fixed effects approach. For our current example, the values contained in Table 14.5 under the column labeled t_i are the same as in Table 14.3 (t_i). The effect size estimate for the first study in our example is 0.2476.

Task 2 (Variation 5):
Calculate a Variance Estimate Within Each Study (v_i^a)

This procedure is similar to the fixed effects approach, except that each variance estimate also contains an estimate of the between-study source of variance σ_θ^2. The variance estimate for each study is represented in Formula 14.15:

$$v_i^a = \hat{\sigma}_\theta^2 + v_i \qquad (14.15)$$

The within-study variance v_i for each study is estimated in the same way that we have described previously (e.g., Formula 14.12). The values for the within-study variance for our example are reported in Table 14.5 under the column labeled v_i (same as Table 14.3, column headed by v_i). The value of v_i for the first study is 0.00286. The between-study variance is estimated by Formula 14.16:

$$\hat{\sigma}_\theta^2 = \frac{[Q - (k-1)]}{c} \qquad (14.16)$$

TABLE 14.5 Data for Meta-Analysis Variation 5 on Random Effects Approach

Study #	t_i ($p_1 - p_2$)	v_i	$\dfrac{w_i}{(1/v_i)}$	$t_i * w_i$	$w_i * w_i$	v_i [a]	w_i [a]	$t_i * w_i$ [a]
1	0.24760	0.00286	349.99176	86.65892	122494.23342	0.03226	31.00082	7.67589
2	0.22705	0.02111	47.36087	10.75343	2243.05164	0.05051	19.79630	4.49481
3	0.20633	0.00507	197.33648	40.71669	38941.68801	0.03447	29.01285	5.98626
4	0.24641	0.02110	47.38401	11.67596	2245.24434	0.05050	19.80035	4.87903
5	0.22583	0.00531	188.35170	42.53578	35476.36179	0.03471	28.81079	6.50639
6	0.42476	0.00806	124.10408	52.71469	15401.82301	0.03746	26.69674	11.33976
7	0.29808	0.01250	80.02163	23.85260	6403.46067	0.04190	23.86827	7.11458
8	0.49619	0.00491	203.58389	101.01639	41446.39838	0.03431	29.14434	14.46114
9	0.63741	0.00173	576.45095	367.43829	332295.69801	0.03113	32.11845	20.47277
10	0.36667	0.01130	88.52459	32.45902	7836.60306	0.04070	24.57226	9.00983
11	0.17391	0.01907	52.44397	9.12069	2750.36952	0.04847	20.63218	3.58821
12	0.29630	0.01626	61.50938	18.22500	3733.40321	0.04566	21.90212	6.48952
13	0.32856	0.00062	1602.43946	526.49928	2567812.23627	0.03002	33.30663	10.94326
14	0.43878	0.00468	213.60386	93.72414	45626.60822	0.03408	29.34138	12.87428
15	0.02174	0.01464	68.32049	1.48523	4667.68983	0.04404	22.70823	0.49366
16	0.02525	0.00221	452.94342	11.43515	205157.73863	0.03161	31.63778	0.79874
17	0.18538	0.01094	91.37201	16.93896	8348.84382	0.04034	24.78667	4.59507
Sum	4.84626	0.16237	4445.74253	1447.25022	3442931.45182	0.66217	449.13617	131.72319
Mean	0.28507	0.00955	261.51427	85.13237	202525.37952	0.03895	26.41977	7.74842

a. Variables have different numeric values, due to adjustments for between-study variance, than the same variable without this notation (i.e., the within-study variance).

In the above expression, the value of Q is obtained from the heterogeneity of variance test performed for the fixed effects example of Table 14.3. Recall for the fixed effects example that $Q = 123.9455$ (Variation 3, Task 8). Formula 14.17 estimates the value of c:

$$c = \sum_{i=1}^{k} w_i - \left(\frac{\sum\limits_{i=1}^{k} w_i^2}{\sum\limits_{i=1}^{k} w_i} \right) = (4445.7425) - \frac{(3442931.4518)}{(4445.7425)} = 3671.3091 \qquad (14.17)$$

The values of w_i are obtained from the fixed effects analysis in Table 14.3 and are repeated in Table 14.5. The value of w_i for the first study is $1/v_i = 1/0.0028 = 349.99176$. The sum of the w_i across all studies $= 4445.7425$. The values in Table 14.5 at the bottom of the column labeled $w_i * w_i$ provide the estimate for the sum of $(w_i)^2 = 3{,}442{,}931.4518$. The value of $c = 3671.3091$.

We can substitute these values of Q and c into Formula 14.16* to estimate σ_θ^2:

$$\hat{\sigma}_\theta^2 = \frac{[Q - (k-1)]}{c} = \frac{[123.9455 - (v_i 17 - 1)]}{3671.3091} = 0.0294 \qquad (14.16^*)$$

The estimated value of the between-study variance is 0.02940, and this number is added to each value of vi to produce an estimate of v_i^a. Variables with the dagger superscript notation (e.g., v_i^a) have different numeric values, due to adjustments for between-study variance, than the same variable without this notation (e.g., v_i), the within-study variance. The values of v_i^a for the between-study variances in our example are reported in Table 14.5. The value of v_i^a for the first study is (0.00286 + 0.02940) = 0.03226.

Task 3 (Variation 5): Calculate the Random Effects Weighting Factor (w_i^a)

This procedure is analogous to the fixed effects approach except that we use $1/v_i^a$. The value for the first study is $w_i^a = 1/0.03226 = 31.0008$ (Table 14.5).

Task 4 (Variation 5):
Adjust Each Study Effect Size by the Weighting Factor ($t_i * w_i^a$)

This procedure is analogous to the fixed effects approach except that we use w_i^a instead of w_i. For Study 1, the resulting value is $t_i * w_i^a = (0.2476 * 31.00082) = (7.6759)$.

Task 5 (Variation 5): Calculate the Average Effect Size $T\bullet$

This average value is obtained from Formula 14.1* except for the use of w_i^a instead of w_i. Note that the obtained value of the random effect size is similar to the fixed effects value of 0.3255.

$$\overline{T\bullet} = \frac{\sum\limits_{i=1}^{k} w_i^a t_i}{\sum\limits_{i=1}^{k} w_i^a} = \frac{(131.6759)}{(449.1362)} = 0.29328 \qquad (14.1^*)$$

Task 6 (Variation 5):
Calculate a Conditional Variance ($V\bullet$)
and Standard Error of Estimate Across All Studies

This estimate is obtained using Formula 14.3* except for the use of w_i^a.

$$V\bullet = \frac{1}{\sum\limits_{i=1}^{k} w_i^a} = \frac{(1)}{(449.13617)} = 0.00223 \qquad (14.3^*)$$

The standard error of estimate $(V\bullet)^{1/2}$ is the square root of 0.00223 = 0.04719. This value is used in calculating the confidence interval and in tests of significance.

Task 7 (Variation 5): Calculate a Confidence Interval for $T\bullet$

We use the value of $T\bullet$ and $(V\bullet)^{1/2}$ to calculate the confidence interval with Formula 14.6*. The value of C_α is the critical value of t (t distribution) when we have a value of alpha = 0.05. The calculations below use data from the previous Task 5 and Task 6, which use w_i^a.

$$[T\bullet - C_\alpha(V\bullet)^{1/2}] \le \delta \le [T\bullet + C_\alpha(V\bullet)^{1/2}]$$
$$[0.2933 - (1.96)(0.00223)^{1/2}] \le \delta \le [0.2933 + (1.96)(0.00223)^{1/2}] =$$
$$[0.2008] \le \delta \le [0.3858] \qquad (14.6^*)$$

Note that the confidence interval in the random effects case goes from 0.2008 to 0.3858 and is substantially larger than in the fixed effects case, where the interval ranged from 0.296 to 0.355 (Variation 3, Task 7).

Task 8 (Variation 5):
Calculate the Heterogeneity of Effect Size Statistic (Q)

Note that this procedure was completed as part of Variation 3 (Task 8) and the value of $Q = 123.9455$.

Task 9 (Variation 5):
Perform a Test of Significance on the Average Effect Size

This calculation, shown in Formula 14.8*, also uses data from Tasks 5 and 6 above.

$$Z = \frac{\left|\overline{T} \bullet\right|}{(V\bullet)^{1/2}} = \frac{|0.2933|}{(0.0022)^{1/2}} = 6.2155: p < .001. \tag{14.8*}$$

The value of Z indicates that the average random effect size is statistically significant so that you would make a similar statistical decision with a random or a fixed effects analysis. However, you might make quite different decisions in your meta-analysis if the effect sizes are smaller, if the sample sizes are smaller, or if the between-study variance is much larger than the current case.

Variation 6: Combining Study Effect Size Differences in Odds Ratios

One of the most useful statistics in healthcare research is the odds ratio. Two different approaches are used to combine odds ratios depending on the number of studies and the sample sizes of the studies. When you have large sample sizes and a small number of studies, you would use the log odds ratio (see Fleiss, 1981; Shadish & Haddock, 1994). However, you would use the Mantel-Haenszel (MH) procedure when you have a larger number of studies to combine, but the sample size for each study is small (Fleiss, 1981). Both of these methods are valuable approaches, and we will demonstrate each of them in the variations that follow.

For this example, we will use data that have been artificially generated to support a hypothetical meta-analysis from randomized controlled clinical trials. The purpose of these trials was to test the efficacy of a new bacteriocidal antibiotic (D-71) for adult and elderly patients (age range: 55 to 95 years) diagnosed with chronic *E. coli pyelonephritis*. The control group was treated with a traditional bacteriostatic antibioic (*Y*). Seventeen RCTs met our validation criteria, and the hypothetical data are displayed in Table 14.6. "Infection Cleared" indicates that catheterized urine showed no growth 2 weeks after 16 weeks of treatment and again at the 3- and

TABLE 14.6 Computation for Variation 6 Using Odds Ratios for Hypothetical Pyelonephritis Population (RCT) Testing New Antibiotic

| Study # | Sample (n) | Treatment (New Antibiotic D-71) | | Control (Traditional Antibiotic Y) | | Odds Ration (OR) | Log Odds (Natural Log) $t_i = \ln(OR)$ | v_i | $w_i (1/v_i)$ | $w_i * t_i$ | $w_i * t_i * t_i$ |
		Infection Cleared A	Infection Same B	Infection Cleared C	Infection Same D						
1	153	22	58	2	71	13.4655	2.6001	0.5768	1.7338	4.5080	11.7214
2	41	8	10	5	18	2.8800	1.0578	0.4806	2.0809	2.2012	2.3284
3	148	21	40	12	75	3.2813	1.1882	0.1693	5.9072	7.0190	8.3402
4	41	17	5	10	9	3.0600	1.1184	0.4699	2.1280	2.3799	2.6618
5	143	58	12	44	29	3.1856	1.1586	0.1578	6.3377	7.3432	8.5081
6	110	49	26	8	27	6.3606	1.8501	0.2209	4.5268	8.3751	15.4950
7	50	9	15	2	24	7.2000	1.9741	0.7194	1.3900	2.7439	5.4167
8	145	49	26	11	59	10.1084	2.3134	0.1667	5.9978	13.8751	32.0982
9	262	97	4	52	109	50.8317	3.9285	0.2887	3.4636	13.6069	53.4552
10	60	14	16	3	27	7.8750	2.0637	0.5043	1.9830	4.0922	8.4450
11	46	10	13	6	17	2.1795	0.7791	0.4024	2.4850	1.9360	1.5084
12	54	20	7	12	15	3.5714	1.2730	0.3429	2.9167	3.7128	4.7263
13	2,011	1,098	429	189	295	3.9949	1.3850	0.0119	83.8744	116.1675	160.8940
14	217	108	60	10	39	7.0200	1.9488	0.1516	6.5977	12.8574	25.0561
15	89	33	33	11	12	1.0909	0.0870	0.2348	4.2581	0.3705	0.0322
16	435	125	78	137	95	1.1113	0.1055	0.0386	25.8758	2.7299	0.2880
17	77	45	7	17	8	3.0252	1.1070	0.3489	2.8661	3.1727	3.5122
Sum	4,082	1,783	839	531	929	130.2413	25.9383	5.2856	164.4226	207.0916	344.4871
Mean	240.118	104.88235	49.352941	31.235294	54.647059	7.6613	1.5258	0.3109	9.6719	12.1819	20.2639

6 months posttreatment period. "Infection Same" indicates that urine grew more than 100,000 colonies per milliliter (ml) of the same coliform strain at any time two weeks after the 16-week treatment period and prior to the 6-month posttreatment follow-up.

The same sequence of tasks used in the previous variations will be used for odds ratios as well. Table 14.6 contains all the computations for the example, and the tasks are again listed below for your convenience.

Task 1 (Variation 6):
Calculate an Effect Size Index Within Each Study (t_i)

The values considered to be the effect size from each study are not the odds ratios themselves but rather the natural log (ln) of the odds ratios (Shadish & Haddock, 1994). The odds ratios are calculated using Formula 14.18 based on the data in Table 14.6. We can use Table 14.6 to illustrate the computations. The frequency in each cell of a two-by-two table are here labeled, respectively, *A, B, C,* and *D*. Calculation of the odds ratio uses Formula 14.18:

$$\text{Odds Ratio} = (A * D)/(B * C) \tag{14.18}$$

The results of the calculations for the odds ratio for each study are listed under the column titled "Odds Ratio" in Table 14.6. For Study 1, the odds ratio would be the following:

$$\text{Odds Ratio} = 22 * 71/58 * 2 = 1562/116 = 13.466$$

The natural logs of the odds ratios are presented in the column labeled as "Log Odds." Calculating the natural logs (ln) of each of these odds ratios can be done on a regular spreadsheet or by looking them up in a table. It is easier to perform the operation on a spreadsheet by selecting ln transformation functions in the spreadsheet; each required ln number will be calculated and inserted into the space. The resulting value is the effect size (t_i).

Task 2 (Variation 6):
Calculate a Variance Estimate Within Each Study (v_i)

Formula 14.19 is used to calculate the variance of the odds ratio for each study. In this expression, we demonstrate the calculation of values for Study 1 in Table 14.6.

$$v_i = \frac{1}{A_i} + \frac{1}{B_i} + \frac{1}{C_i} + \frac{1}{D_i}$$

$$v_1 = \frac{1}{22} + \frac{1}{58} + \frac{1}{2} + \frac{1}{71} = 0.5768 \tag{14.19}$$

Task 3 (Variation 6): Calculate the Weighting Factor (w_i) for Each Study

The value of w_i can be obtained for each study by calculating $1/v_i$, Formula 14.2*, as in the previous examples. For the first study, this calculation yields a value of 1.734. The values for all studies are presented under the column headed w_i.

Task 4 (Variation 6): Adjust Each Study Effect Size by the Weighting Factor ($w_i * t_i$)

We have adjusted the log odds ratio in each study with the study variance by multiplying the log odds value times the weighting factor, w_i. This value for Study 1 is $(2.600 * 1.734) = 4.508$. The values for the remaining studies are presented under the column headed $t_i * w_i$.

Task 5 (Variation 6): Calculate the Average Effect Size $T\bullet$

We obtain an average log odds ratio using Formula 14.1* in two steps. First, we sum across all of the weighted log odds ratios (i.e., the sum of the column headed by $t_i * w_i$. The resulting value is 207.0916. Next we divide this value by the sum of the w_i or 164.42. The resulting division $(207.0916)/(164.42) = 1.259$. Thus, the average odds ratio is 1.260.

$$\overline{T\bullet} = \frac{\sum\limits_{i=1}^{k} w_i t_i}{\sum\limits_{i=1}^{k} w_i} \tag{14.1*}$$

Task 6 (Variation 6): Calculate a Conditional Variance ($V\bullet$) and Standard Error of Estimate Across All Studies

The conditional variance ($V\bullet$) for the log odds ratio is calculated using Formula 14.3*. The standard error $(V\bullet)^{1/2}$ is the square root of this number. We compute this number from the sum of the variance estimates from each study (i.e., the numbers in Table 14.6 under the column headed (w_i)), and then we divide 1 by this number.

$$V\bullet = \frac{1}{\sum\limits_{i=1}^{k} w_i} = \frac{1}{\sum\limits_{i=1}^{k} (1/v_i)} \qquad (14.3^*)$$

The sum of the weighting factor (w_i) is 164.42, thereby making the conditional variance computation, $V = (1/164.42) = 0.006$. We convert these into a standard error of estimate by calculating the square root of this number, and the result is 0.0780.

Task 7 (Variation 6): Calculate Log Odds Ratio (T•) Confidence Interval

This procedure is accomplished using Formula 14.6*. The value of C_α in this formula is the critical value in the sampling distribution that includes alpha proportion of the sampling distribution. For a two-tailed test for the normal distribution with an alpha = 0.05, the value of $C_\alpha = 1.96$.

$$[T \bullet -C_\alpha(V\bullet)^{1/2}] \le \delta \le [T \bullet +C_\alpha(V\bullet)^{1/2}] =$$
$$[1.260 - (1.96)(.006)^{1/2}] \le \delta \le [1.260 + (1.96)(.006)^{1/2}] =$$
$$[1.108] \le \delta \le [1.411] \qquad (14.6^*)$$

Thus, we can say with 95% certainty that the value of the odds ratio lies between 1.108 and 1.411 if the average odds ratio was 1.260, calculated in Task 5 for this variation.

Task 8 (Variation 6):
Calculate Log Odds Ratio Heterogeneity of Effect Size Statistic (Q)

We calculate a log odds heterogeneity statistic to evaluate the plausibility of the hypothesis that all of the studies in the data set come from the same population. The statistic is calculated using Formula 14.7*, and the relevant values are presented in Table 14.6. We obtain the values of $w_i * t_i * t_i$ from the column with the same heading. The sum is 344.4871.

$$Q = \sum_{i=1}^{k} w_i t_i^2 - \frac{\left(\sum_{i=1}^{k} w_i t_i \right)^2}{\sum_{i=1}^{k} w_i}$$

$$= (344.4871) - \frac{(207.0916 * 207.0916)}{(164.4226)}$$

$$= 83.6356 \qquad\qquad (14.7^*)$$

This value Q is distributed as a $\chi 2$ statistic with $k - 1$ degrees of freedom. With 16 degrees of freedom, this value of 83.6356 is statistically significant ($p < .001$). The results suggest that the 17 studies were not sampled from the same population.

Task 9 (Variation 6):
Perform a Test of Significance on Log Odds Ratio Average Effect Size

The formula to be used for testing the statistical significance of an odds ratio is Formula 14.8*, similar to a traditional Z or t test. The numerator contains the absolute value of the mean effect size, and the denominator is the square root of the pooled variance estimate.

$$Z = \frac{|T \bullet|}{(V \bullet)^{1/2}} = \frac{|1.259|}{(0.0061)^{1/2}} = 16.15: p < .001 \qquad\qquad (14.8^*)$$

These results are consistent with the hypothesis that the probability of success in the treatment condition is higher than the probability of success in the control condition.

Variation 7: Combining Study Effect Size Differences in Odds Ratios With Small Sample Sizes (Mantel-Haenszel)

The Mantel-Haenszel method for combining odds ratio effect sizes is useful when the sample sizes are smaller. The computations are done across studies, so the sequence of steps differs from the above examples as we start off immediately computing an average effect size across studies, formerly Task 5. Note that in Variation 7, there are only five tasks for this method.

Task 1 (Variation 7): Calculate the Average Effect Size T•

A computationally convenient form of the MH (average effect size across stud-ies) is based on cell frequencies where n_i is the total number of research participants in each study, and the values of *A, B, C,* and *D* are defined in Table 14.7a. The value for MH indicates that the probability of success in the treatment condition was 3.76 times as likely as in the control condition for the data in Table 14.7b and calculated using Formula 14.20.

$$\overline{O}_{MH} = T\bullet = \frac{\displaystyle\sum_{i=1}^{k}(A_i D_i / n_i)}{\displaystyle\sum_{i=1}^{k}(B_i C_i / n_i)} \tag{14.20}$$

Task 2 (Variation 7):
Calculate a Conditional Variance (V•)
and a Standard Error of Estimate Across All Studies

The variance expression for this formula is quite complex (Robins, Breslow, & Greenland, 1986). The values for *P, Q, R,* and *S* are defined below, and we report the values of P, Q, R, and S for the first study presented in Table 14.7a. *(Note that the Q listed in Formula 14.21 and 14.23 is not the same variable that is a test for heterogeneity.)*

$$V\bullet = \frac{\displaystyle\sum_{i=1}^{k} P_i R_i}{2\left(\displaystyle\sum_{i=1}^{k} R_i\right)^2} + \frac{\displaystyle\sum_{i=1}^{k}(P_i S_i + Q_i R_i)}{2\left(\displaystyle\sum_{i=1}^{k} R_i\right)\left(\displaystyle\sum_{i=1}^{k} S_i\right)} + \frac{\displaystyle\sum_{i=1}^{k} Q_i S_i}{2\left(\displaystyle\sum_{i=1}^{k} S_i\right)^2} \tag{14.21}$$

$$P_i = \frac{(A_i + D_i)}{n}; P_1 = \frac{(22+71)}{153} = 0.608 \tag{14.22}$$

$$Q_i = \frac{(B_i + C_i)}{n}; Q_1 = \frac{(58+2)}{153} = 0.392 \tag{14.23}$$

$$R_i = \frac{(A_i * D_i)}{n}; R_1 = \frac{(22*71)}{153} = 10.209 \tag{14.24}$$

$$S_i = \frac{(B_i * C_i)}{n}; S_1 = \frac{(58*2)}{153} = 0.758 \tag{14.25}$$

The value of $V\bullet$ is obtained from Formula 14.21. In Table 14.7b, we present the calculations for the products of P_iR_i, P_iS_i, Q_iR_i, and Q_iS_i for each of the studies. Below are the calculations for $V\bullet$, and the summation values are obtained from Table 14.7.

$$V\bullet = \frac{(236.668)}{2(348.951)^2} + \frac{(170.339)}{2(348.951)(92.715)} + \frac{(34.660)}{2(92.715)^2}$$

$$= \left(\frac{1}{2}\right) * [(0.002) + (0.005) + (0.004)] = 0.006$$

This finding, then, indicates that the average variance across studies is 0.006.

Task 3 (Variation 7): Calculate a Confidence Interval for $T\bullet$

Following procedures recommended by Shadish and Haddock (1994), we would create a lower limit of the confidence intervals using Formula 14.26. Note that "exp" means *antilog*.

$$\varpi_L = \exp[\ln(T\bullet) \pm 1.96 * (V\bullet)^{1/2}] \tag{14.26}$$

This expression indicates that we take the reverse (antilog) of the natural log (ln) to determine the lower limit of the confidence interval at the alpha = 0.05 level. Using the values calculated above, this expression would be as follows:

$$\varpi_L = \exp[\ln(3.763) - 1.96 * (.006)^{1/2}]$$

$$= \exp[(1.324) + (0.152)]$$

$$= \exp[(1.324) - (0.152)]$$

$$= \exp(1.172) = 3.23$$

The upper confidence interval can be obtained by adding the second half of the expression. Using the values obtained above, the upper limit is as follows:

TABLE 14.7a Computation of Variation 7 (Columns 1–12 of 24) Combining Effect Size Differences in Odds Ratios With Small Sample Sizes (Mantel Haenszel)

Study #	Sample (n)	Risk Present (A)	Risk Absent (B)	Disease Present (C)	Disease Absent (D)	(A * D)/n	(B * C)/n	P (A + D)/n	Q (B + C)/n	R (A * D)/n	S (B * C)/n
1	153	22	58	2	71	10.2092	0.7582	0.6078	0.3922	10.2092	0.7582
2	41	8	10	5	18	3.5122	1.2195	0.6341	0.3659	3.5122	1.2195
3	148	21	40	12	75	10.6419	3.2432	0.6486	0.3514	10.6419	3.2432
4	41	17	5	10	9	3.7317	1.2195	0.6341	0.3659	3.7317	1.2195
5	143	58	12	44	29	11.7622	3.6923	0.6084	0.3916	11.7622	3.6923
6	110	49	26	8	27	12.0273	1.8909	0.6909	0.3091	12.0273	1.8909
7	50	9	15	2	24	4.3200	0.6000	0.6600	0.3400	4.3200	0.6000
8	145	49	26	11	59	19.9379	1.9724	0.7448	0.2552	19.9379	1.9724
9	262	97	4	52	109	40.3550	0.7939	0.7863	0.2137	40.3550	0.7939
10	60	14	16	3	27	6.3000	0.8000	0.6833	0.3167	6.3000	0.8000
11	46	10	13	6	17	3.6957	1.6957	0.5870	0.4130	3.6957	1.6957
12	54	20	7	12	15	5.5556	1.5556	0.6481	0.3519	5.5556	1.5556
13	2,011	1,098	429	189	295	161.0691	40.3187	0.6927	0.3073	161.0691	40.3187
14	217	108	60	10	39	19.4101	2.7650	0.6774	0.3226	19.4101	2.7650
15	89	33	33	11	12	4.4494	4.0787	0.5056	0.4944	4.4494	4.0787
16	435	125	78	137	95	27.2989	24.5655	0.5057	0.4943	27.2989	24.5655
17	77	45	7	17	8	4.6753	1.5455	0.6883	0.3117	4.6753	1.5455
Sum	4,082	1,783	839	531	929	348.9514	92.7145	11.0034	5.9966	348.9514	92.7145
Mean	240.118	104.882	49.3529	31.2353	54.6471	20.5266	5.4538	0.6473	0.3527	20.5266	5.4538

TABLE 14.7b Data for Meta-Analysis Variation 7 (Columns 13–24 of 24)

(PS + QR)	(Q * R)	(P * R)	(Q * S)	E	(A + C)	(B + D)	(A + B)	(C + D)	N²(N − 1)	V	(O − E)
4.4644	4.0036	6.2056	0.2973	12.5490	24.00	129.00	80.00	73.00	3558168	5	9.45098
2.0583	1.2849	2.2272	0.4462	5.7073	13.00	28.00	18.00	23.00	67240	2	2.2927
5.8428	3.7390	6.9028	1.1395	13.6014	33.00	115.00	61.00	87.00	3219888	6	7.3986
2.1386	1.3653	2.3664	0.4462	14.4878	27.00	14.00	22.00	19.00	67240	2	2.5122
6.8526	4.6062	7.1560	1.4459	49.9301	102.00	41.00	70.00	73.00	2903758	7	8.0699
5.0240	3.7175	8.3098	0.5845	38.8636	57.00	53.00	75.00	35.00	1318900	6	10.1364
1.8648	1.4688	2.8512	0.2040	5.2800	11.00	39.00	24.00	26.00	122500	2	3.7200
6.5567	5.0876	14.8503	0.5033	31.0345	60.00	85.00	75.00	70.00	3027600	9	17.9655
9.2497	8.6255	31.7295	0.1697	57.4389	149.00	113.00	101.00	161.00	17916084	15	39.5611
2.5417	1.9950	4.3050	0.2533	8.5000	17.00	43.00	30.00	30.00	212400	3	5.5000
2.5217	1.5265	2.1692	0.7004	8.0000	16.00	30.00	23.00	23.00	95220	3	2.0000
2.9630	1.9547	3.6008	0.5473	16.0000	32.00	22.00	27.00	27.00	154548	3	4.0000
77.4265	49.4981	111.5710	12.3903	977.2496	1287.00	724.00	1527.00	484.00	81286632	85	120.7504
8.1344	6.2613	13.1488	0.8919	91.3548	118.00	99.00	168.00	49.00	10171224	9	16.6452
4.2620	2.1997	2.2497	2.0164	32.6292	44.00	45.00	66.00	23.00	697048	4	0.3708
25.9165	13.4925	13.8063	12.1416	122.2667	262.00	173.00	203.00	232.00	82123650	26	2.7333
2.5210	1.4572	3.2181	0.4817	41.8701	62.00	15.00	52.00	25.00	450604	3	3.1299
170.3386	112.2836	236.6678	34.6596	1526.7630	2314.00	1768.00	2622.00	1460.00		191.8571	256.2369
10.0199	6.6049	13.9216	2.0388	89.5096	136.12	104.00	154.24	85.88		11.2857	15.0728

$$\omega_U = \exp[\ln(3.763) + 1.96*(0.006)^{\frac{1}{2}}$$
$$= \exp[(1.324) + (0.152)]$$
$$= \exp(1.476) = 4.38.$$

The 95% confidence interval for this example ranges from 3.23 through 4.38. This interval does not contain the value 1.00, so we can use this confidence interval to provide evidence permitting us to reject the null hypothesis that the probability of success is the same in the treatment as in the control condition.

Task 4 (Variation 7):
Calculate Odds Ratio Heterogeneity of Effect Size Statistics (Q)

We can use the same procedure in the Mantel-Haenszel as we used in the log odds procedure for Variation 6, Task 8.

Task 5 (Variation 7):
Perform Significance Test on Odds Ratio Average Effect Size

To test the significance of this overall Mantel-Haenszel odds ratio, you would use Formula 14.27:

$$\chi^2 = \frac{\left[\left|\sum_{i=1}^{k}(O_i - E_i)\right| - 0.5\right]^2}{\sum_{i=1}^{k} V_i}. \tag{14.27}$$

The values for O_i, A_i, E_i, and V_i are defined in Formulas 14.28 through 14.30 (see Shadish & Haddock, 1994).

$$E_i = \frac{(A_i + C_i)*(A_i + B_i)}{n_i}. \tag{14.28}$$

Although this expression looks somewhat complicated, we can understand what it represents by using our asbestos example. First, note that $(A + C)/n$ is the proportion of all individuals at risk who later had the disease, and $(A + B)$ is the number who had the disease. If the null hypothesis is correct, then you would expect the proportion of individuals who were at risk to have the disease—that is, the $(A)/(A + B)$

groups—to be the same proportion as those who were not a risk to have the disease—that is, the $(C)/(C + D)$ groups.

$$\frac{A_i}{(A_i + B_i)} = \frac{C_i}{(C_i + D_i)} = \frac{(A_i + C_i)}{n_i} \tag{14.29}$$

The value of E, then, is the expected number of successful team treatment patients in the condition, and the value $(O - E)$ is the difference between observed and expected values. The value of 0.5 in Formula 14.27 is subtracted from the value of $\Sigma(O_i - E_i)$ to improve the accuracy of the χ^2 approximation. If the null hypothesis is false, we would expect this value to be relatively large. The value of V_i (Formula 14.30) for each sample is the variance of the expression $(O_i - E_i)$, which can be written as the product of the four marginals (the row and column totals) divided by $n_i^2 * (n_i - 1)$ (Shadish & Haddock, 1994):

$$V_i = \frac{(A_i + C_i)(B_i + D_i)(A_i + B_i)(C_i + D_i)}{n_i^2(n_i - 1)} \tag{14.30}$$

Procedure C. Conduct a Sensitivity Analysis

As described previously under theoretical considerations (Section G, Chapter 13), a secondary or sensitivity analysis involves evaluating your synthesis results or outcomes. This is a method for exploring the impact of uncertainties, assumptions, and judgments on the conclusions of your analysis. Eddy et al. (1992, p. 310) describe three basic approaches you might consider in Tasks 1, 2, and 3.

TASKS FOR CONDUCTING A SENSITIVITY ANALYSIS

1. Examine and modify distribution assumptions
2. Repeat analysis using different estimation assumptions
3. Use analysis of covariance

Ideally, you should apply all three of these tasks. However, which tasks are done in a sensitivity analysis is arbitrary because each question and synthesis is different. Therefore, you might find it more appropriate to complete only one or two. In any event, sensitivity analysis is an important final function in conducting your overall meta-analysis.

Task 1: Examine and Modify Distribution Assumptions

This approach involves modifications of the parameter estimation process by varying the types of distributions assumed for the process being studied. For example, the investigator might examine the effects of assuming an underlying Poisson rather than a normal distribution.

Task 2: Repeat Analysis Using Different Estimation Assumptions

This approach (Eddy et al., 1992, p. 311) involves repeating the analysis using different assumptions about independent and dependent variables.

Consider Including or Excluding Successive Evidence. First, the investigator may successively include or exclude particular pieces of evidence. For example, he or she might successively include studies in which the independent or dependent variables deviate from the prototypic study. One strategy is to examine results from small samples versus large samples to see if the results differ.

Consider Adjusting for Combinations of Biases. Second, the investigator might include or exclude adjustments for various combinations of biases (e.g., contamination and dilution with or without sampling bias estimates).

Consider Different Adjustment Methods. Third, the investigator might select different approaches to incorporate adjustments for biases (weighting strategies vs. psychometric methods vs. Bayesian approaches).

Consider Assuming Fixed Values for Bias Magnitude. Fourth, the analyst can assume a fixed value for the magnitude of the bias but incorporate estimates of the degree of uncertainty about the presence or absence of the bias. In other words, a study might be coded as possibly having a 25% dilution rate in the treatment condition. There can be uncertainty about whether this dilution actually occurred. Thus, the possibility of this dilution might be considered to be of very low, moderate, or high likelihood.

Consider Reanalysis Incorporating Expert Judgment. Fifth, the problem might be reanalyzed with the judgment of experts used as a source of data. The experts can provide subjective judgments for particularly important parameters in the problem. If the experts disagree about any of the parameter values, the meta-analysis can be conducted under the competing sets of beliefs.

Consider Parameter Estimates Using Fixed or Random Effects Models. Sixth, the investigator can calculate parameter estimates for the effects using either the fixed or random effects model.

Task 3: Use Analysis of Covariance

Another widely used approach in meta-analysis is to use an analysis of covariance to evaluate the stability of the observed effects. This method is particularly useful when the test for heterogeneity of effect sizes is significant. In this analysis, the effect size index for the individual studies is used as the dependent variable, and possible sources of variation among studies are used as covariates. For example, the investigator might use the year of publication, the size of a clinic in which the study was conducted, the proportion of patients with comorbid conditions, the experience of clinicians, or other variables as possible covariates explaining the variation in effect sizes. If, by using a covariate, the variance among effect sizes is reduced to zero, then we have found a possible explanation.

An Example in Education. Bryk and Raudenbush (1992) describe an interesting application of this procedure. The teacher expectancy effect is a widely known phenomenon in education settings. The hypothesis states that teachers' expectations can influence students' intellectual development, but the research on this topic is quite controversial (Rosenthal & Rubin, 1978, 1980). A series of experiments have tested this hypothesis. In the experiments, teachers are randomly assigned to expect either "high ability" for some students or control conditions in which no expectations are created. Subsequently, students' achievement test performance is collected as the main dependent variable. The research hypothesis states that the achievement test performance of the "high-expectancy" group will be greater than the control condition. Raudenbush (1984) found 18 experiments to test teacher expectancy effect. The effect sizes in this research varied from -0.32 to +1.18 (see Bryk & Raudenbush, 1992, p. 162). The average effect size was 0.083, which was not significantly different from 0.00. The test for heterogeneity of effect sizes was statistically significant $\chi^2_{(18)} = 35.85$, $p < 0.009$.

Bryk and Raudenbush (1992) explored the idea that the variation in effect size might be explained by the teachers' prior experience with their students. If teachers have extensive prior knowledge of the students before the introduction of the experimental treatment, these teachers may not be influenced by the experimental variation. For each study in their data set, the researchers were able to identify the length of contact between students and the teacher. This variable, then, only assessed between-study information; it did not assess the covariate within each study. By using the between-study measure of teachers' prior experience as a covariate, Bryk and Raudenbush determined that teachers' expectancies influence performance for unfamiliar students but did not determine performance with those for whom they had prior experience. For example, they estimated that the largest effect size in these studies occurred for teachers who had no prior experience with students (effect size = 0.407), $t = 4.67$. However, with each week of contact, the estimated effect size decreased by an amount equal to 0.157. In studies in which the prior contact occurred for 2 weeks or longer, the average effect size was not significantly different from 0.00. Thus, the covariate of prior contact helped to account for the heterogeneity of effects across studies. Furthermore, the between-study assessment of student teacher contact added an additional finding about the expectancy effect that was not tested within any of the studies.

By using teachers' prior experience as a covariate, Bryk and Raudenbush (1992) determined that teachers' expectancies influence performance for unfamiliar students but did not determine performance with those for whom they had prior experience.

Summary

The procedures we introduce in this chapter enable you to perform a variety of meta-analyses. We outline the specific tasks to be completed for the quantitative analysis of your data set. We organize these procedural tasks into three major functions—namely, (a) develop a strategic plan, (b) implement your plan, and (c) complete a sensitivity analysis. We present examples of meta-analyses procedures for correlation coefficients, differences in proportions (or mean differences), quality-weighted solutions, random effects models, and analyses of odds ratios. These are illustrated step-by-step for the nine basic tasks of a meta-analysis, completed separately for each of seven variations of a quantitative synthesis. Finally, we describe methods for performing sensitivity analyses to examine the robustness of the findings obtained.

CHAPTER 15

Evaluation and Improvement
of Stage IV Results

I n Stage IV, each of our four basic assessment areas will be discussed. Recall that these are the following: (a) adequate documentation, (b) clinical significance, (c) scientific soundness, and (d) cost-effectiveness. For each of these areas, we suggest you use a procedural checklist to help you judge the adequacy of the meta-analytic processes that you have now completed.

PROCEDURES TO EVALUATE AND IMPROVE STAGE IV RESULTS

Assess and enhance:
    A.   Documentation adequacy
    B.   Clinical importance
    C.   Scientific soundness
    D.   Cost-effectiveness

Procedure A. Assess and Enhance Documentation Adequacy

**TASKS TO ASSESS AND
ENHANCE DOCUMENTATION ADEQUACY**

1. Recognize the importance of meta-analysis documentation
2. Determine the detail necessary for meta-analysis documentation
3. Establish a customized documentation checklist

Task 1: Recognize Importance of Meta-Analysis Documentation

The ability to judge any synthesis is dependent on the thoroughness of the documentation. In terms of the synthesis stage itself (i.e., the actual statistical combinations and calculations), documentation becomes increasingly important. The principle goal is to compile enough information so that another colleague can evaluate, augment, or even replicate the synthesis. In Stage V, when you are developing your manuscript, it may be necessary to be exceptionally parsimonious with space, especially if you are publishing your synthesis in a journal article. Though you may not be able to include the fine detail, this information should be available if you are contacted in the future by colleagues who, for example, may want to update your work.

Equally important is the fact that online publications now provide a media for facilitating a continual updating of information from their published articles. For example, the Cochrane Library includes a formal review of each systematic review in its collection. By this means, it becomes immediately evident if there is insufficient documentation to judge a synthesis on any of its explicit criteria of quality.

Likewise, the *British Medical Journal's* online publications, although not providing a formal review, do publish the reactions of the scientific community to each article. For example, they include "letters to the editor" that often provide valuable criticism as well as praise. Many of the comments relate to inadequate documentation, which becomes evident in the published author's replies to outside criticism.

Unfortunately, a rather large proportion of research does not produce useable numbers, in many cases, not because the work is invalid but because there is insufficient detail to evaluate its scientific soundness (Williamson et al., 1986).

Task 2: Determine Detail Necessary for Meta-Analysis Documentation

Ideally, we suggest the meta-analysis documentation required is that which would facilitate a qualified colleague to replicate your synthesis. For this purpose, information is needed not only to document methods and results but also to communicate the logic underlying your analysis, including why some choices were not selected.

However, it may be feasible only to provide sufficient documentation for facilitating editorial peer review, as opposed to more formal evaluation of a meta-analysis. The Cochrane Library provides valuable information about the parameters it considers as well as evaluating systematic reviews that it includes in its library, as a full report or as an abstract. In Appendix 18.3, Chapter 18, we provide lists of criteria for evaluating systematic reviews—criteria sets that we have screened that show an evolution between 1977 and 2000. Each of these sets provides important information for you to consider in deciding how much detail you want in your own synthesis documentation, as well as in your own evaluation of your final product.

Task 3: Establish a Customized Documentation Checklist

For applying the results of Task 2, we suggest that you develop your own list of documentation criteria that are reasonable for your synthesis purpose and application. To facilitate this suggestion, we provide a simple checklist (Form 15.1) at the end of this chapter that summarizes what we consider important information to include. Furthermore, the documentation you do compile will require astute judgment about what to include in a publication as opposed to what should remain in your own files.

Form 15.1 can provide a starting checklist on which you may establish your own documentation criteria. As previously mentioned, you have our full authorization to copy and modify any of the forms found in this book.

Procedure B. Assess and Enhance Clinical Importance

TASKS TO ASSESS AND ENHANCE CLINICAL IMPORTANCE

1. Reevaluate the form of your meta-analysis question
2. Consider how you will communicate meta-analysis results

In Stage IV, *clinical importance* of an information synthesis refers to the degree that its results and conclusions are applicable to clinical practice. Two aspects of a synthesis are important to consider here.

Task 1: Reevaluate the Form of Your Meta-Analysis Question

The form of the synthesis question has significant impact on its clinical importance and usefulness. Initially, the question is developed in Stage I in the form of a model conceptually representing the phenomena of interest. Because your synthesis design is a meta-analysis, then at the time of synthesizing your data, your model can be reduced and precisely specified. This precision may be very useful to the clinician because variables are exactly defined (e.g., obesity may be defined as a body mass index [BMI] $\geq$ 30 kg/square meter, or the elderly may be defined as anyone older than age 72). However, such precision may be detrimental to clinical usefulness if the definition of the variables of interest is not clinically significant, is expressed in vague biological terms, or is about topics that are extremely rare. Usually, clinicians want to know how close the characteristics of their own patients are to those encompassed by your synthesis. In other words, to what degree does the population in the synthesis resemble the population whose healthcare these clinicians are managing? In addition, to what degree are the measurement units similar to those units they use in practice? We recommend that as part of a systematic evaluation, an effort should be made to address these aspects of the synthesis. Attributes we suggest you include are listed in Form 15.2.

Task 2: Consider How You Will Communicate Meta-Analysis Results

The next aspect of clinical importance relating to Stage IV, in preparation for Stage V, is the manner in which you will report your meta-analysis results. How you communicate quantitative results may well determine whether or not your synthesis will be applied so as to facilitate improving healthcare outcomes.

Reports of statistical significance alone are usually not interpretable to a practicing clinician. Results should be expressed in terms such as the **number needed to treat** to prevent one event (NNT) and the number needed to treat to cause one harmful event due to treatment (NNH). On the other hand, Smeeth, Haines, and Ebrahim (1999) caution that "numbers needed to treat" that are derived from meta-analysis are sometimes informative but usually misleading due to heterogeneity of data pooled. (See Chapter 13 for an extensive discussion on avoiding such biases.)

Graphs, figures, effect tables, and expressing confidence intervals and control group event rates are all very useful and easy to interpret. They should be employed frequently. Reporting the same results in more than one way may be redundant but necessary to be most helpful to the reader. This principle will be discussed in more detail in Procedure C, Chapter 17 and in Appendix 18.2, Chapter 18 when you are developing your manuscript from the point of view of facilitating the reader's application of your results.

Procedure C. Assess and Enhance Scientific Soundness

Scientific soundness refers to the degree to which the methods and results of the synthesis lead to valid conclusions. Cook and Campbell (1979) discuss three aspects of validity—namely, statistical validity, internal validity, and external validity. When these principles are applied to information syntheses and the synthesis process itself, the following issues must be reemphasized in this Stage IV evaluation.

TASKS TO ASSESS AND ENHANCE SCIENTIFIC SOUNDNESS

1. Reanalyze and improve internal validity
2. Reanalyze and improve external validity
3. Reanalyze and improve statistical validity

Task 1: Reanalyze and Improve Internal Validity

Review the Concept of Internal Validity. This term refers to the strength of the inference that can be drawn from the study's evidence. Because meta-analysis is essentially retrospective research, it is subject to all of the biases inherent in descriptive research. As an author of a meta-analysis, you are attempting to take a few samples (effect sizes) and generalize to a larger population. No formal manipulation or random assignment is done regarding kinds of settings, variations in the independent variable(s), or authors of studies. Consequently, the concept of **internal validity** can only be applied to the subjects and studies specifically included. Generalizability encompasses different variables and will be discussed in regard to external validity. If internal validity is seriously inadequate, estimating external validity is moot.

Understand and Manage Bias Most Related to Internal Validity. There is no guarantee against bias, which, in reality, cannot be totally eliminated. Your task is to understand and minimize those sources of bias that will most likely influence your conclusions. It is incumbent on you to delineate for your readers the most serious sources of these biases and the means you applied to minimize them. In Stage IV, biases arise when (a) the quality of the original studies is not systematically analyzed in the synthesis process; (b) the coding process is not systematic, thorough, or unambiguous; (c) missing data are mismanaged thoroughly and systematically; (d) there is a lack of power to identify significant differences that may exist; (e) correlated or inappropriate effect sizes are used; or (f) if heterogeneity between studies is not sufficiently addressed. Form 10.1 (Section A, Chapter 10) lists items to consider when evaluating internal validity of your meta-analysis.

Task 2: Reanalyze and Improve External Validity

Review the Concept of External Validity. Assuming adequate internal validity, external validity refers to the degree to which conclusions can be generalized to other persons, settings, treatments, outcomes, and times. In this regard, issues of representativeness and prototypicality of individual study populations become central. In addition, the consistency and comprehensiveness of the independent variable across studies are also important. In other words, the population universe to be sampled must be described in detail. The methods used to sample that universe must be appropriate and conducted correctly. The difficulty in making this assessment for one study is a problem in itself, but making the same assessment for a group of studies becomes even more difficult. Again, review Chapter 13 for ways of coping with these issues.

Identify and Manage Bias Most Related to External Validity. To test assumptions related to bias, multiple sensitivity analyses are extremely important. Sensitivity analyses assess the robustness of the results relative to contextual features of the primary studies. By conducting systematic sensitivity analyses, you can test some of the key assumptions underlying your work. Form 10.1 (Section D, Chapter 10) provides a checklist for these issues.

Task 3: Reanalyze and Improve Statistical Validity

Statistical validity refers to the degree to which the data analyses comply with essential statistical assumptions. Although there are many assumptions that are relevant to a meta-analysis, a few rank as relatively more important. These include issues of correlated or nonindependent effect sizes, heterogeneity of effect sizes, the misuse of fixed or random effects models, and the lack of statistical power. Form 10.1 (Section B, Chapter 10) provides a checklist for these issues.

Procedure D. Assess and Enhance Cost-Effectiveness

Cost-effectiveness evaluation in Stage IV involves a simple determination of total fiscal and time costs of implementing this stage of the synthesis. Perhaps a team consensus might be achieved in terms of whether the resulting synthesis results were worth the effort and resources expended. The main benefit of this exercise would be in the consensus discussion, where lessons learned could be noted to enhance the cost-effectiveness of future Stage IV accomplishments. About the only opportunity for enhancement of cost-effectiveness of your current synthesis at this point is to improve the meta-analysis results in terms of accuracy by rechecking the processes completed and perhaps in terms of applicability if additional subgroup analyses might add to the clinical importance of synthesis results.

At this point, the bulk of the work has been completed, and the next major goal will be putting it all together in writing your final report of the synthesis. The authors need to reaffirm exactly who will do the write-up and who will be responsible for such tasks as editing, finding missing references, and obtaining permissions from authors of material used that goes beyond "fair use." "The doctrine of *fair use* was originally developed by judges as an equitable limit on the absolutism of copyright. Although incorporated into the new copyright law, the doctrine still does not attempt to define the exact limits of the fair use of copyrighted work" (Grossman, 1993, p. 145; see pp. 143-150 for a cogent discussion of the doctrine of "fair use").

Summary

In this chapter, we review the procedures for conducting an evaluation of Stage IV. The focus of this evaluation is meta-analysis; however, the principles apply to all types of syntheses as well. Four areas of evaluation are reviewed, including documentation, clinical significance, scientific soundness, and cost-effectiveness.

In the domain of *clinical significance,* the focus is on the specification of a question in clinically relevant terms, both for the measurement and the variable model. In addition, reporting the data in terms relevant to healthcare providers is also stressed.

In terms of *scientific soundness,* the issues of internal, external, and statistical validity are addressed. A number of potential biases are discussed.

To enhance documentation, a checklist is provided of the items thought to be useful to a reader and important for another researcher. This checklist provides a guide to what should be reported.

Cost-effectiveness at this stage can be addressed simply in terms of assessing the remaining resources and time for the tasks that need to be completed.

FORM 15.1: DOCUMENTATION CHECKLIST REGARDING
THE STAGE IV META-ANALYTIC PROCESS

Date: _____

Recorder: _____

> **Instructions:** Have search team agree that the following information is available. (If two different types of information are requested, both requirements must be met for a Yes):

1. Was the type of combination model used, and reasons why, reported? ____Yes ____No

2. Did you record the names and versions of computer programs used? ____Yes ____No

3. Were assumptions reported regarding fixed or random effects? ____Yes ____No

4. Did you conduct and report power analyses? ____Yes ____No

5. Were methods and results of testing for heterogeneity reported? ____Yes ____No

6. Did you report variance-component estimates, especially for random effects models? ____Yes ____No

7. Did you describe your methods of handling missing data? ____Yes ____No

8. Was missing data management evaluated by sensitivity analyses? ____Yes ____No

9. Did you report coding reliabilities and complete sensitivity analyses on those items with low reliability? ____Yes ____No

10. Were degrees of freedom, p values, confidence intervals or standard errors and statistical results reported for every test? ____Yes ____No

11. Did you identify and report evidence of publication bias? ____Yes ____No

12. Were general sensitivity analyses done, and reasons why, reported? ____Yes ____No

13. Did you differentiate between subgroup analysis done á priori from those done á posteriori? ____Yes ____No

14. Was (if possible) a cumulative meta-analysis by year reported? ____Yes ____No

FORM 15.2: ATTRIBUTES OF CLINICAL SIGNIFICANCE IN STAGE IV

Date: _____

Recorder: _____

Item	Description	Yes	No
Independent variable ("IV")	Do you report and discuss what is known regarding the range of studies used in Stage IV, the consistency of its manipulation across studies, and its relationship to actual clinical decision making (including reasons why the focus may be different in this analysis)?		
Dependent variables ("DVs")	Do you report how measurement of the "DVs" varies across different clinical situations; what range of values are clinically relevant; and evidence for a dose–response relationship between the "IV" and the "DVs" (including issues of mediation, changes in the relationship across time, disease severity, and issues of how the results might vary in terms of populations, settings, and disease staging)?		
Timely	Is the issue of clinical timeliness addressed and presented so that it would be of interest now?		
Application maturity	Do you discuss to what degree the findings are immediately applicable to practice?		
Readable results	Are results presented in a manner easily understood by a clinician with little statistical background (are units for reporting quantitative findings being presented in clinically relevant terms)?		

SYNTHESIS REPORT COMPLETION AND EVALUATION

CHAPTER 16

Synthesis Manuscript Preparation Primer

Having compiled a reasonably thorough and valid information database and completed your analysis and synthesis, you are ready to write your synthesis report. This discussion is rather basic, so experienced authors might choose to move on to Chapter 17. Two procedures (A and B) will apply to both journal articles (including technical reports) and books (including monographs). One procedural section (C) will cover both the front and trailing matter for a journal article. The final section (D) will cover front and trailing matter for a book.

PROCEDURES FOR SYNTHESIS MANUSCRIPT PREPARATION

A. Prepare to write synthesis manuscript
B. Write the body of synthesis report
C. Write the front and trailing matter for a journal article
D. Write the front and trailing matter for a book

Procedure A. Prepare to Write Synthesis Manuscript

Task 1: Compare Original and Final Synthesis Plan

The content of the original plan includes the title, purpose, goals, target audience, likely use by reader, database development, validation, analysis and synthesis of salient material, and, finally, your budget and timetable. Your original synthesis plan may remain the same, but more likely it will evolve during the subsequent stages of your project. By comparing your original with your final plan, you can identify any major differences in terms of topic, purpose, goals, your intended readers, the needs your synthesis will meet, and the status of your time and fiscal budget. If the content of your final plan is substantially different from your original, you must determine whether the change was intentional or unintentional and whether your remaining resources are sufficient to cover Stage V costs.

Task 2: Organize Material for Initial Write-Up

Recognizing that how you organize your material for write-up is somewhat arbitrary, we would suggest that you compile your material in the same order as the five stages of your synthesis development. For each stage, be sure you have a clear statement of purpose and a compilation of all products, including search plans, relevance-coded citations and reference lists, the electronic master list indicating both relevance and validity ratings, and complete documents rated A+, A, and A-, together with their data coding forms. (Ideally, all of the above materials are in digital form.) Perhaps most important, you should check the adequacy of the methods documentation and statistical counts of methods results. If you keep in mind your final readers and their likely application of your synthesis, you should be ready to prepare your report.

Task 3: Select Manuscript Format and Style

The following are a few considerations you might find useful in managing the daunting task of developing your final manuscript.

Finding Help for Selecting the Format of Your Report. A first task is to select the form that will be most appropriate for your final synthesis (e.g., a journal article, technical report, book, or monograph). Each of these forms requires a somewhat different outline. If your synthesis will be a technical report for internal corporate use, you would follow the standard style of previous documents. However, there are instances when you will be able to choose the format that suits you personally. There are several published articles, including two consensus statements, regarding manuscript writing with which you should be familiar.

STANDARDS FOR WRITING REVIEWS, CONTROLLED TRIALS, AND ABSTRACTS

International Committee of Medical Journal Editors (2000): Uniform requirements for manuscripts submitted to biomedical journals

Moher et al. (1994): Improving the quality of reports of meta-analysis of randomised controlled trials: The QUORUM statement

Altman (1996): Better reporting of randomized controlled trials: The CONSORT statement

Begg et al. (1996): Improving the quality of reporting randomized controlled trials—the CONSORT statement (Consolidated Standards of Reporting Trials) (also see Moher, 1998)

Maxwell and Cole (1995): Tips for writing (and reading) methodological articles

Bailar (1986): Reporting statistical studies in clinical journals

DerSimonium and Laird (1986): Meta-analysis in clinical trials

Mosteller (1986): Writing about numbers

Ad Hoc Working Group for Critical Appraisal of the Medical Literature (1987): A proposal for more informative abstracts of clinical articles

See also Appendix 18.3 for a listing of systematic review assessment criteria as they have evolved from 1977 to 2000.

Selecting the Style of Your Manuscript. Note that the final style you will use will likely depend on the requirements of whomever agrees to publish or print your work. Issues of style of scientific writing have a long history. One early example is that of Bruner (1942). By checking with the publishers of various journals or books, you will see the variety of different styles that may be required. However, to maintain consistency in developing your manuscript, you should select a tentative style and obtain a style manual, such as the *Publication Manual of the American Psychological Association* (American Psychological Association, 2001), as a guide. If new to publishing, you may be shocked at the level of detail demanded by an appropriate style. This is especially so for references. For example, the style for citing a work having a single author is somewhat different from that with two or three authors. Many documents may have an organization as the author and possibly the same organization as the publisher as well. Each of these different cases will require that you follow a different set of style rules.

Writing a Meta-Analysis. One of the more authoritative guides for writing a quantitative synthesis is by R. Rosenthal (1995), a highly respected expert on meta-analysis at Harvard University. He provides a very valuable article describing what should be included in the introduction, method, results, and discussion sections of a systematic review. His 10-page report highlights the most important elements to be emphasized in developing a manuscript for a meta-analysis. If you are developing a quantitative synthesis, we refer you to this article for help when you reach Stage V.

Understanding Use of Abstracts, Their Value, and Deficiencies. With many if not most articles, the abstract may be the section of the paper most frequently read. To help improve the utility of abstracts, in 1987 the Ad Hoc Working Group for Critical Appraisal of the Medical Literature reported a consensus-developed, structured outline for writing abstracts for biomedical research.

Use of structured abstracts is a positive step forward, if well written. Because the abstract is the part of an article that is most often read, it has the potential for being seriously misleading to the reader. Pitkin, Branagan, and Burmeister (1999) found that "data in the abstract that are inconsistent with or absent from the article's body are common, even in large-circulation general medical journals" (p. 1110). They found 18% to 68% of 264 abstracts from our most prestigious journals (e.g., *JAMA, BMJ, Lancet, NEJM*) "had data in the abstract that were either inconsistent with, or absent from, the main body of the article" (p. 1111).

There has been a recent movement to require structured abstracts in medical journals. However, even this approach has its critics. In a randomized controlled trial, Pitkin and Branagan (1998) tested the efficacy of providing specific instructions to authors for writing the abstract. There was no difference in abstract quality in either the experimental or control group. Pitkin et al. (1999) found no difference in deficiencies comparing structured and nonstructured abstracts. Scherer and Crawley (1998) applied a criterion-based evaluation of 125 clinical trials in ophthalmology, finding no difference between structured and nonstructured journal abstract content quality.

On the other hand, Winker (1999), in her editorial in *JAMA,* reported 10 quality criteria for assessing abstracts. Use of these criteria in a pilot evaluation indicated considerable improvement when they were used. Also, abstracts developed by expert panels (e.g., *ACP Journal Club*) provide meta-validated information that would seem far more trustworthy.

Reporting Biomedical Research: Use of Official Consensus Formats. On the other hand, the International Committee of Medical Journal Editors (1997; 2000) developed "Uniform Requirements for Manuscripts Submitted to Biomedical Journals." It is noteworthy that these requirements include the following: "Authors submitting review manuscripts should include a section describing the methods used for locating, selecting, extracting, and synthesizing data. These methods should also be summarized in the abstract" (p. 929).

If publishers wish to endorse these standards, it is mandatory that they state this fact in the "Advice to Authors" section. *JAMA,* in its "Instructions for Authors," states that use of these uniform requirements is optional. The *NEJM's* "Information for Authors" section states that its guidelines are "in accordance with the 'Uniform Requirements for Manuscripts Submitted to Biomedical Journals'" (most recently in *NEJM,* June 2000), which it endorses.

In any event, if your synthesis will be reviewed for publication, you must carefully read and follow the publisher's instructions to authors. In journals, these instructions are available in specific issues during the year. For books, special instructions in booklet form must be requested from the publisher, as each might have unique requirements that must be followed precisely.

Reporting RCTs: Use of Official Consensus Formats. The Consolidated Standard of Reporting Trials (CONSORT) group has an officially developed format for reporting randomized controlled clinical trials (RCTs). Begg et al. (1996) report that over the past 30 years there has been "a wide chasm between what a trial should report and what is actually published" (p. 637). The CONSORT group developed a consensus set of criteria for evaluating reports of such trials. CONSORT is both evolving and being widely adopted. There are approximately 70 journals that endorse these standards.

Task 4: Outline Proposed Manuscript

The following outline is a brief synopsis of suggestions for developing your overall manuscript.

ILLUSTRATIVE OUTLINE OF AN ARTICLE (RESEARCH REPORT)

a.   Front matter
Title page
Title
Author(s)
Abstract
Full journal reference (for this article)
Footnote
Institutions where authors work
Name and address of author(s)
Source of funding
Responsibility for correspondence

       Responsibility for reprints
       Disclaimers (if any)
       Short running head
   b. Body of report
       Introduction (background)
       Methods
       Results
       Discussion
       Conclusions
   c. Trailing matter
       Acknowledgments
       Staff
       Source of funding (if not in footnote on title page)
       Appendixes (if any)
       References

Task 5: Reaffirm Authorship Criteria

In the planning stage, you should have established the criteria for authorship (i.e., who qualifies to be an author and in what order they will be listed). Ideally, this decision should be made at the time you plan the project as a whole. As your manuscript nears completion, you might reanalyze authorship to be certain you have followed the agreed-on criteria. If these criteria are not developed until the end of your project, there may be serious conflict among the authors when it comes time for assigning credits. See Section G, Chapter 2, for a more detailed discussion of official scientific authorship criteria from recent literature.

We advocate that the authors be listed in the order of their substantive contributions. It is up to the principal investigator, ideally with input and agreement of all the synthesis team, to make the final decision as to who should be included as authors and in what order. Clerical, copyediting, and review staff are usually mentioned in the acknowledgments and not listed as authors.

Procedure B. Write Body of Synthesis Report

Task 1: Write Introduction (or Background)

Though arbitrary, we suggest that the introduction (or background) of your article or book include at least four elements—namely:

State Purpose and Goals of Your Project. The purpose (i.e., research question) of your synthesis should be stated up front, before the reader gets into the details of your report. This simple statement of what you are trying to accomplish by this project might be a single sentence. This can be followed by a list of the specific goals to be accomplished to achieve that purpose. Too often, the statement of purpose is omitted completely, is buried in one of the multiple paragraphs of the introduction, or is somewhere in the report itself. It is a disservice to your readers to have them spend time searching your synthesis report for a statement of purpose and then discover that your subject is not relevant to their needs.

Explain Importance to Whom and for What Use. The rationale or reason for writing this synthesis is explained by its importance to whom and for what application. This is the initial statement of your project's contribution in adding to healthcare knowledge and facilitating improvement of healthcare outcomes. This element should indicate your target audience rather precisely, including how these readers might benefit from this review. As we mention later on, consideration of these potential applications can be of help for integrating and formatting your paper. For example, if the results of your synthesis will directly facilitate clinical diagnostic decision making, this fact should be stated in the introduction. If your material can be applied directly to the development of healthcare improvement resources (such as electronic alerts or guidelines), this also needs to be made explicit. The diffusion of innovation is usually slow, often taking years or, in some cases, decades. Whatever you can contribute, not only in content (e.g., to help prove the superiority of Intervention A over Intervention B) but also in facilitating its dissemination, will enhance a more timely impact of your effort.

Briefly Describe Your Project Content. Your project content is essential for both understanding and evaluating your synthesis. In writing a synthesis, you must abstract information from a range of single studies for each factor you need to describe.

   Element (1): Title of Synthesis. The title provides the most abstract description of your subject matter. Taken alone, it may be misleading and provide very little information about the content of a synthesis. We suggest that a title should be descriptive rather than a catchy phrase.
   Element (2): Research Question, Model, and Assumptions. These important factors should be briefly highlighted because the details will be provided in subsequent sections of the body of your report. The research question defines the issue you want to resolve by your investigation. This question must be explained in terms of your research model, which then defines your causal assumptions and mediator and moderator variables. The model determines your study design and helps focus your project. Study designs might include experimental (e.g., randomized controlled clinical

trials), quasi-experimental trials, descriptive (e.g., simple epidemiological surveys), or methodological types. From this model, you then define the relevance criteria for searching and compiling your database.

Element (3): Criteria of Relevance. These criteria provide a cryptic but all-inclusive description of content searched in your multiple information sources. They should be briefly summarized, highlighting major inclusions and exclusions for your topic. The following aspects of your topic might be briefly summarized.

Study populations encompassed. The demographics or epidemiological profile of your study populations is essential information for your readers to know. This description explains the range of populations encompassed by the many research studies you synthesized. Sampling methods used provide a more precise description of each population denominator and numerator included. In a meta-analysis, these details are even more important.

Health problem(s) or disease(s) involved. Most information syntheses in the health field will relate directly or indirectly to a given health condition or spectrum of such conditions. Use of the *International Classification of Disease—9* Clinical Modification (*ICD-9* CM) codes are recommended as one of the more concise descriptions of health conditions. This resource is available through the U.S. Department of Health and Human Services (HHS), the Centers for Disease Control and Prevention (CDC), and the National Center for Health Statistics (NCHS). *ICD-10* CM will most likely be a future publication. Likewise, diagnosis-related group codes (DRGs) are familiar to most healthcare organizations, especially hospitals. HHS sponsors this coding standard for health policy and research. These codes are applied in its ongoing Healthcare Cost and Utilization Project (HCUP-3).

Care setting(s) that apply. These represent the sites where care was provided in the various studies included in your synthesis. Studies in ambulatory care settings may not compare to studies in acute hospital settings or long-term care facilities. Inclusion of only those studies having a common care setting might prove more meaningful than including those where the care settings are mixed. Finally, it is important to know setting characteristics, such as urban or rural, hospital, and office or home.

Care providers included. Your write-up should include an adequate description of the providers encompassed in your final database, especially if your topic is a specific health problem. For example, several studies of presurgical instructions might provide quite different conclusions if the practitioners involved vary from educational specialists to nurses or physicians. Competence depends on the health problem involved and on the domain of training and experience of the care providers. These factors can be strikingly different among the studies included in your synthesis, requiring that these differences be managed or at least described.

Care interventions used. Variations in diagnostic and therapeutic interventions should be briefly mentioned. For example, you should specify the diagnostic interventions applied, such as history and physical or laboratory tests done. Likewise, you should delineate the therapeutic interventions: pharmacological, surgical, rehabilitation, mental health counseling, and psychotherapy. This information is helpful in judging homogeneity or heterogeneity of the healthcare outcomes achieved, especially in regard to the evidence for efficacy of the interventions used.

Element (4): Outcomes Measured and by What Means. The definition and description of healthcare outcomes must also include the instruments used for their measure. The eight generic clusters of outcomes outlined in Figure 2.4, Chapter 2, can provide a quasi-comprehensive overview of outcomes measured. When a project focuses on a healthcare process, the implications may apply to several of the eight clusters of final outcomes. For example, a topic such as "improving the effectiveness of family support groups" could affect not only the patient's health but also the economic costs to the patient's family, as well as job satisfaction of the provider.

Analyze Previous Reviews on This Topic. It is helpful to the reader to know if other investigators have developed an information synthesis, or at least a traditional review, on your topic. In your final database, you most likely will have retrieved several such articles. In our judgment, it is essential that you briefly describe these literature studies to provide a basis for establishing how your synthesis is different and what unique contribution your work makes to the review literature related to your subject.

Outline Remaining Sections of Report (Optional). If your synthesis outline follows the classic form (introduction, methods, results, discussion, summary, and conclusions), it is likely this final paragraph of your introduction may not be necessary. However, if your conceptual framework is different or more complex, a rationale for your unique outline and a description of the remaining sections might be considered. This paragraph will be helpful in keeping your readers oriented to the structure of your synthesis report.

Task 2: Describe Synthesis Methods

In writing a research report, few scientists would argue that the methods section is critical for interpreting the results. However, authors of review articles consistently omit essential details about how they conducted their review. Their methods section may be as meager as this statement: "A thorough review of the literature was accomplished." The senior author of this book has commented on the importance of review documentation since the 1970s (Williamson, 1977), and the general scientific community is now recognizing this problem. Groups such as the Cochrane Collaboration and the evidence-based practice centers (EPCs) of the Agency for Health

Care Policy and Research have embarked on an effort to emphasize the considerable importance of detailing the methods used in literature reviews.

Procedure A, Chapter 4 provides suggestions for assessing adequacy of documentation of a synthesis report. Unfortunately, lack of adequate funding, poor planning of available time, and failure to recognize the importance of synthesis documentation might lead to the omission of the necessary information required to review your final product. One possible consequence is that publishers may not accept your work for publication, as might happen with a manuscript of a controlled clinical trial that omits, or skimps, on methods documentation.

Task 3: Describe Synthesis Results

After completing the description of your synthesis methods, you are ready to report results. As shown above, reporting synthesis results requires two independent subtasks.

Report Search Methods Results. The search statistics aggregated from each of your search iterations are reported in this section of the manuscript. For example, such items as the total number of citations screened—together with their relevance-coding profile, the total A (A+, A, A-) citations or abstracts searched, and the number of articles retrieved with their coding profile—can be meaningful. The number of A and B citations in your master list should be mentioned, together with the number of A (A+, A, A-) references cited in those articles. Including the proportion of A+ and A articles that should have been validated and the number that actually were, together with the profile of validation codes thus identified, is also important.

Report Substantive Results. Research results can be reported using a wide variety of different styles. We suggest that you consider the style most understandable to your intended audience and their likely use of your material.

Your synthesis database will consist of a compilation of complete research reports, published or unpublished, and in some instances expert consensus statements. These documents will have been rated for both relevance and validity and will have received ratings above a specified inclusion threshold.

Task 4: Prepare Tables, Figures, and Graphs

Although text is helpful in describing substantive results, tables, figures, and graphs are often more helpful in conveying the meaning of the data compiled. Understanding your readers and how they might use your results can help determine how to present your textual, tabular, and graphic data. Appropriate graphics can be essential to the communication effectiveness of your synthesis. If your results might

Risk Ratio 95% CI

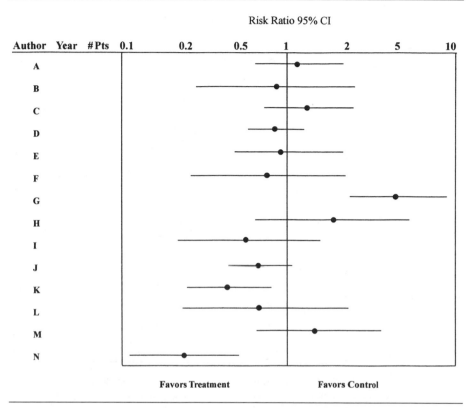

Figure 16.1. Odds Ratio (95% CI) Arranged Alphabetically by Author

provide input into a decision analysis, using branching logic and causal diagrams with probability data can all be helpful.

It is usually important to include evidence tables and/or graphics in your report. These devices document the synthesis and enhance its communication effectiveness. As mentioned earlier, Light, Singer, and Willet's (1994) chapter in the *Handbook of Research Synthesis* is a helpful resource for this purpose. However, although tables and graphics can help elucidate the meaning of evidence, if done poorly, they may be a source of confusion and misinterpretation. We strongly suggest that Light et al.'s guidelines be reviewed and considered in the write-up of quantitative synthesis reports.

In reporting effect sizes in tabular form, Light and Pillemer (1984) point out that individual study effect sizes are often listed chronologically by date of publication or alphabetically by author (see Figure 16.1). At first glance there does not appear to be a significant treatment effect because most of the means favor the controls.

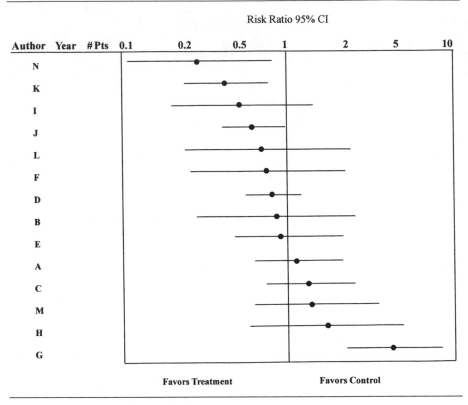

Figure 16.2. Odds Ratio (95% CI) Arranged by Magnitude of Effect Size

If the reader is to adequately interpret such tables, it is far more meaningful to array them by the measured effect size or by effect size within each mediating variable (e.g., gender), as shown in Figure 16.2. This array seems to favor the controls or at least indicates an effect somewhere between favoring treatment and controls.

Expressing cumulative results may also be meaningful as shown in Figure 16.3, where it is very clear that a statistically significant treatment effect has occurred. This method clearly indicates to the reader that the effect favors the treatment, in terms of the cumulative means and standard deviations.

In these illustrations, we emphasize the necessity of using tables and graphs that more adequately communicate the meaning of your data.

Task 5: Discuss Synthesis Findings

Relate Substantive Findings to Synthesis Goals. This element explains the extent to which your synthesis achieved its purpose, particularly in relation to the goals set

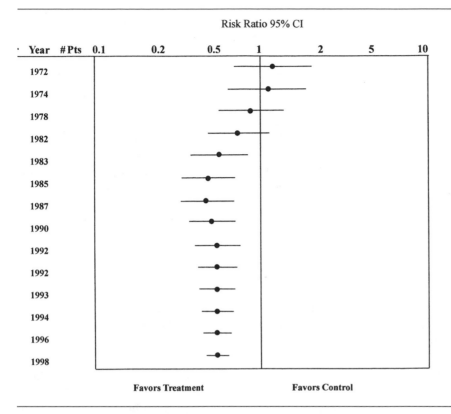

Risk Ratio 95% CI

Figure 16.3. Cumulative Odds Ratio (95% CI)

forth in the introduction. The findings will rarely be conclusive but usually tentative, depending on the extent to which each goal was accomplished. Your reader will be less than impressed if you set forth five goals and only discuss three of them or, even worse, only have data for three. If the latter is true, novice investigators can learn an important lesson about limiting their purpose and goals at the planning stage.

Suggest Use of Synthesis Findings to Improve Healthcare Outcomes. Your synthesis may suggest several important implications for the reader, particularly for quality management personnel and clinicians, to improve healthcare outcomes. These should be described together with a discussion of the potential benefits to be gained by use of your validated findings. For example, suppose your purpose is to synthesize evidence regarding the reliability, validity, and cost-effectiveness of a new guideline for management of simple depression in primary practice. Suppose also, based on many sound studies, the evidence supports the value of this guideline to help primary practitioners diagnose and treat simple depression in their local practice population. Because of your validated review, quality management professionals might be convinced to facilitate use of these guidelines in their community, possibly resulting in health status improvement of their local patients.

Discuss Limitations Restricting Synthesis Applicability. It is rare, if not impossible, for an information synthesis to be flawless. For example, if you plot a funnel display of effect sizes against sample size, and the funnel proves truncated in the lower left quadrant of your graph, it might indicate publication bias, or missed "fugitive literature" that reports negative results. As a consequence, your database might overrepresent "positive" studies, leading to an inaccurate conclusion.

On the other hand, problems such as budget and time limitations may preclude your identifying new "invisible colleges" whose research might contradict those in your current database. If such studies are located and retrieved but resources do not allow an adequate validation analysis, this fact must be explained in the "limitations" section of your discussion.

Describe Synthesis Methods "Lessons Learned." The field of systematic validated reviews is relatively new in healthcare and therefore requires that authors learn from each other, as well as from experts in this field. For example, if an author discovers a research historian for a given topic who is maintaining a "bibliography of bibliographies" on the management of hip fractures, this would be an important finding for future researchers interested in that particular field. Recent advances in "meta-analysis" methods would be valuable to readers interested in conducting quantitative syntheses. These syntheses are usually complex, and authors may make mistakes that they, or editorial peer reviewers, do not recognize. If an author of a meta-analysis finds a serious or unique methods problem in his or her synthesis, especially one that may not be easily solved, such a finding might be reported in the manuscript discussion section so others can learn from the author's experience.

Suggest Future Research Required on Your Topic. In conducting a research synthesis, there will be frequent gaps in current knowledge on various topics. By reporting these gaps, others might be motivated to confirm them and, if they concur, make this topic a high priority for future studies. On the other hand, if a certain topic reveals a large volume of studies, with few reviews or syntheses, this might motivate other authors to analyze and synthesize this research to transform such data into information and knowledge of value for improving future healthcare outcomes.

The description of "research gaps" is an important element of the synthesis report. This finding can also be of value to practitioners who must often base patient management decisions on causal relations that may not be supported by adequate evidence. By describing these gaps, a synthesis report provides needed information regarding the limits of current clinical knowledge. The synthesis write-up may describe dry research areas in terms of causal pathway graphics. This technique readily identifies which links are based on solid evidence and which have little or no scientific data supporting them. Equally pertinent is the listing of references supporting inferences regarding mediating and moderating variables, such as the demographics of subpopulations, economic considerations, and other elements related to answering the targeted research question.

Task 6: Write Synthesis Conclusions

To prepare your conclusions, you should review your final research question and hypothesis. Your conclusions will be based on the results of your evaluation findings in relation to the limitations of your database, analysis, and synthesis methods. This information shapes your final answers to the synthesis question(s). Conclusions should include the most meaningful implication of your work for improving future healthcare, research, or information synthesis methodology.

In the past, this final section consisted of a summary and conclusions. More recently, publishers require an abstract on the first page of the article, which substitutes for a summary. However, some authors may have an abstract initially and, at the end of the article, a summary that may include conclusions.

One of the hazards of writing conclusions is that authors tend to generalize beyond their data. For example, if a study focused on one or even a group of small community hospitals, and the conclusions were written to imply the results could be generalized to all such hospitals, the author's judgment might be suspect. If you are conservative in the implications of your work, then the readers are responsible if they generalize beyond the data supporting your conclusions.

Procedure C. Write Front and Trailing Matter for a Journal Article

Task 1: Write Article Front Matter (First Page)

Having completed the body of the article, writing the front matter is relatively easy and takes little time, assuming you have been adhering to the style and formatting required by your potential publisher if your article will be submitted for publication. Most journals have an "Instructions for Authors" in each volume (or in specified volumes during the year) that list each publisher's formal requirements. Some even have a maximum letter count for the title and abstract that must be strictly followed.

Finalize Title. The title of an information synthesis to be published as a journal article should be a concise statement of the content of your review. This facilitates relevance coding by your colleagues in their future literature searches and also helps readers more quickly determine whether your article might meet their needs.

On title content, you can use your own discretion as to whether your title is a vague, eye-catching title, such as "The Web: Where's the Spider?" or is more content-specific such as "Physicians' Use and Misuse of Internet for Pharmaceutical Decisions." We strongly suggest the latter content-specific titles. To anyone who has screened an electronic (e.g., MEDLINE) printout of citations on any topic, the weak relationship between the title and the content of the article is often striking and misleading.

You should state in your title, or subtitle, that your final product is an information synthesis. Even better, if you have produced a quantitative synthesis, terms such as *meta-analysis* are important to highlight. These types of review articles are often highly valued by both clinicians and researchers. In any event, your title should be an accurate indicator of what your synthesis is about; it may determine who reads your report and, consequently, what impact it might ultimately have on improving healthcare.

List Authors. The authors are usually listed in order of the contribution they make to the substance of the article. The first or senior author is usually the one who first conceived the idea of the project, secured the funding, or took the major responsibility for completing the research and writing the manuscript. As discussed earlier, it is important to have criteria agreed on as to who qualifies for authorship and in what order their names will be listed in the final article.

There are numerous styles for listing authors of a publication. For example, the American Psychological Association requires that you list an author's first name, middle initial followed by a period, and last name followed by a comma but with no author titles or academic degrees indicated (e.g., James L. Scott, John H. Hilliard). This is in contrast to articles in the *Journal of the American Medical Association* (*JAMA*) that require a similar format, only adding academic degrees, with no periods (e.g., PhD or MD), and followed by a semicolon (e.g., James L. Scott, MD; John H. Hilliard, PhD). Each journal may have its own format standards that must be followed. The *New England Journal of Medicine* (*NEJM*) requires a similar format plus academic degrees with periods, followed by a comma when necessary (e.g., James L. Scott, M.D., John H. Hilliard, Ph.D.).

Write Abstract. Authors of journal articles must usually write an abstract that briefly describes their synthesis report. The abstract provides potential readers with the information they need to decide whether to invest time reading the synthesis. The exact format of your abstract will depend, again, in part, on the journal to which you submit your manuscript. For example, *NEJM* requires the standard format shown below:

THE STANDARD *NEW ENGLAND JOURNAL OF MEDICINE* ABSTRACT FORMAT

1. Background
2. Methods
3. Results
4. Conclusions

Other journals may have their own elaboration of the above basic elements. For example, *JAMA* requires the following elements in journal article abstracts:

THE STANDARD *JOURNAL OF THE AMERICAN MEDICAL ASSOCIATION* ABSTRACT FORMAT

1. Context
2. Objective
3. Design
4. Setting
5. Participants
6. Main Outcome Measures
7. Results
8. Conclusions

Prepare Footnotes. Many journals request a footnote on the front page of an article indicating (a) the authors' occupational affiliations, (b) sources of project support (some journals, e.g., *JAMA* or *NEJM,* list financial support followed by acknowledgments at the end of the article, preceding the reference list), and (c) the name and address (or e-mail address) of the author to whom reprint requests should be sent.

Task 2: Write Article Trailing Matter

Acknowledgments. Most synthesis or research projects usually involve many individuals who contribute their time in helping the project succeed (e.g., colleagues who review the final manuscript and make suggestions for changes or additions). There are usually many ancillary staff paid to do specific tasks, such as literature searching, coding, or helping to prepare front or trailing matter. These individuals usually deserve to be mentioned in the acknowledgment section. It is even better to make a brief mention of their specific contributions to the project, rather than just listing their names.

Project Fiscal Support. Most projects receive monetary support from several sources, usually grants and contracts. Those contributing, either directly or in-kind, must be mentioned in the article. Your reader often checks this statement to determine whether there is a real or apparent conflict of interest or a bias in favor of the group providing money. Most journals place this statement after the acknowledgments; however, some may include this statement in the footnotes on the first page of the article.

Conflict of Interest Statement. The disclosure of author's conflict of interest in published (and unpublished, we might add) reports is becoming more important to the integrity of science, let alone the author's reputation. Smith's (1998) editorial for the *British Medical Journal* provides an important description of this concept:

> Conflict of interest has been defined as "a set of conditions in which professional judgment concerning a primary interest (such as patients' welfare or the validity of research) tends to be unduly influenced by a secondary interest (such as financial gain)." [Thompson, 1993] It is a condition not a behavior, and there is nothing wrong with having a conflict of interest. It is common.

Smith goes on to list research that suggests that conflict of interest is becoming a much more serious problem. For example, 70 articles on calcium channel blockers were reviewed with the findings that 96% of supportive researchers had financial relationships with manufacturers, compared to 60% of neutral authors and 37% of critical authors. He then recommends that conflict of interest usually cannot be prevented, but it must be disclosed. The Cochrane Collaboration has established this requirement as policy so that authors of Cochrane-approved systematic reviews must sign two statements disclosing any conflict of interest (Clarke & Oxman 1999, Section 2.2.3). We strongly support this policy and suggest that such disclosure will strengthen the credibility of an information synthesis and reflect favorably on the authors as well.

Appendixes. On occasion, detailed data tables, methods descriptions, or supplementary texts cannot be included in the body of the article due to space restrictions. Some journals allow a condensed version to be appended at the end of the article (e.g., the *New England Journal of Medicine* will sometimes have an appendix listing numerous members, such as consortia, a big study group, a corporation, or a government agency, involved with a large project).

References. The reference list is one of the most important aspects of the synthesis documentation. The main caution with the bibliography is that it should consist of primary references that the authors have read and quoted correctly. Too often, secondary references are listed that authors have not read but merely noted from the reference list of a primary article source. If a secondary source is listed, a note should be appended to the citation, such as, ". . . found in Jones (1989, p. 76)."

The second major caution relates to the style of the reference. Each publisher may use a standard style manual, such as the *Publication Manual of the American Psychological Association* (American Psychological Association, 2001), or may require a unique style. One journal may require an author listed as "Jones DW," whereas another would insist on listing this author as "Daniel W. Jones, MD." Fortunately, each publisher provides style requirements in its "Instructions for Authors," published periodically in its journal.

Whatever style you use, it is essential to copyedit your final manuscript to be sure all references in your bibliography are cited in the text, and all references cited in the text are in your reference list.

Procedure D. Write Front and Trailing Matter for a Book

Task 1: Write Book Front Matter

In writing a synthesis manuscript for publication as a book, it is necessary to include several unique sections that are printed prior to Chapter 1. The authors themselves usually write these materials; however, in the case of the forward or a preface, an outside guest author(s) is sometimes invited to contribute these sections.

The following eight tasks might be considered in writing book front matter. We list these tasks as a checklist from which you can select those that best meet your needs.

Prepare Title Page. Your title page will include title, subtitle, authors, publisher, and city of publication. The style for listing the authors' names differs among publishers. Some require the authors' academic degrees and organizational affiliations listed on the title page. Others require this information be listed on the back of the title page or elsewhere. (See a discussion of different styles for listing authors, located in Task 1, Procedure C of this chapter in the "Article Front Matter.")

Be Familiar With Back of Title Page. The publisher prepares this material so it usually does not require your input. The back of the title page includes information about date(s) of publication, copyrights, "Library of Congress Cataloging-in-Publication Data," information regarding the publisher, where the book was published, and on some occasions relevant extracts of editorial policy and a publisher disclaimer for errors and omissions.

Write Dedication Statement (Optional). These optional statements are usually personal, mentioning family members or honoring a special colleague. Sometimes the publisher's "Instructions for Authors" may address this topic. However, many books have no dedication.

Prepare Forward. A book may have a forward, a preface, or both. An outside authority in your subject area can be invited to write a forward. This section may include the strengths of the book, as well as negative comments or cautions for the reader. In some cases, there may be more than one forward, one of which may be written by the author(s).

Write Preface. A preface and/or a forward may be written. The preface is more often written by the author(s) of the synthesis and may discuss the importance of the work, its rationale, context, and intended target audience, including potential benefits for readers.

Write Acknowledgments. Contributors not listed as authors often deserve recognition for their special contributions to your book. Ideally, these statements should describe the specific contribution made by each individual. Financial as well as other contributors may also be acknowledged in this section.

Prepare Table of Contents. The table of contents is often a final element of the front matter or may be placed before the forward or preface. This element outlines the organization of the book in relation to the author's theoretical framework. It is customary to limit the table of contents to less than three or four levels of organization. The first level can be merely the chapters of the book. In a slightly more complex manuscript, the first level can be the chapters, and the second level can be chapter sections. An even more complex book might be divided into major themes or parts, with the second level being chapter headings and the third level consisting of chapter sections and subsections. In our experience, if your outline becomes more complex than this, you will likely confuse your readers.

The page numbers for each of the table of contents listings will be done later when the manuscript is in final form. Although you should always double check listed page numbers, keep in mind that the publisher will do the final repagination of the book prior to publication.

Prepare Lists of Tables, Graphs, and Figures. Lists of tables, graphs, and figures are usually standard in most books in the scientific literature. Sequentially numbered and titled, tables, graphs, and figures will provide an index when, for example, the reader needs material from an earlier table he or she cannot easily find. A code for these, which signifies the chapter by number or appendix by letter, followed by a decimal and two digits for each table or figure, is useful. Careful copyediting is required to verify that the tables and figures listed are actually in the book, that they are numbered correctly, and that the tables and figures within each chapter are actually listed in this part of the front matter.

Task 2: Write Book Trailing Matter

Your book publisher's "Information for Authors" or "An Author's Guide" provides specific details to help you cope with their format and style requirements for the above sections.

Develop Reference List. Your database consists of a subset of data, relevance-rated as A+ or A, that meets threshold levels of scientific validity. These subsets of articles are those that you will synthesize. However, your remaining references might be valuable to others or to you in the future, and you might want to include them in an ancillary reference list categorized by relevance and validity ratings. For example, you might list your A- relevance-coded articles. This information might provide valuable leads to related, but different, topics your readers may wish to study.

As with any document citation lists, the style for listing these references, as well as where in the text they are cited, is particularly important. Before submitting your manuscript, you should decide on what style you will use and obtain a manual for that style (e.g., *Publication Manual of the American Psychological Association*). You should also check with prospective publishers for their style requirements to ensure that your material will be in the correct format. Multiple meticulous copyedits of all references is essential to verify the fine details of correct citation listings.

Add Appendixes or Attachments. The synthesis report should include copies of project planning forms, data-gathering instruments, relevance criteria logs (which detail the evolution of your topic inclusions and exclusions), rating and consensus forms (from which you calculate your Kappa statistics), data analysis forms, and the final preexternal peer review forms. These forms also assist in judging the adequacy of your report's documentation. This information clarifies what was done and also provides the documentation needed to improve future syntheses. Books will provide more page space for these materials, so you might include as many of them as is reasonable. We also suggest that you inform your readers that more detailed materials are available from you if needed.

Compile Alphabetic List of Cited Authors. This section follows the appendixes. Most readers will need to obtain specific references from your report by looking up the authors you have cited. This is especially of value should you choose to use a unique format for your bibliographic listings, such as in footnotes on each page, at the end of each chapter, or in numbered notes and commentary at the end of the book, before the index. The author listing is also of value when you cannot recall a citation but can remember the author's name.

Produce Glossary (Optional). Often, technical subject matter contains complex healthcare jargon, acronyms, and other technical terms or phrases that need to be defined in an alphabetic listing, to facilitate the readers' understanding of the text. Though it is optional whether or not you include such a reading aid, we suggest that a glossary is important for any technical writing, especially information syntheses. Definitions of words used in the text can be unknown to many readers outside a given specialty area. A well-written glossary can provide these needed definitions. As mentioned before, although some authors may place their glossary with the front matter, most place it in the trailing matter right before the index.

In providing glossary definitions, you must check to be sure that the same term defined in the glossary is not used in other contexts with a different meaning for the same word. If this is the case, two definitions for that term should be included. For example, words such as *quality* and *outcome* may have very different connotations depending on the author or the context in which they are used. Some authors use the term *outcome* to mean only patient health results of healthcare. As you have read in this book, we use this term in a far more generic sense to mean any class of healthcare results (health, economic, and satisfaction for consumers and/or providers) of any process and structure measured at one point in time (see Section F, Chapter 2).

Develop Acronym List. It is possible that the reader may have more occasions to look up acronyms or abbreviations than glossary words. Thus, you can help your reader by placing these acronyms, with the complete words or phrases they denote, in a special list just for this purpose.

In the health field, with its literature explosion of articles by specialists and subspecialists, each group produces a litany of acronyms they use in everyday communication with their peers. The database of an information synthesis may contain an acronym list that can be placed before or after the glossary either in the front or trailing matter.

Prepare Author and Subject Indexes. The author and subject indexes are important and are usually placed in the final section of the trailing matter. The author index will often be used by readers to identify a key article whose reference list might indicate other relevant material written by that professional or his or her colleagues in an "invisible college." Because the word-processing software command "Find" makes it so easy to identify authors or key words cited in your text, it is relatively easy to compile this reading aid.

Your subject index should cover the major concepts in the manuscript. As you read each section of your synthesis, you might, at the same time, highlight jargon, technical terms, acronyms, and subject matter to be listed or indexed. Word-processing software may have the capability to auto-index your final manuscript as you produce each chapter and section. When your work is final, the publisher need only fill in the correct page numbers where indicated. The subject index, author index, glossary, and acronym lists require careful copyediting to be sure the listings are accurate. In other words, each term listed or indexed should be found in the text; likewise, each such term found in the text should also be found in a list or index.

Summary

This chapter provides a brief, and admittedly simplistic, procedural guide for beginners to produce a synthesis manuscript. Chapter 16 consists of four parts: (a) preparation for writing your manuscript, (b) producing the body of your synthesis report, (c) writing the front and trailing matter for a journal article, and (d) writing the front and trailing matter for a book. In each section, we provide task-by-task suggestions for writing each part of your final synthesis.

Finally, this chapter, together with Chapter 17, will improve the probability that your work will be read, understood, and put to effective use in improving healthcare outcomes.

CHAPTER 17

Applying Synthesis Results for Healthcare Outcomes Improvement

The purpose of this chapter is to present several factors that, in our judgment, have at least moderate evidence for facilitating healthcare outcome improvement. We are sharing the results of our own training, experience, and judgment by presenting this series of statements regarding elements of the problem of effecting behavioral change in healthcare.

PROCEDURES FOR APPLYING SYNTHESIS RESULTS FOR HEALTHCARE OUTCOMES IMPROVEMENT

    A.   Coping with the difficulty of behavioral change and diffusion of innovation

    B.   Avoiding conflicts of interest and hazards of science propaganda

    C.   Achieving healthcare outcomes improvement

Procedure A: Coping With the Difficulty of Behavioral Change and Diffusion of Innovation

To facilitate improvement, you must be aware that effecting behavioral change and diffusing innovations are likely the most difficult tasks in the field. In the following subsections, we will discuss a few of the more important factors to be considered in these endeavors.

Task 1: Understand Difficulty of Behavioral Change

You will have spent substantial energy and resources developing a relevant and scientifically valid information synthesis whose use could be healthcare improvement. On the other hand, all of your hard work may be the development of just another document to be filed away and rarely seen again if certain tasks are not accomplished. Before reading Chapter 18 (evaluation of the synthesis as a whole), we suggest you think about some implicit assumptions you may have regarding your project. If you are a beginner in this field, you may have presumed that by being rigorous in developing a relevant and scientifically sound systematic review, your resulting information will be ready for immediate application in the community. Furthermore, you may also have assumed that to effect outcomes improvement, all you need to do is report your work at a prestigious conference or publish and distribute your synthesis, and improvements will happen.

Such assumptions are often naive. Your greatest challenge lies ahead as you try to make your manuscript understandable and motivate your readers to try applying your synthesis to enhance healthcare outcomes. We hope that some of the ideas shared in this chapter will help you cope better with this difficult challenge.

Before you can achieve this goal of effecting behavioral change, you require substantial information about your targeted audience. Who are they? What are they like? What are their values? What is their role in the healthcare field? In what environment do they work? What are the consumer or provider issues that frustrate them the most? What healthcare information or actions might motivate behavioral change?

With such information, some creative problem solving will be needed to determine how best to help your readers enhance the outcomes of the healthcare they provide or influence. It is equally important that you help them establish evidence that their interventions are related to whatever outcomes improvement they may claim. If you have had much personal experience with the problems of effecting behavioral change, you will not be surprised by our assumption that effecting and maintaining such change are among the more difficult of professional endeavors.

Task 2: Recognize Similar Difficulties in Diffusion of Innovation

Rogers's (1983) classic research on the diffusion of innovation is highly relevant to this problem. He was one of the early research pioneers in this subject. He portrays the rate of adoption using an "S" curve, with the x-axis being time and the y-axis being percent adoption (p. 11). He formulated the now-familiar categories of adopters: (a) innovators, (b) early adopters, (c) early majority, (d) late majority, and (e) laggards (i.e., late adopters) (p. 22).

Equally important, Rogers (1983, p. 20) portrays five steps in the adoption process: (a) knowledge, (b) persuasion, (c) decision, (d) implementation, and (e) confirmation. He explains that the knowledge step begins with awareness of a useful innovation (because the learner often does not know what he or she does not know) or awareness of the need for change. Next, data gathering leads to a favorable or unfavorable attitude and expectations regarding outcomes, which, in turn, lead to a choice to adopt or reject this new advance. If adopted, techniques for using the innovation are learned, work processes are adjusted, and policies change. Then a determination is made whether to keep using or to reject this technology or knowledge. For example, suppose a nurse learns of a new computerized program to assess patient acuity that will compute the information automatically. He or she will begin to read about it, might try out a demonstration, and may talk to others who have used it. Once a decision is made, the nurse may purchase it to try it out on one ward. Once individuals start learning how to use it, adjustments have to be made in their workflow. They may have to collect some information before the morning report instead of after in order for the program to be useful for patient assignments. Once adjustments have been made, a decision will be made to continue. In this case, the innovation cues his or her awareness of a need, referred to in Rogers's (1983) step (a) (i.e., knowledge or awareness). This might then lead to Rogers's steps (b), (c), (d), and (e).

Conversely, if the individual is already aware of a need, then this might motivate a search process, which in turn leads to the discovery of an innovation to meet that need. If subsequent inquiry stimulates a positive attitude, this could result in a decision to obtain this resource. After a trial period, the decision will either be confirmed or lead to a disappointment. Again, Rogers's (1983) cycle is completed.

Understanding principles of effecting behavioral change and of diffusion of innovations can be helpful to you in coping with these issues. We will discuss these principles briefly.

Task 3: Prepare to Manage the Problems of Change

There has been much research in the area of behavioral change. The disciplines of psychology, education, quality management (both healthcare and industrial), and business (marketing, accounting, organizational change, and systems analysis) have all contributed substantial theory and often demonstrated evidence of successful change (improvement). For example, the field of advertising is based on sound market research to better understand market segments and the customers themselves. Their success in changing market behavior is known to all. Those desiring to effect improvement in healthcare can learn much from such relevant disciplines. For example, Bucher, Weinbacher, and Gyr (1994), and Naylor, Chen, and Straus (1992) studied how methods of reporting scientific studies influence prescribing behavior. Likewise, Lilford, Pauker, Braunholtz, and Jiri (1998) explored decision analysis methods for getting research findings into practice.

The following areas are especially helpful.

Understand Principles of Adult Learning. **Ethnography educational theory** has been evolving for centuries. In the past several decades, leaders in the field have developed many contrasting theories and have reported considerable research to support their ideas. A Sci-Search, through the Institute for Science Information (ISI), of such classic works as the following could bring you up-to-date on modern concepts in this field: Knowles's (1970*) The Modern Practice of Adult Education,* Knox's (1977*) Adult Development and Learning,* and Cross's (1981) *Adults as Learners.*

Recognize Paradox in Current Continuing Education. Presently, healthcare professionals are coping with the increasing quantity of technology and literature and the problems of relevance and validity in the information they obtain (Williamson et al., 1989). The seeming paradox is that we have progressed substantially in learning what educational modalities in healthcare seem to work and then spend much of our continuing education budgets on those interventions that randomized controlled educational trials have shown to have little impact on either behavior or outcomes (Davis et al., 1984; Davis, Thompson, Oxman, & Haynes, 1992; Davis et al., 1995). Recently, Oxman et al. (1995) evaluated 102 carefully selected randomized controlled educational trials and very aptly concluded, "There are no 'magic bullets' for improving the quality of healthcare" (p. 1423). Bero et al. (1998) reviewed systematic reviews on this subject and found that those published after 1991 were of better quality. Five reviews cited by her were formal meta-analyses (Austin, Balas, Mitchell, & Ewigman, 1994; Beaudry, 1989; Gyorkos et al., 1994; Silagy, Lancaster, Gray, & Fowler, 1995; Waddell, 1991). There are, however, wide ranges of interventions available that are derived from the best available evidence, which, if used appropriately, could lead to substantial improvements in clinical care (Bero et al., 1998). Davis, Thompson, Oxman, and Haynes (1995) analyzed 99 randomized controlled educational trials. (Note: We have not determined the overlap of Davis et al.'s trials with those analyzed by Oxman et al. [1995] as they all seem to be in the same "invisible college"; e.g., Davis was also a coauthor of Oxman's study.) In any event, Davis et al. concluded, "Widely used CME delivery methods such as conferences have little direct impact on improving professional practice. More effective methods, such as systematic practice-based interventions and outreach visits, are seldom used by Continuing Medical Education (CME) providers" (p. 700). Based on our own experience, we strongly agree with these findings.

Coping with these problems requires a new educational paradigm for which traditional continuing education methods (conferences, lectures, seminars, and film or paper media [e.g., medical journals]) are clearly ill equipped.

Use Technology of Evidence-Based Learning. Preparing to cope with innovation and change will depend on accessing relevant and scientifically sound facts, especially regarding the efficacy and cost-effectiveness of any learning experience. In our judgment, such outcomes should be measured in terms of clinician and patient results in such areas as health, satisfaction, and economics, to name a few.

CAUTION

The terms *evidence based* and *systematic reviews* are becoming widely used internationally. Unfortunately, they are also becoming buzzwords (i.e., words that many people use without really understanding what they imply, how important these implications are, or how complex a process is required to meet even mediocre thresholds of acceptability). This is much like what happened to the term *quality* since the 1980s.

More and more institutions are claiming that they use "evidence-based medicine," "evidence-based guidelines" or "evidence-based education," to name but a few such terms. Consequently, the reader must be cautious in that "all evidence that glitters may not be gold." In one large multihospital network, "evidence-based" guidelines were made policy; a directive was given from the executive head that "systematic literature reviews" be done immediately to produce evidence for use in their guidelines. Nowhere was such a "systematic review" explained. In a single seminar, an outside expert showed employees dozens of overheads and filled the room with confusing new jargon. These selected employees were then told they were ready to develop "evidence-based" guidelines.

Thus, it is important to be very cautious and carefully analyze the methods section of any so-called "systematic review" that supposedly produces evidence-based data, let alone "mature" information for immediate use in healthcare (see Badgett, O'Keefe, & Henderson, 1998).

Keeping up with the explosion of healthcare technology and knowledge requires a rapidly growing capability for producing relevant, valid, understandable, and applicable information syntheses. Put in more modern jargon, this concept requires "evidence-based learning." Perhaps the leading proponents of this approach are Sackett, Haynes, Davis, Oxman, Guyett, and other colleagues (Cook, Greengold, Ellrodt, & Weingarten, 1997; Ellrodt, Cho, Cush, Kavanaugh, & Lipsky, 1997; Greenhalgh & Douglas, 1999; Haynes, Sackett, Gray, Cook, & Guyatt, 1997; Haynes, Sackett, Guyatt, Cook, & Gray, 1996, 1997). These pioneers have spent a major part of their careers in furthering these concepts. We suspect that few researchers in the healthcare and adult education field have accepted what we personally judge to be a core concept of future quality improvement and continuing education. Both healthcare education and quality management require validated evidence that their precepts are scientifically sound and that their claims for outcomes improvement are **evidence based**. The Dr. Fox studies of Ware and Williams (1975) were among the earlier research reports to emphasize this need. They illustrated how "self-perceived" learning had little relationship to "objectively measured" (i.e., evidence-based) learning. Grimshaw and Russell (1993) wrote a systematic review of "rigorous evaluations" of guidelines. More recently, Onion and Walley (1998) have questioned whether guidelines should be restricted to being evidence based. Grimshaw, Watson, and Eccles (1998) then wrote an interesting commentary on their article.

In the future, however, with increased financing of the Cochrane Collaboration and multiple nations developing centers for development and dissemination of information syntheses (e.g., the U.S. and Canadian governments' investment in evidence-based practice Centers), a new day may be dawning for the emergence of evidence-based learning. This would require funding new controlled educational trials to more objectively evaluate our most promising new methods of effecting behavioral change. Using such evidence, we might then experience a substantially greater impact of continuing education on outcomes for both the providers and consumers of healthcare.

Procedure B. Avoiding Conflicts of Interest and Hazards of Science Propaganda

As an author of a systematic review, you would be well served taking a few moments to reflect on unintentional negative effects your synthesis might have. Think of yourself as a reader of your work and ask what hazards you might be concerned about in that role. In this procedure, we will outline a few of the serious ways your synthesis could be misleading, so that you might correct them now, while your manuscript is still in draft stage.

Task 1: Follow the Money to Understand Incentives

With the present state of our healthcare system, you will be bombarded with many conflicting and immature statements of what "the latest research shows." Great benefits are predicted, with little mention of the fact that these benefits may be 10 to 20 years in the future. With our competitive grant and contract funding system, the future of many researchers' careers and earnings may depend on their reporting not only "positive findings" but findings that have the potential for widespread beneficial impact. Most research funding in this country is for doing research, not writing grants, and often not writing papers. Many academic faculties, as well as private corporation officials, are impressed by the length, rarely the quality, of your personal bibliography (publish or perish). Finally, as much as we do not like to admit it, there is also some fraud and deception in healthcare, as well as in research (Broad & Wade, 1982; Wise, 1998). In our judgment, these problems are real and extremely difficult to solve.

What can you do to cope with these issues? Perhaps the adage "follow the money" might lead to some clues. It can be informative to know the sources of an investigator's funds. For example, certain groups in the pharmaceutical industry pay large sums for "independent" research in their field. Serious bias can result from this practice. Some corporations pay funds to medical journals to facilitate publication of a supplement to be developed in their area of interest. Scientists who happen to share a corporate bias may be invited to contribute. Yet some still contend that any mention of financial support by an author should be voluntary, if permitted at all (Krimsky & Rothenberg, 1998).

There may be monetary influences where "publication bias" exists. Frank Davidoff, M.D., editor *of Annals of Internal Medicine,* stated, "Scientific journals and publishers have always had different agendas. The fundamental issues of generating revenues and meeting the scientific responsibilities and standards are not new, but the stakes have increased on both sides" (quoted in Mitka, 1999, pp. 622-623). Richard Glass, *JAMA* interim coeditor, stated, "It's an old conflict between commercialism and professionalism and seems to reflect a trend that's going on in medicine in general" (quoted in Mitka, p. 623).

There may be other clues regarding conflict of interest. Do authors of information syntheses include a "funnel plot" of their literature database, comparing effect size against sample size? (A truncated plot might indicate serious bias, particularly "publication bias.") Do the investigators often give lectures at conferences where they report findings favorable to the sponsor's interest? Does a meta-analysis have a weak literature search strategy that produces mainly articles favorable to the investigator's interest?

Is there evidence of political bias in government research funding, especially in times of conflict regarding a topic of interest to Congress? Special interest lobbyists have made a science of how best to influence state and federal leaders in such matters. The impact of lobbyists is often clearly in the financial interest of the groups who hire them and the politicians involved.

Task 2: Check for Nonfinancial Conflicts of Interest

As discussed for implementing Task 1 on financial conflict of interest, this issue is likely the most common bias. However, there are many other author interests and, as Thompson (quoted by Smith [1998], the editor of the *British Medical Journal*) points out, all authors have both primary interests, such as the patient's welfare or scientific validity of research, as well as secondary interests, such as financial gain. However, authors can be motivated by many other influences than money. There is a series of editorials and correspondence in the *New England Journal of Medicine* (*NEJM*) that illustrates this point. Kassirer (then editor of the *NEJM*) and Angell (1993) also refer to Thompson's (1993) article, stating that conflict of interest is a subtle matter of unconscious bias, as opposed to dishonesty. They go on to state this as a major reason for having authors disclose, rather than omit, any possible source of bias that they might have. This is policy at the *NEJM*.

However, Kassirer and Angell (1993) go on to point out other sources of bias not necessarily related to finances. For example, nearly all researchers share an "intellectual" conflict of interest to publish important results and to make a contribution. This bias can also produce even more serious conflicts when the author does not submit negative randomized clinical trials (RCTs) for publication or have them listed on a register. Religious conflicts of interest can be equally as subtle, especially when an investigator prides himself or herself as an objective scientist. It is possible that peer reviewers may give greater weight to studies whose results support their own theories than to those that do not, regardless of methodological rigor. By making a conscientious attempt to disclose such nonfinancial biases or conflicts, the scientific community will surely benefit, and the quality of reviews based on those studies will likely improve, especially if reviewers sign an appropriate disclosure statement themselves.

Task 3: Verify Evidence, Especially in Systematic Reviews

There are a wide variety of criteria that can be applied to discern valid research findings for use in an information synthesis, particularly a meta-analysis. Often the criteria are left unstated, and they vary widely in their stringency and rigor. Criteria should be referenced, specific, and relevant to the area of study. On the other hand, if an extensive validation effort is applied, such as that of the RAND Corporation (Chassin et al., 1986), the cost may be out of reach. We suggest that the criteria applied by the editors of the *ACP Journal Club* might be an acceptable compromise. They are subject-specific and not design specific, though research design can be inferred. Their strength is in the fact that their criteria can be supported by their considerable experience and previous publications. Refer to such material as the "Users' Guide to the Medical Literature" series published in *JAMA* (see Oxman et al. [1993] for the first article of this series, and Guyatt, Rennie, & Hayward [2001a; 2001b]). However, validity of research sources is but one dimension of evidence to be checked.

Determining how representative the final literature "database" is of a systematic review can be just as difficult. In our experience, a sloppy, brief, and poorly documented literature search may yield a bias that is often in the author's favor, in addition saving considerable funds required by a sound search strategy. In earlier times, documenting a search in detail was unknown. Usually, the reference list of any scientific paper was merely a numerator of an unknown denominator of literature. Thus, it was impossible to determine the quality of the review strategy itself. However, again there is a wide range of strategies to identify relevant research material. For instance, is there any attempt to identify invisible colleges or fugitive literature, including unpublished studies? These search goals are important for single investigative reports but far more important for information syntheses. Again, as with validation assessment, representativeness of the final database may be substantially restricted by lack of funds or expertise. If such is the case, then reader beware.

We will not go into further detail on assessing how sound research evidence may be identified because one of the purposes of this book is to facilitate achieving an adequate standard in this regard.

Task 4: Don't Be Misled by Inappropriate Alpha or Beta Values

We assume you are aware of 2×2 contingency table applications in research. If not, Appendix 12.1 in Chapter 12 might help you become more familiar with these important concepts. In this section, we will highlight ways where alpha and beta values might be misleading.

Understanding Implications of Alpha and p Values. The setting of alpha values is a judgment call that investigators make to help them interpret results. An alpha value is agreed on prior to a research trial, quality improvement (QI) assessment, or clinical work-up. In contrast, *p* values are calculated after a study, when the findings are known. If a *p* value is statistically larger or, in some cases, smaller than your alpha threshold, specific action implications should be clear. In most research, a *p* value is the lowest acceptable probability of a **Type I error**. For example, in a controlled trial, a Type I error is when you find a difference between the experimental and the control group that, in reality, does not exist. Clinical researchers generally establish an alpha of 0.05 (1 in 20, or a 5% probability that any difference found will be due to chance alone).

These alpha values are threshold levels that you set, depending on your values, local circumstances, whether you are testing for diagnostic accuracy and therapeutic efficacy or making a clinical decision, and your estimate of the likely cost or harm of a Type I error. However, they should not be regarded as firmly fixed at 0.05 or 0.01. Chalmers and Lau (1993) at the Harvard School of Public Health state,

> In clinical trials of new interventions, attempting to disprove the null hypothesis may be inappropriate because past data so often suggest or even establish that it is not true. Furthermore, we need to recognize that trends (p greater than 0.05) can be both clinically and statistically important, and we must abandon the notion that if p is not less than 0.05, the treatment is ineffective. (p. 161)

Thus, it is important to understand that there is no absolute alpha or p value that everyone should accept for every research or decision purpose, every time.

Furthermore, Type I and Type II errors are somewhat inversely related. (A **Type II error** occurs, e.g., when you incorrectly rule out a positive effect that actually exists.) If you minimize Type I errors, you may increase Type II errors or vice versa, so you have to use astute judgment that is often heavily influenced by the question you are asking and by your local circumstances.

Understanding Beta Values.   Often of much greater concern is the beta value (i.e., the risk of a Type II error, or a false negative rate). In a therapeutic example of this type of error, your beta value would be the proportion of all patients having a positive effect who were missed by the RCT—in other words, of the total cases where, in reality, exercise program R is more efficacious than exercise program S, the proportion that the clinical trial found *not* to be better is the beta value. Or in a pharmaceutical clinical trial, a beta value would indicate the probability that research would find no difference between the experimental and control group when, in fact, there was a significant difference. On the other hand, power (1 - beta) indicates the probability that a trial will identify a significant difference should it exist.

This concept has the important implication that a study sample may be too small to identify a real difference that does, in fact, exist. This fact is a major rationale for doing a meta-analysis where pooled results may have greater power for detecting a significant difference. Although in clinical research, an alpha = 0.05 (i.e., 1 in 20, or 5%) is the traditionally acceptable risk of a measured difference being due to chance, it has also been traditional to accept a beta value of 0.20 (i.e., 1 in 5, or 20%) likelihood that a positive result will be due to chance (Sackett et al., 1991, p. 201). In this instance, the power (1 - beta) would indicate an 80% probability of finding a difference that in fact really exists. Naturally, if a Type I error merely results in lost money, and a Type II error results in lost life, their threshold percentages should be adjusted accordingly.

Misleading Implications of Inadequate Statistical Power. Power is directly related to sample size—the larger the sample, the greater the power to detect a small significant difference that really exists. Power is computed as (1 - beta). This attribute is important to recognize when a researcher or QI professional claims there is no significant difference, say, between intervention L and M. When it is important to be sure of this claim, you must check the sample size to determine how small a difference can be detected by that power. This distinction is especially important in studies of causality where pooling of effect sizes, for example, by meta-analysis might increase the power to better detect true differences that, in fact, exist.

But even here, statistical significance and clinical significance may be in conflict. For example, a large population sample could yield a statistically significant difference that is clinically not significant. To illustrate, a study may be conducted to determine the difference between exercise programs for blood pressure. A sample size might be so large as to have the power to detect differences of 1 or 2 points between those doing the exercise and those not doing the exercise. This small drop in blood pressure, though statistically significant, is hardly significant clinically, especially if the new program costs large amounts of money.

Who Benefits From Inappropriate Alpha or Beta Values? For either alpha or beta values, there are some circumstances in which the investigator must be more rigorous and other circumstances where he or she can be less so. The significance level you set for either alpha or beta threshold values is a judgment call and depends on your values, the circumstances, and the likely cost of a Type I or Type II error. However, there are times when inappropriate levels might benefit either the provider or the patient but at the expense of the other. The following examples illustrate this principle.

A QI project was conducted at an inner-city, university-affiliated, for-profit health maintenance organization (HMO). The HMO QI Board set its beta value at 0.27. In other words, the Board agreed that improvement action would not be warranted unless primary care clinicians were missing the diagnosis of treatable depression in more than 27% of adolescents and adults found to be seriously depressed by independent psychiatric examination. This beta value seemed to be a rather high acceptable risk because in this case, Type II errors could result in avoidable suicides. The final measured result indicated that primary physicians were missing the diagnosis in 85% of depressed patients. This error could save the HMO substantial expense, and the patients could avoid suffering pain and possibly death (Williamson, 1978a, pp. 269-274).

This somewhat self-serving acceptance of a high beta error in HMO management of depressed patients may still be of concern. In another for-profit HMO, to keep costs down, administrative approval was required for any prescription of expensive serum serotonin reuptake inhibitors (SSRIs). Furthermore, the HMO would not allow hospitalization of depressed patients unless approved by a case manager nearly 1,800 miles away. Unutzer et al. (2000) reported that only 4% to 7% of depressed elderly (older than age 65) patients in a large staff model HMO were receiving treatment. Of those who were treated, only 30% were receiving adequate antidepression medication.

In clinical decision making, it is our judgment that the patient and his or her doctor should agree on, or at least discuss, what is an acceptable risk of Type I and Type II errors in terms of health, economic, and satisfaction outcomes (see Glasziou et al., 1998, p. A-16).

Task 5: Don't Be Misled by Large Relative Risk Reductions

In 1988, Forrow, Taylor, and Arnold (1992) published an article titled "Absolutely Relative: How Research Results Are Summarized Can Affect Treatment Decisions." In this study, results from an actual RCT testing the efficacy of Drug X for health problem A were presented in a questionnaire to approximately half of 235 Harvard Medical Center physicians, including faculty, fellows, epidemiologists, and research methods specialists. The study results indicated that these clinicians would not use Drug X on reading that the **absolute risk** reduction (ARR) was 0.4%. However, when given the same results presented as a **relative risk reduction** (RRR) of 24%, they would use the drug. The other half of the group went through the same exercise, only this time results were from an RCT for Drug Y for an entirely separate topic, and again the same pattern of response was found. The clinicians would not prescribe Drug Y when reading that the ARR was only 1.5%. When the same results were presented as an RRR of 20.3%, they would prescribe this drug.

Clearly, on the questionnaire, these participants were far more inclined, after reading the RRR, to prescribe the experimental drug by a factor of nearly 10 (p = .0001). Even more amazing, there was no difference in "prescribing" response on the questionnaire among those physicians with epidemiological or research methods background, as compared to those clinicians without such quantitative training or experience.

Bobbio, Demichelis, and Giustetto (1994) drew similar conclusions from their questionnaire studies, only they elicited the intent to prescribe from 148 primary practitioners who were shown results of a single RCT measuring 5-year mortality and cardiac events for an experimental drug versus a placebo. However, in this questionnaire study, the same RCT results were presented in five different ways, each as if derived from a different study of the same drug. These reporting methods included relative risk reduction, absolute risk reduction, differences in event-free patients, number needed to treat to prevent one event, events reduction, and mortality. In this study, for example, the RCT results indicated an RRR of mortality as 34% versus an

ARR of 1.41%. Again, by a very wide margin, physicians would prescribe when seeing RRR, as opposed to reading the same results as presented in all other formats. They concluded, "The method of reporting trial results and the completeness of information in the case of controversial results affects physicians' willingness to prescribe" (p. 1209). (Also see Naylor, Chen, and Strauss, 1992.)

Feinstein, as quoted in Bobbio et al. (1994), stated, "As [Feinstein] recently pointed out, the best methods to describe differences do not depend on statisticians but on description and substantive perception" (p. 1211). The title of Feinstein's (1988) article says it all: "Fraud, Distortion, Delusion, and Consensus: The Problems of Humans on Natural Deception in epidemiologic science."

With pharmaceutical advertising, it is common policy to stress the relative improvement of a product over a competing product while keeping the absolute improvement obscure or not mentioned at all. If isolated RRR is used, the statistics can be misleading if there is no concurrent mention of ARR. For example, if the risk of gastric bleeding associated with experimental Drug E were decreased by 100% (RRR) over traditional Drug T, a physician might be motivated to prescribe, or a patient might be motivated to accept Drug E. However, if the absolute risk of gastric bleeding was 1 in 1,000 with Drug E, as opposed to 2 in 1,000 with Drug E (ARR), this 100% increased benefit, even if statistically different, would hardly be considered clinically significant. Even worse, if the cost of Drug E was substantially higher than that of Drug T, the miniscule gain in possible benefit might be considered economically harmful, all other factors being equal.

When you report the results of your own systematic review of RCTs, try to avoid the human tendency to report an exciting RRR and not the unimpressive ARR.

Task 6: Look for Investigators Overgeneralizing Results

Hypothetically, suppose a poorly documented but superbly implemented double-blind controlled clinical trial compared the side effects of two pharmaceuticals, Drug X and Drug Y. It was found that Drug Y had much less potential for life-threatening arrhythmias than Drug X. Naturally, this fact is stressed in the investigator's conclusions. What is often not mentioned is the fact that this difference can be generalized only to middle-aged, healthy, adult American males because this demographic group made up 85% of the population sample studied. Unfortunately, it might also be discovered later that the risk of arrhythmias of Drug Y in middle-aged pregnant women was far greater than in nonpregnant females and caused life-threatening complications for the fetus. In this hypothetical example, not accounting for this epidemiological bias, though in the investigator's favor, would result in placing an important subpopulation at great risk.

The implication of such a research report to the unwary clinician is that Drug Y must be much more efficacious for all people everywhere, regardless of their age, health, gender, or geography. The point we wish to make is that researchers should be very conservative in establishing limits for generalizability of their findings. Furthermore, these limits should be clearly stated in their study conclusions if they are claiming a significant effect size. The implication of overgeneralizations for those developing information syntheses is equally grave.

Task 7: Check for Biased and Untrustworthy Information on the Internet

In the current rush to develop Web sites, both commercial and academic leaders are often providing information of questionable validity. Impicciatore, Pandolfini, Casella, and Bonati (1997) published a study of the reliability of health information on the Internet related to management of childhood fever. Of 41 Net pages analyzed, only 4 adhered closely to five generally accepted criteria from published guidelines. They concluded, "Only a few Web sites provided complete and accurate information for this common and widely discussed condition. This suggests an urgent need to check public oriented healthcare information on the Internet for accuracy, completeness, and consistency" (p. 1875). This complete article can be obtained from the following Web site (last updated ??, copyright 1997):

> www.bmj.com/cgi/content/full/314/7098/1875?view=full&pmid=
> 9224132.

(Also see Lightner et al., 1996.)

McClung, Murray, and Heitlinger (1998) corroborated the above findings. The Web recommendations were compared to the guidelines developed by the American Academy of Pediatrics (AAP). They concluded,

> As demonstrated by information supplied on World Wide Web sites by traditional medical sources, recommendations for the treatment of acute diarrhea shows a low percentage of concurrence with the AAP guidelines. Major medical institutions, schools, and hospitals need to devise ways to carefully monitor and establish quality control of what is being distributed from their home pages. Patients must be warned about the voluminous misinformation available on medical subjects on the Net. (p. e2)

This complete article can be located at the following Web site (last updated ??, copyright 1998): www.pediatrics.org/cgi/content/full/101/6/e2.

Finally, we abstracted the following information from the *Public Citizen Health Research Group Health Letter,* edited by Sidney Wolfe (1999, pp. 10-11). There it was reported that the *New York Times* (April 19, 1999) carried a full-page ad from Aetna U.S. Healthcare, congratulating InteliHealth for being voted the "Best Health Web site" by the International Academy of Digital Arts and Sciences. Then it was explained in the bulletin that InteliHealth is a media company in a joint venture with Aetna U.S. Healthcare and the Johns Hopkins University. Furthermore, it was reported that the *New York Times* ad stated, "Its [InteliHealth] two million pages of thoroughly researched, continuously updated health information . . . offers a complete range of online services . . . because we believe in giving you the information you need when you need it." The *Public Citizen* bulletin continues, "We printed the information for five drugs from the InteliHealth Web site [www.InteliHealth.com] and found that for these drugs the information was incomplete, out-of-date, inaccurate, and thus potentially dangerous" (Wolfe, 1999, p. 55). It was noted that InteliHealth did not mention that the drug PROPULSID has caused life-threatening heart arrhythmias and 38 deaths, including deaths of children, and so is contraindicated for that age group (the death count as of June 2000 is more than 100 and climbing, so the Food and Drug Administration has directed that this drug be removed from the market). After Wolfe pointed this out, the labeling for this drug was changed to read, "Safety and effectiveness [of CISAPRIDE] in pediatric patients under the age of 16 years have not been established for any indication." (We might add that the relabeling is both euphemistic and misleading in not mentioning the potential danger to children.) Wolfe continues, noting that InteliHealth stated in its Web site that PROCARDIA can be used to treat high blood pressure. Wolfe notes that the capsule form (PROCARDIA) of the drug (PROPULSID) has never been approved for this use. Again, after Wolfe pointed this out, the drug was relabeled to read, "Procardia capsules should not be used for the control of essential hypertension." He reported finding similar potentially life-threatening problems on this InteliHealth Web site for the other three drugs studied. The bulletin then continues, "So much for InteliHealth and the Johns Hopkins University . . . thoroughly researched, continuously updated health information" and, in reference to the *New York Times* ad, "So much, also for the conflict of interest that is implicit in a company's buying ads to congratulate a corporate creature of its own." As an aside, Wolfe further reported that Johns Hopkins did respond to *Public Citizen,* claiming that this Web site would be updated by July 1, 2000. We concur with Wolfe that such information, so freely available on the Internet, can, indeed, be dangerous to your health.

In the next section of this chapter, we will discuss several of many generic methods for applying information syntheses to improve healthcare outcomes. This is not a comprehensive overview, but rather highlights several developments, together with their advantages and disadvantages, that seem promising for effecting healthcare outcomes improvement.

Procedure C. Achieving Healthcare Outcomes Improvement

Task 1: Communicating Quantitative Research Results

Each of the three clusters below covers a number of statistical concepts that are important to understand if you are to accurately communicate quantitative research results to either a clinical or lay audience. Each term refers to a specific statistical formula portraying a mathematical relationship of variables. The terms are roughly ordered by increasing complexity of the concepts involved. Although it is not our purpose to teach research nomenclature or statistical formulae, we do wish to highlight the concepts you need to understand in communicating quantitative synthesis results. We divide these concepts into three clusters: (a) fundamental concepts, (b) concepts related to diagnostic accuracy, and (c) concepts related to therapeutic efficacy and effectiveness.

COMMUNICATING QUANTITATIVE RESEARCH RESULTS

Cluster a. Fundamental Concepts
- (1) Rates
- (2) Ratios
- (3) Confidence intervals (CI)
- (4) Total population (*N*)
- (5) Sampling frame
- (6) Sample population
- (7) Sampling methods
- (8) Sampling error
- (9) Incidence
- (10) Prevalence

Cluster b. Terms Used for Diagnostic Accuracy
- (11) True positive (TP)
- (12) False positive (FP)
- (13) True negative (TN)
- (14) False negative (FN)
- (15) True-positive rate (TPR)
- (16) False-positive rate (FPR)
- (17) True-negative rate (TNR)
- (18) False-negative rate (FNR)
- (19) Sensitivity rate
- (20) Specificity rate
- (21) Positive predictive value (PPV)
- (22) Negative predictive value (NPV)
- (23) Positive likelihood ratio (+LR)
- (24) Negative likelihood ratio (-LR)

Cluster c. Terms Used for Therapeutic Efficacy
- (25) Risk
- (26) Absolute risk (AR)
- (27) Relative risk (RR)

(28) Experimental event rate (EER)
(29) Control event rate (CER)
(30) Experimental relative risk (ERR)
(31) Control relative risk (CRR)
(32) Relative risk reduction (RRR)
(33) Absolute risk reduction (ARR)
(34) Number needed to treat (NNT)
(35) Number needed to harm (NNH)
(36) Odds
(37) Odds ratios
(38) Effect sizes (ES)

There are numerous sources for learning to understand the above concepts. If available, we recommend the book *Clinical Epidemiology: A Basic Science for Clinical Medicine* (Sackett et al., 1991) as an exceptional reference covering most of the above concepts with clear illustrations of contingency tables that facilitate understanding. Chatellier, Zapletal, Lemaitre, Menard, and Degoulet (1996) present a simple nomogram to estimate "the number needed to treat." Another good source available on the Web is the *Cochrane Reviewers' Handbook Glossary, Version 4.0* (last updated May 1999) available by linkage (click "Browse the Handbook Online") through the following Web site (site last updated May 2001): www.cochrane.org/cochrane/hbook.htm.

Another approach is by accessing *JAMA*'s series (1993-1999) titled "Users' Guides to the Medical Literature." (See the initial article of the series, Oxman et al., 1993.) As of February 2000, at least 19 articles had been published in this series. Much of the essential information from this series is now available in book form, which includes a CD-ROM version in hypertext. In the following Web site, they state, "As the culmination of nearly two decades of teaching and research, all of the Users' Guides to the Medical Literature products provide the most detailed yet clinician-friendly exposition of the concepts necessary to use the medical literature to solve patient problems" (last updated August 2001; see www.usersguides.org). Another important source is the American College of Physicians' *ACP Journal Club*'s rather frequent editorials on concepts contained in the *JAMA* series (e.g., Guyatt, Jaeschke, & Cook, 1995; Sackett & Haynes, 1997; Sackett & Straus, 1998). It is not surprising that all or most of the above references are by members of the "invisible college" that includes D. L. Sackett, R. B. Haynes, D. A. Davis, and G. H. Guyatt, among many others of the Cochrane Collaboration.

Quantifying and communicating quality of life outcomes of healthcare is another area of importance to all practitioners of the health professions. The exceptional work of Ware and colleagues is vital in this regard (Ware, 1998; Ware, Keller et al., 1999; Ware & Sherbourne, 1992).

Task 2: Using Ethnographic Educational Methods

ETHNOGRAPHIC EDUCATIONAL METHODS

Ethnography is a concept emanating from cultural anthropology, sociology, and social psychology. In an educational context, this concept requires the ethnographer to assume several roles—namely, a "participant–observer," an interviewer, a learning facilitator, and an evaluator. This person must combine expertise in the subject content with ethnographic skills, applied in the learner's own work environment. This theory assumes that the learner may not be ideally suited to know what he or she doesn't know and therefore may have difficulty in identifying important personal learning needs. The ethnographer and the learner establish priorities for these needs, formulate required learning experiences, and perform an evaluation of educational impact.

This concept assumes that a healthcare professional's working environment is a unique mini-culture and that the most important learning must involve a "participant-observer" who interacts with the learner and provides timely, expert, on-the-job feedback, based on direct observations, questionnaires, and "artifacts" (e.g., a job description, a corporate employment contract, or other official documents). The concept of "on-the-job" training is not new by any means. However, an **ethnographic approach** differs by taking a more holistic view of a work environment as a "culture," which is the focus of study and feedback rather than of specific skills to be learned and used sometime in the future.

An ethnographic educational modality that has been applied with substantial success in medicine requires the use of participant-observers, such as the following: (a) "academic detail" people, (b) opinion leaders who are familiar with the local healthcare environment, and (c) trained simulated patients (SP) who come into the office as patients and, after the visit, record details of the care observed and received in terms of the physician's technical quality, physician's communication skills, and feeling responses experienced by the SP. (In a later meeting, they provide direct feedback to the clinician.) The Bayer Pharmaceutical Company has developed a network of doctor-patient communication learning centers throughout the United States. As a standard part of their training, physicians interact with trained "simulated patients" and receive immediate feedback after they participate in a role-play exercise (Bayer Institute for Health Care Communication, 1995a).

The Harvard Medical School is now using this approach. It has trained numerous simulated patients, as well as faculty members, to act in the capacity of a participant learner. If substantiated, the efficacy of this approach will undoubtedly facilitate diffusion of this educational innovation to other medical schools. Though not using the technical ethnographic jargon, residencies and fellowships have used this approach for more than a century. Before that, mentors or apprenticeships provided a similar training environment.

Ethnographic education is being used increasingly in the military, especially the U.S. Army. They term this method the "Lessons Learned" program (Hecht 1998; Henderson & Sussman, 1996). The U.S. Department of Veterans Affairs has also adopted this program.

Business has picked up the idea for many applications—one known as "ethnographic marketing," developed by such organizations as PortiCo Research associated with New York University. The company does ethnographic marketing research with a number of companies. For example, Helene Curtis, Inc. is one of its clients. In this example, we can imagine one of its beautician participant-observers going to the home of a customer to watch how this customer uses the products. Both the observer and the "observed" learn from the encounter. The benefit to the customer is the feedback from the expert and "hands-on" demonstrations to facilitate the client obtaining improved benefit from a given line of products. The benefit to the company is the valuable information from participant-observer feedback to improve its products as well as its marketing. The Web site home page for PortiCo Research, as well as access to a description of business use of ethnography, is (last updated ??) porticoresearch.com.

Ware, Tugenbert, Dickey, and McHorney (1999) applied ethnographic principles in their study, "An Ethnographic Study of the Meaning of Continuity of Care in Mental Health Services." They conclude, "Ethnography promises to be a valuable methodological tool in constructing valid and reliable measures for use in mental health services research" (p. 395). As author of a systematic review, you might provide ideas in your report about how your readers could apply these ethnographic education methods to facilitate diffusion of your findings. This ethnographic education approach complements the provision of quantitative measures of benefit and harm discussed above, as well as those to be discussed below.

Anthropologist H. P. Lundsgaarde (1992) gave a paper on clinical "knowledge engineering and ethnography" at the annual meeting of the American Anthropological Association. He spent several years working with the Department of Medical Informatics at the University of Utah, where knowledge engineering is a major department activity. He concluded that knowledge engineering (e.g., as used for developing computerized expert systems) could be substantially improved by using the principles of ethnography. This subject seems like an important focus for an information synthesis.

We suggest that ethnographic education is a field of substantial promise for learning both how to do systematic reviews and how to apply such material in the healthcare community. For example, participant-observers could be trained to facilitate medical guideline development and use. The Department of Veterans Affairs has adopted these methods in the Health Services Administration implementation of its computerized patient-record program use of "clinical coordinators." There are numerous other areas where ethnography could be used to apply information syntheses for improving clinical care and outcomes.

Task 3: Applying Healthcare Teleinformatics

Systematic reviews of research, reporting experience with "teleinformatics" (telemedicine, telepsychiatry, telepediatrics, and teledermatology, to name but a few), are still in an early stage of development. This topic provides a rich area of current synthesis development to establish a firm evidence-based foundation for this important technology.

HEALTHCARE TELEINFORMATICS

Healthcare teleinformatics is a generic term encompassing an integrated computer-driven technology having a broad infrastructure to facilitate inter- and intrafacility communication. It focuses on text, data, images, sound, and tactile sensations for use in healthcare, education, quality management, research, and particularly guideline development and application.

The infrastructure is based on use of integrated multimedia computer workstations, each having a multi-gigabyte hard drive; a large high-definition monitor; a stereo sound system with microphones; a video camera and peripherals, including a color printer, scanner, and external data storage; and it is hoped, data warehouse availability having multi-terrabyte capacity. With the advent of robotic distant surgery, we should also add equipment for tactile capture and transmission.

Intra-institutional connectivity can be by fiber-optic cable and a local-area network (LAN); interinstitutional and intergeographic connectivity can be by a wide-area network (WAN) using copper phone lines or fiber-optic cable with required modems or satellite.

Each of the teleinformatics elements mentioned above has been developed and tested. However, there are very few large integrated hospital computer networks currently operating. The Veterans Integrated System Architecture (VISTA) network of the U.S. Department of Veterans Affairs, Veterans Health Administration probably comes closest, as it is integrating 172 facilities with such capability.

One of the more important modes of a teleinformatics infrastructure is to provide access to expert systems. To illustrate such a broad-based integrated computer system, we provide an example from Intermountain Health Care's Latter Day Saints (LDS) Hospital's Health Evaluation Through Logical Processing (HELP) system in Salt Lake City, Utah. This system was initiated primarily by Gardner, Pryor, and Warner (1999). It has proven highly successful for improving healthcare processes and outcomes (Haug et al., 1994). For example, Tate and Gardner (1993) found that 11.4% of patients experienced one or more life-threatening conditions during their hospital stay. To cope with this problem, they tried a simple computer alert system, with a later follow-up clinician alert review, to measure response. If a test indicated a patient was in a life-threatening situation, the nurse would post the patient's room number on the computer screen. There was only a 41.4% physician acknowledgment rate and an average response time of 38.7 hours. When the alerts were digitized and posted with the patient's electronic laboratory test reports, acknowledgment of the alert improved to 94.6%, with an average response time of 3.6 hours. Next, flashing lights were attached to the nurses' computers to indicate one of these life-threatening events; then the nurse was supposed to contact the doctor. Acknowledgment rose to more than 99%, with an average response time of 6 minutes (Tate, Gardner, & Scherting, 1995). However, response retention was not maintained because the nurses became so distracted by flashing lights that they often disconnected the alerts (R. M. Gardner, personal communication, fall 1998). This was euphemistically stated in the paper as "the flashing light used in the original CLAS [Computerized Laboratory Alerting System] was very unpopular with users" (Tate et al., 1995, p. 168).

Next, they tried computer alerts by means of direct transmission to a nurse's digital pager (Tate et al., 1995, p. 165). The nurse would read the complete message on the computer screen and acknowledge receiving the alert. If the alert were not acknowledged within 15 minutes, it would then be transmitted to the pager of the charge nurse. Next, the nurse or charge nurse would "chase down" the physician to stimulate a response. Based on follow-up questionnaires, these alerts proved clinically valid 92% of the time; the critical laboratory values were presented to the doctor 100% of the time, with an average response time of 38.6 minutes, 51% being received within 12 minutes. The primary care nurse responded 76% of the time. (It is assumed the charge nurse responded most of the remaining times.)

The U.S. Department of Veterans Affairs (1996; or see Demakus et al., 1996) has also developed an integrated multihospital computer system. Its Center for Cooperative Study in Health Services completed a multisite study of computer-generated reminders to improve ambulatory healthcare. Based on validated literature review information and consensus of local experts, they programmed 10 ambulatory care alerts, which were agreed on as important, efficacious, and reasonable. This controlled clinical trial revealed that the experimental group had a statistically significant increase in adherence to these 10 consensus standards, from 53% at baseline to a 58.8% peak during the computer reminder activation period. This is a 10.9% relative increase or a 5.8% absolute increase. The controls went from 55.3% at baseline to 53.5% adherence in the period of trial activation. This is a 3.3% relative decrease, or a 1.8% absolute decrease. "The adherence rates dropped from a 95.2% relative advantage of the reminder system across the first three months of the study (reminder group 24.2%; control group 12.4%) to a 22.9% relative advantage by the final months (reminder group 13.4%; control group 10.9%)" (U.S. Department of Veterans Affairs, 1996, p. 14). Thus, despite the continued use of these alerts, much, if not most, of this learning effect was extinguished within 1 year.

Like results from a lot of other literature, we are reminded that alerts have not been altogether successful in effecting continuing performance improvement. If alerts are to be used, we suggest that those whose behavior will be affected must be in on the planning phase, especially in terms of practice standards consensus. Next, the alert context and content must be very carefully considered in light of the experience at LDS Hospital in Salt Lake City, Utah. On the other hand, alerts at the time the physician has the intention to act are usually successful—for example, letting the doctor know, while writing the prescription, that he or she has mistakenly ordered a fatal dose of a certain drug by misplacing the decimal point (Tate & Gardner, 1993). R. M. Gardner, chairman of the Department of Medical Informatics, University of Utah School of Medicine, notes that computer alerts can work very well "if they are done right" (R. M. Gardner, personal communication, fall 1998). From his experience, "doing it right" is usually difficult and quite different in different settings.

McMaster (2000) reports that a "unique computer database provides quick answers to crucial questions, helping health professional save lives" (p. 1). This development is at the University of Alberta Hospital in Canada. This resource consists of a network of new clinical integrator (CLINT) computer stations that facilitates staff obtaining both local patient data (e.g., laboratory results) as well as sound scientific information in real time from select sources such as *the New England Journal of Medicine*. They claim that their Centers for Health Information separates "the good stuff from the junk." However, it is likely unwarranted to assume their information is truly "evidence based" at the present time. This presumption in no way detracts from the value of this innovative approach, which, in our judgment, is certainly an important step in the right direction.

Task 4: Developing and Applying Sound Guidelines

Defining Guidelines. Guidelines are proving to be one of the most promising modalities for applying information syntheses to affect healthcare outcomes, especially if they are in an electronic format. But first, what is a guideline?

DEFINING GUIDELINES

The National Guideline Clearinghouse (NGC) uses the definition of clinical practice guidelines developed by the Institute of Medicine, Committee on Clinical Practice Guidelines (1992): "Clinical practice guidelines are systematically developed statements to assist practitioner and patient decisions about appropriate healthcare for specific clinical circumstances" (p. 38).

The authors of this book view guidelines as a subset of decision support technology (DST) that is logic based and integrated with relevant, scientifically sound information and knowledge. Used in this broad, generic way, guidelines could include algorithms, clinical pathways, decision support systems, expert systems, logic-based alert systems, practice parameters, practice protocols, practice policies, and many other forms of artificial intelligence.

SOURCE: Institute of Medicine, Committee on Clinical Practice Guidelines (1992).

Guidelines are being applied much more frequently, with some proving successful (Bergman, 1999; Cook et al., 1997; Hoyt, 1997; Woolf, Grol, Hutchinson, Eccles, & Grimshaw, 1999) and many others proving less than successful (Ellrodt, Conner, Riedinger, & Weingarten, 1995; Rhew et al., 1998; Worrall, Chaulk, & Freake, 1997). Consequently, you have to make sure your information synthesis base for such a guideline is sound and, equally important, that the way the guideline is developed and reported meets National Guideline Clearinghouse (NGC) standards of acceptability.

Developing Guidelines. There are many resources to facilitate improved guideline development (Greengold & Weingarten, 1996; Stokes, Shukla, Schober, & Baker, 1998). You, as a potential author of an information synthesis, should be familiar with these materials if you intend to structure your synthesis for that purpose. As we have mentioned before, ideally, sound guidelines should involve the end user early in the planning stage and be evidence based and applied in electronic form, providing immediate feedback to the physician in real time as he or she makes decisions. They should be sponsored by professional medical organizations for greater credibility, though according to J. P. Kassirer (former *NEJM* editor) and M. Angell (current *NEJM* executive editor, 2000), in some instances the commercial influence on these noteworthy organizations may make even them suspect (in Mitka, 1999). In any event, syntheses must be validated by experts and be updated as often as warranted by the research activity in the subject field.

However, this field is growing rapidly, and many new reviews are appearing in the literature. For example, Bauchner and Simpson (1998) wrote a review article that stresses the need for patients to be more involved in guideline dissemination and adoption. Cook, Greengold, Ellrodt, and Weingarten (1997) wrote a review article emphasizing the use of systematic reviews as a basis for guideline development. The existence of such reviews indicates maturation of this research field.

New ideas are being reported to facilitate guideline development. For example, Hayward, Hogeterp, Langton, Summerell, and Roizen (1995) report a computer-assisted design tool to develop "evidence-based automated questionnaires that may assist health practitioners to implement clinical practice guidelines" (p. 934). Owens (1998) stated, "Differences in patients' preferences may lead to differences in the preferred therapy; a clinical practice guideline that does not consider patients' preferences may provide recommendations that are not optimal" (p. 1073). Nijs, Blecker, Van der Waal, and Casparie (1998) stress the need for expert panel consensus as a basis for guideline or protocol development. Browman et al. (1998) conclude, "The changes made to the EBRs [evidence-based recommendations] in response to feedback suggest that practitioners' opinions can be valuable in shaping evidence-based guidelines" (p. 1226). In our judgment, clinical end users of guidelines are essential for guideline development.

The use of guidelines has been accepted in many healthcare facilities, including at a community health level (Gyorkos, Tannenbaum, Abrahamowicz, Bédard, et al., 1994; Gyorkos, Tannenbaum, Abrahamowicz, Oxman, et al., 1994). Fang, Mittman, and Weingarten (1996) surveyed the directors of physician medical groups and independent practice associations. They found that 87% of the physician organizations were reported to be developing or implementing clinical guidelines. Unfortunately, 19% of these organizations threatened sanctions on physicians who did not use guidelines. The evidence of their efficacy, like that for alerts, is mixed. Hadorn, Baker, Hodges, and Hicks (1996), in their article "Rating the Quality of Evidence for Clinical Practice Guidelines," describe the many serious biases found in evaluating the Agency for Health Care Policy and Research (AHCPR, now AHRQ) guidelines. To validate these guidelines, Hadorn et al. (1996) developed a seven-level criteria hierarchy that provides data and information for validation by the evaluation panels. These criteria range from evidence from well-conducted randomized controlled trials that include 100 patients or more (Level 1) through the use of expert opinion alone (Level 7).

LEVELS OF EVIDENCE FOR GUIDELINE RECOMMENDATIONS

1. Supportive evidence from well-conducted randomized controlled trials that include more than 100 patients
   (a) Evidence from a well-conducted multicenter trial
   (b) Evidence from a meta-analysis that incorporated quality ratings in the analysis and included a total of 100 patients in its estimate of effect size and confidence intervals
2. Supportive evidence from well-conducted randomized controlled trials that include fewer than 100 patients
   (a) Evidence from a well-conducted trial at one or more institutions
   (b) Evidence from a meta-analysis that incorporated quality ratings in the analysis and included fewer than 100 patients in its estimate of effect size and confidence intervals
3. Supportive evidence from well-conducted cohort studies
   (a) Evidence from a well-conducted prospective **cohort study** or registry
   (b) Evidence from well-conducted retrospective cohort studies

     (c) Evidence from a well-conducted meta-analysis of cohort studies
4. Supportive evidence from a well-conducted case-control study
5. Supportive evidence from poorly controlled or uncontrolled studies
     (a) Evidence from randomized clinical trials with one or more major or three or more minor methodological flaws that could invalidate the results
     (b) Evidence from **observational studies** with high potential for bias (such as case series with comparison to historical controls)
     (c) Evidence from case series or case reports
6. Conflicting evidence with the weight of evidence supporting the recommendation
7. Expert opinion

SOURCE: Hadorn et al. (1996).

The use of computer expert systems that apply both Boolean and Bayesian logic, such as Iliad (Lau & Warner, 1992), seems promising for improving diagnostic accuracy and therapeutic appropriateness. Such systems require input of local disease prevalence statistics (i.e., á priori probabilities) for each different health condition in its database, as well as expert judgment (through the process of "knowledge engineering") regarding probabilities not available from data, notes, and other information to be programmed into the system. However, evaluation studies of Iliad have been mixed. There is suggestive evidence that Iliad can improve medical students' diagnostic skills (Lincoln et al., 1991), as well as those of nurse practitioner students (Lange et al., 1997). Also, it can enhance Professional Review Organization (PRO) care problem screening accuracy (Lau & Warner, 1992). Heckerling, Elstein, Terzian, and Kushner (1991), although confirming the seeming diagnostic accuracy of Iliad (Version 2.01) when the unknown diagnosis was in Iliad's knowledge base, found this expert system to be potentially misleading when the unknown condition was not in its database. Several studies of Iliad by Elstein et al. (1996) have not been altogether promising in their results. Murphy et al. (1996) could not confirm the structural validity of this system and concluded that "the quality of Iliad's diagnostic advice in terms of the presence of the correct diagnosis, is no better for consultations done by students or residents compared to attendings [senior physician supervisors]" (p. 219). Wolf et al. (1997), in a subsequent preliminary study of Iliad (Version 4.2) based on 16 subjects, were unable to demonstrate structural validity or any significant findings on such variables as whether consultations with this expert system proved at all helpful. However, more recently, Friedman et al. (1999) concluded, "Our study supports the idea that 'hands-on' use of diagnostic Decision Support Systems (DSSs) can influence diagnostic reasoning of clinicians. The larger effect for students suggests a possible educational role for these systems" (p. 1851).

Because most of these studies have been done by the same group with a small number of subjects and/or have been preliminary in nature, the jury is still out regarding the accuracy and **utility** of Iliad as an expert system. It is our judgment that expert systems will improve with time. The following enhancements will likely be required: (a) enlargement of its database, (b) use of more "commonsense knowledge" (Bouhaddou, Lambert, & Morgan, 1995), (c) use of ethnographic principles for knowledge engineering, (d) better validation of the database of these systems, and (e) use of locally and nationally available disease prevalence statistics for á priori probability estimates.

Several other "if-then" logic systems are also of interest. Berne, Jackson, and Algina (1996) provide a comparative analysis between Dxplain, Meditel, and QMR and also include Iliad. In relation to pediatrics, Johnson and Feldman (1995), at Johns Hopkins in Baltimore, provide an overview of Meditel, Quick Medical Reference, Dxplain, Iliad, and PEM-DXP, including "virtues and problems . . . current controversies and future goals for computer-based decision support" (p. 1371). This whole field of decision support systems is ripe for information syntheses, both qualitative and quantitative. The results could be mature information for immediate healthcare improvement applications.

Ensuring Guidelines Are Evidence Based.   You will find, in the past decade, that guideline usage and literature have rapidly increased. Both those who develop and those who accredit guidelines are beginning to emphasize an evidence-based foundation (Bowers, 1998; Cook et al., 1997; Ellrodt et al., 1997). Although some authors do not seem to comprehend what *evidence based* implies, we still applaud this direction for improving future guidelines. This trend will likely stimulate familiarity with the requirements of a health science information synthesis or systematic review. Although few would question that articles or reviews, which meet the above criteria, are evidence based, some question the wisdom of such a stringent restriction for all guidelines (Onion & Walley, 1998).

However, accepting the value of evidence-based guidelines, you must realize an important distinction. It is one thing for a guideline to be evidence based because it was developed from systematic reviews, and it is quite another thing for it to be evidence based from having been tested by RCTs with guidelines being the experimental intervention and health outcomes as the measure of success. Hackner's (1999) 25-year review of pulmonary medicine guideline applications stresses this point, which has been a focus of Weingarten et al. (Weingarten, Conner, et al., 1995; Weingarten, Ellrodt, Riedinger, & Huang, 1993; Weingarten et al., 1996; Weingarten, Riedinger, Conner, Johnson, & Ellrodt, 1994; Weingarten, Stone, et al., 1995).

The U.S. Department of Veterans Affairs (1998) mandated that the Health Services Research and Development Service (HSR&D) sponsor the development of "evidence-based practice guidelines that can improve health care outcomes and efficiency for our patient population" (p. 1). HSR&D further stated, "Evidence-based guidelines represent a systematic rational approach to medicine because they are more rigorously grounded in science" (p. 3). As part of this mandate, the HSR&D was asked to develop a primer to facilitate development of this program. "This Primer was developed to help a broad audience, including clinicians, health care managers, and policy makers—both within and outside the VA" (p. 1). Indeed, this guide provides an excellent knowledge foundation to support evidence-based healthcare guideline development.

This VA program includes participation of the San Antonio VA Cochrane Center at the Audie L. Murphy Memorial Veterans Hospital in Texas. With this strong affiliation, systems implementation, and ongoing research and evaluation in multiple VA hospitals throughout the country, this program might be one of the more valuable guideline development studies of which we are aware.

Validating Guidelines. The American Medical Association (AMA, 1994) originated a clearinghouse for guidelines and published the *Directory of Practice Parameters, Titles, Sources, and Updates.* It was among the earliest to outline criteria (attributes) that are necessary for a guideline to be considered sound and potentially successful. The main question this raises is the level of validation stringency required. This could range from subjective structural validity ("Given its design and development, it should work") through to its being successfully implemented ("It worked") (Weir, Lincoln, Roscoe, & Moreshead, 1995) through to validation by RCTs where the experimental variable was the guideline ("A systematic review shows that the evidence is clear that healthcare outcomes were improved and causality to the guideline established") (Hackner, 1999). Below, we have paraphrased the AMA's early set of conformance standards. Note that we have substituted *guideline* for the term *practice parameter*, which the AMA used at that time.

AMA ATTRIBUTES TO FACILITATE DEVELOPMENT OF GUIDELINES CHARACTERISTICS OF CONFORMANCE

1. *Authority*   Guidelines are developed by, or in conjunction with, a physician organization; the sponsoring organization is characterized by scientific and clinical expertise in the content area of the guideline.

2. *Evidence-Based*   Guidelines are based on reliable methodologies that integrate relevant research findings and appropriate clinical expertise. The evidence upon which they are based is described, as is the expert clinical judgment/review process; the qualifications of the reviewers/clinical experts are provided.

3. *Comprehensive, Clinically Specific*   Guidelines are comprehensive and have specific clinical management strategies noted in the guideline itself.

4. *Updated Every 3 Years*   Guidelines are based on current information and have been written, reviewed, or revised within the last three years.
5. *Widely Disseminated; Have Publication Plans*   Guidelines are to be widely disseminated, and plans to have them published in peer-reviewed or other widely circulated publication(s) are noted.

SOURCE: American Medical Association (1994).

NOTE: We substitute "guidelines" for "Practice Parameter"

Recently, the AMA has partnered with AHRQ (formerly AHCPR) and the American Association of Health Plans (AAHP) in maintaining this service under the title of the NGC, having the following Web site address (last updated May 2000): www.ngc.gov.

Note that the words *systematic* and *evidence based,* currently used by the NGC, refer to data and information from a systematic review (i.e., an information synthesis in our terminology). The following is an official list of NGC criteria for an acceptable guideline. To be included in its clearinghouse, guidelines must meet all of the following criteria.

The bolded headings in parentheses are our modifications. Recall that we use the term *mature* to mean immediately applicable for healthcare outcome improvement, being efficacious, cost-effective, and acceptable to both consumer and provider of care.

NATIONAL GUIDELINE CLEARINGHOUSE ACCEPTANCE CRITERIA (UNITED STATES)

1. **(Mature Clinically Oriented Information)** The clinical practice guideline contains systematically developed statements that include recommendations, strategies, or information that assists physicians and/or other healthcare practitioners and patients to make decisions about appropriate healthcare for specific clinical circumstances.
2. **(Official Sponsorship)** The clinical practice guideline was produced under the auspices of medical specialty associations; relevant professional societies, public or private organizations; government agencies at the federal, state, or local level; or healthcare organizations or plans. A clinical practice guideline developed and issued by an individual not officially sponsored or supported by one of the above types of organizations does not meet the inclusion criteria for the National Guideline Clearinghouse.
3. **(Systematic Review Based)** Corroborating documentation can be produced and verified that a systematic literature search and review of existing scientific evidence published in peer reviewed journals was performed during the

guideline development. A guideline is not excluded from the National Guideline Clearinghouse if corroborating documenta-tion can be produced and verified detailing specific gaps in scientific evidence for some of the guideline's recommendations.

4. **(Up-to-Date)** The guidelines are in the English language, current, and the most recent version produced. Documented evidence can be produced or verified that the guideline was developed, reviewed, or revised within the last 5 years.

NOTE: Federal Register, U.S. National Archives and Records Administration (1998, pp. 18065-18066).

Working with the Institute of Medicine and the National Institutes of Health Committee on Clinical Practice Guidelines (National Academy of Sciences, 1992), this group produced the monograph *Guidelines for Clinical Practice: From Development to Use.* This document included the following criteria (attributes) for sound guidelines:

DESIRABLE ATTRIBUTES OF CLINICAL PRACTICE GUIDELINES

Validity

Strength of evidence

Estimated outcomes

Reliability/reproducibility

Clinical applicability

Using Guidelines to Affect Healthcare Outcomes. In the past decade, an increasing number of authors are recognizing guidelines as one of the more effective means of improving healthcare quality (Bergman, 1999; Chassin, 1990; Cook et al., 1997; Ellrodt et al., 1997; Gray, Haynes, Sackett, Cook, & Guyatt, 1997; Grimshaw & Hutchinson, 1995; Grimshaw & Russell, 1993; Hoyt, 1997; Leape, 1990; Woolf, 1993; Woolf et al., 1999). However, the serious problem of whether or not these guidelines can be used effectively and have an impact on healthcare outcomes depends on many factors that must be understood. We have discussed how "computer alerts" can be sabotaged or ultimately disregarded altogether (Lundsgaarde & Williamson, 1987; Tate et al., 1995). Lundsgaarde and Williamson (1987, p. 14) list four barriers to the diffusion of healthcare decision support technology (DST) in order of importance:

1. Lack of consistent and coordinated strategies for development and dissemination of DST;

2. Lack of resources, encompassing personnel, financial, and technical support;

3. Lack of attention to the selection and testing of DST;

4. Lack of attention to the attitudes and preferences of professionals who might be expected to use the new DST (see Armstrong, Fry, & Armstrong, 1994).

On the other hand, Worrall et al. (1997), in a systematic review of randomized controlled clinical trials (RCCTs) regarding guideline effects on patient outcomes, concluded,

> There is very little evidence that the use of CPGs [clinical practice guidelines] improve patient outcomes in primary medical care, but most studies published to date have used older guidelines and methods, which may have been insensitive to small changes in outcomes. Onion and Walley's (1998) evocative article questioned whether being entirely evidence-based may result in more difficult application and less compliance. Thus, research is needed to determine whether the newer, evidence-based CPGs have an effect on patient outcomes. (p. 1705)

It is our assumption that systematic reviews can provide a needed foundation for developing sound guidelines. Studies on guideline development methods can be synthesized to facilitate making better guidelines. For example, what criteria have proven valid for evaluating guideline development? Analyzing the criteria by Hadorn et al. (1996) shown previously (Task 4, Procedure C, in this chapter), you may infer that there is a growing consensus as to what factors are required for developing sound guidelines. See the Cochrane Library for a valuable bibliography of studies on research methods for leads to this literature (last updated ??): www.update-software.com/cochrane.htm.

However, one of the most cogent articles we have read that summarizes and documents the potential benefits and harms of clinical guidelines is that of Woolf (1998) and Woolf et al. (1999). This group has been studying guidelines for more than a decade. In this article, they highlight an important fact—that the success of guidelines depends on who develops them, for what reason, and how they are implemented. For example, guidelines forced on clinicians by managers and administrators, to control costs or increase profits, likely will be met with resentment and resistance by clinicians. We quote their conclusion as an excellent summary on the impact of guidelines:

Clinical guidelines are only one option for improving the quality of care. Too often, advocates view guidelines as a 'magic bullet' for healthcare problems and ignore more effective solutions. Clinical guidelines make sense when practitioners are unclear about appropriate practice and when scientific evidence can provide an answer. They are a poor remedy in other settings. When clinicians already know the information contained in guidelines, those concerned with improving quality should redirect their efforts to identify the specific barriers, beyond knowledge, that stand in the way of behaviour change. (p. 530)

If you choose not to develop or apply guidelines, you should at least seek evidence-based clinical interventions (Van Weel & Knotterus, 1999).

One of the authors in Woolf's group, with a colleague (Grimshaw & Russell, 1993), wrote an information synthesis of 59 published "rigorous evaluations" of the clinical impact of guidelines. They concluded "that explicit guidelines do improve clinical practice, when introduced in the context of rigorous evaluations. However, the size of the improvements in performance varied considerably" (p. 1317).

Task 5: Minimizing External Motivation for Behavior Change

As alluded to previously, when developing strategies to apply information syntheses or guidelines, perhaps the most efficient but least desirable way to change behavior is by external motivation. For example, a direct executive order, a monetary threat or reward, and legal means are but a few. As an example how external motivation can counteract guideline benefit, Rhew et al. (1998) report a prospective, nonrandomized, intervention trial to study the effects of length-of-stay guidelines. There was no significant change in guideline compliance and no statistically significant effects on patient outcomes. Inadequate lengths of stay remained unchanged and seemed related more to external economic factors than guideline recommendations to improve quality of care.

However, there are some circumstances when such incentives are warranted. An example occurred recently in a large multihospital organization installing a paperless clinical record system, with computerized order entry by doctors and nurses. The reaction was that many physicians procrastinated or outright refused to learn how to type, let alone use a computer keyboard. The regional hospital director sent the physicians a letter indicating that use of computer systems was essential to the future of the organization. His reasoning was that use of these computers requires typing ability, which would substantially speed up healthcare processes and allow for use of computer guidelines and other quality improvement methods. The director then, in very diplomatic language, indicated that physicians' employment in their organization might depend on their having this typing skill. The result was that most, if not all, of these physicians learned how to type very soon thereafter.

Although external incentives do work, and often quickly, they can have a heavy price. There is no better way to lower morale and build resentment than to use force or threat of force. From the Lundsgaarde and Williamson (1987) article, previously referenced, employees can passively, if not actively, resist such change. Phillip Crosby, an international quality management guru (cited in Brown, Hitchcock, & Willard, 1994), stated,

> The governments have the illusion that they can make up rules about quality so they have an International Standards Organization (ISO) and the Baldridge criteria but they adopt the philosophy that if companies follow these, they will become world-class quality companies, but it's just not so. Europeans are trying to make other people as inefficient as they are, by using ISO 9000. (p. 56)

(ISO 9001 is their most recent notation for their healthcare accreditation system, similar to that which they apply to business and industry.) Brown et al. (1994) also wrote a subsection of their book, labeled "Common Mistakes That Waste Time and Money" (p. 57), to show how many institutions invest in quality management methods that focus on the wrong outcomes. They identify several behavioral change strategies that are counterproductive because instead of improvement, they "emphasize the wrong indicators, reinforce the wrong behavior, and encourage the wrong attitude" (p. 57). They emphasize the folly of collecting data on the following indicators:

- the time staff applies to "training" each year,
- the number of quality management teams in place,
- the percentage of staff involved on these quality assurance (QA) teams,
- the proportion of the staff who can recite the organization's mission and values,
- the number of processes for which process models have been developed,
- the number of improvement suggestions turned in,
- the number of quality-related awards given out.

Such indicators are very common in healthcare quality management, using such forced mandates as accumulating continuing education (CE) units. For example, to ensure quality, a large number of states have laws forcing their healthcare professionals to attend certified continuing education programs to maintain their licenses. Here again, politicians are insisting on easily measured processes (hours of attendance, or CE units) instead of outcomes (improved performance and enhanced patient health status). Healthcare providers, to meet these political directives, spend multimillions, if not billions, of dollars each year.

Another disadvantage of external motivation is that care providers start "gaming" the system. Some show up at conferences, missing or sleeping through lectures and filling out rather meaningless evaluation forms to earn their CE credits. This is not to say that most attendees are not conscientiously attending every lecture or that they are not learning much from socializing with geographically distant colleagues.

Finally, there are circumstances when externally motivated behavior change is indicated. One is when there is a tight time constraint, such as under emergency conditions. Another is as an intervention of last resort when all else has failed.

Task 6: Achieving Improved Healthcare Outcomes Is Attainable

By this time, you may be very discouraged about evidence-based reviews of anything. If so, you too might be a victim of overgeneralization or suffering from "medical student's disease." Now that you have learned how many things can go wrong in developing systematic reviews and guidelines, you must also remember how many new resources are available to help you cope with these problems. With modern informatics tools and evidence-based knowledge developing, as well as new understanding of effecting successful behavioral change, information syntheses can be an exciting and professionally rewarding endeavor.

Perhaps most important is the opportunity for you, as a healthcare professional, scientist, or author, to participate in contributing to this new era by generating and/or applying systematic reviews yourself. Most important of all will be to motivate your own readers to apply the new information you produce in such modalities as automated expert systems. We will then await studies of postimplementation evaluations that may demonstrate the success of these newer methods for disseminating innovations, enhancing the quality of care, and improving healthcare outcomes. The challenge to contribute is yours.

Summary

Procedure A. In this section, we discuss what might be the most difficult function of all: applying systematic review findings to improve healthcare performance and outcomes. Few will question the fact that effecting behavioral change, especially among professionals, is clearly possible but a slow and complex matter. Likewise, few question the known fact that diffusion of innovation is likewise slow and difficult. (There are dramatic exceptions such as insulin, penicillin, and other antibiotics.) However, with the use of systematic reviews and effective electronic guidelines, it is becoming possible to provide needed patient findings or scientific information at the point of decision making. These new resources and knowledge offer promise for substantial outcome improvements, if they are sound.

Procedure B. Here we discuss the unpleasant fact that sound information and valid systematic reviews may be a conflict of interest to certain groups. When compiling your database, this fact requires that you be aware of conflicting incentives from those who financially support research and research syntheses. Also, you must learn to identify sound versus sloppy systematic reviews. The quality of your synthesis may help motivate your readers to apply your findings in the meaningful ways you suggest. Finally, we pointed out several hazards in reporting your results, such as stating relative risk reduction in the absence of absolute risk reduction. Likewise, it is important that you detect overgeneralizations in the studies you synthesize and, more important, avoid this hazard in reporting your own systematic reviews, whether qualitative or quantitative.

Procedure C. To help you with this task, we suggest that several important theoretical considerations be understood and applied. The first is the need for you to communicate to your readers complex statistical concepts, especially results of randomized controlled clinical trials. You may need a consult to help with this task. In this procedure, we list more than 30 basic terms that are important in this regard. Second, we introduce the concept of ethnographic education, using "participant-observers" who spend time in a healthcare worker's own environment, helping the learner identify and meet his or her most urgent educational needs on-the-job. Third, we discuss the coming world of teleinformatics, which will provide the infrastructure for instant communication of new knowledge, transmission of images locally or at a distance, and incorporation of electronic guidelines that are evidence based and have been proven cost-effective. Fourth, we delve into the current state of the science of guideline development, use, and impact on patient and provider performance, as well as on healthcare outcomes. An assortment of "official criteria" for validating guidelines is presented as raw material to assist you in developing your own local set of criteria. Fifth, and finally, we discuss the use of external motivation to effect behavior change. We look at the advantages (rapid, inexpensive staff performance improvement) and the disadvantages (low morale, resentment, and passive-aggressive behavior). There are times when this "top-down" approach is essential, but we hope it would usually be an action of last resort.

Finally, by the end of Procedure C, we hope you will be excited by the potential for achieving outcomes improvement by producing sound information syntheses, following the principles in this book and using the growing availability of evidence-based, computerized information resources.

CHAPTER 18

Evaluation and Refinement of Synthesis Report

Introduction

The purpose of this Stage V evaluation is to determine whether your manuscript is developed sufficiently to be submitted for publication or distribution to whomever your target audience might be. At this point, your information synthesis is all but final. You have a manuscript in hand that is a product of five completed stages. Your next task is to select qualified reviewers who are willing to read your synthesis and provide feedback for a final revision. Because these reviews may not be returned for 4 to 8 weeks, your task, in the meantime, is to attend to several critical time-consuming final details. At the end of this chapter, Form 18.1 lists our suggestions for a procedural checklist of items that must be done prior to submission or distribution.

Assuming you obtained an adequate overall review of your manuscript by the independent reviewers you selected, we have included a brief form for a team consensus session related to each of the four major quality criteria suggested. However, as all of the team members have been working very hard, it might be of interest to spend half an hour to one hour to determine whether, in your collective judgment, your synthesis meets the original criteria listed in Section E, Chapter 1.

Finally, in the appendixes, we provide more detailed discussion and suggestions for doing your own review: Appendix 18.1 for assessing the adequacy of your manuscript documentation, Appendix 18.2 for assessing the communication effectiveness of your manuscript, and Appendix 18.3 to review the formal information synthesis evaluation criteria that have evolved over the past 25 years.

Procedure A. Understanding Considerations for Project Finalization

Definitions and Concepts

The terms *externally* and *internally selected reviewers* require an explanation. They both refer to experts who are independent of the project team and staff but agree to critique your manuscript. The main difference is in who selects these experts. If selected by you, then the following definition pertains.

INTERNALLY SELECTED REVIEWERS

Internally selected reviewers are qualified independent colleagues, not currently involved with your project, who agree to read your manuscript and provide critical feedback. These reviewers can be considered surrogate members of your project team who work with you to improve your manuscript for publication submission or other external review.

If professionals outside your team or professional network select the reviewers, the following definition pertains.

EXTERNALLY SELECTED REVIEWERS

Externally selected reviewers are review panels selected by professionals who are independent of your project team and staff. They are often associated with or employed by outside organizations. For example, with book or journal editors, their editorial boards and review panels must decide whether or not to publish your work. Editorial peer review is the classic type of critique using externally selected reviewers. The same pertains to formal corporate review by outside experts as to whether or not your manuscript should be one of their officially printed technical reports. Another example is when professional organizations have their experts decide whether or not your paper should be presented in a conference or other formal meeting.

One of the main goals of this manual is to help you prepare an information synthesis of sufficiently high quality to be submitted for critique by externally selected reviewers, as defined above. The most stringent review process usually occurs if you elect to submit your manuscript for publication in a peer-reviewed journal or as a book or monograph produced by a respected publisher. In some instances, less stringency may be applied when your report is submitted for printing as a corporate technical report or for presentation at a professional meeting. If you are a member of a Cochrane Collaboration Centre, your team products, such as systematic reviews, will be evaluated by independent members of the collaboration who have been specially trained for this task. In our judgment, these reviewers are the equivalent of "externally selected" experts because they are independent of the particular Cochrane center that generated the review.

Internal Review Issues

The first consideration in arranging for an evaluation by internally selected reviewers is to develop an instrument to elicit feedback. Obtaining consultation from experienced evaluation specialists in your field to help you design this form is of considerable value if you are inexperienced with this task.

The design of your instrument might well determine your response and completion rates. Some reviewers will not take the time to complete a questionnaire if it is long and requires considerable time and effort. If your survey form fits on one page, or both sides of one page, and does not use a font smaller than 10 points, you will be much more successful in securing needed feedback from the reviewer.

The second consideration is selecting reviewers whose knowledge, experience, and judgment are respected by their colleagues. The feedback they provide will likely enhance the value of your synthesis. If you elect to do a quantitative synthesis, you will require not only experts on the subject content of your synthesis but also experts who are methodologically skilled and keep up with advances in the quantitative sciences. For example, the field of meta-analysis is rapidly advancing to overcome serious methods problems that often made earlier and many current quantitative syntheses questionable, even misleading (Bailar, 1998).

The third consideration is persuading these skilled and overworked colleagues you have selected to donate the time and effort required for this difficult review.

Perhaps the strongest motivation will be their professional interest in the subject matter and curiosity about the possible contribution your work could make.

If you intend to place your synthesis on the Internet, such as on a Web site, without a critique by internal or external reviewers, this fact should be made known to the reader. Knowing this, he or she must take final responsibility for a decision to read and/or apply the results of your work. We suggest that your synthesis would be premature without any form of peer review, and wide distribution may be a disservice to the scientific community. We also remind you to include the names of those who critique your synthesis in your "Acknowledgment" paragraph, both to give them credit and to improve the credibility of your own work.

Final Synthesis Assessment

Once your manuscript is completed, even if you are fairly certain it will be accepted for publication (if that is your goal), an objective assessment of the impact of your project is not possible. Such a final objective evaluation can only be done when your findings are implemented in the community and when sound evidence is compiled establishing healthcare outcomes improvement. Even then, you must verify that the improvement can be reasonably attributed to your synthesis. Thus, the final results of your work cannot be determined until months or years after its dissemination. In the meantime, you can only weigh probabilities. If your synthesis meets the four major criteria suggested in Section E, Chapter 1, you have taken a major step toward ultimate healthcare outcomes improvement.

It is possible at this point to establish at least some consensus as to the judgment of a group you respect regarding the clinical significance, scientific soundness, adequacy of documentation, and cost-effectiveness of your final product. The bottom line will be to estimate whether the benefits that may occur as a result of implementing your findings will outweigh the costs and possible harm that occur as a result.

Procedure B. Finalizing Synthesis Project

The final preparation of the manuscript can require as much work as writing the text, as it should include incorporating reviewer feedback, analyzing the overall conceptual framework of the synthesis for consistency in labeling sections and procedures, checking for sections or tasks that might be missing, and especially checking for redundancy. To assist with this, we suggest the following four procedures: synthesis internal review and revision, final manuscript cleanup and copyedit, consideration of a final "expert review," and preparation for publication.

Task 1: Synthesis Internal Review and Revision

Internally selected reviewers who are willing to read your synthesis and provide feedback will do the most valuable assessment of your manuscript. The following tasks are suggested to facilitate this procedure.

State Goals of Your Internal Review. Your team will have read the manuscript many times and will have a fairly accurate intuitive judgment about the main flaws of your synthesis. Perhaps you can conduct a modified nominal group technique with your team to produce a weighted list of factors for which you need expert feedback (see Appendix 2.1, at the end of Chapter 2, titled "A Scientific Group Consensus Process"). This will help your internally selected reviewers to focus their time on questions or issues of high priority, as they will not be able or willing to spend much time with your synthesis.

At this time, you must also decide whether you require feedback in terms of the communication effectiveness of your manuscript. The above experts may provide a few suggestions, but they are not likely to be the audience that will finally read and use the material in your synthesis. This assessment may require a different group of readers. If you decide to conduct a communication check of your writing, you need to use a somewhat different approach, described in Appendix 18.2.

Prepare Internal Review Instrument. Reviewers should be provided a one-page worksheet that, on the front, asks for brief overall comments. On the back of this page, they might be asked to answer the weighted list of factors developed in the preceding task of this worksheet. Another approach might be to have them comment on how well your synthesis met each of the four overriding criteria for success, itemized in Form 18.2 at the end of this chapter. Or, you can request information on any number of issues such as technical factors, formatting issues, or communication effectiveness. As long as this worksheet is limited to one page, you are more likely to achieve a high response and completion rate, as well as thoughtful feedback. However, do not be surprised if your reviewer ignores your questionnaire. Instead, many times they will write comments on your manuscript and mail it back. Or they may write a critique in their own format and send it to you.

Select and Recruit Reviewers. Selecting your reviewers can be a difficult balancing act. On one hand, you want experts in your subject matter who are highly respected. However, these are usually the people who are most overburdened with work and can least afford to take on this onerous review. On the other hand, if you seek experts who are young or new in the field and have time to do a thoughtful review of your manuscript, they might be too inexperienced or not have enough of a reputation to give you much help.

We still recommend that, if you are convinced your synthesis is important, you contact the professionals who have done the most research on your topic. If they are intensely interested in your topic, you might be surprised when they agree to be reviewers. However, if they do so, they will likely take a long time to complete their review and mail it back. More promising would be to seek an older retired professional who is well known in your field. These individuals might have the interest, knowledge, reputation, and time to provide insightful feedback.

Revise Manuscript Based on Feedback. The main consideration in applying the feedback from your internal reviewers is the time and resources that might be required to improve your manuscript. Depending on how substantive the criticism, the amount of effort might be more than you can afford. At the other extreme, many reviewers will do copyediting and pick up spelling errors, wrong citations, or lack of a reference from a work you quoted heavily. This last flaw could result in legal repercussions. These latter errors are usually readily fixed because they take so little time. Then there are the majority of suggested changes that are between the above two extremes. Your whole team should read all the feedback; they can be especially helpful for those issues in the gray zone.

Task 2: Final Manuscript Cleanup and Copyedit

After sending your manuscript to the internally selected reviewers, there are numerous tasks to be completed and incorporated into your manuscript. Because the reviewers will take 1 to 2 months, this is a good time to complete final details required. On the other hand, at this point, your team is likely exhausted and frustrated with the project. Unfortunately, there is still much work to be done, with several tasks being time-consuming and requiring attention to detail. It is hoped that your staff will be motivated by the fact that the project is drawing to a close and your synthesis will soon be ready to submit for publication or for whatever end product you have chosen.

List All Remaining Tasks to Be Completed. This task will involve the entire project team. Assuming the main body of your manuscript is complete, the front and trailing matter must be prepared, which will consume considerable time. Next, a number of factors will require time and effort from your assistants. If you have a publisher selected for consideration, obtain their "Instructions to Authors" as a prerequisite checklist of specific cleanup items. Form 18.1 might also be helpful in this regard.

Complete "Final Assignments" Worksheet. Although the need for this assignment sheet seems self-evident, with the energy of your team wearing down, specific deadlines often have to be imposed or the project might go on indefinitely. In Form 18.1, we list a few illustrative tasks, divided into three categories, according to the level of staff expertise each requires: authors, research assistants, and clerical assistants. You may make a copy of our form, or merely use it as a checklist to create your own where you can customize the instrument according to your own needs, and at the same time take into account the publisher's "Instructions for Authors," if this is available.

With the worksheet complete, authors and team should agree on which assignments are given to whom and for what. Some of the completion dates might have to be negotiated, but when finished, this form should be similar to a contract to which each member makes a personal commitment.

Complete and Critique All "Final Assignments." It is hoped that your staff will come through and complete the tasks and produce the final products necessary to finish this synthesis. If anyone falls behind, the whole project may be delayed. The worst-case scenario is having several of your team members quit working, continually delay getting assignments done or have to be constantly reminded to complete them, and provide excuses rather than products. The remaining team (usually key authors) will be left doing their own work plus that of those who find no further interest in the project. Equally hazardous is having some of the staff do sloppy work, with omissions and errors (e.g., inconsistent outlines, relying on secondary references, failing to provide glossary definitions, failure to have their work checked, failure to provide "camera-ready" figures and graphs). Each of these problems will then have to be corrected by others. This occurrence not only lengthens the time but also can generate considerable resentment. If authors themselves are errant in this, it is even worse; their tasks have to be redone by others or left out entirely.

Task 3: Preparation for Publication

Much earlier in your project, the process of contacting numerous publishers to find one interested in your work might have been a long and frustrating task. If you were successful and if your manuscript is finally accepted for publication, there are a number of papers to be completed, such as a contract to be negotiated, your suggestions for people who might provide a written endorsement of your work, a clear description of the market (including its size) of those who might be interested, and participation in developing advertising material. One caution—your contract will have to be signed by all authors, and the shares of whatever royalties that are accrued must be agreed on in writing. Furthermore, the number of pages of your final book must be estimated fairly accurately.

It is still not time to celebrate, because because there is considerably more work to be done as your manuscript is being prepared for publication. The publisher's editors, especially their copy editors and production editors, will be in contact with you for many questions or decisions that have to be made. The mock-up of your book in print will have to be studied very carefully. The publisher will cover most minor adjustments. However, if there is some major rewriting or changing of tables and figures, you will likely be responsible for these costs.

Procedure C. Self-Assessing the Final Synthesis

If it is not possible to complete a critique of your manuscript by internally selected reviewers, we suggest the following four tasks for a final review by your own team. Perhaps you can assign a different team member to each one of these final review tasks.

Task 1: Review Synthesis Purpose, Audience, and Likely Use

Throughout this synthesis project, your purpose, goals, and procedures will have evolved to some extent. At this point, you should check the consistency with which each of your stages has been revised to reflect this evolution. It is possible that some chapters might still reflect your former, rather than your current, purpose and goals. This error could be overlooked unless brought to your attention by internal reviewers.

Task 2: Assess Stage Evaluation Results in Chapters 4, 7, 11, and 15

Each of Chapters 4, 7, 11, and 15 reflects the quality and adequacy of Stages I, II, III, and IV, respectively. Now that you are nearing the end of your manuscript preparation, this might be the last chance to identify those errors that can still be remedied. For example, in Chapter 11 (evaluation of Stage III), if you now identify a set of important articles that have not been validated, you will need to decide if time and fiscal resources allow this task to be done. Next, you might repeat your "file drawer" analysis to estimate how many additional negative articles would be required to reverse your synthesis conclusions. If the number of negative articles among those that were missed is sufficient to overturn your current conclusions, as estimated by the "file drawer" calculation, you should validate these missed studies and recalculate your synthesis data. If warranted, you may need to rewrite your discussion and conclusions.

Task 3: Assess Manuscript Completeness and Documentation

This procedure involves reviewing Chapter 16 (manuscript preparation), using it as a checklist to be sure you have not left out important sections, such as your glossary or acknowledgments. If such sections are missing, this augmentation will have to be accomplished before submitting the manuscript for independent review.

Next, manuscript documentation must be briefly reviewed. A first step might be rereading your "methods" section to determine whether, for each stage of the synthesis, the procedural steps were explained and related documentation included. For example, in Criterion A, Chapter 7, Stage II, the following questions need to be asked: Is the search documentation complete? Are the formal relevance criteria clear? Are the results of the calibration sessions included? Are search statistics shown (e.g., how many citations were screened, how many were coded A+ through C, and how many A+, A, A- were searched and retrieved)? Similar documentation for Stage III (validation) should be recorded, especially study design definitions, validation criteria for each type of design, and validation statistics, including how many articles were validated and with what results. See Appendix 18.1 for further discussion on documentation assessment and procedural steps.

It could prove helpful to review the items from the various criteria as shown at the end of Appendix 18.3. Ask yourself, would these reviewers approve your information synthesis?

Task 4: Make Final Revisions, Deletions, or Augmentation

It is hoped that at this point in completing your manuscript, this final evaluation confirms that you have been thorough in preparing your synthesis for independent review. If this is the case, you are ready to do a final copyedit for consistency in style, voice, and person and for a check of spelling, glossary, references, and attachments.

On the other hand, if major omissions, errors, and/or redundancies are found, you will have to make a cost-benefit estimate in terms of the extent of revision required and the resources now available. The minimum that must be done is copyediting. For example, if you have many references that are not mentioned in your text, or many text references that are not found in your reference list, this must be corrected before submission for publication review. On checking your "invisible college" analysis described in Section C, Chapter 5, suppose you find that you did not follow up on one or more missed "colleges" previously identified. If resources allow, this would be an important lead to follow. If resources do not allow, this is a serious threat to the soundness of your synthesis and must be stated in your report.

Or suppose your earlier file drawer results (Stage II) implied you would need a substantial number of null studies to reverse your conclusions. In this instance, if you decide you have represented the major invisible colleges, you likely could be assured that your findings are on solid ground. On the other hand, if your previous file drawer analysis indicates only a few negative studies are required to reverse your conclusions, then it is probably too late to do anything about it, except to state this fact in your "limitations" section.

Procedure D. Has Your Final Product Been Worth the Effort and Cost Involved?

When your manuscript is complete, you might consider a final brief assessment of the overall quality of your work after it has been submitted for publication or other form of external review. This exercise would be quite different from when you asked internally selected outside experts to help you finalize your manuscript by more detailed feedback. The purpose of this last assessment is to estimate how well your product met the four criteria for overall evaluation, including the cost-effectiveness of your project as a whole. Though we have not emphasized this, the data for the cost-effectiveness analysis could also provide a basis for estimating "opportunity costs." What might have been a better use of funds and personnel time expended for this synthesis?

This final critique is for your own benefit and provides an opportunity to estimate the strengths and weaknesses of the synthesis as a whole. Obviously, this will be based almost entirely on subjective professional judgments. The principle involved is that, although any such overall critique by a single individual might be of little value, the median judgment of a group, if accomplished by following "scientific consensus" procedures, has been shown to be surprisingly good (Dalkey et al., 1972; Delbecq et al., 1975; Murphy et al., 1998; Sackett, 1997).

To conduct this simple evaluation with any credibility, it is necessary to organize another group of interested specialists who are internally selected to participate in this structured group judgment exercise. For this purpose, we suggest a modified nominal group judgment task involving use of Form 18.2. Timewise, this task can be accomplished by means of a single meeting that should last less than 1 hour. This, of course, does not include the time that independent colleagues would require to read your report or at least an abstract of your report (see Appendix 18.3 to scan the various criteria that have been applied over the past decade for evaluating reviews).

If such a review were not feasible, another option would be to have your own project team participate, as a final wrap-up meeting. We consider this exercise optional, as the whole team may be so exhausted that the results may not seem worth the time, whether accomplished by experts or your team alone. However, it can be a satisfying task to complete, and you all may learn something for future syntheses.

Summary

We divide this chapter into three sections to facilitate completing and evaluating your final synthesis.

In Section A, we discuss the theoretical considerations at this end stage of your synthesis project. We explain the concept of internally selected and externally selected reviewers. To facilitate a review by internally selected experts, we outline development of a brief one-page form that can be completed in a few minutes after consultants have screened your manuscript. We discuss the theoretical considerations related to final revision, copyediting, and other tasks required prior to sending your manuscript for external review (e.g., to a publisher). Because achievement of your ultimate purpose, health outcomes improvement, cannot usually be measured until after dissemination of your work, you can still estimate probabilities.

In Section B, we discuss the specific procedures required to finalize your manuscript, in light of the above theoretical discussion. This involves arranging for and completing a review by internally selected experts, stressing again the brevity of a structured form to facilitate this achievement. We next discuss the tasks for cleanup and copyediting of your work. We suggest that you might have many additional rounds of copyediting at this point. Every change you make in response to your expert reviewers may require addition or removal of certain literature references, changing the focus of such phrases as "see paragraph . . ." that refer to other parts of your work that may now be different in content and/or placement.

In Section C, we discuss methods for self-assessing your final synthesis. We suggest four tasks such as having your team review your synthesis purpose, audience, and likely applications through to making final revisions. Next, we suggest you estimate how well your project met suggestions in the evaluation chapters for Stages I (Chapter 4), II (Chapter 7), III (Chapter 11), and IV (Chapter 15) of this book. Finally, assess the manuscript completeness and documentation and the revisions you made.

In Section D, we suggest that you consider an optional task of estimating the extent to which your synthesis product is worth the effort and cost you have expended. We provide Form 18.2 as a simple means to answer this question, whether by a colleague's or merely by your own team's judgment. Ideally, this could be accomplished by a modified nominal group technique in a meeting of less than 1 hour or by just completing half of Form 18.2, which takes 3 to 5 minutes. If independent colleagues participate, this time estimate does not include the time required to read your report or read a Cochrane-type review abstract of your report.

APPENDIX 18.1
Assessing Synthesis Documentation

This appendix provides a more detailed procedural guide for screening your manuscript documentation. Overall, by providing adequate synthesis methods documentation, an interested and qualified colleague, at a minimum, should be able to critique your review and, more ideally, update if not replicate your synthesis with a minimum of duplicative effort.

We suggest four steps that might be considered for this purpose:

PROCEDURES FOR ASSESSING SYNTHESIS DOCUMENTATION

A. Recheck adequacy of synthesis topic and purpose description
B. Recheck adequacy of "search methods" documentation
C. Review documentation of validation, analysis, and synthesis
D. Recheck adequacy of "documentation limitations" statement

Procedure A. Recheck Adequacy of Synthesis Topic and Purpose Description

The manuscript should clearly describe (a) synthesis purpose, (b) target audience, and (c) how the audience will use this information. Many authors do not state these factors until well into the text, forcing the reader to search for a clear statement of the synthesis topic and its purpose. For journal articles, we suggest that the above three elements be stated up front in the introduction or background section. Likewise, a clear statement of purpose should be the leading sentence in any abstract. For books, we suggest that the initial section of the front matter (i.e., preface or forward) lead out with a statement of the topic, purpose, and intended audience for this particular information synthesis.

Procedure B. Recheck Adequacy of "Search Methods" Documentation

Look for obvious omissions that require a more adequate explanation. For example, is your search scope adequately described, including such factors as the search time frame or language limitations? Does the list of relevance criteria clearly indicate both the inclusions and exclusions? Is there evidence that information sources were adequately screened, including contacting experts, using electronic bibliographic databases, and searching for fugitive literature? Electronic database screening should include a study of the official list of index terms. For MEDLINE, this should include screening official MeSH descriptors, including the volume listing dates for when these descriptors were first indexed or terminated by the National Library of Medicine. (There is a considerable body of classic literature that is published before being officially indexed into a given electronic database.) A final tally of the number of references screened and relevant documents obtained should be stated in the search statistics. In addition, search team training and calibration methods should be reported.

Procedure C. Review Documentation of Validation, Analysis, and Synthesis

The credibility of your final synthesis depends heavily on the scientific soundness of your final database and conclusions; consequently, it is important to recheck documentation of these procedures one final time before your manuscript is complete. You might review such issues as whether each study in the database is classified by research design. Is the validation protocol adequate for each design, and is the internal and external validation assessment complete, with a profile of the results specified?

Procedure D. Recheck Adequacy of "Documentation Limitations" Statement

Recheck your synthesis "limitations" statement in the discussion section of your manuscript to be sure these problems have been adequately described. There are many legitimate reasons why you may not have implemented your synthesis as rigorously as first intended. This can be true of all scientific studies and syntheses. However, what is more important is that you clearly document these limitations and briefly state the implications of these errors for your readers' application of your findings. Failure to do so can be both self-serving and misleading to your target audience. For example, if a physician makes erroneous assumptions about the validity of your synthesis, there might be unacceptable consequences for his or her patients.

APPENDIX 18.2
Assessing Synthesis Communication Effectiveness

Relevant and valid reviews, including meta-analyses, may be read but go unheeded or, worse, not be read and merely added to our current accumulation of unused literature. This sad fact may be due to lack of communication effectiveness of the author's final report. Your original goal and target audience will likely evolve as your project progresses, making it essential that you clearly identify and understand your **synthesis audience**. Lacking this, you may produce a report that is too technical to understand or too simple to be of interest. If you are concerned about the communication effectiveness of your manuscript, we suggest you read this appendix for ideas about how you can assess this important factor.

PROCEDURES FOR EVALUATING COMMUNICATION EFFECTIVENESS

A.   Reanalyze target audience
B.   Ensure consistency of voice and person
C.   Pilot test draft copy with intended readers and revise
D.   If required, retest manuscript with similar readers and revise

Procedure A. Reanalyze Target Audience

We suggest that you first examine Stage I documentation to compare your original with your final synthesis purpose, goals, and audience. Your final plan is the result of an evolutionary process while doing your search (Stage II) and database validation (Stage III). This should help you focus and increase your understanding of the readers your final synthesis will address. In Stage IV, you selected a synthesis method that would best meet your intended purpose and your readers' needs. A synthesis report contributing to new knowledge by use of a meta-analysis most likely would be highly technical and aimed at fellow scientific colleagues. For health education purposes or for public education aimed at a lay audience, a simple narrative synthesis may be much less complex. Targeting lay audiences requires much simpler language, minimal scientific jargon, and clear illustrated explanations of technical concepts necessary for them to understand. In any event, you must understand your readers and write at their level of technical comprehension.

Procedure B. Ensure Consistency of Voice and Person

In writing your manuscript, you may often, unintentionally, change the voice or person of your text at different times in writing the manuscript. This is especially true if different authors each write independent chapters. A copy editor, if available, can help ensure consistency of voice and person. Otherwise, the author(s) must give the manuscript a special reading specifically for this purpose. Most editors prefer an active rather than a passive voice. Whether you write in first person (I, me/we, us), second (you/you), or third (he, she, it, one/they), person is arbitrary. If addressing beginners, second person is often more personal and appealing to the reader. If addressing a more sophisticated audience, third person is often used.

Microsoft Word and other software tools also can be used to check reading difficulty. A weakness of these systems is that they do not necessarily work as well for scientific or healthcare material as they do for business documents. However, these tools do provide an alternative to help facilitate checking your language level. If you are communicating with fellow scientists familiar with the jargon terms in the field, the language level can be technical, making your task much easier.

Procedure C. Pilot Test Draft
Copy With Intended Readers and Revise

The final test for adequacy of your language level is to ask representatives of your target-readers to read parts of or, ideally, all of your manuscript. If your target audience will be young graduate students or fellows, one language level might be fine, but if you are addressing practicing physicians, nurses, or clinical social workers, another level might be more appropriate. Finally, if you are addressing researchers with a strong statistical background, a more sophisticated language level will be required. These reviewers can make notes and give you feedback on your communication effectiveness. The more questions they have, the more you may have to revise. In conducting this pilot test, it is important to provide a structured feedback instrument to ensure a thorough and consistent review. For example, you should seek feedback on your graphics and tables to be sure they contribute to the clarity of your manuscript. Tables and graphics can facilitate communication effectiveness substantially and may help maintain the readers' interest. Such graphics and tables force you to be much more careful in conceptualizing and communicating the important message of your data synthesis. This is especially true if you are submitting your manuscript for publication.

Procedure D. If Required, Retest Manuscript With Similar Readers and Revise

Depending on the results of the above pilot test of your manuscript, you may have to revise your language level, assuming that your voice and person are consistent. On the other hand, it is possible that your text may require little or no change. The final test and revision of your communication level are vital if your synthesis is to achieve its intended impact for improving healthcare. If your pilot test reveals serious problems that require major revision, you might consider repeating this assessment.

APPENDIX 18.3
Recent Criteria Sets for Validating Systematic Reviews (1977-2000)

There are numerous criteria in the literature for evaluating an information synthesis. The following are examples of such criteria that have evolved during my own experience over the past 25 years. They are quoted directly from the various publications mentioned, with the possible exception of the numeration and a few clarifying bracket inserts of our own. (Note spelling differences for the United States and the United Kingdom. For example, *analyze* in the United States, is spelled *analyse* in the United Kingdom.) These criteria sets primarily provide an overview of the recent evolution of methods for analyzing reviews. They also provide ideas to help you establish a custom set of your own criteria for validation assessment of a systematic review.

CRITERIA SET A. CRITERIA FOR ASSESSING A REVIEW

1. Are the limits of the topic made explicit so the reader can understand what was included and what was excluded?
2. Is the extent of the information search described explicitly in terms of the time period covered, sources checked, and specific illustrative search descriptors indicated? (The denominator for any information search must be described for valid interpretation of [numerator] results.)
3. Are the information sources included adequately documented?
4. What indication does the author give regarding [assessment of] references in terms of quality?

SOURCE: Williamson (1977, p. 8).

CRITERIA SET B. CHECKLIST FOR EVALUATING REVIEWS

1. What is the precise purpose of the review?
2. How were the studies selected?
3. Is there publication bias?
4. Are treatments similar enough to combine?
5. Are control groups similar enough to combine?
6. What is the distribution of study outcomes?
7. Are outcomes related to research design?
8. Are outcomes related to characteristics of programs, participants, and settings?
9. Is the unit of analysis similar across studies?
10. What are guidelines for future research?

SOURCE: Light and Pillemer (1984).

CRITERIA SET C. CRITERIA FOR ASSESSING REVIEW ARTICLES

1. Were the questions and methods clearly stated?
2. Were comprehensive search methods used to locate relevant studies?
3. Were explicit methods used to determine which articles to include in the review?
4. Was the validity of the primary studies assessed?
5. Was the assessment of the primary studies reproducible and free from bias?

6. Was the variation in the findings of the relevant studies analysed?
7. Were the findings of the primary studies combined appropriately?
8. Were the reviewers' conclusions supported by the data cited?

SOURCE: Oxman and Guyatt (1988).

CRITERIA SET D. ASSESSING SCIENTIFIC QUALITY OF RESEARCH OVERVIEWS

1. Were the search methods reported?
2. Was the search comprehensive?
3. Were the inclusion criteria reported?
4. Was selection bias avoided?
5. Were the validity criteria reported?
6. Was validity assessed appropriately?
7. Were the methods used to combine studies reported?
8. Were the findings combined appropriately?
9. Were the conclusions supported by the reported data?
10. What was the overall scientific quality of the overview?

SOURCE: Oxman et al. (1991); Oxman and Guyatt (1993).

CRITERIA SET E. CRITERIA FOR ASSESSING REVIEW ARTICLES

1. What is the precise purpose of the review?
2. How were studies selected?
3. Is there publication bias?
4. Are treatments similar enough to combine?
5. Are control groups similar enough to combine?
6. What is the distribution of study outcomes?
7. Are outcomes related to research design?
8. Are outcomes related to characteristics of programs, participants, and settings?
9. Is the unit of analysis similar across studies?
10. What are the guidelines for future research?

SOURCE: Oxman and Guyatt (1991).

NOTE: These criteria are almost identical to Criteria Set B by Light and Pillemer.

CRITERIA SET F. BIASES THAT THREATEN META-ANALYSIS VALIDITY

1. Patient-selection bias
2. Population biases
3. Confounding factors
4. Contamination and dilution
5. Differences in the intensity of the independent variable
6. Errors in measuring outcomes
7. Errors in ascertaining exposure to an intervention
8. Loss to follow-up
9. Length of follow-up

SOURCE: Eddy, Hasselblad, and Shachter (1992).

CRITERIA SET G. SOURCES OF AND METHODS FOR PROTECTING AGAINST BIAS IN REVIEW ARTICLES

Problem formulation
  Is the question clearly focused?
Study identification
  Is the search for relevant studies thorough?
Study selection
  Are the inclusion criteria appropriate?
Appraisal of studies
  Is the validity of included studies adequately assessed?
Data collection
  Is missing information obtained from investigators?
Data synthesis
  How sensitive are the results to changes in the way the review is done?
Interpretation of results
  Do the conclusions flow from the evidence that is reviewed?
  Are recommendations linked to the strength of the evidence?
  Are judgments about preferences (values) explicit?
  If there is "no evidence of effect," is caution taken not to interpret this as "evidence of no effect"?
  Are subgroup analyses interpreted cautiously?

SOURCE: Oxman (1994); see also Oxman, Cook, and Guyatt (1994).

CRITERIA SET H.   ASSESSING THE QUALITY OF A SYSTEMATIC REVIEW

1. Did the review address a focused question?
2. Is it likely that important, relevant studies were missed?
3. Were the inclusion criteria used to select articles appropriate?
4. Was the validity of the included studies assessed?
5. Were the assessments of the studies reproducible?
6. Were the results similar from study to study?
7. What are the overall results and how precise are they?
8. Will the results help in caring for patients?

SOURCE: Hunt and McKibbon (1998).

CRITERIA SET I.   INCREASING RELIABILITY OF A SYSTEMATIC REVIEW

Use of explicit criteria for inclusion and exclusion; these should specify the population, the intervention, the outcome, and the methodological criteria for the studies included in the review

Use of comprehensive search methods to locate relevant studies, including searching a wide range of computerized databases using a mixture of appropriate key words and free text

Assessment of the validity of the primary studies; this should be reproducible and attempt to avoid bias

Exploration of variation between the findings of the studies

Appropriate synthesis and, when suitable, pooling of primary studies

SOURCE: Sheldon, Guyatt, and Haines (1998).

CRITERIA SET J.   COCHRANE COLLABORATION (2000)
(United Kingdom)

The Cochrane Collaboration Centres and teams have developed and applied formal protocols for evaluation of systematic reviews. Their protocols can be surmised as applied to their collection of "complete reviews" and "abstracts of quality-assessed systematic reviews." The formal protocols do not seem to be publicly available at this time. Based on their extensive experience in the field of information synthesis, their protocols are likely among the best being applied today.

CRITERIA SET K.   NATIONAL HEALTH SERVICE CRITICAL APPRAISAL SKILLS PROGRAM (2000) (United Kingdom)

The National Health Service's Critical Appraisal Skills Programme (CASP) offers "10 questions to help you make sense of a review." Its questions were adapted from Oxman (1994), as reported above in Criteria Set G. The unique contribution of this CASP criteria set is the way the criteria are organized and annotated to make them exceptionally clear. CASP also adds three important items to explore how likely the review will be applied (locally), the first questions of this type among any of the above criteria sets. We suggest that you would be well served, especially if you are a beginner in systematic reviews, to obtain CASP's questionnaire. As of May 2001, CASP suggests you contact Ann Davis through e-mail (ann.davis@ phru.anglox. nhs.uk) to request a formal copy that includes the question annotations that are so cogent.

CASP Questions for Assessing a Review Article

A.   Are the results of the study valid?

    1.   Did the review address a clearly focused research question?
    2.   Did the review include the right type of studies?
    3.   Did the reviewers try to identify all relevant studies?
    4.   Did the reviewers assess the quality of the included studies?
    5.   If the results of the studies have been combined, was it reasonable to do so?

B.   What are the results?

    6.   What are the main results of the review?
    7.   Could these results be due to chance?

C.   Will the results help locally?

    8.   Can the results be applied to the local population?
    9.   Were all important outcomes considered?
    10.   Should policy or practice change as a result of the evidence contained in this review?

SOURCE: CASP, Institute of Health Sciences, Old Road, Headington, Oxford, OX3 7LF. The Web site (last updated July 2000) is www.public-health.org.uk/casp/review.html.

FORM 18.1: FINAL TASK ASSIGNMENTS TO COMPLETE MANUSCRIPT

Instructions: The first step is to read your publisher's "Instructions to Authors" and then revise this assignment sheet as needed, adding or deleting any items warranted. The next step is to make all assignments and fill in the dates when they are due. The final step is to have each team member in the three professional levels complete his or her assignment.

	Name	Date Due	Date Received
AUTHORS			
Original material to be added			
Write introduction	_____	_____	_____
Write preface	_____	_____	_____
Write acknowledgments	_____	_____	_____
Other: (List _____)	_____	_____	_____
Heavy editing or rewrite			
e.g., Chapter X (pp. 113–114) rewrite	_____	_____	_____
e.g., Chapter Y (p. 56) missing paragraph	_____	_____	_____
Substance edit (reread manuscript)	_____	_____	_____
Check jargon list and definitions	_____	_____	_____
Check glossary definitions	_____	_____	_____
RESEARCH ASSISTANTS			
Substantive consultations with experts			
Check unclear concepts or jargon terms	_____	_____	_____
Check meta-analysis methods	_____	_____	_____
Check with science writer (Chapters X and Y)	_____	_____	_____
Mathematical formulas			
Define math and statistical terms (e.g., $\wedge$ = circumflex)	_____	_____	_____
Apply publisher-required type fonts (e.g., Times New Roman font, boldface, and italics)	_____	_____	_____

Tables, forms, figures, graphs, and charts

    Prepare each on a separate page
        (ensure each is "camera ready")   _____   _____   _____

    "Table X About Here" inserts (this
        includes tables, forms, figures,
        graphs, and charts)   _____   _____   _____

References

    Find missing references   _____   _____   _____

    Find secondary reference originals   _____   _____   _____

    Delete references not in text   _____   _____   _____

    Edit for required style (e.g., APA)   _____   _____   _____

    Develop cited author list   _____   _____   _____

Complete glossary and acronym list

    Fill in definitions from book text   _____   _____   _____

    Delete terms or definitions not in text   _____   _____   _____

    Complete acronym definition list   _____   _____   _____

Copyedit

    Edit "jargon" list (all text jargon in quotes)   _____   _____   _____

    Use publisher's style preference (e.g.,
        *Publication Manual of the American
        Psychological Association*)   _____   _____   _____

    Consistent person, gender, and tense   _____   _____   _____

    Spelling, grammar, and punctuation   _____   _____   _____

Page numbers, table of contents, and index terms

    Finalize table of contents   _____   _____   _____

    Fill in page numbers   _____   _____   _____

    List key concepts and terms to be indexed
        (e.g., *Chicago Manual of Style*)   _____   _____   _____

    Fill in index page numbers   _____   _____   _____

CLERICAL ASSISTANTS

Obtain written approval of copyright material   _____   _____   _____

Retrieve missing information (e.g., references)   _____   _____   _____

Prepare alphabetical list of referenced authors   _____   _____   _____

Develop tabular list of tables, forms, and
    figures   _____   _____   _____

Be sure listed tabular numbers are in text   _____   _____   _____

Be sure tabular numbers in text are on list   _____   _____   _____

FORM 18.2: OVERALL SYNTHESIS ASSESSMENT BY CONSENSUS

> **Instructions:** This assessment uses a modified nominal group technique involving your team or, ideally, 5 to 11 topic experts who have read your synthesis report. This exercise is done face-to-face, by telephone, or through e-mail. The meeting requires about 1 hour.

Round 1: At this meeting, the team is given the enclosed Round 1 question form. The discussion consists of only questions for clarification and lasts about 10 minutes. Each member then completes the form and gives it to the leader to calculate average group scores.

Example of Calculations by Leader

Suppose your team consists of seven members, whose total team score for Criterion A is 42. Dividing 42 by 70 (7 × 10, i.e., the total possible raw score for the team as a whole) equals 0.60, multiplied by 100, yields a percentage of 60% of the total possible adjusted group weight for that group.

Round 2: At this point, the leader feeds back the team's Round 1 results. These are then openly discussed for up to 30 to 40 minutes, especially those criteria on which the team members widely disagree. The discussion is limited to factual input and experience, not unsupported opinions. With the new information from the discussion, each member completes the Round 2 form, and the exercise is finished. Waiting to see the final scores is arbitrary.

Synthesis Assessment Criteria Round 1
(Prediscussion, Except for Questions of Clarification)

Circle one number per criterion. Note that "1" means *poor* and "10" means *excellent.*

Criterion A: Is your synthesis adequately documented?

(Consider documentation of Stage I planning process, Stage II database process, Stage III coding and validation, Stage IV analysis and synthesis, and Stage V write-up process.)

1   2   3   4   5   6   7   8   9   10

Criterion B: Is your synthesis clinically significant?

(Consider clinical importance, i.e., population net benefit and information maturity.)

1   2   3   4   5   6   7   8   9   10

Criterion C: Is your synthesis scientifically sound?

(Consider internal, external, construct, and statistical validity.)

1   2   3   4   5   6   7   8   9   10

Criterion D: Was your synthesis cost-effective?

(Consider whether the time and dollars spent were acceptable, whether the likely net benefit [benefit minus harm] would be substantial, and whether the product would be worth the cost.)

1   2   3   4   5   6   7   8   9   10

Synthesis Assessment Criteria Round 2
(Postdiscussion)

Circle one number per criterion. Note that "1" means *poor* and "10" means *excellent.*

1   2   3   4   5   6   7   8   9   10

Criterion A: Is your synthesis adequately documented?

(Consider documentation of Stage I planning process, Stage II database process, Stage III coding and validation, Stage IV analysis and synthesis, and Stage V write-up process.)

1   2   3   4   5   6   7   8   9   10

Criterion B: Is your synthesis clinically significant?

(Consider clinical importance, i.e., population net benefit and information maturity.)

1   2   3   4   5   6   7   8   9   10

Criterion C: Is your synthesis scientifically sound?

(Consider internal, external, construct, and statistical validity.)

1   2   3   4   5   6   7   8   9   10

Criterion D: Was your synthesis cost-effective?

(Consider whether the time and dollars spent were acceptable, whether the likely net benefit [benefit minus harm] would be substantial, and whether the product would be worth the cost.)

1   2   3   4   5   6   7   8   9   10

Compendium of Internet Sources and Addresses for Information Synthesis

R elevant government sites are arranged by organizational hierarchy; non-government sites are arranged by degree of relevance to evidence-based material.

For a detailed listing of the compendium's contents, see the synopsis, p. 667.

Introduction

The purpose of this compendium is to provide a brief guide to the major organizations that are financing, producing, analyzing, synthesizing, and disseminating information to improve healthcare outcomes in the immediate future.

The most important goal of this compendium is to help you see a broader range of information resources than you might otherwise consider when you plan your synthesis or seek sound information for immediate decision purposes. This material ranges from a listing of completed and assessed "systematic reviews" or their abstracts to registries of randomized controlled trials (including a registry of registries) to raw statistical data where, for example, you can learn about prevalence of various health conditions in different geographic areas in the world, such as the northeastern region of the United States, Western Europe, or South Africa.

(Note that Uniform Resource Locator [URL] addresses are provided to facilitate your contacting and keeping up with the various Internet Web sites included.)

TO FACILITATE USE OF URL ADDRESSES SHOWN

(1) The following Internet and Web site addresses have been checked for accuracy just prior to publication. At that time, the month and year when that site explicitly stated to have been last updated or reviewed is enclosed in parentheses. For example: (last updated May 2001). If that date is not visible on the Internet site, double question marks (??) are shown.

If no update is stated, then the last Internet or Web page copyright is shown, if available. If the term "at least . . ." is given, the date is our inference, perhaps from the latest reference citation.

(2) When an Internet or Web site address is changed, the old address is usually made available for a limited time informing you of the new URL. After a time, you will be required to link to the new address from its home page. It is wise to save a new bookmark or favorite address on your computer at that time. If you cannot link to the home page, you can try "www.(their name).com." Rather than ".com" for commercial, the final part of the address may be ".org" for a nonprofit organization, ".edu" for an educational or academic location, ".gov" for a government location, or ".mil" for a military site. These are called "root domain names," of which there may be hundreds. Names of organizations are often abbreviated or run together as one word with no periods. If this approach fails, then you will likely have to start from the beginning with your local browser or become acquainted with searching by use of numeric "domain names."

(3) Note that long quotations from an Internet site are indented and in blocked style. These quotes do not have quotation marks per the American Psy-

chological Association (APA) style manual (American Psychological Association, 2001).

(4) If on your manuscript you insert an address that does not open (or gives a message that "Internet is unable to open this address," or "The Internet site reports that the item you requested could not be found," or, even worse, your browser crashes, don't panic. This is a common happening, especially with overseas URLs. The address may be perfectly valid, but you have to use a few tricks to make it connect. If the Internet does not crash, click on the address again once or twice until it opens. If this fails, or your browser does crash, open it again, copy the troublesome address into the space labeled "Location" (Netscape) on your browser home page, and click "Go" or hit "Enter" on your keyboard.

If this fails, it is advisable to insert the root of your address, not the entire address again. Also, many sites are only available by linking through their home page and cannot be accessed directly by their complete URL address. For example, in June 2000, the Institute of Medicine (IOM) sites were often of this type and had to be opened by linking to the home page of their sponsor, the National Academies (United States).

(5) We strongly urge that after opening an important Internet site, you immediately make a "bookmark" or "favorites" to save that URL in your browser memory. In this way, you can organize these addresses in any outline form you find useful.

(6) If your computer is connected to the Net, you can type URL addresses in the text of electronic word-processed documents. By clicking on those addresses, as shown below, you can hyperlink directly to a Net site. To do this using Word, click on the hyperlink button on the "Insert" menu. A simple short-cut is to place your cursor after the last letter or digit of the URL address you entered in your text, then hit your spacebar. If the address turns blue (and likely underlined in blue), you have made a direct hyperlink connection in your Word document. On occasion, if the address does not turn blue, you may have to erase that final space mark and try again one or two times. From then on, after you click on that address, it will turn magenta and open up that Internet site. However, if you do link correctly and go to another site, you can still go back and click on the magenta-colored address and link back again to that site you originally typed into your text.

(7) Finally, to learn more about searching the Web, we recommend guidebooks such as Glossbrenner and Glossbrenner's (1999) *Search Engines for the World Wide Web.*

The next goal of this compendium is to help you develop your database, after your project plans are established. Reviewing the literature is an inductive process of managing many clues to establish a meaningful and representative information base for your synthesis. This particular process is one that many reviewers fail to manage adequately. The result can be introduction of serious bias, such as missing major "invisible colleges" that may produce research results on your topic that are substantially different from those you might find readily through current electronic bibliographic databases and indexes.

The rationale for usually arranging these Internet sources by sponsoring organizations is the fact that Internet addresses may change rather frequently, making it difficult to keep up with them. However, when you have a need to find their most current versions, it is better to start at the top-or home page or root address-of the sponsoring organization that finances those sites you require. For example, one major root for U.S. government health information is the Department of Health and Human Services, which can be located at the following Web site (last updated May 2001):

www.dhhs.gov

From there you can link down to the material you need, even if the database name and Internet address may have changed. In this way, even if government or corporate departments, administrations, agencies, and centers change their names occasionally, their parent group most likely will remain stable. The groups are listed in order of the approximate size of the populations they serve.

Finally, the particular organization sponsors we mention are more likely than most to provide sound information that has had some validation assessment, such as meta-validation by two independent groups.

There are a number of organizations, both government and private, that have active programs to research and improve methods for identifying and certifying sound health information on the Net. See Berland et al., 2001.

The U.S. Agency for Healthcare Research and quality has one such site that lists these criteria:

www.ahcpr.gov/data/infoqual.htm

AHRQ is working in collaboration with Mitretek Systems to further develop such criteria.

See the following URL address to access the Mitretek System's Healthcare Division's Health Summit Working Group policy paper, "Criteria for Assessing the Quality of Health Information on the Internet" (last updated ??, copyright 1998):

hitiweb.mitretek.org/iq/

CRITERIA FOR EVALUATING INTERNET HEALTH INFORMATION*

Credibility: includes the source, currency, relevance/utility, and editorial review process for the information.

Content: must be accurate and complete and an appropriate disclaimer provided.

Disclosure: includes informing the user of the purpose of the site, as well as any profiling or collection of information associated with using the site.

Links: evaluated according to selection, architecture, content, and back linkages.

Design: encompasses accessibility, logical organization (navigability), and internal search capability.

Interactivity: includes feedback mechanisms and means for exchange of information among users.

Caveats: clarification of whether site function is to market products and services or is a primary information content provider.

*Health Summit Working Group

Another group, the U.K. Centre for Health Information Quality, together with the Health Education Authority and "Showme" Multimdia, Ltd., is developing "QUICK" (the Quality Information Checklist) as a guide for healthcare consumers to determine health information quality on the Web.

Their teachers' guide Web site (updated December 1999) is

www.quick.org.uk

Section A. World Health Organization

WHO Mission

WHO (World Health Organization) is the integrating organization for improving health outcomes throughout the world. This organization is important to those interested in systematic reviews because of their extensive international healthcare information connections to nearly all countries. Although, as of May 2000, its electronic databank is relatively small, it will likely be growing rapidly as it establishes more Internet links, which for most it provides free access.

The WHO's home page and site index (last update May 2001) is

www.who.int

Its official mission statement is quoted as follows:

The objective of WHO is the attainment by all peoples of the highest possible level of health. Health, as defined in the WHO Constitution, is a state of complete physical, mental and social well-being and not merely the absence of disease or infirmity. WHO also proposes conventions, agreements, regulations and makes recommendations about international nomenclature of diseases, causes of death and public health practices. It develops, establishes and promotes international standards concerning foods and biological, pharmaceutical and similar substance.

The reference for this quote (as of May 2001) is the following Web site (last updated ??):

www.who.int/aboutwho/en/mission.htm

Perhaps their most relevant site for healthcare information synthesis use is its Annual Reviews in Medicine, maintained with the collaboration of Stanford University in the United States and having multiple links to many other useful resources. The URL address for this Web site (last updated May 2001) is

med.AnnualReviews.org

WHO Library

This library supports the work of the World Health Organization by offering its knowledge bank of supportive evidence and global information resources to all. The entire collection of the library is referenced in its electronic database, available worldwide via the Web.

The library's home page (last updated ??, copyright 2000) is

www.who.int/hlt

WHOLIS (Library Catalog)

The electronic database catalog to the entire WHO Library's collection is available through the WHOLIS Web*Cat* search engine (developed by Sirsi Corporation) at the following address (last updated ??, copyright 2000):

saturn.who.ch/uhtbin/cgisirsi/UGHdalACS9/16624013/60/30007

WHOLINK (Library Virtual Reference Desk)

The WHO Library and Information Networks for Knowledge (WHOLINK) is the library's Virtual Reference Desk.

The Virtual Reference Desk provides links to electronic resources in an attempt to assist WHO staff and others, in quickly locating information to assist them in their daily work. Whenever possible, sources of an international scope are included, as well as multi-language links. The Virtual Reference Desk complements the library's physical holdings and *those using these links should keep in mind that information, in any format, should be critically assessed for authority, accuracy, currency and reliability.* (emphasis added)

The reference for the quotes and access to the LINK Web site (last updated January 2001) is

www.who.int/library/index.en.shtml

WHO.INT: WHO Program Web Sites
With Access to Full-Text Documents

Although WHO has an extensive databank, due to licensing restrictions, only limited parts are available without cost. Some databases can only be accessed from computers located in the WHO Library. However, some databases are available, free-of-charge, on the Internet. This site provides an index of health topics to which you can directly link.

The linkage to its databases is at the following Web site (last updated March 2001):

www.who.int/library/index.en.shtml

WHOSIS (WHO Statistical Information System)

This database is from WHO's Global Programme on Evidence for Health Policy. It maintains one of the largest health and health-related statistics databanks anywhere. Its purpose is quoted as follows:

The purpose of this WHOSIS website (WHO Statistical Information System) is to describe-and to the extent possible provide access to-statistical and epidemiological data and information presently available from the World Health Organization and elsewhere in electronic or other forms. Most WHO technical programmes make information available to the public. The WHOSIS allows the user to search by keywords through the entire WHO website, and globally throughout the WWW.

The following Web site is the reference for the above quote and home page for WHOSIS and provides many different linkages of value to information synthesis (last updated ??):

www.who.int/whosis/

WHO Reproductive Health Library

This material is compiled by Update Software, with input of systematic reviews from the Cochrane Collaboration. This is one of WHO's newer additions to evidence-based information. This library is described in more detail below in Section E under Update Software.

Section B. United States Library of Congress

Introduction

One of the most useful introductions to the United States Library of Congress (LC) is the Web site titled "Using the Library of Congress-Collections and Services." This site is a key to understanding and accessing the vast resources of this amazing collection of information. For purposes of information synthesis, we suggest that this is a major source to identify "fugitive literature" related to medical research and health care.

For an introductory overview of the library, access the following Web site address (update February 2001):

www.loc.gov/library

Online Catalog

The LC Online is a database of approximately 12 million records representing books, serials, computer files, manuscripts, cartographic materials, music, sound recordings, and visual materials in the library's collections. The Online Catalog also provides references, notes, circulation status, and information about materials still in the "acquisitions" stage.

Its Net site (update March 2001) is

catalog.loc.gov

LC New Online Catalog

This catalog "is a database of approximately 12 million records representing books, serials, computer files, manuscripts, cartographic materials, music, sound recordings, and visual materials in the Library's collections." The Internet reference for this quote (last updated April 2001) is

lcweb.loc.gov/catalog

This is a recent edition of the Library of Congress catalog that likely includes all of the material in the above "old" catalog. This version went online January 18, 2000; it contains bibliographies, research guides, and "finding aids." This site provides a search engine that covers the entire book collection of the LC and provides many aids for locating information. For example, they have an interesting guide on locating information in medicine. To illustrate, one quote related to fugitive literature is as follows: "Other print sources for health-related articles are 'General Science Index' and 'Readers' Guide to Periodical Literature.'" There are also other compact disk products for health literature that a local library may have, such as "Health Index" and "Health Reference Center," or the more general disk, "Magazine Index." A description is quoted as follows:

> As an integrated database, the Online Catalog includes 12 million catalog records. This source contains about 3.1 million records from an earlier database of books and serials from between 1898 and 1980. These sources are being edited to comply with current cataloging standards and to reflect contemporary language and usage.

The reference to this quote (last updated August 1999) is

catalog.loc.gov/libinfo.htm

Z39.50 Gateway

"This is the Library of Congress Page for gateway access to LC's catalog and those at many other institutions."

The URL address (updated May 2001) is

lcweb.loc.gov/z3950

Z39.50 is a national standard defining a protocol for computer-to-computer information retrieval. Z39.50 makes it possible for a user in one system to search and retrieve information from other computer systems (that have also implemented Z39.50) without knowing the search syntax that is used by those other systems. Z39.50 is an American National Standard that was originally approved by the National Information Standards Organization (NISO) in 1988.

The reference for this quote and access to its search engine is at the following Net site (updated May 2001):

lcweb.loc.gov/z3950/gateway.html#about

Use of this form results in a search of the LC Voyager database (well over 12 million records). This database contains records in all bibliographic formats (i.e., books, serials, music, maps, manuscripts, computer files, and visual materials), and includes the retrospective, unedited older bibliographic records known as the PreMARC File. LC name and subject authority records cannot be searched.

Reference to this quote can be accessed through the above Net site by clicking on "Simple Search."

Services for Researchers

This is the home page to a rich source of information aids for the most effective use of the Library of Congress' complete collection.

It is available (updated May 2001) at

lcweb.loc.gov/rr/

Research Tools

The Library of Congress offers a wide variety of online databases and Internet resources to the public via the Net, including its own online catalog. In addition, LC provides an easy-to-use gateway for searching other institutions' online catalogs and extensive links to resources on the Internet.

Category H (Medical Sciences) may prove useful for synthesis development.

The reference for this quote and access to these research tools (updated March 2001) is

lcweb.loc.gov/rr/tools.html

Access to Periodical Articles

Abstracts, Indexes, and Bibliographies For Finding Citations to Periodical Articles. . . . This guide was prepared to help researchers find periodical articles on subjects within the general areas of humanities and social sciences. Its scope, while very broad, is limited to reference material located within the reading rooms of the Humanities and Social Sciences Division. Such reference works may be identified from the Table of Contents, or the Subject Index at the end.

This source indexes articles from both scientific and some popular periodicals such as the *New York Times, Wall Street Journal,* and the *Saturday Review of Literature Indexes.* It covers such relevant bibliographies as those on library and information science, medicine, medical ethics, and psychology, to name a few. One example covers the entire Index Medicus. However, this source is a long shot, valuable mainly for heuristic reasons, with most of this material available only at the Library of Congress Reading Room.

The reference for the above quotes and access to this index is by way of the following Net site (last updated September 1998):

lcweb.loc.gov/rr/main/ab_index.html

Search-Browse

The search engine for this databank allows you to search the Library of Congress Net sites alphabetically or using key words. The Internet address for this site (last updated June 1998) is

lcweb.loc.gov/harvest/query-lc.html

Section C. United States Department of Health and Human Services

The Department of Health and Human Services is the U.S. government's principal agency for protecting the health of all Americans and providing essential human services, especially for those who are least able to help themselves. They sponsor more than 300 programs and encompass the largest granting agency in the health field. The programs described below are among the more relevant for development of healthcare information syntheses. The key to the multiple administrations, agencies, and centers within HHS is a Directory of HHS Data Resources, which provides links to somewhere between 100 and 200 Internet database addresses arranged by the organizational structure of this department. The Internet address for this site (last updated May 2000) is

aspe.hhs.gov/datacncl/datadir/

The Internet address, which provides direct links to the organizational offices and personnel of HHS and allows free text browsing using Boolean operators, is (last updated July 2001)

waisgate.hhs.gov/search

National Library of Medicine (NLM)

Search Engines and Electronic Information Sources

These are described on the NLM's home page. This site is key to the rich resources and multiple search engines and databanks of the NLM as of May 2000 is the following (last updated ??):

www.nlm.nih.gov/nlmhome.html

PubMed. This is a powerful search engine developed within the framework of the Unified Medical Language System®. The NLM categorizes PubMed as a "server farm" because it provides such broad access to so many of the NLM's major databanks for both molecular biological sciences (through Entrez) and the healthcare sciences.

Its overview Web address (last updated September 2001) is

www.ncbi.nlm.nih.gov:80/entrez/query/static/overview.html

Gateway. This is an important recent development by NLM to facilitate access to multiple databases from one Web site (a server farm). NLM states that Gateway is your entrance to the knowledge resources of the National Library of Medicine. Most of the individual databases mentioned below will remain as separate entities, one exception being OLDMEDLINE. Note that the data server Grateful Med has been retired. Gateway will undoubtedly become the "meta-server" that will eventually encompass a substantial proportion of NLM's extensive online library. The following quote provides the current (as of September 2001) description of this source:

> The NLM Gateway allows users to search in multiple retrieval systems at the U.S. National Library of Medicine (NLM). The current Gateway searches MEDLINE/PubMed, OLDMEDLINE, LOCATOR*plus,* MEDLINEplus, DIRLINE, AIDS Meetings, Health Services Research Meetings, Space Life Sciences Meetings, and HSRProj.

This remarkable search engine will enable "one-stop shopping" as it will search both the journal file of MEDLINE/PubMed and also books, consumer information, drug files, and a directory of health organizations. Full-text articles are available by clicking on a LinkOut button to more than 1,600 journals. Complete hard copy documents can be obtained by the direct link to Loansome Doc® and a participating medical library. Gateway will have additional databases added in the near future.

The home page and source of the above quote (last updated ??, at least August 2001) is

http://gateway.nlm.nih.gov/gw/Cmd

The primary fact sheets for NLM databanks can be found at the following site (last updated October 2001):

www.nlm.nih.gov/pubs/factsheets/factsubj.html

To keep current on the description and contents of NLM databanks and to access them, refer to the following Web address (last updated October 2001):

www.nlm.nih.gov/databases/databases.html

LOCATORplus. This is the National Library of Medicine's "catalog of books, journals, and audiovisuals and access points to other medical research tools. Select from the following menu choices to access a variety of medical information." One problem, however, is that once you locate the book you need, you likely will have to check with your local medical library and/or arrange an interlibrary loan.

The reference for the above quote (last updated ??) is

locatorplus.gov/

MEDLINEplus. This is

> . . . for anyone with a medical question. Both health professionals and consumers can depend on it for accurate, current, medical information. This service provides access to extensive information about specific diseases and conditions and also has links to consumer health information from the National Institutes of Health, dictionaries, lists of hospitals and physicians, health information in Spanish and other languages, and clinical trials. There is no advertising on this site, nor does MEDLINE*plus* endorse any company or product.

The Web site for this quote (last updated January 2001) is

www.nlm.nih.gov/medlineplus/aboutmedlineplus.html

The home page for MEDLINE*plus* (Net page last updated ??) is

medlineplus.gov

DIRLINE® (Directory of Information Resources Online). This database

> . . . focuses primarily on health and biomedical information resources including organizations, government agencies, information centers, professional societies, voluntary associations, support groups, academic and research institutions, and research facilities and resources. Records contain resource names, addresses, phone numbers, and descriptions of services, publications, and holdings.

This is a good site for exploring the "fugitive literature" by networking with other professionals and organizations listed. This resource can be accessed through Gateway or LOCATOR*plus*.

The DIRLINE fact sheet Net address (last updated July 2000) is

www.nlm.nih.gov/pubs/factsheets/dirlinfs.html

National Information Center on Health Services Research and Health Care Technology (NICHSR). This center coordinates the development of information products and services related to health services research. Three of their most relevant databanks for synthesis use are HealthSTAR, HSTAT, and DIRLINE (the latter described above).

The home page for this site (last updated March 2001) is

www.nlm.nih.gov/nichsr/nichsr.html

HSTAT (Health Services/Technology Assessment Text). This provides access to full-text documents useful for clinical decision making. It includes clinical practice guidelines, quick-reference guides for clinicians, consumer brochures, evidence reports, and technology assessment reports sponsored by the Agency for Healthcare Research and Quality (AHRQ, previously AHCPR), NIH consensus development reports, and other such clinical decision-related information.

Its home page (last updated May 2001) is

text.nlm.nih.gov

Other NICHSR Related Health Services Research Web Sites. This is a Web site that indexes much material directly relevant to systematic review activity.

> It lists valuable information on health services research topics, including links to fugitive literature information. Content coverage includes "Federal Agencies, Associations, Data Sets/Data Sources, Epidemiology/Health Statistics, Evidence Based Medicine/Health Technology Assessment, Funding, Health Policy/Health Economics, Information Systems, Public Health, Rural Health, State Resources."

The reference to the above quotes and Web address (last updated December 2000) is

www.nlm.nih.gov/nichsr/hsrsites.html

Evidence-Based Medicine and Health Technology Assessment. This site has recently added this heading for links to highly relevant material for information synthesis retrieval and development. As of October 2001, we had difficulty opening several of their listings, but this may be a temporary problem. The quality of listings in terms of Cochrane criteria of "evidence based" is somewhat mixed at this time. However, this is a promising source for readily obtaining material of value for information synthesis.

Lister Hill National Center for Biomedical Communications (LHNCBC)

"We conduct R & D for the broad purpose of improving health-care information dissemination and use." This program is administered through NLM and sponsors research that is fundamental to healthcare informatics. Perhaps its most important work relates to the Unified Medical Language System (UMLS) Project. This work is fundamental for understanding health science knowledge structures. Its purpose is to facilitate electronic translation of information into a common language in digital form. By means of their UMLS Metathesaurus, data and text from hundreds of unique sources can be translated into strings, terms, and concepts (including those in certain foreign languages) that provide a universal language for such purposes as text translation and Internet communications. The most important NLM search engines (PubMed and GATEWAY) build on a UMLS foundation.

The Lister Hill Web site (last updated July 2001) is

www.lhncbc.nlm.nih.gov

Natural Language systems have been a major focus for research programs to improve information access. They developed the Visible Human Project for creating anatomical images of the male and female body. The HSTAT (Health Services/Technology Assessment Text) program facilitates access to most of the databanks of AHRQ.

This Lister Hill Net site for the above quotes (site last updated ??) is

tlc.nlm.nih.gov/abouttlc/description/description.html

The Learning Center for Interactive Technology is now closing after 16 years of operation. It was a laboratory for the exploration of network-based applications of information and education technology in the health

The Collaboratory for High Performance Computing and Communication is a recent development at Lister Hill. The work being done will provide innovative methods for application of information syntheses, particularly in distance-learning modalities. It

. . . is part of the National Library of Medicine's Office of High Performance Computing and Communication (OHPCC). While it is a focal point for the office's internal research and development activities, it also a venue for integrating selected technologies and applications from R & D projects that the office has funded externally. Internal R and D activities often involve working with others in the field, and online collaboration tools are not only part of the physical infrastructure of the collaboratory, their development and use for medical consultation and distance learning is an important area of research.

The Web site for this quote (last updated ??) is

http://collab.nlm.nih.gov

DXPNET (Digital X-ray Prototype workstations linked via Internet) program "relates to archiving and accessing high-resolution (2048 ∗ 2560 pixels) x-ray images and text from nationwide surveys."

The source of this quote is the following (Net site last updated September 1996):

archive.nlm.nih.gov/proj/dxpnet/dxpnet.html

Radiographs (about 17,500) from the phases of the National Health and Nutrition Examination Survey (NHANES) survey that are already completed and an additional 10,400 X-rays from a subsequent phase make up its current file. "The radiographs are of cervical and lumbar spine, and hands and knees." These surveys are of adults 25 to 75 and older.

The source of this quote is Net site (last updated September 1996) is

archive.nlm.nih.gov/nhanes/nhanes.html

(Because this survey is being conducted in collaboration with the National Center for Health Statistics, we would imagine that its sample is representative of a major portion of the U.S. population.)

NLM Extramural Programs (EP)

This division provides funding for small and large research and education programs, including book projects. It

. . . funds projects in areas defined by NLM as important to its mission. As the nation's premier repository of biomedical information, NLM has a vital interest in information management and in the enormous utility of computers and telecommunication for improving storage, retrieval, access, and use of biomedical information. NLM provides extramural support through grants-in-aid and, less commonly, contracts.

The Web address for this quote (last updated October 2001) is

www.nlm.nih.gov/pubs/factsheets/extrapro.html

You can find what its current priorities are for grant and contract applications, as well as lists of grants and contracts funded in the past 5 years or so.

The following Web site provides direct research priority information related to NLM extramural funding (last updated May 2001):

www.nlm.nih.gov/ep/extramural.html

DOCLINE® (Automated Interlibrary Loan Request Routing and Referral System)

DOCLINE is the National Library of Medicine's automated interlibrary loan (ILL) request routing and referral system. The purpose of the system is to provide efficient document delivery service among libraries in the National Network of Libraries of Medicine® (NN/LM). DOCLINE serves over 3,000 United States and Canadian medical libraries at no cost. Some selected national and major medical libraries in other countries also have DOCLINE access. Health sciences libraries and libraries at institutions with a health sciences mission are eligible to apply for access to the DOCLINE system. Libraries may join DOCLINE as part of their affiliation with the NN/LM as either a full member or affiliate member.

The Web site for the above quotes can be found on its home page, plus a link to its "Fact Sheet" (last updated October 2001):

www.nlm.nih.gov/docline/newdocline.html

Loansome Doc®

Loansome Doc is a means for an individual to order complete medical literature documents over the Internet by means of a one-time registration with the National Library of Medicine (NLM) and a local university medical library. This service is available to those using PubMed or GATEWAY from the NLM. Articles can be faxed, mailed, or picked up at the local library. There is a nominal per page fee involved.

At this site, you can learn more about Loansome Doc® (last updated May 2001):

www.nlm.nih.gov/pubs/factsheets/loansome_doc.html

Agency for Healthcare Research and Quality (AHRQ)

Legislation passed in November 1999 established AHRQ as the lead federal agency on quality research. The purpose of this agency is as follows:

> The Agency for Healthcare Research and Quality (AHRQ) research provides evidence-based information on health care outcomes; quality; and cost, use, and access. Information from AHRQ's research helps people make more informed decisions and improve the quality of health care services. AHRQ was formerly known as the Agency for Health Care Policy and Research.

The Web site for this quote (last updated Mar 2001) is

www.ahrq.gov/about/profile.htm.

The AHRQ home page address is (last updated ??) is

www.ahrq.gov

EPCs (Evidence-Based Practice Centers)

The purpose of these centers is to synthesize scientific evidence to improve quality and effectiveness in clinical care.

> The EPCs will review all relevant scientific literature on assigned clinical care topics and produce evidence reports and technology assessments, conduct research on methodologies and the effectiveness of their implementation, and participate in technical assistance activities. Public and private sector organizations may use the reports and assessments as the basis for their own clinical guidelines and other quality improvement activities.

The Web site for this quote is (last updated October 2001)

www.ahrq.gov/clinic/epc

This is a highly relevant source of information for purposes of developing mini-syntheses or complete systematic reviews. However, only 40 "Evidence Reports" (EPs) have been developed as of May 2001. On their first round, AHRQ contracted for 40 reports, including meta-analyses and cost analyses. We hope this number will increase in the near future, although that may depend on congressional appropriations.

AHRQ Databanks and Databases

These sites are especially relevant to systematic reviews in terms of both background information and potential topics.

The Healthcare Cost and Utilization Project (HCUP)

This is an important database for U.S. economic outcome data. The use for data from this project is quoted as follows:

> HCUP data are used for research on hospital utilization, access, charges, quality and outcomes. The data are used to describe patterns of care for uncommon as well as common diseases, analyze hospital procedures, including those that are performed infrequently, and study the care of population sub-groups such as minorities, children, women, and the uninsured.

The Web site for this reference and access to its file (last updated September 2001) is

www.ahcpr.gov/data/hcup/hcupnet.htm

Data and Surveys. This is an AHRQ databank that provides access to numerous other databases on economic information (including HIV and AIDS) and on healthcare informatics standards. It has links to the Medical Expenditure Panel Survey (MEPS) and to the Healthcare Cost and Utilization Project (HCUP).

The Internet Home Page address (last updated ??) is

www.ahrq.gov/data

MEDTEP (Medical Treatment Effectiveness Program)

> . . . Projects in the Medical Treatment Effectiveness Program (MEDTEP) are designed to determine the strategies that are most effective and cost effective for preventing, diagnosing, treating, and managing clinical conditions.
>
> MEDTEP has four essential elements: research, development of data for research, development of clinical practice guidelines, and dissemination of information to health care practitioners, consumers, insurers, employers, policymakers, and others.

The Web site for this quote (last updated ??) is

www.ahcpr.gov/clinic/medtep/#over

MEDTEP Update is another MEDTEP databank, which includes links to seven relevant databases: (a) PORTs (Patient Outcomes Research Teams), (b) PORT-IIs (the next generation of MEDTEP research), (c) MEDTEP research centers on minority populations, (d) research on pharmaceutical therapy and outcomes, (e) clinical practice guideline development and evaluation, (f) performance indicators and quality of care, and (g) outcomes measurement, research methods, and data.

The Web site for MedTep Update (last updated ??, at least 1995) is

www.ahcpr.gov/clinic/medtep

Healthfinder.™ This is a consumer health information Web site from the U.S. government. It can lead you to select online publications, databases, Web sites, and support and self-help groups, as well as the government agencies and not-for-profit organizations that produce reliable health information for the public.

It covers questions consumers frequently ask, consumer versions of clinical guidelines, and information on common preventive health style practice.

The URL address (last updated ??) is

www.ahcpr.gov/consumer

National Guideline Clearinghouse (NGC)

The NGC has the mission to provide physicians, nurses, healthcare providers, purchasers, and others an accessible mechanism for obtaining objective, detailed information on clinical practice guidelines and to further their dissemination, implementation, and use.

The home page (last updated October 2001) is

www.guideline.gov/body_home_nf.asp?view=home

NGC provides guideline abstracts, utilities for comparing if not combining the guidelines, complete systematic reviews, and bibliographies. The review provides the evidence base on which the guideline was structured. This information is even more valuable than an EPC Evidence Report in that the authors provide not only an information synthesis but also a ready-made framework for its implementation in the community. The AHRQ, the American Medical Association, and the American Association of Healthplans are the three sponsors of NGC.

Another access to NGC is the following Web site (last updated October 2001):

www.guideline.gov

Academic Healthcare Informatics Centers

This is a group of academic informatics programs that are funded by the National Library of Medicine. They are important to the field of information synthesis because they can be a source of informatics expertise that might be required in your own synthesis projects. Its Web site is (last updated October 2001)

www.nlm.nih.gov/ep/curr_inst_grantees.html

"Funding Opportunities"

These are shown on the following index page. This source includes sections on "Contract Solicitations," "Grant Announcements," and "Policy Notices" listing certain programs that have been deactivated and other areas receiving greater emphasis, as well as "Future Year Commitments on AHRQ Grant Awards."

The URL address (last updated ??) is

www.ahrq.gov/fund

Centers for Disease Control and Prevention (CDC)

The mission of CDC is "to promote health and quality of life by preventing and controlling disease, injury, and disability." (Note that its acronym remains CDC, even though its official name is now the Centers for Disease Control and Prevention.) There are 11 centers, an institute, and offices that make up this complex, including the National Center for Health Statistics (NCHS), National Center for Infectious Diseases (NCID), and the National Institute for Occupational Safety and Health (NIOSH). It is one of the largest organizations, with the most databanks in HHS.

The Web site for the above quote, overview, and links to all of its member sites (last updated September 2001) is

www.cdc.gov/aboutcdc.htm

The CDC home page address (last updated October 2001) is

www.cdc.gov/

One of the most valuable Internet addresses in CDC provides access to the major health surveys and provides information on how to access "public use" resources such as data tapes from a survey for the years requested.

The Net site (last updated ??, at least 1999) is

aspe.os.dhhs.gov/datacncl/datadir/cdc3.htm

National Center for Health Statistics (NCHS)

This center is the federal government's principal vital and health statistics agency. Since 1960, when the National Office of Vital Statistics and the National Health Survey merged to form NCHS, the agency has provided a wide variety of data with which to monitor the nation's health.

The Web site for this quote and overview of the center (last updated May 2001) is

www.cdc.gov/nchs/about.htm

Its home page Web site (last reviewed October 2001) is

www.cdc.gov/nchs/default.htm

Its search engine for obtaining health statistics is at the following Web site (last updated ??):

www.fedstats.gov/programs/health.html

National Ambulatory Medical Care Survey (NAMCS)

This national survey

. . . is designed to meet the need for objective, reliable information about the provision and use of ambulatory medical care services in the United States. Findings are based on a sample of visits to nonfederally employed office-based physicians who are primarily engaged in direct patient care. Physicians in the specialties of anesthesiology, pathology, and radiology are excluded from the survey. The survey was conducted annually from 1974 to 1981, in 1985, and annually since 1989.

The Internet address for this quote (last updated May 2001) is www.cdc.gov/nchs/about/major/ahcd/namcsdes.htm

This database is important because it can provide useful data and ideas to formulate topics for information syntheses. For example, NAMCS is one of the only surveys that includes coded "reason for visit" in terms of chief complaints and symptoms, as well as *ICD-CM* coded diagnoses. This makes it possible to identify a profile of reasons for visit for any single diagnosis, as well as a profile of diagnoses for any single reason for a visit. This can provide numerous clues to possibly missed diagnoses or misdiagnoses. Such evaluation of diagnostic accuracy is often limited to presurgical versus postsurgical pathology, or premorbid versus autopsy validated diagnoses. Furthermore, this survey is an important source of prevalence of conditions seen in the physician's office. Such national or regional statistics can provide á priori probabilities essential for determining diagnostic accuracy or improvement of diagnostic accuracy by means of computerized expert systems.

The following Internet site map address provides links to the many statistical compilations from NAMCS (last updated October 2001):

www.cdc.gov/nchs/about/major/ahcd/ahcd1.htm

Federal Electronic Research and Review Extraction Tool FERRET is a resource developed by "a collaborative effort between NCHS and the Bureau of the Census. The Census' FERRET system will provide full access to complex large data sets through the Internet."

The reference for this quote and access to this data warehouse (last updated June 2001) is

www.cdc.gov/nchs/datawh/ferret/ferret.htm

ClinicalTrials.gov

This resource

. . . provides patients, family members, health care professionals, and members of the public easy access to information on clinical trials for a wide range of diseases and conditions. The United States National Institutes of Health (NIH), through its National Library of Medicine (NLM), has developed this site in close and ongoing collaboration with all NIH Institutes and the Food and Drug Administration (FDA).

The Web site for this quote (last updated ??) is

clinicaltrials.gov

Food and Drug Administration (FDA)

The mission of this administration is explained in the following quote:

For it is FDA's job to see that the food we eat is safe and wholesome, the cosmetics we use won't hurt us, the medicines and medical devices we use are safe and effective, and that radiation-emitting products such as microwave ovens won't do us harm. Feed and drugs for pets and farm animals also come under FDA scrutiny. FDA also ensures that all of these products are labeled truthfully with the information that people need to use them properly.

The reference for this quote (updated July 2001) is

www.fda.gov/opacom/hpview.html

The Web site index with links to their information resources (updated September 2001) is

www.fda.gov/opacom/hpchoice.html

The National Institutes of Health (NIH)

The NIH mission is to uncover new knowledge that will lead to better health for everyone. NIH works toward that mission by: conducting research in its own laboratories; supporting the research of non-Federal scientists in universities, medical schools, hospitals, and research institutions throughout the country and abroad; helping in the training of research investigators; and fostering communication of biomedical information.

The reference for the above quote (prepared as a Web site in August 1999) is

www.nih.gov/about/nihnew.html

The home page for this biomedical research complex (last updated ??, at least May 2001) is

www.nih.gov/index.html

Consensus Development Program of NIH

This is a source of meta-validated information based on agreement of panels of the leading experts on the topic addressed. It is one of the more relevant sources of sound information for systematic reviews, particularly mini-syntheses.

Its home page is at the following Net site (last updated ??, at least December 2000):

odp.od.nih.gov/consensus

NIH Consensus Development Conferences are convened to evaluate available scientific information and resolve safety and efficacy issues related to biomedical technology. The resultant NIH Consensus Statements are intended to advance understanding of the technology or issue in question and to be useful to health professionals and the public.

The reference for the above quote and index listing of available consensus statements, by date or by subject, is at the following Net site (last updated ??):

odp.od.nih.gov/consensus/cons/cons.htm

Some Technology Assessment Conferences and Workshops adhere to the NIH Consensus Development Conference (NIH CDC) format because the process is altogether appropriate for evaluating highly controversial, publicized, or politicized issues. In the CDC format, NIH Technology Assessment Statements are prepared by a non advocate, non-Federal panel of experts.

Likewise, the reference for the above quote and Net site for the NIH consensus statements on healthcare technology assessment (last updated ??, after January 2000) is

odp.od.nih.gov/consensus/ta/talist.htm

Consumer Information

This is a "consumer-friendly" Web site to access the NIH index to information for patients and their families. It highlights three specific databases: (a) MEDLINE*plus* from the National Library of Medicine, (b) an index to healthcare conditions, and (c) a link to research involving patients. It also provides links to many other sites of interest to consumer.

This Web site (last updated August 2001) is

www.nih.gov/health

Sourcebook: Office of Intramural Research (OIR)

The OIR "is responsible for oversight and coordination of intramural research, training, and technology transfer conducted within the laboratories and clinics of the National Institutes of Health (NIH)."

This quote and an overview of its activity can be found at the following Web site (updated August 2001):

www1.od.nih.gov/oir/sourcebook/oir/oir-staff.htm#Overview

To directly access its sourcebook and learn more about its programs and administrative structure, link to (last revised January 2000)

www1.od.nih.gov/oir/sourcebook/

This source is of interest as background information, particularly in regard to laboratory molecular biology. Thus, it is somewhat peripheral to the needs of information synthesis.

Extramural Funding Programs

This source may be one of the largest that funds basic molecular biological and clinical research in the health field. Its programs are somewhat peripheral to health services research but have some overlap that, in certain cases, like reports of randomized clinical trials (RCTs), are worth checking. In terms of funding, it is doubtful that it would fund systematic reviews for immediate application in the community.

Its Internet address (last updated ??) is

grants.nih.gov/grants

NOTE

Although, organizationally, the NLM is located within the NIH family, we describe it in Section C of this compendium. We judge it to be among the most relevant U.S. government organizations to both the field of systematic information reviews and of healthcare informatics. NLM provides access to relatively mature material that can be immediately useful for improving healthcare outcomes in the community.

National Center for Biotechnology Information (NCBI)

> Established in 1988 as a national resource for molecular biology information, this Center is administered by the National Institutes of Health through the National Library of Medicine. NCBI creates public databases, conducts research in computational biology, develops software tools for analyzing genome data, and disseminates biomedical information—all for the better understanding of molecular processes affecting human health and disease.

We give this site an independent subsection due to its cutting-edge importance to the future of healthcare, although, at present, it is somewhat peripheral or premature to the content focus of this book.

The reference for this quote and home page (last updated October 2001) is

www.ncbi.nlm.nih.gov

Section D. United Kingdom National Health Service

The National Health Service's information sources have been world leaders for some time with its adoption of evidence-based medical projects and products. The following four sources are but an introduction to its rich literature of meta-validated information. Its interaction with the Cochrane Collaboration was likely seminal in having the British government and associated universities invest so heavily in developing systematic reviews, learning resources, and methods research for healthcare information syntheses. Based on the Cochrane example, its information is usually not only relevant and scientifically sound but often mature for immediate use in practice and quality improvement activity.

Centre for Evidence Based Medicine (CEBM)

This centre is sponsored by Oxford University.

> The Centre has been established in Oxford as the first of several centres around the country whose broad aim is to promote evidence-based health care and provide support and resources to anyone who wants to make use of them. Our prospectus outlines the specific aims of the Centre and the goals we have identified, as well as the means we propose to use in achieving those goals.

The reference for the above quote and access to its contents (Net site last updated ??, at least 1998) is cebm.jr2.ox.ac.uk/docs/adminpage.html

The home page for this center (last updated October 2001) is

cebm.jr2.ox.ac.uk

This NHS program is exceptionally relevant to anyone interested in or developing information syntheses. Useful tools, teaching materials, evidence-based journals, and other materials are made available to assist in learning about evidence-based medicine. In our section below, covering the United Kingdom Centre for Reviews and Dissemination, is a valuable enumeration of principles and a glossary for developing systematic reviews. It even has a Net address for medical students. This group is obviously in the same "invisible college" as the Cochrane group, which likely facilitated this site.

EBOC (Evidence-Based on Call)

"This is a project to create accurate, up-to-date evidence-based information for clinicians."

Its home page and reference for this quote (last updated ??, copyright 2000) is

cebm.jr2.ox.ac.uk/eboc/ebocDemo/index.htm

Its introduction explains,

Decisions about managing patients require the integration of the best available external evidence with clinical expertise, and the patients' rights, values and expectations. Accordingly the recommendations in each chapter are not a cookbook of what to do, but a summary of what to think about when caring for patients.

"Levels of evidence" provide a more objective empirical approach for establishing soundness of research studies of various designs. This site provides an interesting visual as an overview of this method, including references that describe its early origins by Cochrane systematic review specialists.

The reference for the quote (last updated ??, at least 1996) is

http://cebm.jr2.ox.ac.uk/eboc/ebocDemo/content/levels.html

The EBOC sponsors or collaborates with the following evidence-based journals:

Evidence-Based Medicine

Evidence-Based Nursing

Evidence-Based Mental Health

Evidence-Based Dentistry

Journal of Evidence-Based Health Care

Each of these journals is produced by its own center or institute, with the exception of nursing, which is collaborating with the Royal College of Nursing. The *Journal of Evidence-Based Health Care* targets administrators and managers with the best evidence available about financing, organization, and delivery of healthcare.

NHS Centre for Reviews and Dissemination (CRD)

This center is sponsored by the University of York.

The NHS Centre for Reviews and Dissemination (CRD) was established in January 1994 to provide the NHS with important information on the effectiveness of treatments and the delivery and organisation of health care. The CRD, by offering rigorous and systematic reviews on select topics, a database of good quality reviews and a dissemination service, is helping to promote research-based practice in the NHS.

Within the NHS R&D programme, the CRD is the sibling organisation of the UK Cochrane Centre. The UK Cochrane Centre is part of an international network, the Cochrane Collaboration, committed to preparing, maintaining and disseminating systematic reviews of research on the effects of health care. The CRD will play an important role in disseminating the contents of Cochrane reviews to the NHS. The CRD collaborates with a number of health research and information organisations across the world and is a UK member of the International Network of Agencies for Health Technology Assessment (INAHTA).

The Web site for the above quote and site access to it (last updated ??) is

www.york.ac.uk/inst/crd/centre.htm

The NHSCRD home page is at the following Web site (last updated September 2001):

www.york.ac.uk/inst/crd/welcome.htm

DARE (Database of Abstracts of Reviews of Effectiveness)

This database is particularly valuable in identifying meta-validated information. With its recent change in policy, now placing major emphasis on systematic reviews, DARE promises to be another of the leading bibliographic sources of systematic reviews. This is a vital Net site to screen, especially if you contemplate doing a mini-synthesis.

This source is updated at the end of every month, and it is free and easily accessed. The home page for DARE (last updated ??) is

nhscrd.york.ac.uk/darehp.htm

DARE is updated monthly and can also be searched via the Internet: users should be aware that the online version of DARE will always have more information than the Cochrane Library version. The Internet version of the DARE database also contains "flag" records with abstracts of Cochrane reviews and protocols, and brief records noting those Cochrane reviews published elsewhere, such as in academic journals.

The above quotes were from the following Net site (last updated ??):

nhscrd.york.ac.uk/faq6.htm

The reports produced by CRD will not be included in DARE automatically. CRD reports will be passed to NICE [National Institutes for Clinical Excellence—ours] for appraisal and incorporation into NICE publications such as guidelines. Please refer to the NICE website for further information.

The reference for this quote is at the following address (last updated ??):

nhscrd.york.ac.uk/dnice.htm

National Health Service Economic Evaluation Database (NHS EED)

This is another valuable database for those interested in developing information syntheses.

Full economic evaluations are studies in which a comparison of two or more treatments or care alternatives is undertaken and in which both the costs and outcomes of the alternatives are examined. Full economic evaluations in the scope of the NHS Economic Evaluation Database are regarded as cost-benefit analyses, cost-utility analyses, and cost-effectiveness analyses. Cost-minimization analyses and cost-consequence analyses are also included. A cost-benefit analysis (CBA) measures both costs and benefits in monetary values and calculates net monetary gains or losses (presented as a cost-benefit ratio). A cost-effectiveness analysis (CEA) compares interventions with a common outcome (such as blood pressure level) to discover which produces the maximum outcome for the same input of resources in a given population. A cost-utility analysis (CUA) measures the benefits of alternative treatments or types of care by using utility measures such as Quality-Adjusted Life Years (QALYs) and may present relative costs per QALYs.

The Net site for the above quote (last updated ??) is

nhscrd.york.ac.uk/nfaq1.htm

NHS R&D Health Technology Assessment Program (HTA)

This is another major government-supported program at the University of York (United Kingdom) that is relevant to healthcare information syntheses. It indexes both evidence-based and non-evidence-based sources. The purpose of this program is to ensure that sound research information on the costs, effectiveness, and impact of health technologies is most efficiently produced for those who use manage and work in the NHS. It is a member of the International Network of Agencies for Health Technology Assessment (INAHTA). It defines healthcare technology and healthcare technology assessment very similar to that group. (See Sections E through G on nongovernment information sources.) The United Kingdom NHS HTA definition is as follows:

Health care technology is defined as prevention and rehabilitation, vaccines, pharmaceuticals, and devices, medical and surgical procedures, and the systems within which health is protected and maintained. Technology assessment studies the medical, social, ethical and economic implications of development, diffusion, and the use of health technology and informs policy decisions. Its aim is to improve the quality and cost-effectiveness of healthcare.

The Internet address for the above quote (last updated ??) is

nhscrd.york.ac.uk./hfaq2.htm

The home page and Internet address for the above quote and access to the database (last updated ??) is http://nhscrd.york.ac.uk./htahp.htm

The program is overseen by the NHS Standing Group on Health Technology (SGHT), analogous to the U.S. National Advisory Council for Health Care Policy, Research, and Evaluation.

National Institute for Clinical Excellence (NICE)

The purpose of this organization is provided in the following quote:

The National Institute for Clinical Excellence was set up as a Special Health Authority on the 1st April 1999 and as such it is a part of the National Health Service (NHS). [It will] . . . provide the NHS in England and Wales with authoritative, robust and reliable guidance on current "best practice." This guidance will cover both individual health technologies and the clinical management of specific conditions. NICE guidance is aimed at both providers and users within the NHS. . . . NICE has asked the HTA programme to ensure that the NICE Appraisals Committee has the evidence and knowledge it requires to inform its advice to the NHS. Other evidence to support the work of the Appraisal Committee is sought by NICE from industry, health professionals and interest groups.

Our only question is the extent to which its information is based on Cochrane standards for evaluating systematic reviews. The reference for the above quotes can be accessed at the NICE home page at the Net site below, by linking to "Background" and finally to "A guide to our work."

The NICE home page is at the following Internet address (last updated ??):

www.nice.org.uk/index.htm

Critical Appraisal Skills Programme (CASP)

The purpose of this program, as quoted from its Web site, is as follows:

CASP's aim is to help health service decision makers and those who seek to influence decision makers to develop skills in the critical appraisal of evidence about effectiveness, in order to promote the delivery of evidence-based health care.

The Internet address for this quote can be accessed through its home page (last updated ??, copyright 2001) by clicking on "About CASP":

www.casp.org.uk/

This is a program to facilitate understanding and applying systematic reviews. This program was initiated in the "Anglia and Oxford" region in 1993. It is part of the United Kingdom's National Health Service, Public Health Resource Unit, at the Institute of Health Sciences in Oxford. The program's approach is by use of an interactive CD-ROM on evidence-based health care and the Open Learning Resource. The latter consists of five units, each having a separate workbook. This group provides both workshops and distance learning educational modalities. These materials are described in the Web site (last updated December 2000) and can be accessed by clicking on "About CASP" and also "Open Learning."

Another advantage of this program is its provision of criteria for evaluating "Randomised controlled trials; economic evaluations; qualitative research studies; and systematic reviews of randomized controlled trials."

The National Research Register (NRR)

This research register provides "raw" data, in terms of clinical trials that might provide material for information syntheses. The format of its database indicates a likely collaboration with the Cochrane group. The following quote describes its purpose and affiliation:

> The National Research Register is assembled and published by Update Software Ltd on behalf of the United Kingdom's Department of Health. The National Research Register is a database of ongoing and recently completed research projects funded by, or of interest to, the United Kingdom's National Health Service.
>
> The current issue #3 contains information on just over 80,000 research projects collected on or before the 29th of June 2001. Projects with an end date later than the 31st of August 2001 have been classified as "Ongoing." All others have been classified as "Complete."

The Web site for this quote, which is available free (last updated September 2001), is

www.update-software.com/National/

Information available from the National Research Register 2001 (Issue 1) includes the following index of resources available in Internet linkage:

(a) National Research Register Projects database
(b) Clinical Trials Directory
(c) Register of Research Registers
(d) Register of Reviews in Progress
(e) Health Research at York Database

Register of Research Registers of Controlled Trials is among the more valuable contributions of the National Research Register, sponsored by the United Kingdom's National Health Service's Department of Health. (This site is made available by Update Software.) The following quote explains more about this resource:

> The mRCT [*meta*Register of Controlled Trials—ours] is a major, searchable international database-a 'register of registers' of ongoing controlled trials-that is provided free of charge. Participating registers are asked to submit details of controlled trials that include some minimum essential items (a process which is automated as far as possible). The list of data items has been expanded recently, following expert advice, and we hope that registers will gradually work towards including this extra information, so that there is consistency of content across all the trial records.
>
> The mRCT is a major new database of ongoing controlled trials. Although the initial emphasis is on controlled trials in progress, information will also be available in future about planned trials and those that have been completed but have not yet been reported. The mRCT will allow users to find out which organisations maintain which registers of controlled trials, and to search all participating registers. The mRCT is also a database (like Medline or Current Contents) to which the participating registers submit a 'citation', ie an entry on each trial that includes some minimum essential fields (a process which will be automated as far as possible). Where entries come from other registers, links are maintained to the original source entries. This basic service is provided by the mRCT free of charge.

The Web site for the above quote (last updated ??, copyright 2000) is

www.controlled-trials.com/

Section E. Nongovernment Evidence-Based Sources

The following sources are especially relevant for developing or retrieving information syntheses or "evidence-based" clinical material. Each of these has as its main purpose the development and/or dissemination of evidence-based information for immediate use in healthcare practice.

CAUTION

As mentioned in the text, you must be very careful about how researchers, writers, and publishers use the term *evidence-based*. It has become a buzzword that has often lost its meaning. To avoid being burned, you must discern exactly what writers mean when they claim their material is "evidence-based." (See Appendix 18.3 (Chapter 18) for the evolution of criteria for evaluating systematic reviews.)

A more practical approach is to check the credentials of the writers. For example, if there is any mention of a connection to the United Kingdom's Cochrane Collaboration, the Canadian Chalmers Centre for Systematic Reviews, or the U.S. Agency for Healthcare Research and Quality's Evidence-Based Practice Centers, you might be much more assured of their information's soundness.

Finally, a quick rule of thumb is that the more detailed their review methods documentation (especially their search strategy and their relevance and validation criteria), the more likely these authors understand what we mean by "evidence based."

By means of these listed sources, you can identify current systematic reviews or link to related online databanks of such material. As noted in the text, the Cochrane Collaboration is the clear leader in this field, having helped start, or collaborating with, most of the other sources listed. Anyone interested in searching for validated systematic reviews or sound articles on information synthesis methods would be wise in starting with the Cochrane Library online. The other sites in Section E likely produce quality mature information that you might find to be highly relevant for developing or retrieving information syntheses.

The Cochrane Collaboration (United Kingdom)

In our judgment, the Cochrane Collaboration is the world leader in the development of systematic reviews related to healthcare. It has 15 centers worldwide that coordinate and support nearly all aspects of the Collaboration's activities. It has more than 50 review groups (as of May 2001), each of which concentrates on a specific health problem, producing, reviewing, abstracting, and keeping up with that subject. Even more important, it has 10 groups that concentrate on systematic review methodology, each focusing on a different aspect. New groups are being added all the time; for example, a new methods team that focuses on quality of life is or has been organized and made part of its network.

Perhaps its paramount contribution is the fact it has taken an international systems framework for the development of a new paradigm in healthcare information. Next, it is building on a foundation of informatics technology to organize and make its resources available to anyone who has a computer and is linked to the Internet. It has pioneered detailed methods, validation criteria (such as their levels of evidence), and recommendations for community education in and implementation of clinical best evidence. It provides training opportunities and tools for those who want to learn more about this subject. If you are interested in becoming involved with this cutting-edge group, link from its home page to "Help for Newcomers," and from there click on "How to become involved." The home page for the Cochrane Collaboration (last updated July 2001) is

www.cochrane.org

The Cochrane Brochure

The Cochrane Brochure provides a description of its organization and activities. The following are two quotes from this online document:

> The Cochrane Collaboration has developed in response to Cochrane's call for systematic, up-to-date reviews of all relevant RCTs of health care. Cochrane's suggestion that the methods used to prepare and maintain reviews of controlled trials in pregnancy and childbirth should be applied more widely was taken up by the Research and Development Programme, initiated to support the United Kingdom's National Health Service. Funds were provided to establish a 'Cochrane Centre', to collaborate with others, in the UK and elsewhere, to facilitate systematic reviews of randomized controlled trials across all areas of health care.
>
> Cochrane reviews (the principal output of the Collaboration) are published electronically in successive issues of The Cochrane Database of Systematic Reviews. Preparation and maintenance of Cochrane reviews is the responsibility of international collaborative review groups. At the beginning of 1997, the existing and planned review groups (over 40) cover most of the important areas of health care. The members of these groups of researchers, health care professionals, consumers, and others share an interest in generating reliable, up-to-date evidence relevant to the prevention, treatment and rehabilitation of particular health problems or groups of problems.

The Internet address for the above quotes from the Cochrane Brochure (last updated August 2001) is

www.cochrane.org/cochrane/cc-broch.htm

We include the following endorsement of the Cochrane group by the United Kingdom's NHS's Centre for Reviews and Dissemination at the University of York:

The Cochrane Library is now the premier resource for information on the effectiveness of healthcare interventions. It is a collection of information put together by the Cochrane Collaboration, the NHS Centre for Reviews and others.

DARE is one of the databases on the Cochrane Library. Other databases include the Cochrane Database of Systematic Reviews (CDSR) which contains the full text of completed reviews carried out by the Cochrane Collaboration, plus protocols for reviews currently in preparation.

The Net site for this quote (last updated ??, at least 2000) is

nhscrd.york.ac.uk/faq6.htm

The Cochrane Library

The Cochrane Library is an electronic publication designed to supply high-quality evidence to inform people providing and receiving care and those responsible for research, teaching, funding, and administration at all levels. It is published quarterly on CD-ROM and the Internet and is distributed on a subscription basis. The abstracts of Cochrane Reviews are available without charge and can be browsed or searched.

The Cochrane Library includes the following:

The Cochrane Database of Systematic Reviews: Regularly updated reviews of the effects of health care

Database of Abstracts of Reviews of Effectiveness: Critical assessments and structured abstracts of good systematic reviews published elsewhere

The Cochrane Controlled Trials Register: Bibliographic information on controlled trials

Other sources of information on the science of reviewing research and evidence-based health care

The reference Internet address for the above quote and access to the Cochrane Library and the above listed resources (last updated ??, copyright 2001) is

www.update-software.com/cochrane/

Guidelines, Manuals, and Software

The Collaboration is developing, identifying, and making accessible a wide variety of resources of value to both beginners and advanced individuals interested in systematic reviews and randomized controlled clinical trials. A few of them are described below. The Web site for linking to these resources (last updated September 2000) is

www.cochrane.org/cochrane/resource.htm

The Cochrane Reviewers' Handbook. This handbook is a guide for helping qualified reviewers screen systematic reviews sent to be included in the file of the Cochrane Library. Only those that meet their threshold of quality are accepted.

The Reviewers' Handbook is the official document that describes in detail the process of creating Cochrane systematic reviews. It is revised frequently to ensure that it remains up-to-date. The current version is 4.0, updated July 1999.

The reference for the above quote and home page for the handbook (last updated September 2001) is

www.cochrane.org/cochrane/hbook.htm

Cochrane Manual. This is a key document for understanding the organization, policies, and operations of the Cochrane Collaboration. To illustrate, the manual's outline is quoted as follows:

1. Central Organisation
    Description of the Cochrane Collaboration
    Communication
    Support

2. Collaboration Policies
    Conflicts of interest
    Publication policy

3. Operations
    Steering Group
    Election Procedures
    Collaborative Review Groups
    Centres
    Methods Groups

Fields
Consumer Network

The source of this quote and linkage to its manual content (last updated May 2001) is

www.cochrane.org/cochrane/cc-man.htm

Review Manager (RevMan). This is another contribution of the Collaboration. However, its helpful resources are only available to members of an official Cochrane Review Group (CRG) because they do not work with individuals outside of these groups. The following quote answers the question, "What is RevMan?"

> RevMan is the Cochrane Collaboration's program for preparing and maintaining Cochrane reviews. RevMan allows you to enter protocols, as well as complete reviews, including text, characteristics of studies, comparison table, and study data. It can perform meta-analysis of the data entered, and present the results graphically using MetaView. RevMan is developed through a continuing process of consultation with its users. Note that RevMan is mainly useful once you are well on the way to develop a review. RevMan is currently developed at The Nordic Cochrane Centre.

This quote and links to RevMan can be found at the following Net site (last updated December 2000):

www.cochrane.org/cochrane/revman.htm

This Internet site also provides suggestions for becoming involved with the Collaboration and perhaps joining one of its review groups.

Cochrane Internet Resources

This Net site address provides linkage to all Collaboration Net sites, as well as Cochrane Library Net sites and the Cochrane FTP (File Transfer Protocol) sites. This URL address (last updated August 2001) is

www.cochrane.org/cochrane/ccweb.htm

Thomas C. Chalmers Centre for Systematic Reviews

This relatively new (1998) Centre was inspired and facilitated by Thomas C. Chalmers, one of the pioneers in analysis and methods development of randomized clinical trials. This organization, to date, has focused on "the majority of child health areas and in vascular disease" (see URL address below). In their "About Us" Web site they state:

> The Thomas C. Chalmers Centre for Systematic Reviews was Ontario, but draws on the talents of a geographically diverse team of researchers. An advisory board deals with the governance and future directions of the Centre.
>
> We have three foci: conducting high quality systematic reviews and meta-analyses, researching optimal approaches to conducting reviews, and training clinicians and future analysts.

The URL address for this site (last updated December 1999) is

www.cheori.org/tcc

Users' Guides to Medical Literature (*JAMA*-United States)

This is a unique and especially valuable resource for practicing "Evidence-Based" medicine. Likewise, its use for developing information syntheses is equally valuable. This material is edited by Drs. Gordon Guyatt, Drummond Rennie, and Robert S. A. Hayward. These are among the leading experts in the field of medicine and information synthesis. For example, Dr. Guyatt coined the term "Evidence-based Medicine" and has led the "Evidence-Based Medicine Working Group" in formulating principles of evidence-based practice. He has worked closely with the Cochrane Collaboration in pioneering information synthesis methodology.

The following quotation is their introductory paragraph

> *Evidence-Based Medicine* From the popular <u>Users' Guides</u> series in JAMA come three state-of-the-art products on evidence-based clinical practice, edited by Drs Gordon Guyatt, Drummond Rennie, and Robert Hayward with contributions from more than fifty of the most renowned evidence-based medicine (EBM) educators and practitioners in the world. As the culmination of nearly two decades of teaching and research, all of the Users' Guides to the Medical Literature products provide the most detailed yet clinician-friendly exposition of the concepts necessary to use the medical literature to solve patient problems.

This Web page quote goes on to describe their textbooks and CD-ROM.

Textbooks

> *Users' Guides to the Medical Literature: A Manual for Evidence-Based Clinical Practice*; and *Users' Guides to the Medical Literature: Essentials of Evidence-Based*

Clinical Practice Together with the practical glossary, index, appendix of calculations, and laminated quick reference cards, each *Users' Guides to the Medical Literature* book and CD-ROM constitutes a comprehensive toolkit to support a clinical rounds presentation on evidence-based medicine. Explore both text and CD-ROM of *Users' Guides to the Medical Literature* textbooks to learn:

Textbooks

- Why framing the right question is so important
- How to find and distinguish between strong and weak evidence
- What's needed to critically appraise the best evidence
- How to weigh the risks and benefits that precede medical management decisions
- How to individualize evidence to each patient

CD-ROM (included FREE with either text)

- Fully hyperlinked and searchable text and graphics
- Organized, classified, and coded to support electronic outlining, content filtering, and full-text searching
- Contains the full text of both books in a hypertext form optimized for electronic viewing and in a print-ready form that exactly matches the content of the books

The above quote is found at the following URL address (last updated Aug. 2001)

www.usersguides.org/

The Centres for Health Evidence.net in Canada are collaborating with AMA in maintaining this "Users Guide" Web site and also an *Interactive Users' Guide,* available at a reduced rate to all who purchase a textbook.

Centres for Health Evidence CHE (Canada)

This group of non-government Canadian centers have the following mission:

The Centres for Health Evidence promote evidence-based health care by presenting knowledge-based resources to health professionals in ways that facilitate their optimum use. The starting point is the information needs of decision makers.

They further state:

Given our focus on teaching evidence-based care in clinical practice environments, we are increasingly drawn to initiatives where virtual learning communities, just-in-time knowledge, and adult learning approaches are deployed to shift the culture of learning in health-related institutions.

These quotes can be located from the CHE home page by clicking on "About Us" at the following Web site (last updated Oct. 2001).

www.cche.net/CHE/home.asp

Users' Guides to Evidence-Based Medicine

CHE works in collaboration with the American Medical Association (AMA) in producing the online version of Users' Guides to the medical literature (available 2002). (For details of these Guides in printed book form see AMA Users' Guides above.) CHE descriptions of this product and online linkage (at no cost) to the original versions of these Users' Guides published in JAMA between 1993 and 1999), see the following CHE Web site (last updated ??, copyright 2001).

www.cche.net/text/usersguides/main.asp

Clinical Evidence Series (*BMJ*-United Kingdom)

This online source is a unique compendium of healthcare information modeled in a question-and-answer format. It provides "high-quality systematic reviews." If these are not available on your topic, then it provides the next most authoritative information, particularly RCTs. After an information synthesis goes online, follow-up RCTs are compiled and provided, starting at the date when the original review left off.

Its search strategies are based on that of Haynes, Wilczynski, McKibbon, Walker, and Sinclair (1994) and that of Dickersin et al. (1994). Dickersin was at McMaster University's Cochrane Center when the 1994 article was published. This is a meta-validated source, again after the Cochrane method. In addition, it has a useful glossary of terms for quantitative analysis of literature. This listing is reasonably thorough and authoritative, after Cochrane.

Its online home page address (last updated ??, copyright 2001) is

www.clinicalevidence.org

To quote its own description:

Clinical Evidence is a six monthly, updated compendium of evidence on the effects of common clinical interventions, produced jointly by the BMJ Publishing Group and the American College of Physicians-American Society of Internal Medicine. It provides a concise account of the current state of knowledge, ignorance, and uncertainty about the prevention and treatment of a wide range of clinical conditions based on thorough searches of the literature. It is neither a textbook of medicine nor a book of guidelines. It summarizes the best available evidence, and where there is no good evidence, it says so.

The reference for this quote (last updated October 2001) is

www.cche.net/CHE/home.asp

Update Software (United States, United Kingdom, Bulgaria)

This is an especially important site for developing information syntheses. The home page for this site (last updated ??, at least 2001) is

www.update-software.com

The most relevant links are the following:

The Cochrane Library

• Cochrane Library has a database of systematic reviews, abstracts of reviews of effectiveness, register of controlled trials, and register of systematic reviews methodology. (The Cochrane Library was described in detail above.)

Metaxis

• Metaxis (available in 2002) is an interactive electronic guide to performing systematic reviews encompassing factors listed in the following quote (numeration ours):

A (1) comprehensive set of linked tasks to guide you through all stages of planning and completing a systematic review; (2) detailed project management to track the progress of all parts of your systematic review; (3) fully integrated reference management; (4) customisable paper and electronic data collection forms produced by a form generator; (5) comprehensive statistical methods for conventional meta-analysis and meta-regression; (6) statistical scripting language that allows adaptation and development of experimental methods; (7) a wide range of sophisticated graphics for printing and plotting; (8) publication quality reports that can be generated in a wide variety of formats; and (9) tasks that can be customised for use in training programmes.

The Web address for Metaxis (last updated ??) is

www.update-software.com/metaxis/default.htm

The WHO Reproductive Library

• The WHO Reproductive Library is a unique source of of information that is sponsored by WHO and produced by Update Software, with input from the Cochrane Collaboration. It provides sound, mature information for immediate decision making.

Now in its fourth edition, this electronic review journal focuses on evidence-based solutions to reproductive health problems in developing countries.

Assembled and produced by Update Software on behalf of the World Health Organisation (WHO), this is the specialised database built around a core of the prestigious Cochrane systematic reviews in the field of reproductive health.

The Internet address for the above quote (last updated ??) is

www.update-software.com/rhl/default.htm

The Cancer Library

• The Cancer Library is another valuable source of "rigorous and unbiased" information on neoplastic disease. Its affiliation with the Cochrane Collaboration again attests to the soundness of the information it provides. A description of this site is displayed in the following quote:

> The core of The Cancer Library is the relevant set of Cochrane systematic reviews. Cochrane reviews aim to incorporate evidence from trials and unpublished material from all over the world, with every attempt made to minimise bias. Cochrane reviews are regularly updated and electronically published to incorporate new evidence as it becomes available.

The Internet address for the above quote (last updated ??) is

www.update-software.com/cancer/default.htm

<u>Gold Nuggets</u>

    • Gold Nuggets is a publication from Update Software that provides a convenient means to keep up with Cochrane reviews of recently developed information syntheses. Again, in view of its editorial policy, the material it provides should be sound and mature for immediate decision making. The following is a quote from its Web site:

> Published quarterly alongside The Cochrane Library, Gold Nuggets provides a fresh way of keeping up to date with new information in the current issue of The Cochrane Library.

This concise booklet provides an invaluable summary of all the new reviews published in each issue of the library. The booklet contains the full abstracts of all new reviews as well as a summary list of all the updated reviews.

The Internet address for the above quote (last updated ??) is

www.update-software.com/Goldnuggets

<u>The National Research Register</u>

    • National Research Register (United Kingdom) states its purpose as follows:

> The National Research Register is a database of ongoing and recently completed research projects funded by, or of interest to, the United Kingdom's National Health Service. The National Research Register is assembled and published by Update Software Ltd on behalf of the United Kingdom's Department of Health.
>
>   *Why would I want to use the NRR?* The NRR has many uses, including the following: identifying unpublished research, particularly important to those undertaking systematic reviews; providing early warning on research that may lead to important findings; helping to improve the uptake and participation in clinical trials; and identifying and bringing together researchers between and across related areas of research, helping to avoid unnecessary duplication in research. The Web site for the above quote is the same as above.

The Web site for the above quote (last updated September 2001) is

www.update-software.com/National/nrr-frame.html

Evidence-Based Medicine Reviews-EBMR (United States)

- The following quote describes this database, which is another source of meta-validated information. It is of particular relevance to development of mini-syntheses, as we describe them in Stage I, Chapter 2.

> Evidence Based Medicine Reviews is a definitive electronic information resource in the Evidence-Based Medicine (EBM) movement. Available online and on CD-ROM, EBMR is a comprehensive database that combines three of the most trusted EBM sources into a single, fully-searchable database. Accessed through Ovid, the EBMR databases, Best Evidence, Cochrane, and DARE link to MEDLINE® and Ovid full text journals but also from the MEDLINE® abstract of the evaluated article to the EBM review. This feature allows the user to restrict retrieval to articles that have been evaluated; the Ovid search engine makes MEDLINE itself an EBM resource.

Its Web site for "Evidence-Based Medicine Reviews" (last update ??, at least 2001) is

www.ovid.com/products/clinical/ebmr.cfm

Bandolier

This online site and printed journal is a relatively recent addition to sources of evidence-based healthcare information. The Internet site is funded privately, although the NHS in the United Kingdom supports the printed version.

Briefly scanning the online version of this source was an interesting, enjoyable experience. The style and readily understandable formatting were exceptional. Our major concern was that the "evidence" for so many of the topics was sparse, often not reviewed. When systematic reviews were available, they were well presented, and some were clearly reviewed using Cochrane criteria for assessing information syntheses. In any event, the educational value of this site seems exceptional for learning basic concepts of evidence-based medicine.

The following quote is Bandolier's own description of this resource:

> Bandolier is a print and Internet journal about health care, using evidence-based medicine techniques to provide advice about particular treatments or diseases for healthcare professionals and consumers. The content is 'tertiary' publishing, distilling the information from (secondary) reviews of (primary) trials and making it comprehensible.

The above quote is from the following Web site (updated October 2001):

www.jr2.ox.ac.uk/bandolier/aboutus.html

This site can be reached at the following Web address (last updated September 2001):

www.jr2.ox.ac.uk/bandolier/index.html

Section F. Nongovernment Partial Evidence-Based Sources

The following sources publish evidence-based materials, but their main emphasis may be on traditional literature. They are worth checking if the government and nongovernment "evidence-based" centers provide little information on your topic. The first two are especially noteworthy in that they focus, among other topics, on nursing literature information syntheses.

Sigma Theta Tau International Honor Society of Nursing

The following quote describes the purpose of this Web site.

> Being committed to nursing scholarship and excellence, this organization has developed an online library that, among other information, allows access to systematic reviews of value to the nursing profession.

The URL for the home page of this society (last updated ??) is

www.nursingsociety.org

The following quote provides more detail about this site:

Online Library

> The Online Library of the International Center for Nursing Scholarship houses the society headquarters and its state-of-the art electronic library, the Virginia Henderson International Nursing Library. Individuals, organizations, schools of nursing and health science libraries can access the library's online service.

The Online Journal of Knowledge Synthesis for Nursing

The Online Journal of Knowledge Synthesis for Nursing, a peer-reviewed full-text electronic journal, gives nurses access to integrative reviews of research pertinent to clinical practice.

Registry of Nursing Research

Registry of Nursing Research, a collection of nursing research data including researchers' demographic information, studies, projects, abstracts, variables studies and scientific results.

Literature Indexes

Literature Indexes, a completely new paradigm that indexes research knowledge, not research articles. It allows the user to go directly to research findings while totally circumventing a traditional bibliographic database search.

The Web site for this quote is the same as above, linking from its home page to "About STTI," then to "Overview."

CINAHL Information Systems (United States)

The index to this database is (last updated ??, at least 2001) is

www.cinahl.com

The Cumulative Index to Nursing & Allied Health (CINAHL) database provides authoritative coverage of the literature related to nursing and allied health. Virtually all English-language publications are indexed along with the publications of the American Nurses Association and the National League for Nursing.

The reference for the above quote is their link through Ovid Technologies at the following Web site (last updated July 2001):

www.ovid.com/documentation/user/field_guide/disp_fldguide.cfm?db=
    nursing.htm

Ovid claims CINAHL to be "the definitive reference tool covering the English language journal literature for nursing and allied health disciplines." This database is updated monthly.

The Web site for this quote (last updated ??) is

www.ovid.com/products/databases/database_info.cfm?dbID=18

The home page for CINAHL (last updated May 2001) is

www.cinahl.com/mainentry.htm

The CINAHL link page to its online database (and from there to its evidence-based site) can be accessed through the above Web site by clicking CINAHL*Sources*).

Ovid Technologies (United States)

This organization provides access to over 80 databases and 350 online journals (as of October 2001). It states the following purpose:

Ovid's mission is to support and improve information access for researchers, clinicians, and students in scientific, medical, and academic communities worldwide by providing innovative and interlinked text retrieval software and database solutions.

The reference to this quote and the home page for this company (last updated ??) is

www.ovid.com/index.cfm

Their search engine can be reached at the following Net site (last updated ??):

www.ovid.com/sales/medical.cfm

This group also services academic, corporate, and medical information. Although Ovid is a rather limited source of evidence-based information, it is becoming a more comprehensive, though expensive, source of general medical literature, particularly with its link to MEDLINE.

However, other new 'mega-sources' are continually being developed, such as "ScienceDirect Family of Products" at the following address (last updated ??, copyright 2001):

www.sciencedirect.com

The following are evidence-based sources available through Ovid.

Evidence-Based Medicine Reviews (EBMR)

This is a product of Ovid Technologies that was described earlier in Section E.

Clinical Evidence

This product is available through Ovid Technologies. It is produced by the British Medical Journal Publishing group. This product was also described earlier in Section E.

Database of Abstracts of Reviews of Effectiveness (DARE)

This source is linked by Ovid from the University of York's National Health Service Centre for Reviews and Dissemination (CRD) in the United Kingdom. See Section D for a more detailed description.

The Web site for this source (last updated ??) is

nhscrd.york.ac.uk/darehp.htm

Centre for Research Support (CeReS, United Kingdom)

This site was started in 1999 by the Welsh Office of Research and Development (WORD). It granted a team at the University of Wales College of Medicine Division of General Practice an award to run a research unit focusing on primary care in Wales. It named this new unit the Centre for Research Support, or CeReS. This is a relative newcomer to the Internet and has proven easy to use and links directly to a number of valuable evidence-based sites. Although this group is committed to improve healthcare in Wales, its scope is clearly international. Its home page Web address (last updated ??, copyright 2000) is

www.ceres.uwcm.ac.uk

The following is a quote of its purpose:

Welcome to the CeReS Web site. CeReS is committed to supporting research in the primary health care field in Wales and see the internet as a powerful tool in facilitating this. This site is the first stage and over the coming months the site will evolve to provide even more services. Have fun exploring the site.

The Web site for the above quote (last updated ??) is

www.ceres.uwcm.ac.uk/frameset.cfm?section=about

The address of its database from which you can link to its numerous sites, including 18 evidence-based data sources (last updated ??, likely in 2000) is

www.ceres.uwcm.ac.uk/frameset.cfm?section=links

TRIP Database. The stated purpose and resources for this CeReS link center are as follows:

Welcome to the 'NEW' TRIP database, which is an amalgamation of 26 databases of hyperlinks from evidence-based sites around the world. At present there are over 10,000 links to evidence based topics, so we have provided a simple search mechanism.

The Web site for this quote is (last updated ??, copyright 2000)

www.ceres.uwcm.ac.uk/section.cfm?section=Trip

It seems as if most of these links are to the home page of these database sources, many of which will not allow you into their library files (e.g., the Cochrane Library) without having a subscription or license. However, this is one of the sites to contact for linkage to evidence-based information.

The Web site that lists its databases (last updated April 2000) is

www.ceres.uwcm.ac.uk/publications.cfm

Section G. Useful Nongovernment, Rarely Evidence-Based Sources

Finally, the following information sources, although not specifically evidence based, do provide important information for developing systematic reviews. This includes meta-validated healthcare and informatics information and expertise that could be immediately applicable to information synthesis development.

The United States National Academies

Overview of the National Academies

The National Academies in the United States consist of the National Academy of Sciences, the National Academy of Engineering, the Institute of Medicine, and the National Research Council. The National Academy of Sciences was created by a congressional charter in 1863 and approved by President Abraham Lincoln. Under this charter, the National Research Council was organized in 1916, the National Academy of Engineering in 1964, and the Institute of Medicine in 1970. The academies are private organizations created by the federal government to be an adviser on scientific and technological matters. The U.S. Congress has no oversight responsibility for them, and provides no financial appropriations for their maintenance. Consequently, they must obtain their own funds, which are obtained primarily through grants and contracts, most of which are with the federal government.

Their home page indicates they have more than 1,500 books online. This Web site (last updated May 2001) is

www.nationalacademies.org

Institute of Medicine (IOM)

In the context of this book, the institute of major interest is the Institute of Medicine, the most recent of the National Academies. You can link to its home page through the above National Academies Web site, or through the following address (last updated ??, copyright 2001):

www.iom.edu

Online access to most of its reports is available from its home page. "The mission of the Institute of Medicine is to advance and disseminate scientific knowledge to improve human health. The Institute provides objective, timely, authoritative information and advice concerning health and science policy to government, the corporate sector, the professions and the public." The Web site for this quote (last updated ??, copyright 2001) is

www.iom.edu/IOM/IOMHome.nsf/Pages/About+the+IOM

The Board of Health Care Services (HCS)

The Board of Health Care Services focuses on issues of health care organization, financing, effectiveness, workforce, and delivery, with special emphasis on quality, costs, and accessibility of care.

The Web site for the above quote (last updated ??, copyright 2001) is

www.nationalacademies.org/IOM/IOMHome.nsf/Pages/Health+Care+Services

National Academy Press (NAP)

This organization is the major publishing arm of the academies. It develops both paper and online publications.

The National Academy Press (NAP) was created by the National Academies to publish the reports issued by the National Academy of Sciences, the National Academy of Engineering, the Institute of Medicine, and the National Research Council, all operating under a charter granted by the Congress of the United States. NAP publishes over 200 books a year on a wide range of topics in science, engineering, and health, capturing the most authoritative views on important issues in science and health policy. The institutions represented by NAP are unique in that they attract the nation's leading experts in every field to serve on their blue ribbon panels and committees. For definitive information on everything from space science to animal nutrition, you have come to the right place.

The Web site for this quote and its online browser (last updated ??, copyright 1999) is

www.nap.edu/about.html

Links to Related Health Services Research Sites

This is one of the more valuable Net sites of the IOM. It links to the following major organizations related to healthcare:

- Health Care Policy Links (from Milbank Memorial Fund)
- Medical Outcomes Trust
- National Institutes of Health

- National Science Foundation
- United States Department of Health and Human Services
- Other electronic information resources (compiled by the NRC Library)

It also provides access to the leading publications for the field of health services research and policy. Through this site, you can link to the Association for Health Services Research; *British Medical Journal; Health Affairs; Inquiry; Institute of Medicine; Journal of the American Medical Association (JAMA); Journal of Health Politics; Policy and Law,* the *Milbank Quarterly;* and *New England Journal of Medicine.*

The Web site for this resource (last updated ??, copyright 2000): is

www.milbank.org/quarterly/links.html

National Certification and Accreditation Organizations

We include these organizations as exceptional people sources in a variety of specialty areas related to your synthesis topics. By this means, you can identify local or national expertise to participate with your project teams in person, by telephone, or by computer conferencing methods. Although we mention U.S. organizations, these are but examples to help remind you of certification or accreditation organizations in other countries for all major healthcare professions.

American Board of Medical Specialties (ABMS)

The mission of ABMS is to maintain and improve the quality of medical care by assisting the Member Boards in their efforts to develop and utilize professional and educational standards for the evaluation and certification of physician specialists. What is the ABMS? The American Board of Medical Specialties (ABMS) is an organization of 24 approved medical specialty boards. The ABMS serves to coordinate the activities of its Member Boards and to provide information to the public, the government, the profession and its members concerning issues involving specialization and certification of medical specialists.

The Net site for this quotation (last updated ??, copyright 2000) is

www.abms.org/default.asp

To learn more about member boards, contact the following site (last updated ??, copyright 2000):

www.abms.org/member.asp

American Board of Quality Assurance & Utilization Review Physicians (ABQAURP)

The primary mission of the American Board of Quality Assurance and Utilization Review Physicians, Inc. is "to improve the overall quality of health care that is provided to the consuming public." Established in 1977, ABQAURP has evolved to become the nation's largest organization of interdisciplinary healthcare professionals, and it remains at the forefront of the health care quality and management (HCQM) field for all medical specialties and professions. ABQAURP is the only HCQM organization with an examination developed, administered, and evaluated through the National Board of Medical Examiners' (NBME's) testing expertise. The NBME's involvement in the certification process serves to reinforce ABQAURP's dedication to establishing HCQM as a specialty with definable standards upheld by knowledgeable experts. In 1999, ABQAURP introduced the National Accreditation Standards for Workers' Compensation and Comprehensive Medical Event Management.

The Internet address for the above quote (last updated ??, at least after 1999) is

www.abqaurp.org

Health Improvement Institute (HII)

The following quote explain the purpose of this organization:

Health Improvement Institute is a non-profit, tax exempt, 501(c)3, educational organization dedicated to improving the quality and productivity of America's health care. The Institute's primary goal is to provide information to patients, providers, payors, purchasers, policy-makers, and the public about available alternatives to ensure that all Americans have the opportunity to make informed health care.

The Web site for the above quote (last updated February 2001) is

www.hii.org/default.htm

Joint Commission on Accreditation of Healthcare Organizations (JCAHO)

This organization is perhaps the oldest U.S. group to focus on hospitals for accreditation purposes, being founded in 1951, and having roots that go back to the era following World War I.

Its home page can be accessed through the following Web address (last updated ??, copyright 2001):

www.jcaho.org

The following quote states its mission:

> The mission of the Joint Commission on Accreditation of Healthcare Organizations is to continuously improve the safety and quality of care provided to the public through the provision of health care accreditation and related services that support performance improvement in health care organizations.
>
> The Joint Commission evaluates and accredits more than 19,500 health care organizations in the United States, including hospitals, health care networks, managed care organizations, and health care organizations that provide home care, long term care, behavioral health care, laboratory, and ambulatory care services. The Joint Commission is an independent, not-for-profit organization, and the world's leading health care standards-setting and accrediting body.

ORYX is the name given to what JCAHO calls "The Next Evolution in Accreditation." This promising new program is to develop unique informatics technology and new criteria to base accreditation on outcomes and other performance measures. This development was initiated in February 1997 and will be a valuable site to access periodically for information that might facilitate future information syntheses. To learn more about this resource, you must link from the JCAHO home page listed above.

Quality Check™ provides a comprehensive guide for interested individuals to learn about the quality standing of nearly 20,000 JCAHO accredited healthcare organizations in the United States. The following quote indicates what it provides.

> The Quality Check listing includes each organization's name, address, telephone number, accreditation decision, accreditation date, and current accreditation status and effective date. For more in-depth quality information, consumers can check the individual performance reports available for many accredited organizations that were surveyed after January 1, 1996. Performance reports provide detailed information about an organization's performance and how it compares to similar organizations.

The reference for this quote, as well as online access to its directory back to January 1, 1996 (and printed copies before that date), is accessible from the JCAHO home page, where you can click on "Quality Check."

From the above JCAHO home page, you can link to a wide number of relevant resources. The JCAHO has its links organized by the type of user you may be. For example, the following two sites can be accessed by clicking on "For the General Public" from the JCAHO home page:

> Helping You Make Health Care Choices is one of several resources the JCAHO has made available to the general public. The purpose of this site is to help laypersons make more informed choices about obtaining quality healthcare for themselves and their family. Several other JCAHO sites for the public can be reached from this link.

> Consumer Health Care Organizations and Information Sources is especially valuable in that it provides linkage to resources on quality healthcare that have been selected as providing useful and sound information for the public. For example, the Mayo clinic database on healthcare information can be reached from here.

National Committee for Quality Assurance (NCQA)

The Web site is sponsored by the National Committee for Quality Assurance (the "NCQA"), which is a private, not-for-profit organization dedicated to assessing and reporting the quality of managed healthcare plans.

Health Plan Report is described as follows:

> The Health Plan Report Card (HPRC), NCQA's online resource for comprehensive, consumer-oriented information about the quality of the nation's health care organizations, now includes PPO plans' NCQA Accreditation status and more detailed information about their performance in the areas of Access and Service and Qualified Providers, the two areas measured under NCQA's PPO Plan Accreditation program.

The URL for the above quote and home page (last updated ??, at least 2001) is

www.ncqa.org/index.htm

NCQA's Health Plan Report Card rates plans in five key areas:

Access and service

Qualified providers

Staying healthy

Getting better

Living with illness

Depending on their performance in these areas, NCQA gives health plans one of the following accreditation outcomes:

****Excellent

***Commendable

**Accredited

*Provisional

Denied

Addition information about the "report card" is in the following quote:

> NCQA's Health Plan Report Card has results on hundreds of health plans that care for commercially insured individuals and Medicare and Medicaid beneficiaries. You can create a customized Report Card that shows results for the health plan or plans you want to know about.

The Web site for this quote (last updated ??) is

hprc.ncqa.org

International Network of Agencies for Health Technology Assessment (INAHTA)

INAHTA is a not-for-profit organization founded in 1993 to provide an international agency to facilitate sharing and cooperation of health technology assessment research and activities. Currently, it has 34 member agencies throughout the world. The secretariat for the organization resides in Sweden. Its own statement of the limits of its science and definition of HTA is as follows:

> Technology is applied science.
>   Healthcare technology is defined as prevention and rehabilitation, vaccines, pharmaceuticals, and devices, medical and surgical procedures, and the systems within which health is protected and maintained.
>   What is technology assessment in health care?

It is a multidisciplinary field of policy analysis. It studies the medical, social, ethical, and economic implications of development, diffusion, and use of health technology.

The Web site for this organization (last updated May 2001) is

www.inahta.org/first.html

The Institute for Scientific Information® (ISI)

Web Site Description

"ISI is a database publisher with a focus on Web-based products that offers scholarly research information in the sciences, social sciences, and arts and humanities." Its main drawback for healthcare researchers is the fact that it covers about 150 disciplines in the general sciences, about 30 of which are relevant to healthcare. Although Current Contents in Clinical Medicine lists 1,107 journals as of March 2000, its main emphasis is on basic and clinical science. Checking its journal list, we were unable to identify any of the evidence-based journal series of meta-validated information.

Its Web site index can be accessed at the following address (last updated ??, copyright 2000):

www.isinet.com/index/index.html

ISI started its collection in 1961, and, as of 15 August 15, 1999, included 8,489 scientific and technical journals, out of more than 16,000 total journals, books, and proceedings. It currently processes more than 12 million articles each year, and screens more than 2,000 new journals for possible addition to its information base. Its main content is cited references, bibliographic information, and some author abstracts.

Its home page can be accessed at the following Web site (last updated ??, copyright 2001):

www.isinet.com/isi/

SciSearch® Online

This database is updated weekly. It has back-year data available to 1974 and covers more than 2,000 journals not covered by the CD-ROM and print versions. The following Web site offers reference searching, as well as optional searchable author abstracts, and allows author key words for searching (last updated ??, copyright 1999):

www.isinet.com/products/citation/citsci.html

Web of Science®

A cited reference search begins with a known, important (or at least relevant) document used as the search term. The search allows one to identify subsequent articles that have cited that document. This feature adds the dimension of prospective searching to the usual retrospective searching that all bibliographic indexes provide.

This quote is from the following address (last updated September 1999):

www.dlib.org/dlib/september99/atkins/09atkins.html

Science Watch® and "Hot" Papers

ISI publishes Science Watch, the subscription newsletter of the Research Services Group which quantitatively analyzes the scientific journal literature and provides science policymakers, research administrators, science journalists, and others with concise overviews of key developments in today's scientific research. Published in print six times a year, Science Watch monitors emerging fields, assesses performance in research, and presents interviews with leading scientists.

The Web site for this quote is the following (last updated ??, copyright 2001):

www.isinet.com/products/rsg/products/sw-hp/

Although ISI's collection of journals is one of the better ones we know, in our judgment, its main value is to identify relevant content as opposed to relevant and valid material. The above-mentioned Science Watch uses a bibliometric approach by which ISI does what it does best (i.e., count citations). It can tell you which journal publishes articles that are most cited, which university department faculty is most cited, and particularly which articles are "HOT," or most cited among the 8,000 journals analyzed, as compared to other papers of the same type and age. Unfortunately, there is little if any solid evidence, of which we are aware, that scientific, or methodological quality correlates with the number of times an article is cited. In our judgment, bibliometrics runs counter to the Cochrane (and our) philosophy as to how to determine scientific soundness. We judge that each article must be validated on its own by analysis of its methods, no matter how outstanding the reputation of the author. Ideally, whether a research report meets accepted standards of scientific soundness must be determined by at least two independent groups (i.e., meta-validated) and, it is hoped, with two or more evaluators in each group.

Elsevier Science (The Netherlands)

This is a publisher whose headquarters is in Amsterdam. It claims to be the "undisputed market leader in the publication and dissemination of literature." It states that its mission is to "to serve the advancement of science, technology and medicine by improving the efficiency and effectiveness of communication among researchers and professionals world-wide and by providing solutions to their information needs." We agree that this is one of the world's paramount leaders in science information dissemination and should usually be included in your search scope, particularly through the online database, EMBASE, as well as its Excerpta Medica classical medical index.

The reference for the above quotes can be located by clicking on "About Us" on Elsevier's home page (last updated ??, copyright 2000) at

www.elsevier.nl

EMBASE, from Elsevier Science in Amsterdam, compiles the European equivalent of MEDLINE in the United States. Its online version was developed in 1974 and has (as of April 2000) indexed more than 8 million articles, from 3,800 journals and other medical serials, from 70 countries. This source is updated weekly. This medical database is one of the many sponsored by Excerpta Medica, which originated in paper form in 1947. EMBASE is available online or on CD-ROM, and covers all areas of human medicine and the biological sciences related to medicine. The CD-ROM version contains more than 3.5 million citations. Woods and Trewheellar (1998) note that MEDLINE and EMBASE complement each other in literature searches, and that it would be a mistake to screen one without the other. Gretz, Schmitt, and Thomas (1996) compared EMBASE, DATA-STAR, DIALOG, DIMDI, and STN using nine standard searches. They found that none of the nine produced the same results, with considerable discrepancies found among some.
The EMBASE STN database summary sheet (this is not a link site) is at the following Net site (last update ??, at least 1998):

info.cas.org/ONLINE/DBSS/embasess.html

Access to its affiliate, STN's online databank (called STN Database Summary Sheets), includes online links to more than 200 databases, of which only about 25 seem related to healthcare and pharmaceutics. It is available at the following Internet address (last updated May 2001):

info.cas.org/ONLINE/DBSS/dbsslist.html

Current Science Group-CSG (United Kingdom)

This is a new group of publishers that provides access to a wide variety of information, from clinical controlled trials to patents, pharmaceutical data, and information for consumers. The following quote can be located by clicking on "About CSG" from the home page address shown below:

> Current Science Group is a group of independent companies that collaborate closely with each other to publish and develop information and services for the professional biomedical community. Our products run the gamut from books and journals to websites, databases, and audiovisuals and cater to clients as various as physicians, scientists, pharmaceutical companies, patients, and students. The Group has its head office in London (UK), with additional offices in Philadelphia, New York and Tokyo.

Its home page, which provides links to each of its many sites (last updated ??, copyright 2000), is

current-science-group.com

The following quotes explain three of CSG's 14 Web sites that represent their collaborating companies. These sources are potentially relevant to developing information syntheses. They each can be accessed by clicking on the list in their "Site Map" linked to their home page listed above.

BioMed Central, Ltd.

> BioMed Central Ltd. was launched in May 2000 as a new 'open' publisher of peer-reviewed original research. BioMed Central fully embraces PubMed Central's vision of barrier-free access to all original research. All research articles published through BioMed Central are available immediately and in full through PubMed Central and are also indexed in PubMed.

The Web site for the above quote (last updated May 2001) is

www.biomedcentral.com/default.asp

We caution the reader that this is not a meta-validated (our own parlance) information source. It seems to use a traditional medical journal peer review process for each entry. The following is a quote from its peer review policy:

> Submitted articles will be reviewed by at least two external experts, usually identified by matching of the submitted paper to recently published papers in the same area of research.
>
> In deciding whether to accept or reject an article, a reviewer asks him/herself whether the scientific community is better served by publishing or not publishing the article. In the absence of compelling reasons to reject, BioMed Central advises that reviewers recommend acceptance, as ultimately the quality of an article will be judged by the scientific community after its publication.

The Web site for this quote and the remaining information about its peer review policy (last updated May 2001) is

www.biomedcentral.com/info/peerreview.asp

We judge that this is a traditional peer review procedure applied by most journal editors in the health field. The fact that these articles are accepted for indexing by PubMed, as well as the team of research methodologists that they use, confirms their review quality might meet or exceed traditional standards. However, these reviewers probably apply implicit criteria, as opposed to the explicit criteria that we and the Cochrane group recommend. In our judgment, such articles are not suitable for inclusion in systematic reviews unless they are corroborated by an independent group of reviewers such as those teams of the Cochrane Collaboration. If this is done acceptably, then the information will be meta-validated and thus suitable for inclusion in a synthesis. (See Appendix 9.1 of this book for an overview of the evolution, between 1977 and 2000, of explicit criteria for reviewing individual research studies.)

On the other hand, by using informatics technology, this group is pioneering relatively new electronic methods of disseminating information. These offer many advantages over paper copy publication methods used since the time of Johann Gutenberg in the 15th century A.D. For example, the rapidity by which they conduct their review process can disseminate much more up-to-date material in a shorter time. Another advantage is that they can be accessed and used without cost. We will follow their progress with great interest.

Current Controlled Trials, Ltd.

The following quote describes the Current Controlled Trials (CCT) database of the Current Science Group (CSG):

> Current Controlled Trials Ltd. is a Web-based publishing company that provides a range of databases, journals and services for scientists, medical practitioners, pharmaceutical companies, patients and others with an interest in controlled trials.

The CSG has its headquarters in London and also has offices in Philadelphia, New York, and Tokyo.

Further information can be obtained by contacting

Anne Greenwood (Managing Director); Claire Marley (Project Manager)
Current Controlled Trials, Ltd.
Middlesex House
34-42 Cleveland Street
London W1P 6LB, UK
Tel: +44 (0)20 7323 0323; Fax: +44 (0)20 7580 1938
e-mail: info@controlled-trials.com or clairem@cursci.co.uk

The Internet home page for this site requires that readers register and state a user name and a password for accessing their material. In so doing, readers agree to follow their policy of restrictions at this address. The Web site for registering or signing in if already registered (last updated ??, copyright 2001) is

www.controlled-trials.com/login.cfm?returnto=frame.cfm

metaRegister of Controlled Trials (mRCT)

This is another Web-based "register of registers," sponsored by Current Controlled Trials, Ltd., which is a database of the CSG. Following a simple registration process, you can access its information free of charge. You can link to 20 healthcare-related registers encompassing 6,441 trials (as of May 2001), and the list will be growing. For example, it recently added the U.S. Department of Veterans Affairs Cooperative Studies Program. Its Web page can be accessed by linking through the home page of Current Controlled Trials, Ltd. and clicking on the "*meta*Register of Controlled Trials (*m*RCT)" (last updated 2001) at

www.controlled-trials.com/home_page.cfm

Consumer Health Care

This is a site of relevance to consumers and patients. The following quote describes this Web site:

> The Consumer Health Care division produces educational websites dedicated to an array of chronic and acute disorders. The sites provide comprehensive, evidence-based consumer health information aimed at facilitating more effective patient-doctor communication, and encouraging patients to participate fully in their own health care decisions. Each disorder-focused site is written by a panel of leading Specialists, GPs, Nurses, Pharmacologists, Nutritionists and Health Writers, all of whom are recognised experts in their chosen fields.

Again, the above quote can be accessed by linking from the above home page of CSG.

American Medical Informatics Association (AMIA)

The American Medical Informatics Association is a nonprofit 501(c)(3) membership organization of individuals, institutions, and corporations dedicated to developing and using information technologies to improve health care. AMIA is one of the premier associations to facilitate the development of medical informatics in the United States and internationally. Its work is fundamental to the development of information syntheses, particularly in the areas of knowledge structures, management, and applications to improve healthcare outcomes worldwide.

Its founders are among the pioneers of the field of informatics. It works closely with such organizations as the United States National Library of Medicine, one of the earliest groups in the health field to develop online bibliographic databanks.

We suggest that AMIA's journal and Web site are among the more valuable means with which to keep up the advances of healthcare informatics. Its Web site permits linkage to the international affiliates that, together with AMIA, are developing this field worldwide.

The home page for this organization (last updated May 2001) is

www.amia.org/index.html

Journal of the American Informatics Association (JAMIA).

AMIA's bimonthly journal, JAMIA, presents peer-reviewed articles that assist researchers, physicians, nurses, and other health care personnel, as well as informatics professionals, develop and apply medical informatics to patient care, teaching, research, and health care administration.

Glossary

ABC convention for relevance coding   An approach for relevance rating that denotes the priority of importance of each citation-abstract (i.e., citation and/or abstract) for subsequent action such as retrieving the complete article or book cited. Citation-abstract relevance can only crudely estimate the value of the complete article retrieved. "A" denotes the highest probability of finding useful data and information when the complete document is retrieved. "B" indicates moderate probability. "C" indicates the lowest if not a nil probability that useful information might be obtained. The A category is further divided into three levels (A+, A, and A-) in order of importance. A+ denotes a validated review, a meta-analysis, or a review article on your exact topic. A denotes a single research study on your topic. Finally, A- denotes an article peripheral to your topic that might yield valuable leads to other relevant information if retrieved.

Absolute risk (AR)   The probability that an individual will experience the specified outcome during a specified period. It lies in the range from 0 to 1. In contrast to common usage, the word *risk* may refer to adverse events (such as myocardial infarction) or desirable events (such as cure).

á posteriori estimate (syn. posterior probability)   A Bayesian term that is a combination of your initial expectation and your actual experience. Your judgment is conditional on your actual experience with the first application.

á priori probability   A Bayesian term that refers to the anticipated results of a test measured in a stated population prior to an intervention.

Application to practice   In the context of this book, this phrase refers to use of the information synthesis findings to influence clinical decision making.

Artifacts   Nonsystematic or random errors in measurement or design that change what results are found. If the study were to be repeated, these artifacts may not be there.

Bias   The deviation of a measurement from the true value. Bias can originate from many different sources, such as allocation of patients, analysis, interpretation, publication, and review of data. In the worst circumstances, it may be systematically associated with the strength of the effect, leading to the wrong conclusions being drawn.

Blinding   The degree to which participants, investigators, and assessors remain ignorant concerning the treatments that participants are receiving. It is done to prevent knowledge of treatment biasing patient response, outcome assessment, and any decisions made within the study. In single-blind studies, only the participants are blind to their allocations, but in double-blind studies, assessors and participants are ignorant of the allocations.

Case-control study   A retrospective study design usually used to investigate the causes of diseases. Study participants who have experienced a disease are compared with participants who have not, in order to detect differences in the hypothesized causal factors.

Ceiling effect   The situation when most of the scores are at the high end of the scale, resulting in very little variation.

Chi-square test   A non-parametric statistical test that tests hypotheses about proportions in a population.

Clinical information maturity   Refers to the extent to which information content is sufficiently developed for immediate application in the community to improve healthcare outcomes.

Clinical significance   The extent to which scientifically valid healthcare information can be applied to a defined population to help improve their health status and quality of life within a relatively short time frame. This concept has two dimensions: clinical importance and information maturity.

Cohen's Kappa statistic   A statistical index of agreement between two or more measures that adjusts for chance agreement. In context of this book, this statistic is most often used to calibrate the search team for agreement on relevance ratings of citation-abstracts or complete documents.

Cohort study   An prospective study design in which groups of individuals are identified who vary in their exposure to an hypothesized causal factor and are compared in terms of outcomes. Association between exposure and outcome is then estimated. Cohort studies are best performed prospectively but can also be undertaken retrospectively if suitable data records are available.

Confidence interval   A boundary surrounding the estimate of the population parameter (the "true" value). It is an estimate of the degree of certainty (e.g., 95% or 99%) of the conclusions.

Confounding   A situation where one or more factors extraneous to the main question are affecting outcomes. The result is a distortion of the true relationship between the independent and dependent variables. Confounding can be avoided through using appropriate study designs and sometimes can be adjusted for by multivariate statistical analysis.

Construct validity   The extent to which the way a variable is measured or manipulated reflects the "true" construct of interest.

Contingency table   The display of data in a tabular form with levels of the independent variable (e.g., risk factor) on one side crossed with levels of the dependent variable on the other side. Frequencies in the cells indicate the number of individuals with corresponding levels of the factors.

Cronbach's alpha   The average of each item's correlation with every other item. It is used to determine the reliability of a scale.

Cumulative meta-analysis   A method of aggregating effect sizes that illustrates the rate of change over time. Effect sizes are averaged after each study is added in chronological order.

Decision analysis   A mathematical process of assigning estimates to information relevant to making a decision and thereby modeling uncertainty.

DerSimonian and Laird model   A meta-analytic method that assumes random effects.

Effectiveness   The extent to which an intervention produces favorable outcomes under usual or everyday conditions.

Effect size   A measure of the overall strength of the effect found in an empirical study. Effects can be reported in terms of odds ratios, mean differences, correlations, or other statistics. The effect size transforms these results into a generalized value.

Efficacy   The degree to which the intervention or treatment produces favorable effects in a laboratory or controlled situation.

Estimate-talk-estimate   A consensus procedure by which the team makes initial independent individual estimate of a value, discusses the variability of the estimates, and repeats the estimates.

Ethnographic approach   An observation method of data collection using qualitative methods of analysis and systematic procedures of observation.

Ethnography educational theory   Assumes that the learner may not be ideally suited to "know what he or she doesn't know" and therefore may be deficient in identifying his or her own learning needs. The ethnographer assumes several roles: a participant–observer, an interviewer, a learning facilitator, and an evaluator. This person must combine expertise in the subject content, with ethnographic skills applied in the learner's own work environment. The ethnographer, together with the learner, establishes priorities for employee learning needs, required learning experiences, and evaluation of educational impact.

Evidence based   Information obtained from well-conducted systematic reviews of valid primary research.

Experimental design   A research protocol that includes the use of a control group, random assignment of subjects to groups, and manipulation of the independent variable.

Externally selected reviewers   Reviewers of a book or journal submitted for publication. Publishers arrange outside review to establish the quality of the material.

External validity   The extent to which findings from a sample can be generalized to the universe or population from which that sample was drawn.

Factor analysis technique   A parametric statistical method that identifies patterns of inter-correlation among a set of items. It provides information about the internal structure of an instrument and is very useful for exploring construct validity. Having the items correlate in sensible patterns supports the overall structure of the assessment instrument.

False-negative coding rate   The proportion of items that signaled a positive result but were wrong. In literature searching, it refers to the proportion of citation-abstracts the gold standard rated as positive (relevant) that your team erroneously coded as negative (irrelevant). A "false-negative" rate is one minus "sensitivity" (i.e., "true positives" divided by the total of "true positives" plus "false negatives," often expressed as percentages).

False-positive coding rate   A proportion that refers to the proportion of those articles that your team rated as relevant (positive) that your gold standard rated irrelevant (negative). In a clinical context, we define a "false-positive" rate as one minus the positive predictive value, as $B/(B + A) \times 100$.

File drawer problem   Refers to the notion that investigators will store the results of studies that do not produce significant effects in their file drawers. Because these articles are never published, their absence creates a bias in the population of available studies.

Final data set   The final set of empirical information abstracted from those database documents that proved to be both relevant and scientifically sound.

Five steps of a search iteration   Step 1: Compile and relevance-code new citation-abstracts; if rated A+, A, or A-, retrieve and code complete documents. Step 2: Relevance-code references in complete documents obtained; if rated A+, A, or A-, retrieve and code documents cited. Step 3: Conduct team calibration session, including interrater reliability, and precision rates, analyzing and improving poor results. Step 4: Update search documentation forms; calculate search statistics for this iteration and file all materials. Step 5: Revise search plan and prepare for the next iteration.

Fixed effects model   A meta-analytical modeling method that assumes one true effect. Variation between studies is assumed to be due to random error and is not assumed to affect the uncertainty of the effect estimate. In this model, the levels of the independent variable (e.g., dosages of drugs, types of treatments, or time spent with patient) exactly reflect the universe of possibilities. Compare with Random effects model.

Floor effect   The phenomenon that occurs when most of the individuals have scores on the low end of the continuum. The result is a significant decrease in variability and a limitation on analysis.

Frequencies or frequency distribution   An analysis of the distribution of variables, the mean, mode, and median, as well as the range and standard deviation.

Fugitive [syn. gray or subterranean] literature   Research that is elusive and difficult to retrieve using standard search methods. It may include both published and unpublished reports (such as information in technical reports, interim reports, unsubmitted papers or manuscripts, presented papers, dissertations, and rejected papers, as well as non-written data on computer printouts or in a researcher's working notes or in his or her head). See File drawer problem.

Funnel plot   A scatterplot display of effect sizes, with effect sizes on one axis and sample size on the other axis. Funnel display or plot graphs are used to estimate publication bias. The principle is that studies with small sample sizes will vary widely in effect sizes. As the sample size gets larger, then the variation in effect sizes is smaller and tends to be closer to the overall mean effect size. If publication bias exists (negative results are not published), it is usually for negative effects that come about from small samples. The result will be a "white-out" of the left-hand side of the funnel where normally negative effect sizes with small samples would be located.

Gold-standard   A set of values that are agreed on by either the scientific community or by experimental measurements that constitute the "true" measure of a variable.

Gray Literature.   See Fugitive literature.

Health   An outcome that includes the physical, mental, emotional, and social well-being of either the consumer or provider.

Healthcare benefit   The extent of outcome improvement accomplished per person times the number of people who might be helped in the population.

Healthcare improvement professionals   Individuals having the responsibility for looking at care across time, patient populations, and service areas. They may have responsibilities for implementing systems for assessment and monitoring patient outcomes.

Healthcare outcome improvement   Both a model of healthcare and a paradigm of thought.

Healthcare outcome improvement cycle   The continuous process of identifying unacceptable outcomes, measuring the extent of the negative outcomes, determining an intervention, instituting that intervention, assessing the results, and then beginning the cycle again.

Heterogeneity   The degree to which the results of studies included in a review are dissimilar. When the differences between studies are large, as assessed by a measure of variability, then the studies are determined to be heterogeneous.

Heuristic validity   The degree to which an article contributes to the overall thought and analysis in the literature on that topic. Some articles may be important to consider in a synthesis because, despite serious quantitative flaws, they have a unique methodological approach, or they may make an especially important contribution to the field.

Hierarchical linear model   A meta-analytical modeling method that assumes random effects for each level of analysis and therefore can provide estimates for each variable. For example, estimates can be provided, such as types of populations examined, components of treatment (if studies are available), or types of settings.

Index terms   It is important to understand the difference between key words and index terms. Official descriptors (e.g., MeSH terms from the National Library of Medicine) are generated by staff of the organization sponsoring these bibliographic databases. These include researching all possible synonyms of your search terms, using descriptors to narrow your search parameters, and using truncation of words.

Information maturity Healthcare personnel in day-to-day practice adequately develop the extent to which information to use. See Clinical information maturity.

Information overload The difficulty inherent in synthesizing the results of a diverse group of publications.

Information synthesis Any formal synthesis of knowledge, including quantitative reviews, qualitative reviews, and structured group judgment reviews.

Internal reviewers Qualified independent colleagues not currently involved with your project but who are willing to read your manuscript and provide critical feedback. You and your project team make the selection of these reviewers.

Internal validity The probability that the independent variable could, believably and logically, have caused the dependent variable. Internal validity refers to the strength of the inferences that can be drawn from the evidence.

Internet The Internet encompasses many "home pages" (or Web pages) of information sites that are connected through a series of hypertext links. Two main Internet purposes are (a) to publish information in an electronic format for consumption by researchers and (b) to provide a way for researchers to retrieve information on a particular topic and obtain access to World Wide Web (WWW or Web) database.

Interrater reliability The degree to which independent coders agree with one another.

Interval scale A type of data in which there is equal distances between numbers.

Invisible colleges Groups of national or international investigators who have similar research subject interests, intercommunicate, often quote each other, or coauthor research papers together. Synonyms are communication networks, solidarity groups, schools, author networks, social circles, and scientific grapevines. Members of these "colleges" or "networks" often use common jargon and possibly similar research designs, and they may or may not produce similar research results. These groups are "invisible" because they do not have a formal name or hierarchy.

Kappa See Cohen's Kappa statistic.

Key words It is important to understand the difference between key words and index terms. To indicate relevant content, authors of a published work usually generate a list of key words.

Knowledge application studies Studies whose purpose is to evaluate applied programs, introduce an intervention in a real-world setting, or improve practice directly.

Mantel-Haenszel model A meta-analytical method originally used to combine odds ratios when the number of studies is small.

Master list A log of citations using computerized bibliographic database management software.

Mediator variables Those factors that are thought to cause the relationship between the independent and dependent variable (e.g., cause the drug to be effective). They specify the mechanism by which the independent variable affects the dependent variable. See Moderator variables.

MeSH   MeSH stands for medical subject heading and is the controlled vocabulary indexing system used by the National Library of Medicine for indexing articles on MEDLINE.

Meta-analysis   The group of statistical methods for pooling research results from many individual studies. It is a subset of the general category of quantitative syntheses.

Meta-validated information   Information that has been validated two or more times by qualified experts, usually including a consensus team or panel of quantitative and qualitative experts who often follow a structured group judgment protocol.

Methods studies   Studies that include the development and assessment of new methods, tools, or instruments and encompasses studies that describe the development of these new methods, as well as evaluation of the reliability and validity of such methods.

Mini-synthesis   The lowest level of a quasi-search, using very few resources and time. A synthesis of syntheses.

Moderator variables   Those factors that change the relationship between the independent and dependent variable (e.g., result in an interaction effect). For example, the relationship between the amount of information given to the patient prior to surgery and anxiety may differ depending on the age of the patient. May include setting, patient acuity, practitioner training, or gender.

μ (pronounced "mu")   This is the mean of the population.

Multivariate questions   Those research questions that consider how a group of independent variables, when considered together, affects one or more dependent variables.

Narrative synthesis   A synthesis of information from either quantitative or qualitative studies in which the results are often subjective and reported in writing, rather than objective based on pooling and synthesis of data from multiple homogeneous studies. Consensus reports are usually of this type, as are mini-syntheses.

Null hypothesis   The hypothesis of no effect. This is the default conclusion if one fails to detect an experimental effect.

Number needed to treat (NNT)   A way of expressing the size of a treatment effect, which is easier to interpret clinically. The NNT is number of patients with a particular condition who must receive a treatment for a prescribed period to prevent the occurrence of specified adverse outcomes of the condition. This number is the reciprocal of the absolute risk reduction.

Observational studies   Epidemiological investigations in which natural variation in exposure is investigated to explore associations between exposures and health outcomes.

Odds ratio   Odds ratios are one way of expressing the size of the effect of a treatment on an event rate. The odds of an event are a ratio of the probability of occurring to the probability of it not occurring. The odds ratio is the ratio of the odds of an event in the treatment (or exposed) group compared to the odds in the control (or unexposed) group.

When the event rates are very low or very high, the odds ratio is very similar to the relative risk.

Operationalization   The process of determining how a conceptual variable can be specifically measured or manipulated. Variables must be defined at a level of precision that is both usable and yet conceptually congruent with the underlying construct.

Outcome assessment   The comparison of a quantitative measure of healthcare outcome (health, economic, or satisfaction) to an accepted threshold standard. The results are usually reported in percentages. The standard may be a calculation of what might be achieved under ideal community practice conditions, for example.

Outcomes   A plural abstract term that refers to the results of any process and structure, measured at one point in time. In healthcare, it is a multidimensional concept that is especially complex and does not relate well to mechanical or industrial outcomes. Healthcare outcomes can be measured at a subatomic level, up to an individual level and through to the total world population. *Outcomes* refers to your initial plan, which includes your initial synthesis question. Outcomes mean any class of healthcare results (health, economic, satisfaction, for either or both consumers and providers).

Parameter   A measure of some aspect of a population.

Path analysis   A form of linear modeling that identifies the strength of the relationship between causal variables, mediator and moderator variables, and the outcomes of interest simultaneously.

Peto model   A method of combining effect odds ratios for meta-analysis. It assumes fixed effects models and is thought to sometimes produce biased results.

Positive predictive value   The proportion of individuals identified as having the disease who really have the disease. The probability that those individuals testing positive are actually positive.

Power (statistical power)   The probability that an effect will be detected if it is indeed there. Power is increased with a larger sample size, a more powerful intervention, a smaller variation, or an increase in alpha.

Precision   See Search precision.

Problem space   The implicit mental construct or model of the research question or problem at hand. It includes associated concepts and variables, ideas about how these elements relate, and the overall context in which they are defined abstractly.

Provider   A term that encompasses the entire range of personnel required to render healthcare, such as clinicians, administrators, manufacturers, suppliers, third-party payers, purchasers, and regulators.

Psychometric approach   A strategy for meta-analysis based on psychometric theory. It provides statistical procedures for estimating the effects of biasing variables such as restriction of range, sampling errors, and unreliability of measurement or the predictive and construct validity of psychological tests.

Publication bias   A type of bias in which the publication of research depends on the strength of the study findings, rather than the quality of the methods by which the study is conducted. It is the tendency for journals to not accept studies that report null results or unique methods that reviewers may reject as being unproven or too nontraditional.

Qualitative research studies   Studies that use grounded or ethnographic research techniques to provide an interpretive explanation, an elaboration of meaning, and a mechanism to enrich human discourse.

Qualitative review   A synthesis of qualitative research studies. They include traditional narrative reviews, as well as methodological reviews, philosophic essays, policy analyses, and meta-ethnographies.

Quality improvement professionals   Individuals in an institution responsible for answering to outside accreditation agencies (e.g., JCAHO).

Quality of care   Any measure that assesses the processes, outcomes, and structure of care.

Quantitative synthesis   The statistical analysis of the pooled data from many individual studies.

Quasi-experimental design   Investigations that are designed to test hypotheses but do not include all of the experimental controls present in an experimental design.

Random effects model   A method of modeling in meta-analysis that assumes the levels of the independent variable are randomly sampled from a universe of levels, and heterogeneity among effect sizes is a function of both variation within studies and between studies. The result is an ability to generalize to all levels of an independent variable (and to all studies in a domain).

Randomized controlled clinical trials   See RCTs.

RCT (randomized clinical trial)   An experimental study in which subjects are randomized to receive either an experimental or a control treatment or intervention. The relative effectiveness of the interventions is assessed by comparing event rates and outcomes in the two groups.

Recall   See Search recall.

Relative risk differences   Commonly called relative risk or relative rate. The relative risk of an event is the risk of the outcome in the treatment group divided by the risk in the control group.

Relative risk reduction (RRR)   The relative reduction in risk associated with an intervention. It is calculated as one minus the relative risk, or 1 - (event rate in treatment/event rate in control).

Relevance coding   Systematic coding of citations for the degree of relevance. Coding refers to the assignment of codes to citation-abstracts or complete documents according to a standard convention. In this book, we suggest the ABC convention specified in five levels: A+, A, A-, B, and C. Conceptually, these relevance ratings refer to the priority of each element (e.g., citation-abstract) for further processing, such as retrieving and coding complete documents.

Relevance criteria   Formal statements of factors by which literature citations, abstracts, and complete articles can be coded as relevant. See Relevance coding.

Reliability   The degree of stability that exists when a measurement is repeatedly made under different conditions or by different observers.

Restriction of range   Refers to a situation where values on a measured variable have a narrow spread. The result of restricted range is a correlation between variables that are attenuated.

Sampling distribution   A theoretical distribution of the statistical values that would be obtained if all possible samples of a given size were drawn from a population, the statistic measured for each sample, and the resultant list of statistics graphed in a frequency distribution.

Scientific soundness   The degree to which the findings and conclusions of a synthesis are valid and reliable. *Validity* refers to many aspects of the synthesis process. Most important, it refers to how representative of current research is the sampling of studies and how nonbiased the synthesis was conducted. *Reliability* refers to the extent a replicated review would identify a similar database and arrive at similar conclusions, as well as the degree of interrater reliability during the synthesis development. Scientific soundness includes internal validity, external validity, construct validity, and statistical validity.

Search engines   Internet tools available to help you find the specific information you require from an electronic database. There are more than 150 different search engines available, among the more popular of which are AltaVista, Excite, Infoseek, Lycos, and Yahoo.

Search precision   This term refers to the proportion of the total number of references that you coded relevant (that were also found relevant by the gold standard test). Precision is an important indicator of the cost-effectiveness of your search, measured in terms of the absence of false-positive references.

Search recall   This term refers to the proportion of gold-standard relevant references that you also coded as relevant. This assumes you were able to test all references in a sample using the gold-standard procedure, a task that is often not feasible. However, this is an extremely important indicator of the search quality measured in terms of the absence of false-negative references.

Sensitivity   The degree to which a test detects those individuals who actually have the disease (the proportion of those detected by the test who truly have the disease).

Sensitivity analysis   A method for an author to systematically test the robustness of his or her findings. By selectively altering different aspects of the question, the number of studies, and the assumptions underlying the synthesis, a clearer understanding of the findings can be achieved.

Social aggregation levels   An abstract dimension ranging from the individual level to the institutional, community, regional, national, and international levels within each generic outcome family. Each level requires different measurement instruments and sampling techniques.

Specificity   The degree to which a test accurately classifies and individual as not having a disease (the proportion of individuals without disease identified by the test as not having the disease).

Standardized mean differences   When outcomes are measured on a variety of continuous scales in different units of measurement, it is not possible to directly combine study results. By expressing the effects as a standardized value (difference in means divided by a pooled standard deviation), the results can be combined because they have no units.

Statistic   Any measurement taken on a sample.

Statistical validity   The degree to which the way the data analysis in a study is valid; for example, it has enough power (sufficient sample size), uses reliable instruments, and does not violate the assumptions of the statistical tests.

Stringency analysis   An analytic procedure to assess how well a validation task was planned, implemented, and evaluated. This is an analysis of the extent to which database article validation meets the accepted standards of quality. This assessment applies to both outcomes and processes of validation.

Structural equations modeling   A multivariate statistical technique that allows for estimates of latent conceptual variables through the use multiple methods of measurement while permitting a path analysis.

Structured group judgment techniques   A systematic method of eliciting and combining expert judgments.

Synthesis audience   The users of healthcare syntheses, including healthcare providers, healthcare improvement professionals, researchers (clinical and health services), policy analysts and administrators, professional educators, and science writers.

Synthesis database   The compilation of relevant research or other information documents from which you will extract and code data required for subsequent document validation and synthesis. This database will include research articles, books, monographs, chapters, technical reports, and "fugitive literature" in any form such as elusive published or unpublished research reports.

Synthesis data set   The coded information extracted from each document in your database. This includes both research content and methods data. To illustrate, "content" would include the description and size of the population studied, the setting of the study, and the results found; "methods" would include the research design, statistical tools used, and levels of significance in terms of the alpha and beta values applied. All of this type of information is coded on a formal code sheet.

Synthesis project   An explicit description of a small aspect of your detailed implicit "problem space" associated with your original synthesis question or topic. A "project model," as defined here, is a verbal, written, or graphical representation of a theoretical relationship between variables. Your model outlines the question, identifies the conceptual variables involved in the question, and specifies possible cause-and-effect relationships.

t **test**   The statistic used to test hypotheses about sample mean differences.

Team calibration The process of measuring the coding agreement among members of the team (i.e., interrater reliability). Team calibration is accomplished by having each team member record his or her relevance codes independently for a common series of citation-abstracts and complete documents. Next, a statistic (e.g., Cohen's Kappa) estimating interrater reliability is applied and compared to a minimum threshold value. This calibration process also facilitates the calculation of citation-abstract relevance-coding precision using the rating of the complete document as a gold standard.

Theoretical development Any empirical work whose purpose is to introduce or extend the development of theory.

Tree structures (of index search terms) A numerically coded hierarchical family of descriptors and other terms under each major subject heading in any standardized thesaurus of index terms for a bibliographic database.

Type I error A theoretical statistical value indicating the probability that the null hypothesis is rejected when it is in fact true. The size of a Type I error is determined by alpha and is usually either .05 or .01.

Type II error A theoretical statistical value indicating the probability that the null hypothesis will be accepted when, in fact, it is false. This probability is indicated by beta and can only be determined when an alternative hypothesis is specified.

Unit of analysis error A bias in analysis of data that is a result of analyzing or grouping data at the inappropriate level. For example, treatments may have been allocated to groups, but the analyses may have been conducted at the level of the individual. Hierarchical linear modeling can correct for this problem.

Univariate questions Questions that focus only on the relationship between one independent variable and one dependent variable.

Utility An assessment of the value of an outcome, usually subjective. These values are most often expressed in terms of proportional weights. Utilities are used in decision analysis.

Validation process (for information synthesis) A process that involves establishing the adequacy and documentation of citation selection procedures, validation procedures, and synthesis methods.

Vote counting A meta-analytical combination procedure that simply involves counting the number of studies in a domain that provide evidence to support, contradict, or is unrelated to a research hypothesis.

Weighted average The usual index of central tendency in meta-analysis and is calculated across all the effect sizes from the individual studies.

World Wide Web (WWW or Web) database One of the databases accessible on the Internet, distinguished by its use of colorful graphics, photographs, and text, usually with multiple links to other Web sites.

References

Adams, C. E., Power, A., Frederick, K., & Lefebvre, C. (1994). An investigation of the adequacy of MEDLINE searches for randomized controlled trials (RCTs) of the effects of mental health care. *Psychological Medicine, 24,* 741-748.

Ad Hoc Working Group for Critical Appraisal of the Medical Literature. (1987). A proposal for more informative abstracts of clinical articles. *Annals Internal Medicine, 106,* 598-604.

Aldag, R. J., & Fuller, S. R. (1993). Beyond fiasco: A reappraisal of the groupthink phenomenon and a new model of group decision processes. *Psychological Bulletin, 113,* 533-552.

Althcide, D. L., & Johnson, J. M. (1994). Criteria for assessing interpretive validity in qualitative research. In N. K. Denzin & Y. S. Lincoln (Eds.), *Handbook of qualitative research* (pp. 485-499). Thousand Oaks, CA: Sage.

Altman, D. G. (1996). Better reporting of randomized controlled trials: The CONSORT statement. *British Medical Journal, 313,* 570-571.

American College of Physicians—American Society of Internal Medicine. (1999). Purpose and Procedure [editorial policy and criteria of article selection]. *American College of Physicians Journal Club, 130,* A-15.

American Medical Association (AMA), Office of Quality Assurance and Medical Review. (1994). *Directory of practice parameters: Titles, sources, and updates.* Chicago: American Medical Association.

American Psychiatric Association. (1994). *Diagnostic and statistical manual of mental disorders* (4th ed.). Washington, DC: Author.

American Psychological Association. (2001). *Publication manual of the American Psychological Association* (5th ed.). Washington, DC: Author.

Antman, E. M., Lau, J., Kupelnick, B., Mosteller, F., & Chalmers, T. C. (1992). Comparison of results of meta-analysis of randomized control trials and recommendations of clinical experts. *Journal of the American Medical Association, 268,* 240-248.

Armstrong, D., Fry, J., & Armstrong, P. (1994). General practitioners' view of clinical guidelines for the management of asthma. *International Journal for Quality in Health Care, 6,* 199-202.

Ashton, R. H. (1986). Combining the judgments of experts: How many and which ones? *Organizational Behavior and Human Performance, 38,* 405-414.

Austin, S. M., Balas, E. A., Mitchell, J. A., & Ewigman, B. G. (1994). Effect of physician reminders on preventive care: Meta-analysis of randomized clinical trials. *In Proceedings of the Annual Symposium on Computer Applications in Medical Care* (pp. 121-124). Washington, DC: American Medical Informatics Association.

Badgett, R. G., O'Keefe, M., & Henderson, M. C. (1998). Using systematic reviews in clinical education. In C. Mulrow & D. Cook (Eds.), *Systematic reviews* (pp. 37-44). Philadelphia: American College of Physicians.

Bailar, J. C., III. (1998). Meta-analyses and large randomized controlled trials [Correspondence to the editor]. *New England Journal of Medicine, 338,* 62.

Bailar, J. C., III. (1986). Reporting statistical studies in clinical journals. In J. Bailar III & F. Mosteller (Eds.), *Medical uses of statistics* (pp. 261-271). Waltham, MA: New England Journal of Medicine Books.

Bailey, K. R. (1987). Inter-study differences: How should they influence the interpretation and analysis of results? *Statistics in Medicine, 6,* 351-358.

Baron, R. M., & Kenny, D. A. (1986). The moderator-mediator variable distinction in social psychological research: Conceptual, strategic, and statistical considerations. *Journal of Personality and Social Psychology, 51,* 1173-1182.

Barratt, A., Irwig, L., Glasziou, P., Cumming, R. G., Raffle, A., Hicks, N., Gray, J. A., & Guyatt, G. H. (1999). Users' guides to the medical literature: XVII. How to use guidelines and recommendations about screening. Evidence-Based Medicine Working Group. *Journal of the American Medical Association, 281,* 2029-2034.

Bauchner, H., & Simpson, L. (1998). Specific issues related to developing, disseminating, and implementing pediatric practice guidelines for physicians, patients, families, and other stakeholders. *Health Services Research, 33,* 1161-1177.

Bayer Institute for Health Care Communication. (1995a). *Physician-patient communication: Faculty workbook.* West Haven, CT: Bayer Institute Publications.

Bayer Institute for Health Care Communication. (1995b). *Physician-patient communication: Workshop syllabus.* West Haven, CT: Bayer Institute Publications.

Beaudry, J. S. (1989). The effectiveness of continuing medical education: A quantitative synthesis. *Journal of Continuing Education Health Professions, 9,* 285-307.

Becker, B. J. (1992). Models of science achievement: Forces affecting male and female performance in school science. In T. D. Cook, H. Cooper, D. S. Cordray, H. Hartmann, L. V. Hedges, R. J. Light, T. A. Louis, & F. Mosteller (Eds.), *Meta-analysis for explanation: A casebook* (pp. 209-281). New York: Russell Sage.

Becker, B. J. (1994). Combining significance levels. In H. Cooper & L. Hedges (Eds.), *Handbook of research synthesis* (pp. 215-230). New York: Russell Sage.

Becker, B. J., & Schram, C. M. (1994). Examining explanatory models through research synthesis. In H. Cooper & L. V. Hedges (Eds.), *Handbook of research synthesis* (pp. 357-382). New York: Russell Sage.

Begg, C. B. (1994). Publication bias. In H. Cooper & L. Hedges (Eds.), *Handbook of research synthesis.* New York: Russell Sage.

Begg, C. B., Cho, M., Eastwood, S., Horton, R., Moher, D., Olkin, I., Pitkin, R., Rennie, D., Schulz, K. F., Simel, D., & Stroup, D. F. (1996). Improving the quality of reporting of randomized controlled trials: The CONSORT statement. *Journal of the American Medical Association, 276,* 637-639.

Begg, C. B., & Mazumdar, M. (1994). Operating characteristics of a rank correlation test for publication bias. *Biometrics, 50,* 1088-1101.

Bender, J. S., Halpern, S. H., Thangaroopan, M., Jadad, A. R., & Ohlsson, A. (1997). Quality and retrieval of obstetrical anaesthesia randomized controlled trials. *Canadian Journal of Anesthesia, 44,* 14-18.

Bentler, P. M. (1995*). EQS: Structural equations programs manual.* Encion, CA: Multivariate Software, Inc.

Bergman, D. A. (1999). Evidence-based guidelines and critical pathways for quality improvement. *Pediatrics, 103*(1, Suppl. E), 225-232.

Berland, G. K., Elliott, M. N., Morales, L. S., Algazy, J. I., Kravitz, R. L., Broder, M. S., Kanouse, D. E., Muñoz, J. A., Purgol, J.-A., Lara, M., Watkins, K. E., Yang, H., & McGlynn, E. A. (2001). Health information on the Internet: Accessibility, quality, and readability in English and Spanish. *Journal of the American Medical Association, 285,* 2612-2621.

Berlin, J. A., & Antman, E. M. (1994). Advantages and limitations of meta-analytic regressions of clinical trials data. *Online Journal of Current Clinical Trials,* Doc. No. 134.

Berlin, J. A., Begg, C. B., & Louis T. A. (1989). An assessment of publication bias using a sample of published clinical trials. *Journal of the American Statistics Association, 84,* 381-392.

Berlin, J. A., Laird, N. M., Sacks, H. S., & Chalmers, T. C. (1989) A comparison of statistical methods for combining event rates from clinical trials. *Statistics in Medicine, 8,* 141-151.

Berne, E. S., Jackson, J. R., & Algina, J. (1996). Relationships among performance scores of four diagnostic decision support systems. *Journal of the American Medical Informatics Association, 3,* 208-215.

Bero, L. A., Grilli, R., Grimshaw, J. M., Harvey, E., Oxman, A. D., & Thomson, M. A. (1998). Closing the gap between research and practice: An overview of systematic reviews of interventions to promote the implementation of research findings. The Cochrane Effective Practice and Organization of Care Review Group. *British Medical Journal, 317,* 465-468.

Berzon, R. A., Simeon, G. P., Simpson, R. L., Jr., Donnelly, M. A., & Tilson, H. H. (1993). Quality of life bibliography and indexes: 1993 update. *Quality of Life Journal, 4,* 53-74.

Berzon, R. A., Simeon, G. P., Simpson, R. L., Jr., & Tilson, H. H. (1992). Quality of life and indexes: 1992 update. *Journal of Clinical Research and Drug Development, 7,* 203-242.

Bhopal, R., Rankin, J., McColl, E., Thomas, L., Kaner, E., Stacy, R., Pearson, P., Vernon, B., & Rodgers, H. (1997). The vexed question of authorship: Views of researchers in a British medical faculty. *British Medical Journal, 314,* 1009-1012.

Bickell, N. A., & Chassin, M. R. (2000). Determining the quality of breast cancer care: Do tumor registries measure up? *Annals of Internal Medicine, 132,* 705-710.

Bobbio, M., Demichelis, B., & Giustetto, G. (1994). Completeness of reporting trial results: Effect on physicians' willingness to prescribe. *Lancet, 343,* 1209-1211.

Borzak, S., & Ridker, P. M. (1995). Discordance between meta-analyses and large-scale randomized, controlled trials: Examples from the management of acute myocardial infarction. *Annals of Internal Medicine, 123*, 873-877.

Bouhaddou, O., Lambert, J. G., & Morgan, G. E. (1995). Iliad and Medical House Call: Evaluating the impact of common sense knowledge on the diagnostic accuracy of a medical expert system. In *Proceedings of the Annual Symposium for Computer Applications to Medical Care* (pp. 742-746). Washington, DC: American Medical Informatics Association.

Bowers, C. W. (1998). Development and implementation of evidence-based guidelines: A multi-site demonstration project. *Journal of Wound Ostomy Continence Nursing, 25,* 187-193.

Breslow, N. E., & Day, N. E. (1980). Statistical methods in cancer research: Vol. 1: The analysis of case-control studies. *IARC Science Publications, 32*, 5-338.

Broad, W., & Wade, N. (1982*). Betrayers of the truth: Fraud and deceit in the halls of science.* New York: Simon & Schuster.

Brook, R. H., Kamberg, C. J., Mayer-Oakes, A., Beers, M. H., Raube, K., & Steiner, A. (1989). *Appropriateness of acute medical care for the elderly: An analysis of the literature.* Santa Monica, CA: RAND.

Browman, G. P., Newman, T. E., Mohide, E. A., Graham, I. D., Levine, M. N., Pritchard, K. E., Evans, W. K., Maroun, J. A., Hodson, D. I., Carey, M. S., & Cowan, D. H. (1998). Progress of clinical oncology guidelines development using the practice guidelines development cycle: The role of practitioner feedback. *Journal of Clinical Oncology, 16,* 1226-1223.

Brown, M. G., Hitchcock, D. E., & Willard, M. L. (1994). *Why TQM fails and what to do about it.* Burr Ridge, IL: Irwin.

Bruner, K. F. (1942). Of psychological writing: Some valedictory remarks on style. *Journal of Abnormal and Social Psychology, 37,* 52-70.

Bryant, F. B., & Wortman, P. M. (1984). Methodological issues in the meta-analysis of quasi-experiments. In W. H. Yeaton & P. M. Wortman (Eds.), *New directions for program evaluation: Issues in data synthesis* (Vol. 24, pp. 5-24). San Francisco: Jossey-Bass.

Bryk, A. S., & Raudenbush, S. W. (1992). *Hierarchical linear models.* Newbury Park, CA: Sage.

Bucher, H. C., Weinbacher, C., & Gyr, K. (1994). Influence of method of reporting study results on decision of physicians to prescribe drugs to lower cholesterol concentration. *British Medical Journal, 309,* 761-764.

Bushman, B. J. (1994). Vote-counting procedures in meta-analysis. In H. Cooper & L. Hedges (Eds.), *Handbook of research synthesis* (pp. 193-215). New York: Russell Sage.

Byrne, B. M. (1998). *Structural equation modeling with LISREL, PRELIS and SIMPLIS: Basic concepts, applications and programming.* Mahwah, NJ: Lawrence Erlbaum.

Campbell, D. T., & Stanley, J. C. (1963). *Experimental and quasi-experimental designs for research.* Chicago: Rand McNally.

Canadian Task Force on the Periodic Health Examination. (1979). The periodic health examination. *Canadian Medical Association Journal, 121,* 1193-1254.

Cappelleri, J. C., Ioannidis, J. P., Schmid, C. H., de Ferranti, S. D., Aubert, M., Chalmers, T. C., & Lau, J. (1996). Large trials versus meta-analysis of smaller trials: How do their results compare? *Journal of the American Medical Association, 276,* 1332-1338.

Castellan, N. J., & Siegel, S. (1988). *Nonparametric statistics for the behavioral sciences* (2nd ed.). New York: McGraw-Hill.

Chalmers, T. C. (1991). Problems induced by meta-analyses [Discussion, pp. 979-980]. *Statistics in Medicine, 10,* 971-980.

Chalmers, T. C., Berrier, J., Sacks, H. S., Levin, H., Reitman, D., & Nagalingam, R. (1987). Meta-analysis of clinical trials as a scientific discipline: II. Replicate variability and comparison of studies that agree and disagree. *Statistics in Medicine, 6,* 733-744.

Chalmers, T. C., Frank, C. S., & Reitman, D. (1990). Minimizing the three stages of publication bias. *Journal of the American Medical Association, 263,* 1392-1395.

Chalmers, T. C., & Lau, J. (1993). Meta-analytic stimulus for changes in clinical trials [Review]. *Statistical Methods in Medical Research, 2,* 161-172.

Chalmers, T. C., Smith, H., Jr., Blackburn, B., Silverman, B., Schroeder, B., Reitman, D., & Ambroz, A. (1981). A method for assessing the quality of a randomized control trial. *Controlled Clinical Trials, 2,* 31-49.

Chassin, M. R. (1990). Practice guidelines: Best hope for quality improvement in the 1990s. *Journal of Occupational Medicine, 32,* 1199-1206.

Chassin, M. R., Kosecoff, J., Park, R. E., Fink, A., Rauchman, S., Keesey, J., Flynn, M. F., & Brook, R. H. (1986). *Indications for selected medical and surgical procedures: A literature review and ratings of appropriateness, angiography.* Santa Monica, CA: RAND.

Chatellier, G., Zapletal, E., Lemaitre, D., Menard, J., & Degoulet, P. (1996). The number needed to treat: A clinically useful nomogram in its proper context. *British Medical Journal, 312,* 426-429.

Clarke, M., & Oxman, A. D. (Eds.). (1999). Cochrane reviewers' handbook 4.0 [updated July 1999], Section 2.2.3. In *Review Manager (RevMan)* [Computer program] (Version 4.0). Oxford, England: Cochrane Collaboration.

Cochrane, A. L. (1972). *Effectiveness and efficiency, random reflections on health services.* London: Nuffiled Provincial Hospitals Trust.

Cochrane Controlled Trials Register. (1997). *Cochrane Library* [CD-ROM and online]. Oxford, UK: Cochrane Collaboration.

Cohen, J. (1968). Weighted kappa: Nominal scale agreement with provision for scaled disagreement or partial credit. *Psychological Bulletin, 70,* 213-220.

Cohen, J. (1988). *Statistical power analysis for the behavior sciences* (2nd ed.). Hillsdale, NJ: Lawrence Erlbaum.

Collen, M. F. (1995). *A history of medical informatics in the United States: 1950 to 1990.* Bethesda, MD: American Medical Informatics Association.

Consumers Union. (1999). *Consumer reports: Home computer buying guide.* Yonkers, NY: Author.

Cook, D. J., Greengold, N. L., Ellrodt, A. G., & Weingarten, S. R. (1997). The relation between systematic reviews and practice guidelines. *Annals of Internal Medicine, 127,* 210-216.

Cook, K. J., Guyatt, G. H., Laupacis, A., & Sackett, D. L. (1992). Rules of evidence and clinical recommendations on the use of antithrombotic agents. Antithrombotic Therapy Consensus Conference. *Chest, 102*(Suppl.), 305S-311S.

Cook, T. D., & Campbell, D. T. (1979). *Quasi-experimentation: Design and analysis issues for field settings.* Chicago: Rand McNally.

Cook, T. D., Cooper, H., Cordray, D. S., Hartmann, H., Hedges, L. V., Light, R. J., Louis, T. A., & Mosteller, F. (Eds.). (1992). *Meta-analysis for explanation: A casebook.* New York: Russell Sage.

Cooper, H. (1998). *Synthesizing research: A guide for literature reviewers* (3rd ed.). Thousand Oaks, CA: Sage.

Cooper, H., & Hedges, L. V. (Eds.). (1994). *The handbook of research synthesis.* New York: Russell Sage.

Cooper, H. M. (1989). *Integrating research: A guide for literature reviews* (2nd ed.). Beverly Hills, CA: Sage.

Cooper, H. M., & Ribble, R. G. (1989). Influences on the outcome of literature searches for integrative research reviews. *Knowledge Creation, Diffusion, and Utilization, 10,* 179-201.

Cooper, H. M., & Rosenthal, R. (1980). Statistical versus traditional procedures for summarizing research findings. *Psychological Bulletin, 87,* 442-449.

Counsell, C. (1998). Formulating questions and locating primary studies for inclusion in systematic reviews. In C. Mulrow & D. Cook (Eds.), *Systematic reviews: Synthesis of best evidence for health care decisions* (pp. 67-79). Philadelphia: American College of Physicians.

Coursol, A., & Wagner, E. E. (1986). Effect of positive findings on submission and acceptance rates: A note on meta-analysis bias. *Professional Psychology, 17,* 136-137.

Crane, D. (1972). *Invisible colleges: Diffusion of knowledge in scientific communities.* Chicago: University of Chicago Press.

Cross, K. P. (1981). *Adults as learners.* San Francisco: Jossey-Bass.

Cuadra, C. A., & Katter, R. V. (1967). Opening the black box of "relevance." *Journal of Documentation, 23,* 291-303.

Dalkey, N. C., Rourke, D. L., Lewis, R., & Snyder, D. (1972). *Studies in the quality of life: Delphi and decision-making.* Lexington, MA: Lexington Books.

Davidoff, F., Haynes, B., Sackett, D., & Smith, R. (1995). Evidence based medicine. *British Medical Journal, 310,* 1085-1086.

Davis, D. A., Haynes, R. B., Chambers, L., Neufield, V. R., McKibbon, A., & Tugwell, P. (1984). The impact of CME–A methodological review of the continuing medical education literature. *Evaluation and the Health Professions, 7,* 251-283.

Davis, D. A., Thomson, M. A., Oxman, A. D., & Haynes, R. B. (1992). Evidence for the effectiveness of CME–A review of 50 randomized trials. *Journal of the American Medical Association, 268,* 1111-1115.

Davis, D. A., Thomson, M. A., Oxman, A. D., & Haynes, R. B. (1995). Changing physician performance: A systematic review of the effect of continuing medical education strategies. *Journal of the American Medical Association, 274,* 700-705.

Dear, K. B., & Begg, C. B. (1992). An approach for assessing publication bias prior to performing a meta-analysis. *Statistical Science, 7,* 237-245.

Delbecq, A. L., & Van de Ven, A. H. (1971). A group process model for problem identification and program planning. *Journal of Applied Behavioral Science, 7,* 466-492.

Delbecq, A. L., Van de Ven, A. H., & Gustafson, D. H. (1975). *Group techniques for program planning: A guide to nominal group and Delphi processes.* Glenview, IL: Scott Foresman.

Demakus, J., Beauchamps, C., et al. (1996). *Multi-site study of computer generated reminders to enhance adherence to standards of ambulatory care* (Final Report #9). Center for Co-operative Studies in Health Services (CCSHS).

DerSimonian, R., & Laird, N. (1986). Meta-analysis in clinical trials. *Controlled Clinical Trials, 7,* 177-188.

Detsky, A. S., Naylor, C. D., O'Rourke, K., McGeer, A. J., & L'Abbe, K. A. (1992). Incorporating variations in the quality of individual randomized trials into meta-analysis. *Journal of Clinical Epidemiology, 45,* 255-265.

Devine, E. C. (1984). Effects of psychoeducational interventions: A meta-analytic review of studies with surgical patients [CD-ROM]. Abstract obtained from *Proquest File: Dissertation Abstracts* (Item: 8404400).

Devine, E. C., & Westlake, S. K. (1995). The effects of psychoeducational care provided to adults with cancer: Meta-analysis of 116 studies. *Oncology Nursing Forum, 22,* 1369-1381.

Dickersin, K. (1990). The existence of publication bias and risk factors for its occurrence. *Journal of the American Medical Association, 263,* 1385-1389.

Dickersin, K. (1994). Research registers. In H. Cooper & L. V. Hedges (Eds.), *Handbook of research synthesis* (pp. 71-84). New York: Russell Sage.

Dickersin, K., Chan, S., Chalmers, T. C., Sacks, H. S., & Smith, H., Jr. (1987). Publication bias and clinical trials. *Controlled Clinical Trials, 8,* 343-353.

Dickersin, K., Hewitt, P., Mutch, L., Chalmers, I., & Chalmers, T. C. (1985). Perusing the literature: Comparison of MEDLINE searching with a perinatal trials database. *Controlled Clinical Trials, 6,* 306-317.

Dickersin, K., Scherer, R., & Lefebvre, C. (1994). Identifying relevant studies for systematic reviews. *British Medical Journal, 309,* 1286-1291.

Dickersin, K., Yuan, I. M., & Meinert, C. L. (1992). Factors influencing publication of research results: Follow-up of applications submitted to two institutional review boards. *Journal of the American Medical Association, 267,* 374-378.

Dolcourt, J. L., & Braude, R. M. (1976). Determination of overlap in coverage of Excerpta Medica and Index Medicus through Serline. *Bulletin of the Medical Library Association, 64,* 324-325.

Donabedian, A. (1966). Evaluating the quality of medical care. *Millbank Memorial Fund Quarterly, 44,* 166-206.

Douglas, G. A., Deeks, J. J., & Sackett, D. L. (1998). Odds ratios should be avoided when events are common [Letter to the editor]. *British Medical Journal, 317,* 1318.

Dumouchel, W. (1995). Meta-analysis for dose-response models. *Statistics in Medicine, 14,* 679-685.

Eagly, A. H., & Wood, W. C. (1994). Using research syntheses to plan future research. In H. Cooper & L. V. Hedges (Eds.), *Handbook of research synthesis* (pp. 485-500). New York: Russell Sage.

Easterbrook, P. J., Berlin, J. A., Gopalan, R., & Matthews, D. R. (1991). Publication bias in clinical research. *Lancet, 337,* 867-872.

Eddy, D. M. (1984). Variations in physician practice: The role of uncertainty. *Health Affairs (Millwood), 3,* 74-89.

Eddy, D. M. (1990). Comparing benefits and harms: The balance sheet. *Journal of the American Medical Association, 263,* 2493-2498.

Eddy, D. M., Hasselblad, V., & Shachter, R. (1990). An introduction to a Bayesian method for meta-analysis: The confidence profile method. *Medical Decision Making, 10,* 15-23.

Eddy, D. M., Hasselblad, V., & Shachter, R., (1992). *Meta-analysis by the confidence profile method: The statistical synthesis of evidence.* San Diego, CA: Academic Press.

Egger, M. (2001). Directions and impact of bias in meta-analysis of controlled trials: Empirical studies of language bias, grey literature bias and MEDLINE bias. In *The Cochrane Methodology Register in the Cochrane Library.* Oxford, UK: Update Software, Ltd.

Egger, M., & Smith, G. D. (1997). Meta-analysis: Potentials and promise. *British Medical Journal, 315,* 1371-1374.

Egger, M., & Smith, G. D. (1998). Bias in location and selection of studies. *British Medical Journal, 316,* 61-66.

Egger, M., Smith, G. D., & Phillips, A. N. (1997). Meta-analysis: Principles and procedures. *British Medical Journal, 315,* 1533-1537.

Egger, M., Smith, G. D., Schneider, M., & Minder, C. E. (1997). Bias in meta-analysis detected by a simple, graphical test. *British Medical Journal, 315,* 629-634.

Eisenberg, M., & Barry, C. (1988). Order effects: A study of the possible influence of presentation order on user judgments of document relevance. *Journal of the American Society for Information Science, 39,* 293-300.

Ellrodt, A. G., Cho, M., Cush, J. J., Kavanaugh, A. F., & Lipsky, P. E. (1997). An evidence-based medicine approach to the diagnosis and management of musculoskeletal complaints. *American Journal of Medicine, 103*(6A), 3S-6S.

Ellrodt, A. G., Conner, L., Riedinger, M., & Weingarten, S. (1995). Measuring and improving physician compliance with clinical practice guidelines: A controlled interventional trial. *Annals of Internal Medicine, 122,* 277-282.

Elstein, A. S., Friedman, C. P., Wolf, F. M., Murphy, G., Miller, J., Fine, P., Heckerling, P., Miller, T., Sisson, J., Barlas, S., Biolsi, K., Ng, M., Mei, X., Franz, T., & Capitano, A. (1996). Effects of a decision support system on the diagnostic accuracy of users: A preliminary report. *Journal of the American Medical Informatics Association, 3,* 422-428.

Ely, J. W., Osheroff, J. A., Ebell, M. H., Bergus, G. R., Levy, B. T., Chambliss, M. L., & Evans, E. R. (1999). Analysis of questions asked by family doctors regarding patient care. *British Medical Journal, 319,* 358-361.

Ely, J. W., Osheroff, J. A., Gorman, P. N., Ebell, M. H., Chambliss, M. L., Pifer, E. A., & Stavri, A. (2000). A taxonomy of generic clinical questions: Classification study. *British Medical Journal, 321,* 429-432.

Emerson, J. D., Burdick, E., Hoaglin, D. C., Mosteller, F., & Chalmers, T. C. (1990). An empirical study of the possible relation of treatment differences to quality scores in controlled randomized clinical trials. *Controlled Clinical Trials, 11,* 339-352.

Emlet, H., Davis, J., & Casey, I. (1971). *Alternative methods for estimating health-care benefits and required resources: Vol. 2. Selecting the estimators* (Report prepared by Analytic Services, Inc., in cooperation with the Johns Hopkins University (JHU) School of Hygiene and Public Health). The Health-Benefit Analysis Project. Falls Church, VA: Analytic Services, Inc.

Emlet, H., Williamson, J., Casey, I., Davis, J., Dittmer, D., Flagle, C., & Miller, G. (1971). *Alternative methods for estimating health-care benefits and required resources: Vol. 1. Summary* (Report prepared by Analytic Services, Inc., in cooperation with the Johns Hopkins University (JHU) School of Hygiene and Public Health). The Health-Benefit Analysis Project. Falls Church, VA: Analytic Services, Inc.

Everitt, B. D., Landau, S., & Leese, M. (2000). *Cluster analysis* (4th ed.). Oxford, UK: Update Software, Ltd.

Eysenck, H. J. (1978). An exercise in mega-silliness. *American Psychologist, 33,* 517.

Fang, E., Mittman, B. S., & Weingarten, S. (1996). Use of clinical practice guidelines in managed care physician groups. *Archives of Family Medicine, 5,* 528-531.

Federal Register, U.S. National Archives and Records Administration. (1998). Reports, forms, and record keeping requirements: Agency information collection activity under Office of Management and Budget [Notice]. *Federal Register, 63*(70), 18065-18066.

Feinstein, A. R. (1979). Methodologic problems and standards in case-control research. *Journal of Chronic Disease, 32,* 35-41.

Feinstein, A. R. (1988). Fraud, distortion, delusion and consensus: The problems of humans on natural deception in epidemiologic science. *American Journal of Medicine, 84,* 475-478.

Feinstein, A. R. (1995). Meta-analysis: Statistical alchemy for the 21st century. *Journal of Clinical Epidemiology, 48,* 71-79.

Feldman, K. A. (1971). Using the work of others: Some observations on reviewing and integrating. *Sociology of Education, 44,* 86-102.

Fink, A. (1998). *Conducting research literature reviews: From paper to the Internet.* Thousand Oaks, CA: Sage.

Fisher, R. A. (1925). *Statistical methods for research workers.* London: Oliver & Boyd.

Flanagin, A., Carey, L. A., Fontanarosa, P. B., Phillips, S. G., Pace, B. P., Lundberg, G. D., & Rennie, D. (1998). Prevalence of articles with honorary authors and ghost authors in peer-reviewed medical journals. *Journal of the American Medical Association, 280,* 222-224.

Fleiss, J. L. (1981). *Statistical methods for rates and proportions* (2nd ed.). New York: John Wiley.

Fleiss, J. L. (1994). Measures of effect size for categorical data. In H. Cooper & L. V. Hedges (Eds.), *Handbook of research synthesis* (pp. 245-260). New York: Russell Sage.

Fleiss, J. L., & Gross, A. J. (1991). Meta-analysis in epidemiology, with special reference to studies of the association between exposure to environmental tobacco smoke and lung cancer: A critique. *Journal of Clinical Epidemiology, 44,* 127-139.

Forrow, L., Taylor, W. C., & Arnold, R. M. (1992). Absolutely relative: how research results are summarized can affect treatment decisions. *American Journal of Medicine, 92,* 121-124.

Forsythe, D. E., Buchanan, B. G., Osheroff, J. A., & Miller, R. A. (1992). Expanding the concept of medical information: An observational study of physicians' information needs. *Computers in Biomedical Research, 25,* 181-200.

Fowkes, F. G. R., & Fulton, P. M. (1991). Critical appraisal of published research: Introductory guidelines. *British Medical Journal, 302,* 1136-1140.

Friedman, C. P., Elstein, A. S., Wolf, F. M., Murphy, G. C., Franz, T. M., Heckerling, P. S., Fine, P. L., Miller, T. M., & Abraham, V. (1999). Enhancement of clinicians' diagnostic reasoning by computer-based consultation: A multisite study of 2 systems. *Journal of the American Medical Association, 282,* 1851-1856.

Gardner, R. M., Pryor, T. A., & Warner, H. R. (1999). The HELP hospital information system: Update 1998. *International Journal of Medical Informatics, 54,* 169-182.

Gehanno, J. F., Paris, C., Thirion, B., & Caillard, J. F. (1998). Assessment of bibliographic databases performance in information retrieval for occupational and environmental toxicology. *Occupational and Environmental Medicine, 55,* 562-566.

Gelman, A., Carlin, J. B., Stern, H. S., & Rubin, D. B. (1995). *Bayesian data analysis.* London: Chapman & Hall.

Glass, G. V. (1976). Primary, secondary and meta-analysis of research. *Educational Research, 5,* 3-8.

Glass, G. V. (1977). Integrating findings: The meta-analysis of research. *Review of Research in Education, 5,* 351-379.

Glass, G. V., McGraw, B., & Smith, M. L. (1981). *Meta-analysis in social research.* Beverly Hills, CA: Sage.

Glasser, B., & Strauss, A. (1967). *The discovery of grounded theory.* Chicago: Aldine.

Glasziou, P., Guyatt, G. H., Dans, A. L., Dans, L. F., Straus, S., & Sackett, D. L. (1998). Applying the results of trials and systematic reviews to individual patients [Editorial]. *American College of Physicians Journal Club, 129,* A15-A16.

Glossbrenner, A., & Glossbrenner, E. (1999). *Search engines for the World Wide Web* (2nd ed.). Berkeley, CA: Peachpit.

Goldman, R. L., Weir, C. R., Turner, C. W., & Smith, C. B. (1997). Validity of utilization management criteria for psychiatry. *American Journal of Psychiatry, 154,* 349-354.

Goldschmidt, P. G. (1986). Information synthesis: A practical guide. *Health Services Research, 21*(2, Pt. 1), 215-237.

Goldschmidt, P. G., & Liao, J. (1998). *Health care quality management resources directory—1998/99.* Bethesda, MD: World Development Group.

Goodman, C., & Baratz, S. R. (Eds.). (1990). *Improving consensus development for health technology assessment: An international perspective.* Washington, DC: National Academy Press.

Goodman, N. W. (1994). Survey of fulfillment of criteria for authorship in published medical research. *British Medical Journal, 309,* 1482.

Gorman, P. N., Ash, J., & Wykoff, L. (1994). Can primary care physicians' questions be answered using the medical journal literature? *Bulletin of the Medical Library Association, 82,* 140-146.

Gray, J. A., Haynes, R. B., Sackett, D. L., Cook, D. J., & Guyatt, G. H. (1997, March/April). Transferring evidence from research into practice: 3. Getting the evidence straight. *American College of Physicians Journal Club, 126,* A14-A16.

Greengold, N. L., & Weingarten, S. R. (1996). Developing evidence-based practice guidelines and pathways: The experience at the local hospital level. *Joint Commission Journal of Quality Improvement, 22,* 391-402.

Greenhalgh, T., & Douglas, H. R. (1999). Experiences of general practitioners and practice nurses of training courses in evidence-based health care: A qualitative study. *British Journal of General Practice, 49,* 536-540.

Greenhouse, J. B., & Iyengar, S. (1994). Sensitivity analysis and diagnostics. In H. Cooper & L. V. Hedges (Eds.), *The handbook of research synthesis* (pp. 383-398). New York: Russell Sage.

Greenland, S., & Robins, J., (1994). Invited commentary: Ecologic studies—biases, misconceptions, and counterexamples. *American Journal Epidemiology, 139,* 747-760.

Greenwald, A. G. (1975). Consequences of prejudice against the null hypothesis. *Psychological Bulletin, 82,* 1-20.

Gretz, M., Schmitt, R. D., & Thomas, M. (1996). EMBASE remains EMBASE—on every host? A comparative analysis of EMBASE on the hosts DATA-STAR, DIALOG, DIMDI, AND STN. *Computers in Biomedical Research, 29,* 494-506.

Grimshaw, J. M., & Hutchinson, A. (1995). Clinical practice guidelines: Do they enhance value for money in health care? *British Medical Bulletin, 51,* 927-940.

Grimshaw, J. M., & Russell, I. T. (1993). Effect of clinical guidelines on medical practice: A systematic review of rigorous evaluations. *Lancet, 342,* 1317-1322.

Grimshaw, J. M., Watson, M. S., & Eccles, M. (1998). A false dichotomy: Commentary on "Clinical guidelines: Ways ahead." *Journal of Evaluation in Clinical Practice, 4,* 295-298.

Grossman, J. (Ed.). (1993). *The Chicago manual of style* (14th ed.). Chicago: University of Chicago Press.

Guyatt, G. H., Drummond, R., & Hayward, R. (Eds.). (2001a). *Users' guides to the medical literature: Essentials of evidence-based clinical practice.* Chicago: American Medical Association Press.

Guyatt, G. H., Drummond, R., & Hayward, R. (Eds.). (2001b). *Users' guides to the medical literature: A manual for evidence-based clinical practice.* Chicago: American Medical Association Press.

Guyatt, G. H., Jaeschke, R. Z., & Cook, D. J. (1995). Applying the findings of clinical trials to individual patients. *American College of Physicians Journal Club, 122,* A12-A13.

Guyatt, G. H., Meade, M. O., Jaeschke, R. Z., Cook, D. J., & Haynes, R. B. (2000). Practitioners of evidence based care: Not all clinicians need to appraise evidence from scratch but all need some skills [Editorial]. *British Medical Journal, 320,* 954-955.

Guyatt, G. H., Sackett, D. L., & Cook, D. J. (1994). Users' guides to the medical literature: II. How to use an article about therapy or prevention. B. What were the results and will they help me in caring for my patients? Evidence-Based Medicine Working Group. *Journal of the American Medical Association, 271,* 59-63.

Guzzo, R. A., Jackson, S. E., & Katzell, R. A. (1986). Meta-analysis analysis. In L. L. Cummings & B. M. Staw (Eds.), *Research in organizational behavior* (Vol. 9). Greenwich, CT: JAI.

Gyorkos, T. W., Tannenbaum, T. N., Abrahamowicz, M., Bédard, L., Carsley, J., & Franco, E. D. (1994). Evaluation of the effectiveness of immunization delivery methods. *Canadian Journal of Public Health, 85*(Suppl. 1), 14S-30S.

Gyorkos, T. W., Tannenbaum, T. N., Abrahamowicz, M., Oxman, A. D., Scott, E. A., Millson, M. E., Rasooly, I., Frank, J. W., Riben, P. D., Mathias, R. G., & Miller, M. A. (1994). An approach to the development of practice guidelines for community health interventions. *Canadian Journal of Public Health, 85*(Suppl. 1), S8-S13.

Hackner, D. (1999). Guidelines in pulmonary medicine: A 25-year profile [Review]. *Chest, 116,* 1046-1062.

Hadorn, D. C., Baker, D., Hodges, J. S., & Hicks, N. (1996). Rating the quality of evidence for clinical practice guidelines. *Journal of Clinical Epidemiology, 49,* 749-754.

Hall, F., Tickle-Degnen, L., Rosenthal, R., & Mosteller, F. (1994). Hypotheses and problems in research synthesis. In H. Cooper & L. V. Hedges (Eds.), *Handbook of research synthesis* (pp. 17-28). New York: Russell Sage.

Halvorsen, K. T. (1986). Combining results from independent investigations: Meta-analysis in medical research. In J. Bailar III & F. Mosteller (Eds.), *Medical uses of statistics* (pp. 392-416). Waltham, MA: New England Journal of Medicine Books.

Hasselblad, V., Mosteller, F., Littenberg, B., Chalmers, T. C., Hunink, M. G. M., Turner, J. A., Morton, S. C., Diehr, P., Wong, J. B., & Powe, N. R. (1995). A survey of current problems in meta-analysis: Discussion from the Agency for Health Care Policy and Research Inter-PORT work group on literature review/meta-analysis. *Medical Care, 33,* 202-220.

Haug, P. J., Gardner, R. M., Tate, K. E., Evans, R. S., East, T. D., Kuperman, G., Pryor, T. A., Huff, S. M., & Warner, H. R. (1994). Decision support in medicine: Examples from the HELP system. *Computers in Biomedical Research, 27,* 396-418.

Haynes, R. B. (1990). Loose connections between peer-reviewed clinical journals and clinical practice. *Annals of Internal Medicine, 113,* 724-728.

Haynes, R. B., McKibbon, K. A., Walker, C. J., Mousseau, J., Baker, L. M., Fitzgerald, D., Guyatt, G., & Norman, G. R. (1985). Computer searching of the medical literature: An evaluation of MEDLINE searching systems. *Annals of Internal Medicine, 103,* 812-816.

Haynes, R. B., Sackett, D. L., Gray, J. A., Cook, D. J., & Guyatt, G. H. (1997, January/February). Transferring evidence from research into practice: 2. Getting the evidence straight [Editorial]. *American College of Physicians Journal Club, 126,* A14-A16.

Haynes, R. B., Sackett, D. L., Guyatt, G. H., Cook, D. J., & Gray, J. A. (1996, November/December). Transferring evidence from research into practice: 1. The role of clinical care research evidence in clinical decisions [Editorial]. *American College of Physicians Journal Club, 125,* A14-A16.

Haynes, R. B., Sackett, D. L., Guyatt, G. H., Cook, D. J., & Gray, J. A. (1997, January/February). Transferring evidence from research into practice: 4. Overcoming barriers to application [Editorial]. *American College of Physicians Journal Club, 126,* A14-A16.

Haynes, R. B., Wilczynski, N., McKibbon, K. A., Walker, C. J., & Sinclair, J. C. (1994). Developing optimal search strategies for detecting clinically sound studies in MEDLINE. *Journal of the American Medical Informatics Association, 1,* 447-458.

Hays, W. (1973). *Statistics.* Austin, TX: Holt, Rinehart and Winston.

Hayes, W. (1997). *Statistics.* 5th ed. New York: Holt, Rinehart and Winston.

Hayward, R. S., Hogeterp, J. A., Langton, K. B., Summerell, D., & Roizen, M. F. (1995). GAP: A computer-assisted design tool for the development and analysis of evidence-based automated questionnaires. *Medinfo, 8*(Pt. 2), 934-937.

Hecht, J. B. (1998). *Ethnographic research* [Syllabus and lecture slides] (Course EAF 410: Research Methodology and Statistics in Education I), Illinois State University.

Heckerling, P. S., Elstein, A. S., Terzian, C. G., & Kushner, M. S. (1991). The effect of incomplete knowledge on the diagnoses of a computer consultant system. *Medical Informatics, 16,* 363-370.

Hedges, L. V. (1992). Modeling publication selection effects in random effects models in meta-analysis. *Statistical Science, 7,* 246-255.

Hedges, L. V., & Olkin, I. (1985). *Statistical methods for meta-analysis.* New York: Academic Press.

Henderson, J. C., & Sussman, S. W. (1996). *Creating and exploiting knowledge for fast-cycle response: An analysis of the center for army lessons learned* (Boston University Working Paper 96-36, Report to National Science Foundation under Grant SBR-9422284). Boston: Boston University System Research Center, School of Management.

Hoen, W. P., Walvoort, H. C., & Overkebe, J. P. M. (1998). What are the factors determining authorship and the order of the authors' names? *Journal of the American Medical Association, 280,* 217-218.

Hoyt, D. B. (1997). Clinical practice guidelines. *American Journal of Surgery, 173,* 32-36.

Hunt, D. L., & McKibbon, K. A. (1998). Locating and appraising systematic reviews. In C. Mulrow & D. Cook (Eds.), *Systematic reviews: Synthesis of best evidence for health care decisions* (pp. 13-22). Philadelphia: American College of Physicians.

Hunter, J. E., & Schmidt, F. L. (1990). *Methods of meta-analysis: Correcting error and bias in research findings.* Newbury Park, CA: Sage.

Hunter, J. E., & Schmidt, F. L. (1994). Correcting for sources of artificial variation across studies. In H. Cooper & L. V. Hedges (Eds.), *Handbook of research synthesis* (pp. 323-336). New York: Russell Sage.

Impicciatore, P., Pandolfini, C., Casella, N., & Bonati, M. (1997). Reliability of health information for the public on the World Wide Web: Systematic survey of advice on managing fever in children at home. *British Medical Journal, 314,* 1875-1879.

Institute of Medicine, Committee on Clinical Practice Guidelines. (1992). *Guidelines for clinical practice: From development to use.* Washington, DC: National Academy Press.

Institute of Medicine, Council on Health Care Technology. (1990). *Improving consensus development for health technology assessment: An international perspective.* Washington, DC: National Academy Press.

International Committee of Medical Journal Editors (ICMJE). (1985). Guidelines on authorship. *British Medical Journal, 291,* 922.

International Committee of Medical Journal Editors (ICMJE). (1997). Uniform requirements for manuscripts submitted to biomedical journals. *Journal of the American Medical Association, 277,* 927-934.

International Committee of Medical Journal Editors (ICMJE). (2000). Uniform requirements for manuscripts submitted to biomedical journals. Update from *Annals of Internal Medicine (1977), 126,* 36-47. Available online (last updated May 2000) at www.icmje.org/

Irwig, L., Tosteson, A. N., Gatsonis, C., Lau, J., Colditz, G., & Chalmers, T. C. (1994). Guidelines for meta-analyses evaluating diagnostic tests. *Annals of Internal Medicine, 120,* 667-676.

Jackson, G. B. (1980). Methods for integrative reviews. *Review of Educational Research, 50,* 438-460.

Jeng, G. T., Scott, J. R., & Burmeister, L. F. (1995). A comparison of meta-analytic results using literature vs. individual patient data: Paternal cell immunization for recurrent miscarriage. *Journal of the American Medical Association, 274,* 830-836.

Johnson, K. B., & Feldman, M. J. (1995). Medical informatics and pediatrics: Decision-support systems. *Archives of Pediatric Adolescent Medicine, 149,* 1371-1380.

Joreskog, K. G., & Sorbom, D. (1988). *LISREL 7: A guide to the program and applications.* Chicago: SPSS, Inc.

Kassirer, J. P., & Angell, M. (1993). Financial conflicts of interest in biomedical research. *New England Journal of Medicine, 329,* 570-571.

Khan, K. S., Daya, S., & Jadad, A. R. (1996). The importance of quality of primary studies in producing unbiased systematic reviews. *Archives of Internal Medicine, 156,* 661-666.

Knowles, M. S. (1970). *The modern practice of adult education.* New York: Association Press.

Knox, A. B. (1977). *Adult development and learning.* San Francisco: Jossey-Bass.

Krimsky, S., & Rothenberg, L. S. (1998). Financial interest and its disclosure in scientific publications. *Journal of the American Medical Association, 280,* 225-226.

Landis, J. R., & Koch, G. G. (1977). The measurement of observer agreement for categorical data. *Biometrics, 33,* 671-679.

Langbein, L. I., & Lichtman, A. J. (1978). *Ecological inference.* Beverly Hills, CA: Sage.

Lange, L. L., Haak, S. W., Lincoln, M. J., Thompson, C. B., Turner, C. W., Weir, C., Foerster, V., Nilasena, D., & Reeves, R. (1997). Use of Iliad to improve diagnostic performance of nurse practitioner students. *Journal of Nursing Education, 36,* 36-45.

La Puma, J., & Lawlor, E. F. (1990). Quality-adjusted life years: Ethical implications for physicians and policymakers. *Journal of the American Medical Association, 263,* 2917-2921.

Lau, J., Antman, E. M., Jimenez-Silva, J., Kupelnick, B., Mosteller, F., & Chalmers, T. C. (1992). Cumulative meta-analysis of therapeutic trials for myocardial infarction. *New England Journal of Medicine, 327,* 248-254.

Lau, J., Ioannidis, J. P., & Schmid, C. H. (1997). Quantitative synthesis in systematic reviews. *Annals of Internal Medicine, 127,* 820-826.

Lau, J., Schmid, C. H., & Chalmers, T. C. (1995). Cumulative meta-analysis of clinical trials builds evidence for exemplary medical care. *Journal of Clinical Epidemiology, 48,* 45-57.

Lau, L. M., & Warner, H. R. (1992). Performance of a diagnostic system (Iliad) as a tool for quality assurance. *Proceedings of the 1992 Symposium on Computer Applications in Medical Care,* 1005-1010.

Leape, L. L. (1990). Practice guidelines and standards. *Quality Review Bulletin, 16,* 42-49.

Leininger, M. (1994). Evaluation criteria and critique of qualitative research studies. In J. M. Morse (Ed.), *Critical issues in qualitative research methods* (pp. 95-115). Thousand Oaks, CA: Sage.

Liberati, A., Himel, H. N., & Chalmers, T. C. (1986). A quality assessment of randomized control trials of primary treatment of breast cancer. *Journal of Clinical Oncology, 4,* 942-951.

Lichtenstein, M. J., Mulrow, C. D., & Elwood, P. C. (1987). Guidelines for reading case-control studies. *Journal of Chronic Disease, 40,* 893-903.

Light, R. J. (1988). A test of missing completely at random for multivariate data with missing values. *Journal of the American Statistical Association, 83,* 1199-1201.

Light, R. J., & Pillemer, D. B. (1984). *Summing up: The science of reviewing research.* Cambridge, MA: Harvard University Press.

Light, R. J., Singer, J. D., & Willett, J. B. (1994). The visual presentation and interpretation of meta-analyses. In H. Cooper & L. V. Hedges (Eds.), *Handbook of research synthesis* (pp. 439-453). New York: Russell Sage.

Light, R. J., & Smith, P. V. (1971). Accumulating evidence: Procedures for resolving contradictions among different research studies. *Harvard Educational Review, 41,* 429-471.

Lilford, R. J., Pauker, S. G., Braunholtz, D. A., & Jiri, C. (1998). Getting research findings into practice: Decision analysis and the implementation of research findings. *British Medical Journal, 317,* 405-409.

Lilford, R. J., Thornton, J. G., & Braunholtz, D. (1995). Clinical trials and rare diseases: A way out of a conundrum. *British Medical Journal, 311,* 1621-1625.

Lincoln, M. J., Turner, C. W., Haug, P. J., Warner, H. R., Williamson, J. W., Bouhaddou, O., Jessen, S. G., Sorenson, D., Cundick, R. C., & Grant, M. (1991). Iliad training enhances medical students' diagnostic skills. *Journal of Medical Systems, 15,* 93-110.

Lipsey, M. W. (1990). *Design sensitivity: Statistical power for detecting the effect of interventions.* Newbury Park, CA: Sage.

Little, R. J. A., & Rubin, D. B. (1987). *Statistical analysis with missing data.* New York: John Wiley.

Louis, T. A., & Zelterman, D. (1994). Bayesian approaches to research synthesis. In H. Cooper & L. V. Hedges (Eds.), *Handbook of research synthesis* (pp. 411-422). New York: Russell Sage.

Lundberg, G. D., Paul, M. C., & Fritz, H. (1998). A comparison of the opinions of experts and readers as to what topics a general medical journal (*JAMA*) should address. *Journal of the American Medical Association, 280,* 288-290.

Lundsgaarde, H. P. (1992). *Knowledge engineering and ethnography.* Paper presented at the the annual meeting of the American Anthropological Association, San Francisco.

Lundsgaarde, H. P., & Williamson, J. W. (1987). Organizational barriers to the diffusion of computer technology. In G. Salvendy, S. L. Sauter, & J. J. Hurrell, Jr. (Eds.), *Social, ergonomic and stress aspects of work with computers.* Amsterdam: Elsevier Science.

Mahoney, M. J. (1977). Publication prejudices: An experimental study of confirmatory bias in the peer review system. *Cognitive Therapy and Research, 1,* 161-175.

Mansfield, R. S., & Busse, T. V. (1977). Meta-analysis of research: A rejoinder to Glass. *Education Research, 6,* 3.

Marcus, S. H., Grover, P. L., & Revicki, D. A. (1987). The method of information synthesis and its use in the assessment of health care technology. *International Journal of Technology Assessment in Health Care, 3,* 497-508.

Marson, A. G., & Chadwick, D. W. (1996). How easy are randomized controlled trials in epilepsy to find on Medline? The sensitivity and precision of two Medline searches. *Epilepsia, 37,* 377-380.

Maxwell, S. E., & Cole, D. A. (1995). Tips for writing (and reading) methodological articles. *Psychological Bulletin, 118,* 193-198.

McAuley, L., Pham, B., Tugwell, P., & Moher, D. (2000). Does the inclusion of grey literature influence estimates of intervention effectiveness reported in meta-analyses? *Lancet, 3561,* 228-231.

McClung, H. J., Murray, R. D., & Heitlinger, L. A. (1998). The Internet as a source for current patient information. *Pediatrics, 101,* e2.

McDonald, S., Taylor, L., & Adams, C. (1999). Searching the right database: A comparison of four databases for psychiatric journals. *Health Library Review, 16,* 151-156.

McIntosh, M. (1996). The population risk as an explanatory variable in research synthesis of clinical trials. *Statistics in Medicine, 15,* 1713-1728.

McMaster, G. (2000). Latest medical cyber-info reaches ER front lines. *University of Alberta Folio, 37,* 1.

McNemar, Q. (1969). *Psychological statistics* (4th ed.). New York: John Wiley.

Meade, M. O., & Richardson, W. S. (1998). Selecting and appraising studies for a systematic review. In C. Mulrow & D. Cook (Eds.), *Systematic reviews: Synthesis of best evidence for health care decisions* (pp. 81-90). Philadelphia: American College of Physicians.

Mehta, C. R., Patel, N. R., & Gray, R. (1985). Computing an exact confidence interval for the common odds ratio in several 2 × 2 contingency tables. *American Statistical Association Journal, 80,* 969-973.

Michels, K. B., & Rosner, B. A. (1996). Data trawling: To fish or not to fish. *Lancet, 348,* 1152-1153.

Miller, N., & Pollock, V. E. (1994). Meta-analytic synthesis for theory development. In H. Cooper & L. V. Hedges (Eds.), *Handbook of research synthesis* (pp. 457-483). New York: Russell Sage.

Miller, T., Turner, C., Tindale, R. S., Posavac, I. J., & Dugoni, B. L. (1991). Reasons for the trend toward null findings on Type A behavior. *Psychological Bulletin, 110,* 469-485.

Mitka, M. (1999). NEJM Editor Jerome P. Kassirer, MD, loses post over "administrative issues." *Journal of the American Medical Association, 282,* 622-623.

Moher, D. (1998). CONSORT: An evolving tool to help improve the quality of reports of randomized controlled trials. *Journal of the American Medical Association, 279,* 1489-1491.

Moher, D., Cook, D. J., Eastwood, S., Olkin, I., Rennie, D., & Stroup, D. F. (1994). Improving the quality of reports of meta-analyses of randomised controlled trials: The QUORUM statement. Quality of reporting of meta-analyses. *Lancet, 354,* 1896-1900.

Moher, D., Fortin, P., Jadad, A. R., Jüni, P., Klassen, T., Le Lorier, J., Liberati, A., Linde, K., & Penna, A. (1996). Completeness of reporting of trials published in languages other than English: Implications for conduct and reporting of systematic reviews. *Lancet, 347,* 363-366.

Moher, D., Jadad, A. R., Nichol, G., Penman, M., Tugwell, P., & Walsh, S. (1995). Assessing the quality of randomized controlled trials: An annotated bibliography of scales and checklists. *Controlled Clinical Trials, 16,* 62-73.

Moher, D., Pham, B., Klassen, T. P., Schulz, K. F., Berlin, J. A., Jadad, A. R., & Liberati, A. (2000). What contributions do languages other than English make on the results of meta-analyses? *Journal of Clinical Epidemiology, 53,* 964-972.

Morgenstern, H. (1982). Uses of ecologic analysis in epidemiologic research. *American Journal of Public Health, 72,* 1336-1334.

Morris, C. N. (1983). Parametric empirical Bayes inference: Theory and applications. *American Statistical Association Journal, 78,* 47-55.

Morris, C. N., & Normand, S. L. (1992). Hierarchical models for combining information and for meta-analyses. In J. L. Bernardo, J. O. Berger, A. P. Dawid, & A. F. Smith (Eds.), *Bayesian statistics 4.* New York: Oxford University Press.

Morton, C. C. (1999, December 17). New guidelines address growing disputes in scientific paper authorship. *Focus* (Harvard Medical, Dental & Public Health Schools Newsletter), p. 3.

Moses, L. E., Shapiro, D., & Littenberg, B. (1993). Combining independent studies of a diagnostic test into a summary ROC curve: Data-analytic approaches and some additional considerations. *Statistics in Medicine, 12,* 1293-1316.

Mosteller, F. (1986). Writing about numbers. In J. C. Bailar III & F. Mosteller (Eds.), *Medical uses of statistics* (pp. 349-369). Waltham, MA: New England Journal of Medicine Books.

Mosteller, F., & Bush, R. (1954). Selected quantitative techniques. In G. Lindsey (Ed.), *Handbook of social psychology: Vol. 1. Theory and method.* Cambridge, MA: Addison-Wesley.

Mulrow, C. (1987). The medical review article: The state of the science. *Annals of Internal Medicine, 106,* 485-488.

Mulrow, C., & Cook, D. (Eds.). (1998). *Systematic reviews: Synthesis of best evidence for health care decisions.* Philadelphia: American College of Physicians.

Mulrow, C. D., Linn, W. D., Gaul, M. K., & Pugh, J. A. (1989). Assessing quality of a diagnostic test evaluation. *Journal of General Internal Medicine, 4,* 288-295.

Murphy, G. C., Friedman, C. P., Elstein, A. S., Wolf, F. M., Miller, T., & Miller, J. G. (1996). The influence of a decision support system on the differential diagnosis of medical practitioners at three levels of training. *Proceedings of the American Medical Informatics Association Annual Fall Symposium,* 219-223.

Murphy, M. K., Black, N. A., Lamping, D. L., McKee, C. M., Sanderson, C. F. B., Askham, J., & Marteau, T. (1998). Consensus development methods, and their use in clinical guideline development [Review monograph]. *Health Technology Assessment, 2,* 1-88.

National Academy of Sciences, Institute of Medicine, Committee on Clinical Practice Guidelines. (1992). *Guidelines for clinical practice: From development to use.* Washington, DC: National Academy Press.

National Institutes of Health, National Heart, Lung, and Blood Institute. (1993). *Emergency department: Rapid identification and treatment of patients with acute myocardial infarction* (National Institutes of Health Pub. No. 93-3278) [Online]. Available: www.nhlbi.nih.gov/nhlbi/cardio/heart/prof/emerdept.txt.

Naylor, C. D., Chen, E., & Strauss, B. (1992). Measured enthusiasm: Does the method of reporting trial results alter perceptions of therapeutic effectiveness? *Annals of Internal Medicine, 117,* 916-921.

Nieminen, P., & Isohanni, M. (1999). Bias against European journals in medical publication databases. *Lancet, 353,* 1592.

Nijs, H. G., Bleeker, J. K., Van der Waal, M. A., & Casparie, A. F. (1998). Need for consensus development in prehospital emergency medicine: Effect of an expert panel approach. *European Journal of Emergency Medicine, 5,* 329-324.

Noblit, G. W., & Hare, R. D. (1988). *Meta-ethnography: Synthesizing qualitative studies.* Newbury Park, CA: Sage.

Normand, L. (1999). Meta-analysis: Formulating, evaluating, combining, and reporting. *Statistics in Medicine, 18,* 321-359.

Nunnally, J. C. (1978). *Psychometric theory.* New York: McGraw-Hill.

Olkin, I. (1995). Statistical and theoretical considerations in meta-analysis. *Journal of Clinical Epidemiology, 48,* 133-146.

Onion, W. R., & Walley, T. (1998). Clinical guidelines: Ways ahead. *Journal of Evaluation in Clinical Practice, 4,* 287-293.

O'Rourke, K., & Detsky, A. S. (1989). Meta-analysis in medical research: Strong encouragement for higher quality in individual research efforts. *Journal of Clinical Epidemiology, 42,* 1021-1024.

Orwin, R. G. (1994). Evaluating coding decisions. In H. Cooper & L. V. Hedges (Eds.), *Handbook of research synthesis* (pp. 139-162). New York: Russell Sage.

Orwin, R. G., & Cordray, D. S. (1985). Effects of deficient reporting on meta-analysis: A conceptual framework and reanalysis. *Psychological Bulletin, 97,* 134-147.

Osheroff, J. A., Buchanan, B. G., Bankowitz, R. A., Blumenfeld, B. H., & Miller, R. A. (1991). Physician's information needs: Analysis of questions asked during clinical teaching. *Annals of Internal Medicine, 114,* 576-581.

Owens, D. K. (1998). Spine update: Patient preferences and the development of practice guidelines. *Spine, 23,* 1073-1079.

Oxman, A. D. (1994). Checklists for review articles. *British Medical Journal, 309,* 648-651.

Oxman, A. D., Cook, D. J., & Guyatt, G. H. (1994). Users' guide to the medical literature: How to use an overview. *Journal of the American Medical Association, 272,* 1367-1371.

Oxman, A. D., & Guyatt, G. H. (1988). Guidelines for reading literature reviews. *Canadian Medical Association Journal, 138,* 697-703.

Oxman, A. D., & Guyatt, G. H. (1991). Validation of an index of the quality of review articles. *Journal of Clinical Epidemiology, 44,* 1271-1278.

Oxman, A. D., & Guyatt, G. H. (1993). The science of reviewing research. *The Annals of the New York Academy of Sciences, 703,* 125-134.

Oxman, A. D., Guyatt, G. H., Singer, J., Goldsmith, C. H., Hutchison, B. G., Milner, R. A., & Streiner, D. L. (1991). Agreement among reviewers of review articles. *Journal of Clinical Epidemiology, 44,* 91-98.

Oxman, A. D., Sackett, D. L., & Guyatt, G. H. (1993). Users' guides to the medical literature: I. How to get started. *Journal of the American Medical Association, 270,* 2093-2095.

Oxman, A. D., Thomson, M. A., Davis, D. A., & Haynes, R. B. (1995). No magic bullets: A systematic review of 102 trials of interventions to improve professional practice. *Canadian Medical Association Journal, 153,* 1423-1431.

Petersen, M. D., & White, D. L. (Eds.). (1989). *Health care of the elderly: An information sourcebook.* Newbury Park, CA: Sage.

Peterson, O. L., Andrews, L. P., Spain, R. S., & Greenberg, B. G. (1956). *An analytical study of North Carolina general practice—1953-1954.* Evanston, IL: American Medical Association.

Petticrew, M., Gilbody, S., & Sheldon, T. I. (1999). Assessing publication bias, and the importance of study quality. In M. Pettigrew (Ed.), *Second Symposium on Systematic Reviews: Beyond the basics.* Oxford, UK: Cochrane Library.

Pigott, T. D. (1994). Methods for handling missing data in research synthesis. In H. Cooper & L. V. Hedges (Eds.), *Handbook of research synthesis* (pp. 163-175). New York: Russell Sage.

Pitkin, R. M., & Branagan, M. A. (1998). Can the accuracy of abstracts be improved by providing specific instructions? A randomized controlled trial. *Journal of the American Medical Association, 280,* 267-269.

Pitkin, R. M., Branagan, M. A., & Burmeister, L. F. (1999). Accuracy of data in abstracts of published research articles. *Journal of the American Medical Association, 281,* 1110-1111.

Popper, K. R. (1968). *The logic of scientific discovery.* London: Hutchinson & Co.

Poynard, T., & Conn, H. O. (1985). The retrieval of randomized clinical trials in liver disease from the medical literature: A comparison of MEDLARS and manual methods. *Controlled Clinical Trials, 6,* 271-279.

Raczek, A. E., Ware, J. E., Bjorner, J. B., Gandek, B., Haley, S. M., Aaronson, N. K., Apolone, G., Bech, P., Brazier, J. E., Bullinge, R. M., & Sullivan, M. (1998). Comparison of Rasch and summated rating scales constructed from SF-36 physical functioning items in seven countries: Results from the IQOLA Project: International quality of life assessment. *Journal of Clinical Epidemiology, 51,* 1203-1214.

Raudenbush, S. W. (1984). Magnitude of teacher expectancy effects on pupil IQ as a function of the credibility of expectancy induction: A synthesis of findings from 18 experiments. *Journal of Educational Psychology, 76,* 85-97.

Raudenbush, S. W. (1994). Random effects models. In H. Cooper & L. V. Hedges (Eds.), *Handbook of research synthesis* (pp. 301-321). New York: Russell Sage.

Ravnskov, U. (1992). Cholesterol lowering trials in coronary heart disease: Frequency of citation and outcome. *British Medical Journal, 305,* 15-19.

Rhew, D. C., Riedinger, M. S., Sandhu, M., Bowers, C., Greengold, N., & Weingarten, S. R. (1998). A prospective, multicenter study of a pneumonia practice guideline. *Chest, 114,* 115-119.

Robins, J., Breslow, N. E., & Greenland, S. (1986). Estimators of the Mantel-Haenszel variance consistent in both sparse data and large-strata limiting models. *Biometrics, 42,* 311-323.

Rogers, E. M. (1983). *Diffusion of innovations* (3rd ed.). New York: Collier Macmillan.

Rosenthal, M. C. (1985). Bibliographic retrieval for the social and behavioral scientist. *Research in Higher Education, 22,* 315-333.

Rosenthal, M. C. (1994). The fugitive literature. In H. Cooper & L. V. Hedges (Eds.), *Handbook of research synthesis* (pp. 85-96). New York: Russell Sage.

Rosenthal, R. (1969). Interpersonal expectations: Effects of the experimenter's hypothesis. In R. Rosenthal & R. L. Rosnow (Eds.), *Artifact in behavioral research* (pp. 181-277). New York: Academic Press.

Rosenthal, R. (1979). The "file drawer problem" and tolerance for null results. *Psychological Bulletin, 86,* 638-641.

Rosenthal, R. (1984). *Meta-analytic procedures for social research.* Beverly Hills, CA: Sage.

Rosenthal, R. (1994). Parametric measures of effect size. In H. Cooper & L. V. Hedges (Eds.), *Handbook of research synthesis* (pp. 231-244). New York: Russell Sage.

Rosenthal, R. (1995). Writing meta-analytic reviews. *Psychological Bulletin, 118,* 183-192.

Rosenthal, R., & Rubin, D. B. (1978). Interpersonal expectancy effects: The first 345 studies. *The Behavioral and Brain Sciences, 3,* 377-386.

Rosenthal, R., & Rubin, D. B. (1980). Further issues in summarizing 345 studies of interpersonal expectancy. *The Behavioral and Brain Sciences, 3,* 475-476.

Rotman, B. L., Sullivan, A. N., McDonald, T. W., Brown, B. W., DeSmedt, P., Goodnature, D., Higgins, M. C., Suermondt, H. J., Young, C., & Owens, D. K. (1996). A randomized controlled trial of a computer-based physician workstation in an outpatient setting: Implementation barriers to outcome evaluation. *Journal of the American Medical Informatics Association, 3,* 340-348.

Runyon, R. P., & Haber, A. (1991). *Fundamentals of behavioral statistics.* New York: McGraw-Hill.

Russett, B. R. (1968). *Methodological and theoretical schools in international relations.* Unpublished paper, Yale University.

Sackett, D. L. (1997). A science for the art of consensus [Commentary]. *Journal of the National Cancer Institute, 89,* 1003-1005.

Sackett, D. L., & Haynes, R. B. (1997). Summarizing the effects of therapy: A new table and some more terms [Editorial]. *American College of Physicians Journal Club, 127,* A15-A16.

Sackett, D. L., Haynes, R. B., Guyatt, G. H., & Tugwell, P. (1991). *Clinical epidemiology: A basic science for clinical medicine* (2nd ed.). Boston: Little, Brown.

Sackett, D. L., Rosenberg, W. M. C., Gray, J. A. M., Haynes, R. B., & Richardson, W. S. (1996). Evidence based medicine: What it is and what it isn't. *British Medical Journal, 312,* 71-72.

Sackett, D. L., & Straus, S. (1998). On some clinically useful measures of the accuracy of diagnostic tests. *ACP Journal Club, 129,* A17-A19.

Sacks, H., Berrier, J., Reitman, D., Ancova-Berk, V. A., & Chalmers, T. C. (1987). Meta-analyses of randomized controlled trials. *New England Journal of Medicine, 316,* 450-455.

Sacks, H. S., Chalmers, T. C., & Smith, H. (1983). Sensitivity and specificity of clinical trials. *Archives of Internal Medicine, 143,* 753-755.

Sarasin, F. P. (1999). Decision analysis and the implementation of evidence-based medicine. *QJM: Monthly Journal of the Association of Physicians [United Kingdom—ours], 92,* 669-671.

Scherer, R. W., & Crawley, B. (1998). Reporting of randomized clinical trial descriptors and use of structured abstracts. *Journal of the American Medical Association, 280,* 269-272.

Sechrest, L., West, S. G., Phillips, M. A., Redner, R., & Yeaton, W. H. (1979). Some neglected problems in evaluation research: Strength and integrity of treatments. In L. Sechrest, S. G. West, M. A. Phillips, R. Rednor, & W. Yeaton (Eds.), *Evaluation studies review annual* (Vol. 4, pp. 15-60). Newbury Park, CA: Sage.

Shadish, W. R., Jr. (1992). Do family and marital psychotherapies change what people do? A meta-analysis of behavioral outcomes. In T. D. Cook, H. Cooper, D. S. Cordray, H. Hartmann, L. V. Hedges, R. J. Light, T. A. Louis, & F. Mosteller (Eds.), *Meta-analysis for explanation: A casebook* (pp. 129-208). New York: Russell Sage.

Shadish, W. R., Jr., & Haddock, C. K. (1994). Combining estimates of effects size. In H. Cooper & L. V. Hedges (Eds.), *Handbook of research synthesis* (pp. 261-284). New York: Russell Sage.

Shadish, W. R., Jr., & Sweeney, R. B. (1991). Mediators and moderators in meta-analysis: There's a reason we don't let dodo birds tell us which psychotherapies should have prizes. *Journal of Consulting and Clinical Psychology, 59,* 883-893.

Shapiro, D. W., Wenger, N. S., & Shapiro, M. F. (1994). The contributions of authors to multi-authored biomedical research papers. *Journal of the American Medical Association, 271,* 438-442.

Shekelle, P. G., & Schriger, D. L. (1996). Evaluating the use of the appropriateness method in the Agency for Health Care Policy and Research clinical practice guideline development process. *Health Services Research, 31,* 453-469.

Sheldon, T. A., Guyatt, G. H., & Haines, A. (1998). Getting research findings into practice: When to act on the evidence. *British Medical Journal, 317,* 139-142.

Silagy, C., Lancaster, T., Gray, S., & Fowler, G. (1995). The effectiveness of training health professionals to provide smoking cessation interventions: Systematic review of randomized controlled trials. *Quality Health Care, 3,* 193-198.

Slavin, R. E. (1986). Best evidence synthesis: An alternative to meta-analytic and traditional reviews. *Educational Researchers, 15,* 5-11.

Slavin, R. E. (1995). Best evidence synthesis: An intelligent alternative to meta-analysis. *Journal of Clinical Epidemiology, 48,* 9-18.

Smeeth, L., Haines, A., & Ebrahim, S. (1999). Numbers needed to treat derived from meta-analyses—sometimes informative, usually misleading. *British Medical Journal, 318,* 1548-1551.

Smith, C. B., Goldman, R. L., Martin, D. C., Williamson, J., Weir, C., Beauchamp, C., & Ashcraft, M. (1996). Overutilization of acute-care beds in Veterans Affairs hospitals. *Medical Care, 34,* 85-96.

Smith, R. (1996). Information in practice [Editorial]. *British Medical Journal, 313,*438.

Smith, R. (1998). Beyond conflict of interest. Transparency is the key [Editorial]. *British Medical Journal, 317,* 291-292.

Smith, T. C., Spiegelhalter, D. J., & Thomas, A. (1995). Bayesian approaches to random-effects meta-analysis: A comparative study. *Statistics in Medicine, 14,* 2685-2699.

Song, F., Eastweed, A., Gilbody, S., & Sutton, A. (1999). Methods for minimising publication bias: Review of methodological studies. In M. Pettigrew (Ed.), *Second Symposium on systematic reviews: Beyond the basics.* Oxford, UK: Cochrane Library.

Stead, W. W. (1998). Medical informatics: On the path toward universal truths. *Journal of the American Medical Informatics Association, 5,* 583-584.

Stock, W. A. (1994). Systematic coding for research synthesis. In H. Cooper & L. Hedges (Eds.), *Handbook of research synthesis.* New York: Russell Sage.

Stokes, T., Shukla, R., Schober, P., & Baker, R. (1998). A model for the development of evidence-based clinical guidelines at local level: The Leicestershire Genital Chlamydia Guidelines Project. *Journal of Evaluation in Clinical Practice, 4,* 325-338.

Straus, S. E., & Sackett, D. L. (1998). Using research findings in clinical practice. *British Medical Journal, 317,* 339-342.

Tabachnick, B., & Fidell, L. (1996). *Using multivariate statistics* (3rd ed.). New York: HarperCollins.

Tate, K. E., & Gardner, R. M. (1993). Development of an effective user interface for a computerized laboratory alerting system. *Proceedings of the 6th Annual IEEE Symposium: Computer-Based Medical Systems, 6,* 183-188.

Tate, K. E., Gardner, R. M., & Scherting, K. (1995). Nurses, pagers, and patient-specific criteria: Three keys to improved critical value reporting. *Symposium of the Computer Applications in Medical Care, 19,* 164-168.

Taveggia, T. C. (1974). Resolving research controversy through empirical cumulating: Toward reliable sociological knowledge. *Sociological Methods and Research, 2,* 395-407.

Thompson, D. F. (1993). Understanding financial conflicts of interest. *New England Journal of Medicine, 329,* 573-576.

Tierney, L. M., Jr., McPhee, S. K., & Papadakis, M. A. (Eds.). (1999). *Current medical diagnosis & treatment* (38th ed.). Stamford, CT: Appleton & Lange.

Tweedie, R. L., & Mengersen, K. L. (1995). Meta-analytic approaches to dose-response relationships, with application in studies of lung cancer and exposure to environmental tobacco smoke. *Statistics in Medicine, 14,* 545-569.

Unutzer, J., Simon, G., Belin, T. R., Datt, M., Katon, W., & Patrick, D. (2000). Care for depression in HMO patients aged 65 and older. *Journal of the American Geriatric Society, 48,* 871-878.

U.S. Department of Veterans Affairs, Center for Cooperative Study in Health Services. (1996). *Multi-site study of computer generated reminders to enhance adherence to standards of ambulatory care* (Study #9, final report). Washington, DC: Veterans Affairs Health Services Research and Development Services.

U.S. Department of Veterans Affairs, Office of Research and Development, Health Services Research and Development Service, Management Decision and Research Center. (1998). *Clinical practice guidelines: Primer.* Unpublished manuscript, Veterans Affairs Health Services Research and Development Services, Washington, DC.

Van Weel, C., & Knotterus, J. A. (1999). Evidence and primary care: Evidence-based interventions and comprehensive treatment. *Lancet, 353,* 916-918.

Vevea, J. L., & Hedges, L. V. A. (1995). A general linear model for estimating size in the presence of publication bias. *Psychometrika, 60,* 419-435.

Waddell, D. L. (1991). The effects of continuing education on nursing practice: A meta-analysis. *Journal of Continuing Education in Nursing, 22,* 113-118.

Ware, J. E., Jr. (1998, July). *Measuring health: Integrating measurement and medical practice.* Paper presented at the meeting of the American Medical Group Association Consortia, Jackson Hole, WY.

Ware, J. E., Jr., Keller, S. D., Hatoum, H. T., & Kong, S. X. (1999). The SF-36 Arthritis-Specific Health Index (ASHI): I. Development and cross-validation of scoring algorithms. *Medical Care, 37*(Suppl. 5), MS40-MS50.

Ware, J. E., Jr., & Sherbourne, C. D. (1992). The MOS 36 Item Short Form Health Survey (SF-36): I. Conceptual framework and item selection. *Medical Care, 30,* 473-483.

Ware, J. E., Jr., & Williams, R. G. (1975). The Dr. Fox effect: A study of lecturer effectiveness and ratings of instruction. *Journal of Medical Education, 50,* 149-156.

Ware, N. C., Tugenbert, T., Dickey, B., & McHorney, C. A. (1999). An ethnographic study of the meaning of continuity of care in the mental health services. *Psychiatric Services, 50,* 395-400.

Weingarten, S., Conner, L., Riedinger, M., Alter, A., Brien, W., & Ellrodt, A. G. (1995). Total knee replacement: A guideline to reduce postoperative length of stay. *Western Journal of Medicine, 163,* 26-30.

Weingarten, S., Ellrodt, A. G., Riedinger, M. S., & Huang, C. (1993). A computerized expert system for outcome-validated medical practice guidelines. *Proceedings of the Annual Symposium of Computer Applications in Medical Care,* 198-202.

Weingarten, S., Riedinger, M., Conner, L., Johnson, B., & Ellrodt, A. G. (1994). Reducing lengths of stay in the coronary care unit with a practice guideline for patients with congestive heart failure: Insights from a controlled clinical trial. *Medical Care, 32,* 1232-1243.

Weingarten, S., Riedinger, M. S., Hobson, P., Noah, M. S., Johnson, B., Giugliano, G., Norian, J., Belman, M. J., & Ellrodt, A. G. (1996). Evaluation of a pneumonia practice guideline in an interventional trial. *American Journal of Respiratory Critical Care Medicine, 153,* 1110-1115.

Weingarten, S., Stone, E., Green, A., Pelter, M., Nessim, S., Huang, H., & Kristopaitis, R. (1995). A study of patient satisfaction and adherence to preventive care practice guidelines. *American Journal of Medicine, 99,* 590-596.

Weir, C., Lincoln, M., Roscoe, D., & Moreshead, G. (1995). Successful implementation of an integrated physician order entry application: A systems perspective. *Annual Symposium of Computer Applications in Medical Care,* 790-794.

Wilcox, L. J. (1998). Authorship: The coin of the realm, the source of complaints. *Journal of the American Medical Association, 280,* 216-217.

Williamson, J. W. (1973). Williamson on effectiveness and efficiency. *International Journal of Health Services, 3,* 105-110.

Williamson, J. W. (1977). *Improving medical practice and health care: A bibliographic guide to information management in quality assurance and continuing education.* Cambridge, MA: Ballinger.

Williamson, J. W. (1978a). *Assessing and improving health care outcomes: The health accounting approach to quality assurance.* Cambridge, MA: Ballinger.

Williamson, J. W. (1978b). Formulating priorities for quality assurance activity: Description of a method and its applications. *Journal of the American Medical Association, 239,* 631-637.

Williamson, J. W. (1991). Medical quality management systems in perspective. In J. B. Couch (Ed.), *Health care quality management for the 21st century* (pp. 23-74). Tampa, FL: Hillsboro.

Williamson, J. W., Alexander, M., & Miller, G. E. (1968). Priorities in patient-care research and continuing medical education. *Journal of the American Medical Association, 204,* 303-308.

Williamson, J. W., German, P. S., Weiss, R., Skinner, E. A., & Bowes, F., III. (1989). Health science information management and continuing education of physicians: A survey of U.S. primary care practitioners and their opinion leaders. *Annals of Internal Medicine, 110,* 151-160.

Williamson, J. W., Goldschmidt, P. G., & Colton, T. (1986). The quality of medical literature: An analysis of validation assessments. In J. Bailar III & F. Mosteller (Eds.), *Medical uses of statistics* (pp. 370-391). Waltham, MA: New England Journal of Medicine Books.

Wilson, L., & Goldschmidt, P. (1995). *Quality management in health care.* Sydney, Australia: McGraw-Hill.

Winker, M. A. (1999). The need for concrete improvement in abstract quality. *Journal of the American Medical Association, 281,* 1129-1130.

Wise, J. (1998). Links to tobacco industry influences review conclusions. *British Medical Journal, 316,* 1554.

Wolf, F. M., Friedman, C. P., Elstein, A. S., Miller, J. G., Murphy, G. C., Heckerling, P., Fine, P., Miller, T., Sisson, J., Barlas, S., Capitano, A., Ng, M., & Franz, T. (1997). Changes in diagnostic decision-making after a computerized decision support consultation based on perceptions of need and helpfulness: A preliminary report. *Proceedings of the American Medical Informatics Association Annual Fall Symposium,* 263-637.

Wolfe, S. M. (Ed.). (1999). Dangerous drug information on the Internet from Aetna/US Healthcare and Johns Hopkins. *Public Citizen Health Research Group Health Letter, 15,* 10-11.

Woods, D., & Trewheellar, K. (1998). Medline and Embase complement each other in literature searches [Letter]. *British Medical Journal, 316,* 1166.

Woolf, S. H. (1993). Practice guidelines: A new reality in medicine: III. Impact on patient care. *Archives of Internal Medicine, 153,* 2646-2655.

Woolf, S. H. (1998). Do clinical practice guidelines define good medical care? The need for good science and the disclosure of uncertainty when defining "best practices." *Chest, 113*(Suppl. 3), 166S-171S.

Woolf, S. H., Grol, R., Hutchinson, A., Eccles, M., & Grimshaw, J. (1999). Potential benefits, limitations, and harms of clinical guidelines. *British Medical Journal, 318,* 527-530.

Worrall, G., Chaulk, P., & Freake, D. (1997). The effects of clinical practice guidelines on patient outcomes in primary care: A systematic review. *Canadian Medical Association Journal, 156,* 1705-1712.

Wortman, P. M. (1994). Judging research quality. In H. Cooper & L. V. Hedges (Eds.), *Handbook of research synthesis* (pp. 97-109). New York: Russell Sage.

Wortman, P. M., & Bryant, F. B. (1985). School desegregation and black achievement: An integrative review. *Sociological Methods and Research, 13,* 289-324.

Wortman, P. M., Smyth, J. M., Langenbrunner, J. C., & Yeaton, W. H. (1998). Consensus among experts and research synthesis: A comparison of methods. *International Journal of Technology Assessment in Health Care, 14,* 109-122.

Wortman, P. M., & Yeaton, W. H. (1987). Using research synthesis in medical technology assessment. *International Journal of Technology Assessment in Health Care, 3,* 509-522.

Yates, F., & Cochran, W. G. (1938). The analysis of groups of experiments. *Journal of Agricultural Science, 28,* 556-580.

Yeaton, W. H., & Wortman, P. M. (1991). *On the reliability of meta-analytic reviews: The role of intercoder agreement.* Unpublished manuscript.

Zelen, M. (1971). The analysis of several 2×2 contingency tables. *Biometrika, 58,* 129-137.

Other References of Note

The following references were not cited in the text of this book. These citations are often for older works, including a few classics, references to systematic reviews by nonphysician clinical professionals, and editorials, commentary, or other less mature studies of synthesis methods. If a single reference is relevant to different chapters, it will be repeated in each.

Chapter 1

Chalmers, I., Dickersin, K., & Chalmers, T. C. (1992). Getting to grips with Archie Cochrane's agenda. *British Medical Journal, 305,* 786-788.

Guyatt, G. H., Meade, M. O., Jaeschke, R. Z., Cook, D. J., & Haynes, R. B. (2000). Practitioners of evidence based care: Not all clinicians need to appraise evidence from scratch but all need some skills [Editorial]. *British Medical Journal, 320,* 954-955.

Lightner, N. J., Bose, I., & Salvendy, G. (1996). What is wrong with the World-Wide Web? A diagnosis of some problems and prescription of some remedies. *Ergonomics, 39,* 995-1004.

Mullins, N. C. (1968, August). *Social origins of an invisible college: The phage group.* Paper presented to the annual meeting of the American Sociological Association, Boston.

Santos, R., Cifaldi, M., Gregory, C., & Seitz, P. (1999). Economic outcomes of a targeted intervention program: The costs of treating allergic rhinitis patients. *American Journal of Managed Care, 5*(Suppl. 4), S225-S234.

Stevens, L. (2000, April 23). Healthcare turns to the Web. *InternetWeek Online* [Online]. Available: internetwk.com/lead/lead042400.htm

Wachter, K. W. (1988). Disturbed by meta-analysis? *Science, 241,* 1407-1408.

Warren, K. S. (Ed.). (1981). *Coping with the biomedical literature: A primer for the scientist and the clinician.* New York, NY: Praeger.

Yeaton, W. H., Smith, D., & Rogers, K. (1990). Evaluating understanding of popular press reports of health research. *Health Education Quarterly, 17,* 223-234.

Chapter 2

Chalmers, I., Dickersin, K., & Chalmers, T. C. (1992). Getting to grips with Archie Cochrane's agenda. *British Medical Journal, 305,* 786-788.

Christensen, C., & Larson, J. R. (1993). Collaborative medical decision making. *Medical Decision Making, 13,* 339-346.

Davis, J. H., & Hinsz, V. B. (1982). Current research problems in group performance and group dynamics. In H. Brandstätter, J. H. Davis, & G. Stocker-Kreichgauer (Eds.), *Group decision making* (pp. 1-20). San Diego: Academic Press.

Deutsch, M., & Gerard, H. B. (1955). A study of normative and informal social influence on individual judgment. *Journal of Abnormal and Social Psychology, 51,* 629-636.

Einhorn, H. J., Hogarth, R. M., & Klempner, E. (1977). Quality of group judgment. *Psychological Bulletin, 84,* 158-172.

Elstein, A. S., Shulman, L. S., & Spraka, S. A. (1978). *Medical problem solving: An analysis of clinical reasoning.* Cambridge, MA: Harvard University Press.

Greenland, S. (1994). Invited commentary: A critical look at some popular meta-analytic methods. *American Journal of Epidemiology, 140,* 290-296.

Guzzo, R. A., Jackson, S. E., & Katzell, R. A. (1986). Meta-analysis analysis. In L. L. Cummings & B. M. Staw (Eds.), *Research in organizational behavior* (Vol. 9). Greenwich, CT: JAI.

Hackman, J. R., & Morris, C. G. (1975). Group tasks, group interaction process and group performance effectiveness: A review and proposed integration. In L. Berkowitz (Ed.), *Advances in experimental social psychology* (Vol. 8, pp. 45-99). New York: Academic Press.

Harmon, J., & Rohrbaugh, J. (1990). Social judgment analysis and small group decision making: Cognitive feedback effects on individual and collective performance. *Organizational Behavior and Human Decision Processes, 46,* 34-54.

Hill, G. W. (1982). Group versus individual performance: Are N + 1 heads better than one? *Psychological Bulletin, 91*(3), 517-539.

Hirokawa, R. Y. (1990). The role of communication in group decision-making efficacy: A task-contingency perspective. *Small Group Research, 21*(2), 190-204.

Hogarth, R. M. (1978). A note on aggregating opinions. *Organizational Behavior and Human Performance, 2,* 40-46.

Institute of Medicine, Council on Health Care Technology. (1990). *Consensus development at the NIH: Improving the program* [Report of a study]. Washington, DC: National Academy Press.

Ioannidis, J. P., & Lau, J. (1996). On meta-analyses of meta-analyses [Letter]. *Lancet, 348,* 756.

Langbein, L. I., & Lichtman, A. J. (1978). *Ecological inference.* Beverly Hills, CA: Sage.

Larson, J. R., Jr., Foster-Fishman, P. G., & Keys, C. B. (1992, August). *Information sharing in decision-making groups.* Paper presented at the meeting of the American Psychological Association, Washington, DC.

Libby, R., & Blashfield, R. K. (1978). Performance of a composite as a function of the number of judges. *Organizational Behavior and Human Performance, 21,* 121-129.

Libby, R., Trotman, K. T., & Zimmer, I. (1987). Member variation, recognition of expertise, and group performance. *Journal of Applied Psychology, 72,* 81-87.

Lilienfeld, A. M., & Lilienfeld, D. E. (1980). *Foundations of epidemiology* (2nd ed.). New York: Oxford University Press.

Lomas, A., Anderson, G., Enkin, M., Vayda, E., Roberts, R., & MacKinnon, B. (1988). The role of evidence in the consensus process: Results from a Canadian consensus exercise. *Journal of the American Medical Association, 259,* 3001-3005.

McGrath, J. E. (1984). *Groups: Interaction and performance.* Englewood Cliffs, NJ: Prentice Hall.

McNemar, Q. (1969). *Psychological statistics* (4th ed.). New York: John Wiley.

Morgenstern, H. (1982). Uses of ecologic analysis in epidemiologic research. *American Journal of Public Health, 72,* 1336-1344.

Petitti, D. B. (1994). *Meta-analysis, decision analysis and cost-effectiveness analysis: Methods for quantitative synthesis in medicine.* New York: Oxford University Press.

Richardson, W. S., Wilson, M. C., Nishikawa, J., & Hayward, R. S. A. (1995, November/December). The well-built clinical question: A key to evidence-based decisions. *American College of Physicians Journal Club,* pp. A12-A13.

Shaw, M. E. (Ed.). (1976). *Group dynamics: The psychology of small group behavior* (2nd ed.). New York: McGraw-Hill.

Sniezek, J. A., & Henry, R. A. (1989). Accuracy and confidence in group judgment. *Organizational Behavior and Human Decision Processes, 43,* 1-28.

Stasser, G. (1988). Computer simulation as a research tool: The DISCUSS model of group decision making. *Journal of Experimental Social Psychology, 24,* 393-422.

Stasser, G. (1991). *Facilitating the use of unshared information in decision making groups.* Paper presented at the 63rd annual meeting of the Midwestern Psychological Association, Chicago.

Stasser, G., Taylor, L. A., & Hanna, C. (1989). Information sampling in structured and unstructured discussion of three- and six-person groups. *Journal of Personality and Social Psychology, 57,* 67-78.

Stasser, G., & Titus, W. (1987). Effects of information load and percentage of shared information on the dissemination of unshared information during group discussion. *Journal of Personality and Social Psychology, 53,* 81-93.

Steiner, I. D. (1972). *Group process and productivity.* New York: Academic Press.

Stumpf, S. A., Freedman, R. D., & Zand, D. E. (1979). Judgmental decisions: A study of interactions among group membership, group functioning, and the decision situation. *Academy of Management Journal, 22,* 765-782.

Thompson, S. G., & Pocock, S. J. (1991). Can meta-analyses be trusted? *Lancet, 338,* 1127-1130.

Wegner, D. M. (1987). Transactive memory: A contemporary analysis of the group mind. In B. Mullen & G. R. Goethals (Eds.), *Theories of group behavior* (pp. 185-208). New York: Springer-Verlag.

Chapter 3

Joy, A. (1989). Using Biblio-link . . . for those other databases. *Database, 12*(1), 26-29.

Knauth, M. (1989). Bibliographies made easy: A look at Pro-Cite. *Computers in Libraries, 9,* 22-24.

Kost, G. J. (1986). Application of program evaluation and review technic (PERT) to laboratory research and development planning. *American Journal of Clinical Pathology, 86,* 186-192.

Novallo, A., Alampi, M., & Nolan, K. L. (Eds.). (1997). *Gale directory of databases: Vol. 1. Online databases.* Detroit, MI: Gale.

Novallo, A., Alampi, M., & Nolan, K. L. (Eds.). (1997). *Gale directory of databases: Vol. 2. CD-ROM, diskette, magnetic tape, handheld, and batch access database products.* Detroit, MI: Gale.

Reed, J. G., & Baxter, P. M. (1994). Using reference databases. In H. Cooper & L. V. Hedges (Eds.), *Handbook of research synthesis* (pp. 57-70). New York: Russell Sage.

Silagy, C. (1993). Developing a register of randomized controlled trials in primary care. *British Medical Journal, 306,* 897-900.

Spilker, B., Simpson, R. L., Jr., & Tilson, H. H. (1992). Quality of life bibliography and indexes, 1991 update. *Journal of Clinical Research and Pharmacoepidemiology, 6,* 205-266.

Whiteley, S. (Ed.). (1994). *The American Library Association guide to information access: A complete research handbook and directory.* New York: Random House.

Chapter 5

Counsell, C., & Fraser, H. (1994). Identifying relevant studies for systematic reviews [Letter]. *British Medical Journal, 310,* 126.

Crumley, E. (2000). Canadian health evidence. *Health Connections, 2*(2&3), 2.

Davidoff, F. (1997). Where's the bias? *Annals of Internal Medicine, 126,* 986-988.

Joswick, K. E. (1994). Getting the most from PsycLIT: Recommendations for searching. *Teaching of Psychology, 21,* 49-53.

Joy, A. (1989). Using Biblio-link . . . for those other databases. *Database, 12*(1), 26-29.

Mullins, N. C. (1968, August). *Social origins of an invisible college: The phage group.* Paper presented at the annual meeting of the American Sociological Association, Boston.

Reed, J. G., & Baxter, P. M. (1994). Using reference databases. In H. Cooper & L. V. Hedges (Eds.), *Handbook of research synthesis* (pp. 57-70). New York: Russell Sage.

Silagy, C. (1993). Developing a register of randomized controlled trials in primary care. *British Medical Journal, 306,* 897-900.

Smith, B. J., Darzins, P. J., Quinn, M., & Heller, R. F. (1992). Modern methods of searching the medical literature. *Medical Journal of Australia, 157,* 603-611.

Spilker, B., Simpson, R. L., Jr., & Tilson, H. H. (1992). Quality of life bibliography and indexes, 1991 update. *Journal of Clinical Research and Pharmacoepidemiology, 6,* 205-266.

Warren, K. S. (Ed.). (1981). *Coping with the biomedical literature: A primer for the scientist and the clinician.* New York: Praeger.

White, H. D. (1994). Scientific communication and literature retrieval. In H. Cooper & L. V. Hedges (Eds.), *Handbook of research synthesis.* New York: Russell Sage.

Whiteley, S. (Ed.). (1994). *The American Library Association guide to information access: A complete research handbook and directory.* New York: Random House.

Chapter 6

Joswick, K. E. (1994). Getting the most from PsycLIT: Recommendations for searching. *Teaching of Psychology, 21,* 49-53.

Smith, B. J., Darzins, P. J., Quinn, M., & Heller, R. F. (1992). Modern methods of searching the medical literature. *Medical Journal of Australia, 157,* 603-611.

Whiteley, S. (Ed.). (1994). *The American Library Association guide to information access: A complete research handbook and directory.* New York: Random House.

Chapter 9

Davidoff, F. (1997). Where's the bias? *Annals of Internal Medicine, 126,* 986-988.

Green, S., Fleming, T. R., & Emerson, S. (1987). Effects on overviews of early stopping rules for clinical trials. *Statistics in Medicine, 6,* 361-367.

Jadad, A. R., & Moore, R. A. (1996). Assessing the quality of reports of randomized clinical trials: Is blinding necessary? *Controlled Clinical Trials, 17,* 1-12.

Lilienfeld, A. M., & Lilienfeld, D. E. (1980). *Foundations of epidemiology* (2nd ed.). New York: Oxford University Press.

Sacks, H., Chalmers, T. C., & Smith, H. J. (1982). Randomized versus historical controls for clinical trials. *American Journal of Medicine, 72,* 233-240.

Schulz, K. F., Chalmers, I., Hayes, R. J., & Altman, D. G. (1995). Empirical evidence of bias: Dimensions of methodological quality associated with estimates of treatment effects in controlled trials. *Journal of the American Medical Association, 273,* 408-412.

Smith, S. J., Caudill, S. P., Steinberg, K. K., & Thacker, S. B. (1995). On combining dose-response data from epidemiological studies by meta-analysis. *Statistics in Medicine, 14,* 531-544.

Villar, J., Carroli, G., & Belizan, J. M. (1995). Predictive ability of meta-analyses of random-ised controlled trials. *Lancet, 345,* 772-776.

Yeaton, W. H., Langenbrunner, J. C., Smyth, J. M., & Wortman, P. M. (1995). Exploratory research synthesis: Methodological considerations for addressing limitations in data quality. *Evaluation in the Health Professions, 18,* 283-303.

Chapter 10

Davidoff, F. (1997). Where's the bias? *Annals of Internal Medicine, 126,* 986-988.

Chapter 12

Fagan, T. J. (1975). Nomogram for Bayes's theorem. *New England Journal of Medicine, 293,* 257.
Siegel, S., & Castellan, N. J., Jr. (1988). *Nonparametric statistics for the behavioral sciences* (2nd ed.). New York: McGraw-Hill.

Chapter 13

Eddy, D. M., Hasselblad, V., & Shachter, R. (1991). *Meta-analysis by the confidence profile method: The statistical synthesis of evidence.* San Diego, CA: Academic Press.
Fagan, T. J. (1975). Nomogram for Bayes's theorem. *New England Journal of Medicine, 293,* 257.
Glesser, L. J., & Olkin, I. (1994). Stochastically dependent effect sizes. In H. Cooper & L. V. Hedges (Eds.), *Handbook of research synthesis* (pp. 261-284). New York: Russell Sage.
Greenland, S. (1994). Invited commentary: A critical look at some popular meta-analytic methods. *American Journal of Epidemiology, 140,* 290-296.
Greenland, S., & Longnecker, M. P. (1992). Methods for trend estimation from summarized dose-response data, with applications to meta-analysis. *American Journal of Epidemiology, 135,* 1301-1309.
Greenland, S., & Salvan, A. (1990). Bias in the one-step method for pooling study results. *Statistics in Medicine, 9,* 247-252.
Guzzo, R. A., Jackson, S. E., & Katzell, R. A. (1986). Meta-analysis analysis. In L. L. Cummings & B. M. Staw (Eds.), *Research in organizational behavior* (Vol. 9). Greenwich, CT: JAI.
Ioannidis, J. P., & Lau, J. (1996). On meta-analyses of meta-analyses [Letter]. *Lancet, 348,* 756.
Jadad, A. R., & Moore, R. A. (1996). Assessing the quality of reports of randomized clinical trials: Is blinding necessary? *Controlled Clinical Trials, 17,* 1-12.
Langbein, L. I., & Lichtman, A. J. (1978). *Ecological inference.* Beverly Hills, CA: Sage.
Oxman, A. D., & Guyatt, G. H. (1992). A consumer's guide to subgroup analyses. *Annals of Internal Medicine, 116,* 78-84.
Petitti, D. B. (1994). *Meta-analysis, decision analysis and cost-effectiveness analysis: Methods for quantitative synthesis in medicine.* New York: Oxford University Press.

Smith, S. J., Caudill, S. P., Steinberg, K. K., & Thacker, S. B. (1995). On combining dose-response data from epidemiological studies by meta-analysis. *Statistics in Medicine, 14,* 531-544.

Thompson, S. G., & Pocock, S. J. (1991). Can meta-analyses be trusted? *Lancet, 338,* 1127-1130.

Wachter, K. W. (1988). Disturbed by meta-analysis? *Science, 241,* 1407-1408.

Villar, J., Carroli, G., & Belizan, J. M. (1995). Predictive ability of meta-analyses of randomised controlled trials. *Lancet, 345,* 772-776.

Yeaton, W. H., Langenbrunner, J. C., Smyth, J. M., & Wortman, P. M. (1995). Exploratory research synthesis: Methodological considerations for addressing limitations in data quality. *Evaluation in the Health Professions, 18,* 283-303.

Chapter 14

Eddy, D. M., Hasselblad, V., & Shachter, R. (1991). *Meta-analysis by the confidence profile method: The statistical synthesis of evidence.* San Diego, CA: Academic Press.

Glesser, L. J., & Olkin, I. (1994). Stochastically dependent effect sizes. In H. Cooper & L. V. Hedges (Eds.), *Handbook of research synthesis* (pp. 261-284). New York: Russell Sage.

Greenland, S., & Salvan, A. (1990). Bias in the one-step method for pooling study results. *Statistics in Medicine, 9,* 247-252.

Guzzo, R. A., Jackson, S. E., & Katzell, R. A. (1986). Meta-analysis analysis. In L. L. Cummings & B. M. Staw (Eds.), *Research in organizational behavior* (Vol. 9). Greenwich, CT: JAI.

Chapter 15

Davidoff, F. (1997). Where's the bias? *Annals of Internal Medicine, 126,* 986-988.

Chapter 16

Galbraith, R. (1988). A note on graphical presentation of estimated odds ratios from several clinical trials. *Statistics in Medicine, 7,* 889-894.

Haynes, R. B., Mulrow, C. D., Huth, E. J., Altman, D. G., & Gardner, M. J. (1990). More informative abstracts revisited. *Annals of Internal Medicine, 113,* 69-76.

Rennie, D. (1996). How to report randomized controlled trials: The CONSORT statement. *Journal of the American Medical Association, 276,* 649.

White, H. D. (1994). Scientific communication and literature retrieval. In H. Cooper & L. V. Hedges (Eds.), *Handbook of research synthesis.* New York: Russell Sage.

Yeaton, W. H., Smith, D., & Rogers, K. (1990). Evaluating understanding of popular press reports of health research. *Health Education Quarterly, 17,* 223-234.

Chapter 17

Burroughs, C. E. (1994). The use of practice guidelines in Wisconsin for liability protection. *Wisconsin Medical Journal, 93,* 69-75.

Chalmers, I., Dickersin, K., & Chalmers, T. C. (1992). Getting to grips with Archie Cochrane's agenda. *British Medical Journal, 305,* 786-788.

Crumley, E. (2000). Canadian health evidence. *Health Connections, 2*(2&3), 2.

Curry, L. (1993). Continuing medical education: The next steps. *Journal of the American Podiatrist Medical Association, 83,* 355-361.

Deutsch, M., & Gerard, H. B. (1955). A study of normative and informal social influence on individual judgment. *Journal of Abnormal and Social Psychology, 51,* 629-636.

Ebel, M. H., Messimer, S. R., & Barry, H. C. (1999). Putting computer-based evidence in the hands of clinicians. *Journal of the American Medical Association, 281,* 1171-1172.

Elstein, A. S., Shulman, L. S., & Spraka, S. A. (1978). *Medical problem solving: An analysis of clinical reasoning.* Cambridge, MA: Harvard University Press.

Galbraith, R. (1988). A note on graphical presentation of estimated odds ratios from several clinical trials. *Statistics in Medicine, 7,* 889-894.

Guyatt, G. H., Meade, M. O., Jaeschke, R. Z., Cook, D. J., & Haynes, R. B. (2000). Practitioners of evidence based care: Not all clinicians need to appraise evidence from scratch but all need some skills [Editorial]. *British Medical Journal, 320,* 954-955.

Harmon, J., & Rohrbaugh, J. (1990). Social judgment analysis and small group decision making: Cognitive feedback effects on individual and collective performance. *Organizational Behavior and Human Decision Processes, 46,* 34-54.

Hirokawa, R. Y. (1990). The role of communication in group decision-making efficacy: A task-contingency perspective. *Small Group Research, 21*(2), 190-204.

Hofmann, P. A. (1993). Critical path method: An important tool for coordinating clinical care. *Joint Commission Journal of Quality Improvement, 19,* 235-246.

Laupacis, A., Sackett, D. L., & Roberts, R. S. (1988). An assessment of clinically useful measures of the consequences of treatment. *New England Journal of Medicine, 318,* 1728-1733.

Lightner, N. J., Bose, I., & Salvendy, G. (1996). What is wrong with the World-Wide Web? A diagnosis of some problems and prescription of some remedies. *Ergonomics, 39,* 995-1004.

Lilford, R. J., & Braunholtz, D. (1996). The statistical basis of public policy: A paradigm shift is overdue. *British Medical Journal, 313,* 603-607.

Lomas, A., Anderson, G., Enkin, M., Vayda, E., Roberts, R., & MacKinnon, B. (1988). The role of evidence in the consensus process: Results from a Canadian consensus exercise. *Journal of the American Medical Association, 259,* 3001-3005.

Ray-Coquard, I., Philip, T., Lehmann, M., Fervers, B., Farsi, F., & Chauvin, F. (1997). Impact of a clinical guidelines program for breast and colon cancer in a French cancer center. *Journal of the American Medical Association, 278,* 1591-1595.

Richardson, W. S., Wilson, M. C., Nishikawa, J., & Hayward, R. S. A. (1995, November/December). The well-built clinical question: A key to evidence-based decisions. *American College of Physicians Journal Club,* pp. A12-A13.

Sackett, D. L., & Cook, R. J. (1994). Understanding clinical trials: What measures of efficacy should journal articles provide busy clinicians? *British Medical Journal, 309,* 755-756.

Santos, R., Cifaldi, M., Gregory, C., & Seitz, P. (1999). Economic outcomes of a targeted intervention program: The costs of treating allergic rhinitis patients. *American Journal of Managed Care, 5*(Suppl. 4), S225-S234.

Steiner, I. D. (1972). *Group process and productivity.* New York: Academic Press.

Stevens, L. (2000, April 23). Healthcare turns to the Web. *InternetWeek Online* [Online]. Available: internetwk.com/lead/lead042400.htm

Turner, C. W., Weir, C., DiGregorio, V., Morf, C., Thraen, I., & Williamson, J. W. (1996). *Aminoglycoside therapeutic drug monitoring: A meta-analysis.* Technical report, Abbott Pharmaceuticals.

Wachter, K. W. (1988). Disturbed by meta-analysis? *Science, 241,* 1407-1408.

Waddell, D. L., & Blankenship, J. C. (1994). Answer changing: A meta-analysis of the prevalence and patterns. *Journal of Continuing Education in Nursing, 25,* 155-158.

Williamson, J. W., & Van Nieuwenhuijzen, M. G. (1974). Health benefit analysis: An application in industrial absenteeism. *Journal of Occupational Medicine, 16,* 229-233.

Yeaton, W. H., Smith, D., & Rogers, K. (1990). Evaluating understanding of popular press reports of health research. *Health Education Quarterly, 17,* 223-234.

Index

Synopsis of Compendium

About the Authors

John W. Williamson is a graduate of the University of California at San Francisco (UCSF) School of Medicine. He was a professor at the Johns Hopkins School of Public Health for nearly 19 years, including 2 years as a visiting professor at the Harvard School of Public Health. Moving to the University of Utah in 1984, he was Professor of Medicine and Professor of Medical Informatics in the School of Medicine. He is currently Professor Emeritus at the University of Utah. During the past 40 years, Dr. Williamson has worked to integrate the areas of continuing education, health services research, and medical informatics as a foundation for future clinical outcomes assessment and improvement. Dr. Williamson's concepts for healthcare outcomes improvement have been applied throughout the world in more than 40 national quality improvement resource centers, developed under the auspices of the World Health Organization's Collaboration Center for Quality Assurance in Health Care, headquartered in the Netherlands. He served on U.S. presidential commissions and committees under four U.S. presidents, including the 1993 "Interagency Task Force for Health Care Reform" led by Hillary Rodham Clinton. He also served as a quality improvement adviser to staff of the U.S. Senate Committee on Veterans Affairs and was a member of the Utah Governor's Commission that facilitated passage of H.B. 305 on health care reform in his home state. Dr. Williamson's honors and awards include his being the recipient of the American College of Medical Quality's J. Shue Hammon, M.D. Award for outstanding contributions to quality assurance; the American Board of Medical Examiners Hubbard Award for excellence in the field of evaluation in medicine; the first Career Quality Achievement Award from the Department of Veterans Affairs; the Utah Medical Association's Distinguished Service Award, cited as one who "made a difference in medicine"; and the 2000 Ernest A. Codman Award sponsored by the Joint Commission on Accreditation of Healthcare Organizations (JCAHO), recognizing his career-long contribution to use performance measures to achieve quality improvement. He has had a deep interest in health science information synthesis throughout his career. This focus is evident from his research report in the 1968 *Journal of the American Medical Association* article titled "Priorities in Patient Care Research and Continuing Education"; his 1977 book titled *Improving Medical Practice and Health Care: A Bibliographic Guide to Information Management in Quality Assurance and Continuing Education; and* his present book, *Healthcare Informatics and Information Synthesis: Generating and Applying Information for Improving Outcomes.*

Charlene R. Weir is currently the Associate Director for Education and Evaluation for the SLC Geriatric Research Center. She received her B.S. degree from the University of Utah, Salt Lake City Utah, in Nursing and Psychology in 1977. She received a master's degree in nursing from the University of Texas at Austin in 1986 and a Ph.D. in psychology from the University of Utah in 1993. Since 1992, she has worked for the Veterans Health Administration in a variety of positions ranging from the Office of Quality Management, the Office Information Services, and the Medical Inspector's Office. She has assisted in conducting several formal information syntheses for internal use of the VA and in applied clinical practice. In addition, she holds adjunct faculty positions at the College of Nursing and Department of Medical Informatics at the University of Utah. She has taught classes in research design, introduction to statistics, clinical informatics, and quality management. Her research interests are in the area of healthcare decision making, quality management, motivation, and behavior change.

Charles W. Turner received his B.S. degree from the University of California, Berkeley, in 1965 where he studied psychology, mathematics, and physics. He received his Ph.D. in psychology from the University of Wisconsin in 1970. He has been a faculty member in the Department of Psychology at the University of Utah since 1970. A major focus of Dr. Turner's work has been in advanced statistical or quantitative methods. He has taught a variety of graduate-level courses in multiple regression, factor analysis, multivariate analysis of variance, structural equations modeling, and time-series modeling at the University of Utah. He was a faculty member of the Master's Degree Program in Applied Statistics at the University of Utah. His early research interests have included the study of aggressive and violent behaviors. This work led to the examination of Type A and hostility as risk factors for cardiovascular disease. This work led to his first exposure to meta-analysis in a paper that examined Type A behavior and cardiovascular disease. One of his major research interests has been family-based interventions for the prevention and treatment of antisocial behavior. This research has focused on the clinical decision-making processes during the intervention settings. His more recent research interest used medical informatics approaches to test and enhance clinical decision-making processes in medicine. As part of this work, Dr. Turner has participated in a number of meta-analytic investigations. He currently is the Project Director for the Center for Substance Abuse Prevention's Data Coordinating Center (CSAP DCC). The CSAP DCC has a major responsibility for conducting cross-program analyses at CSAP using many standard meta-analytic methods.

Michael J. Lincoln is currently Adjunct Associate Professor in the Department of Medical Informatics at the University of Utah Medical Center. His primary research interests are vocabulary development for electronic medical records and development of graphic user interfaces for clinicians. His interests include the design and implementation of undergraduate and postgraduate medical curricula to meet science information needs using informatics appliances and resources. Dr. Lincoln participates in the Government Computerized Patient Record Initiative (GCPR) for the Department of Veterans Affairs.

Keely M. W. Cofrin received her Ph.D. in social psychology from the University of Utah in 1998. She specialized in medical decision making and examined the factors that influence the ways in which physicians and medical students make decisions. During her graduate training, she also worked on several meta-analytic projects within both the psychology and the medical fields. Dr. Cofrin completed an NIDA-funded postdoctoral fellowship with the Center for Family Studies at the University of Miami. Over the course of that year, she received training in a variety of statistical techniques, including hierarchical linear modeling (HLM) and structural equations modeling (SEM). She now works for Informatix Laboratories (ILC) in Salt Lake City, Utah. ILC is currently a subcontractor on the Center for Substance Abuse Prevention's Data Coordinating Center (CSAP DCC). The purpose of the CSAP DCC is to act as a data repository and supply CSAP with cross-program analysis designed to understand the etiology of substance use and track trends across time. Dr. Cofrin serves as a senior analyst on this project and is responsible for identifying common constructs across DCC data sets, creating a conceptual mapping of constructs assessed by those data sets, and working with the analysis team to propose and conduct analysis projects. Dr. Cofrin lives in Salt Lake City with her husband and two children.